Principles of Pulmonary Protection in Heart Surgery

Edmo Atique Gabriel • Tomas A. Salerno
(Editors)

Principles of Pulmonary Protection in Heart Surgery

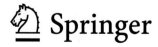 Springer

Dr. Edmo Atique Gabriel
Federal University of Sao Paulo
Sao Paulo
Brazil

Dr. Tomas A. Salerno
University of Miami
Miller School of Medicine
Jackson Memorial Hospital
Miami Florida
USA

ISBN 978-1-4471-5706-9   ISBN 978-1-84996-308-4 (eBook)

DOI 10.1007/978-1-84996-308-4

Springer Heidelberg Dordrecht London New York

A catalogue record for this book is available from the British Library

This book is dedicated to God, to my parents Edmo Gabriel and Maria Lucia Atique Gabriel and my brother Sthefano Atique Gabriel.

This book is dedicated to my wife Helen Salerno, my children Mark and Kim Salerno and to my parents José and Silveria F. Salerno.

Edmo Atique Gabriel
Tomas Salerno

Preface

Over the past fifty years, advanced techniques and strategies have arisen in the field of myocardial protection. Meticulous trials, focusing on pulmonary protection during heart surgery requiring cardiopulmonary bypass (CPB), have been missing. This textbook is intended to serve as a useful tool to spread information on strategies for lung protection during heart surgery with CPB.

Emphasis on pulmonary protection will be turned to lung perfusion as an adjunct for minimizing the deleterious effects of pulmonary ischemia-reperfusion injury in heart surgery. Many renowned authors have contributed by presenting their experience on lung perfusion in basic research and clinical trials. Furthermore, they have enlightened the quality of this textbook with new ideas, concepts, and future perspectives.

The scope of this textbook is of interest to different professionals, such as cardiovascular surgeons, pulmonary surgeons, transplantation physicians, cardiothoracic anesthesiologists, intensive care physicians, cardiothoracic fellows, radiologists, basic sciences physicians, cardiologists, pulmonary medicine physicians, perfusionists, nurses, students, and researchers.

This textbook has 7 sections, aimed at addressing general and specific aspects of pulmonary protection during heart surgery with CPB. The first section on general concepts provides information about anatomic, physiologic, histologic, molecular, and radiologic considerations regarding the lungs.

The second section focuses on ischemia-reperfusion injury and is composed of several interesting chapters, addressing the basic science aspects of pulmonary protection, as well as experimental and clinical experiences from different heart surgery centers worldwide.

It would be unconceivable to comment on pulmonary protection without addressing regarding pulmonary hypertension. We dedicated the third section to describe pathologic mechanisms of pulmonary hypertension, types of pulmonary hypertension, surgical management of chronic thromboembolic pulmonary hypertension, Eisenmenger's syndrome, and disseminated intravascular coagulation. The final part of this section addresses new trends and perspectives for managing pulmonary hypertension.

The following three sections address underlying topics on lung protection, and the fourth section focuses on relationship between CPB and pulmonary injury. In this section, there is special interest emphasis on hemodynamic, gasometric, and inflammatory impact of CPB on pulmonary function. Furthermore, strategies such as ischemic preconditioning, hemofiltration, and ultrafiltration are covered in detail.

The main purpose of this textbook is to highlight the use of controlled lung perfusion during heart surgery with CPB, and this topic is covered in the fifth section. Techniques and principles of controlled lung perfusion are analyzed, based on recent research devised by Gabriel at al.[1] This section provides original discussions on extracorporeal circuit pathways for lung perfusion, how to determine lung perfusion pressure, lung perfusion using arterial and venous blood, and impact of controlled lung perfusion from hemodynamic, gasometric, inflammatory, and radiologic standpoint of view during heart surgery with CPB.

There are many controversial issues related to lung perfusion during heart surgery with CPB, that require new investigation. What is the best strategy: perfusing lungs continuously or intermittently during CPB? Are there indications for lung perfusion using arterial and venous blood? Can brian natriuretic peptide be used as a marker for hemodynamic performance of lung perfusion during CPB? How can we correlate lung perfusion with ECMO? These issues are partially answered in chapter six. This section also gives you an overall view on principles of pulmonary protection during heart surgery with CPB.

Finally, the seventh and last section covers experiences from heart surgery centers on lung perfusion in clinical heart-lung surgery.

We wish to thank all contributors who spent the time and effort to provide information an lung protection during heart surgery with CPB, by writing excellent chapters.

We disclose our gratitude to the publisher, Springer, for giving us this opportunity to writ this book.

Reference

1. Gabriel EA, Locali RF, Matsuoka PK, et al. Lung perfusion during cardiac surgery with cardiopulmonary bypass: is it necessary? *Interact Cardiovasc Thorac Surg.*2008; 7:1089-1095.

Acknowledgments

- Enio Buffolo, MD, PhD, for his mentorship and support during my training career as cardiac surgeon.
- Nipro Brasil for providing resources and supplies for my experimental research.
- Springer for diligent attention and assistance turned to myself and for bestowing countless efforts on this book.

EdmoA tiqueG abriel

Contents

Section I   General Concepts

1 **Anatomy of the Lungs**   3
   Colleen Gaughan and Anthony L. Panos

2 **Respiratory Physiology**   9
   Jesús Armando Sánchez Godoy

3 **Histological Features of Lungs**   27
   Vera Luiza Capelozzi and Edwin Roger Parra

4 **Cellular and Molecular Aspects of Lung Function,
   its Control and Regulation**   33
   Jesús Armando Sánchez Godoy and Alain Riveros Rivera

5 **Imaging Evaluation of the Thorax**   45
   Gilberto Szarf and Henrique M. Lederman

Section II   Ischemia-Reperfusion Injury

6 **Endothelial Protection During Heart Surgery
   and Lung Transplantation**   55
   Qin Yang and Guo-Wei He

7 **Vascular Endothelial Growth Factor and Pulmonary Injury**   67
   Vineet Bhandari

8 **Aprotinin Decreases Lung Reperfusion Injury
   and Dysfunction**   75
   Hartmuth B. Bittner, Peter S. Dahlberg,
   Cynthia S. Herrington, and Friedrich W. Mohr

9 **Effects of Prostaglandin E1 and Nitroglycerin
   on Lung Preservation**   81
   Stefano Salizzoni, Yoshiko Toyoda, and Yoshiya Toyoda

10 **Endothelin and Ischemia-Reperfusion Injury**   91
   Matthias Gorenflo

11   L-Arginine and Ischemia-Reperfusion Injury   97
     Yanmin Yang and Jiming Cai

12   The Role of Nitric Oxide in Pulmonary
     Ischemia-Reperfusion Injury.   107
     Peter Donndorf, Alexander Kaminski, and Gustav Steinhoff

13   Activity of Glutathione-Related Enzymes
     in Ischemia and Reperfusion Injury   113
     Emmanuele Tafuri, Andrea Mezzetti, Antonio Maria Calafiore,
     and Francesco Cipollone

14   Heart Histopathology in Ischemia-Reperfusion Injury.   121
     Paulo Sampaio Gutierrez and Márcia Marcelino de Souza Ishigai

15   Beating Heart Surgery and Pulmonary Ischemia
     and Reperfusion Injury   129
     Tomas A. Salerno, Francisco Igor B. Macedo,
     Maria R. Suarez, and Marco Ricci

Section III   Pulmonary Hypertension

16   Mechanisms of Pulmonary Edema   137
     Si Pham and Eddie Manning

17   Idiopathic Pulmonary Hypertension: New Challenges   147
     Tomas Pulido and Julio Sandoval

18   Chronic Thromboembolic Pulmonary Hypertension
     and Pulmonary Endarterectomy.   159
     Michael M. Madani and Stuart W. Jamieson

19   Eisenmenger Syndrome   171
     Ruchi Gupta, Shirah Shore, Maria M. Rodriguez,
     and Marco Ricci

20   Disseminated Intravascular Coagulation in Cardiac Surgery   179
     Leticia Sandre Vendrame, Helio Penna Guimaraes,
     and Renato Delascio Lopes

21   Pulmonary Arterial Hypertension.   195
     Julie John and Harold Palevsky

Section IV   Cardiopulmonary Bypass and Pulmonary Injury

22   The Extracorporeal Circulation Circuit
     Versus Bioengineering Biomaterials   215
     José Francisco Biscegli, Fábio Nunes Dias,
     Cynara Viterbo Montoya, Sergio Luiz Nogaroto,
     and Edmo Atique Gabriel

23   Ischemic Preconditioning and Lung Preservation   235
David J. Chambers, Hazem B. Fallouh and Nouhad A. Kassem

**24   Impact of Cardiopulmonary Bypass on
Pulmonary Hemodynamic Variables**   235
Edmo Atique Gabriel and Tomas Salerno

**25   Impact of Cardiopulmonary Bypass on
Gas Exchange Features**   239
Edmo Atique Gabriel and Tomas Salerno

**26   Pulmonary Energy Metabolism and
Multiple Inflammatory Repercussions**   245
Edmo Atique Gabriel and Tomas Salerno

27   Benefits of Ultrafiltration for Pulmonary Function   251
Wei Wang and Huimin Huang

28   Principles of Pulmonary Protection During Heart Surgery   263
Mitsugi Nagashima and Toshiharu Shin'oka

Section V   Lung Perfusion – Technique and Principles

29   Determining Hemodynamic Parameters   271
Edmo Atique Gabriel and Tomas Salerno

30   Extracorporeal Circuit Pathways for Lung Perfusion   279
Edmo Atique Gabriel and Tomas Salerno

31   Hemodynamic Performance   287
Edmo Atique Gabriel and Tomas Salerno

32   Quality of Gas Exchange   297
Edmo Atique Gabriel and Tomas Salerno

33   Inflammatory Cell Markers   307
Edmo Atique Gabriel and Tomas Salerno

34   Cytokines and Cellular Adhesion Molecules   323
Edmo Atique Gabriel and Tomas Salerno

35   Macroscopical and Microscopical Findings   333
Edmo Atique Gabriel and Tomas Salerno

Section VI   Lung Perfusion: Issues and Controversies

**36   Continuous or Intermittent Lung Perfusion
with Arterial or Venous Blood**   349
Edmo Atique Gabriel and Tomas Salerno

37 Lung Perfusion and Mechanical Ventilation 351
Edmo Atique Gabriel and Tomas Salerno

38 Pulmonary Hemodynamic Profile and Natriuretic Peptides 359
Edmo Atique Gabriel and Tomas Salerno

39 Low-Frequency Mechanical Ventilation
During Cardiopulmonary Bypass 367
Hajime Imura, Raimondo Ascione, and Gianni D Angelini

40 Inhaled Carbon Monoxide as an Experimental
Therapeutic Strategy of Lung Protection
During Cardiopulmonary Bypass 377
Torsten Loop, Ulrich Goebel, Friedhelm Beyersdorf,
and Christian Schlensak

Section VII   Lung Perfusion in Clinical Heart-Lung Surgery

41 Lung Perfusion and Coronary Artery Bypass Grafting 385
Parwis Massoudy and Heinz Jakob

42 Lung Perfusion in Clinical Mitral Valve Surgery 393
Edmo Atique Gabriel and Tomas Salerno

43 Lung Perfusion in Clinical Aortic Surgery..................... 397
Luca Salvatore De Santo

44 Lung Perfusion in Clinical Heart–Lung Surgery:
Congenital Heart Disease Surgery 407
Takaaki Suzuki

45 Retrograde Pulmonary Perfusion
for Pulmonary Thromboembolism 413
Salvatore Spagnolo, Maria Antonia Grasso,
Paata Kalandadze, and Ugo Filippo Tesler

46 Lung Perfusion in Clinical Heart–Lung Transplantation.......... 417
Bernhard Gohrbandt and Axel Haverich

Section VIII   Final Considerations

47 Principles of Pulmonary Protection During Heart Surgery 431
Chi-Huei Chiang and Fang-Yue Lin

48 Lung Perfusion: Reflections and Perspectives 441
Edmo Atique Gabriel and Tomas Salerno

Index 443

Contributors

Gianni D. Angelini, MD,FR CS
BristolH eartIns titute, BristolU niversity, Bristol, UK

Maria AntoniaGr asso, MD
DepartmentofA nesthesia, Policlinicodi M onza, Monza, Italy

Jesús ArmandoSán chezG odoy, MD,M Sc
Pontificia Universidad Javeriana, Universidad Militar "Nueva Granada",
BogotáD .C., Colombia

Vincenzo Arone, MD
DepartmentofC ardiacS urgery, PoliclinicodiM onza, Monza, Italy

Raimondo Ascione, MD,FR CS
BristolH eartIns titute, BristolU niversity, Bristol, UK

Edmo AtiqueGabr iel, MD,PhD
FederalU niversityofSa oP aulo, SaoP aulo, Brazil

Luciano Barbato, MD
DepartmentofC ardiacS urgery, PoliclinicodiM onza, Monza, Italy

Friedhelm Beyersdorf, MD
Department of Cardiovascular Surgery, University Medical Center,
Freiburg, Germany

Vineet Bhandari, MD,D M
YaleU niversity Schoolo fM edicine, NewH aven, CT, USA

Hartmuth B. Bittner, MD,PhD
Division of Cardiovascular Surgery and Thoracic Transplantation,
HeartC enterofthe U niversityof Le ipzig, Leipzig, Germany

Jiming Cai, MD,M Sc
Department of Cardiovascular and Thoracic Surgery, Shanghai Children's
Medical Center, School of Medicine, Shanghai Jiaotong University
Shanghai, Shanghai, China

Vera Luiza Capelozzi
Department of Pathology, University of Sao Paulo School of Medicine,
SaoP aulo, Brazil

David Chambers, PhD
Cardiac Surgical Research, The Rayne Institute (King's College London),
Guy's and St Thomas' NHS Foundation Trust, St Thomas' Hospital, London, UK

Chi-Huei Chiang, MD,FC CP
Pulmonary Division of Immunology and Infectious Diseases, Chest Department,
TaipeiV eteransG eneralH ospital, Taipei, Taiwan

Francesco Cipollone, MD
Abruzzos ection, ItalianSoc ietyforthe StudyofA therosclerosis, Chieti, Italy

Peter S. Dahlberg, MD,PhD
CardiothoracicA ssociates, Minneapolis Minnesota, USA

Renato DelascioL opes, MD,PhD ,M HS
Division of Cardiovascular Medicine, Duke University Medical Center, Duke
ClinicalR esearchIns titute, Durham, NC, USA

Peter Donndorf, MD
DepartmentofC ardiacSur gery, UniversityofR ostock, Rostock, Germany

Hazem B. Fallouh, MD,M RCS
Cardiac Surgical Research/Cardiothoracic Surgery, The Rayne Institute (King's
College London), Guy's and St Thomas' NHS Foundation Trust, St Thomas'
Hospital, London, UK

Ugo FilippoT esler, MD
DepartmentofC ardiacSur gery, PoliclinicodiM onza, Monza, Italy

José Francisco Biscegli
DanteP azzaneseIns tituteofC ardiology, SaoP aulo, Brazil

Colleen Gaughan, MD
Division of Cardiothoracic Surgery, Miller School of Medicine,
UniversityofM iami,J acksonM emorialH ospital, Miami FL, USA

Bernhard Gohrbandt, MD
Division of Thoracic and Cardiovascular Surgery, Hannover Medical School,
Hannover, Germany

Matthias Gorenflo, MD,PhD
Department of Paediatric Cardiology, UZ Leuven Campus Gasthuisberg,
KatholiekeU niversiteitLe uven, Leuven, Belgie

Ulrich Goebel, MD
Department of Cardiovascular Surgery, University Medical Center,
Freiburg, Germany

Ruchi Gupta, MD
DepartmentofPe diatrics, Universityof Miami, Miami FL, USA

Paulo Gutierrez, MD,PhD
Laboratory of Pathology – Heart Institute, Hospital das Clinicas,
SchoolofM edicine,U niversity ofSã oP aulo, SãoP aulo, Brazil

Axel Haverich, MD,PhD
Department of Cardiothoracic, Transplantation, and Vascular Surgery,
HannoverM edicalSc hool, Hannover, Germany

Guo-Wei He, MD,PhD ,D Sc
Department of Surgery, The Chinese University of Hong Kong, Hong Kong,
China AlbertSta rrA cademicC enter, ProvidenceH earta ndV ascularI nstitute,
PortlandO R, USA
DepartmentofSur gery, OregonH ealtha ndSc ienceU niversity, Portland, OR,
USA TEDAInte rnationalC ardiovascularH ospital, MedicalC ollege,
NankaiU niversity, Tianjin, China

Huimin Huang, MD,Ph D
Department of Pediatric Thoracic and Cardiovascular Surgery, Shanghai Jiaotong
University, School of Medicine, Shanghai Children's Medical Center, Shanghai,
China

Cynthia S. Herrington, MD
Pediatric Cardiac Surgery and Transplantation, Childrens Hospital Los Angeles,
California, USA

Hajime Imura, MD
Department of Surgery, Division of Cardiovascular Surgery,
NipponM edicalSc hool, Tokyo, Japan

Márcia Marcelinode Souz a Ishigai, MD,PhD
DepartmentofP athology, FederalU niversityof Sa oP aulo, SaoP aulo, Brazil

Heinz Jakob, MD
Department of Thoracic and Cardiovascular Surgery, West German Heart Center,
Essen, Germany

Stuart W.J amieson, M B,FR CS
Division of Cardiothoracic Surgery, University of California, San Diego Medical
Center, SanD iegoC A, USA

Julie John, MD
DepartmentofM edicine, PennsylvaniaH ospital, Philadelphia PA, USA

Paata Kalandadze, MD
DepartmentofC ardiacS urgery, PoliclinicodiM onza, Monza, Italy

Alexander Kaminski, MD
Department of Cardiac Surgery, Medical Faculty, University of Rostock,
Rostock, Germany

Nouhad Kassem, PhD
Cardiac Surgical Research/Cardiothoracic Surgery, The Rayne Institute
(King's College London), Guy's and St Thomas' NHS Foundation Trust,
StThoma s'H ospital, London, UK

Henrique M. Lederman, MD,PhD
Department of Radiology, Federal University of Sao Paulo, Sao Paulo,
Brazil FleuryD iagnosticC enter, SaoP aulo, Brazil

Fang-Yue Lin, MD,PhD
CardiovascularSur gery, TaipeiV eteransG eneralH ospital, Taipei, Taiwan

Torsten Loop, MD
Department of Cardiovascular Surgery, University Medical Center,
Freiburg, Germany

Sergio LuizN ogaroto
NiproM edicalLtda , Sorocaba SaoP aulo, Brazil

Francisco Igor B. Macedo, MD
UniversityofPe rnambuco,Sc hoolofM edicine, Brazil

Michael M.M adani, MD,F ACS
Division of Cardiothoracic Surgery, University of California, San Diego Medical
Center SanD iegoC A, USA

Eddie Manning, MD
UniversityofM iami, JacksonM emorialH ospital, Miami FL, USA

Antonio MariaC alafiore, MD
PrinceSulta nC ardiacC enter, Riyadh, KingdomofSa udiA rabia

Parwis Massoudy, MD
Department of Thoracic and Cardiovascular Surgery, West German Heart Center,
Essen, Germany

Andrea Mezzetti, MD
Abruzzos ection, ItalianSoc ietyforthe StudyofA therosclerosis, Chieti, Italy

Friedrich W. Mohr, MD,PhD
Division of Cardiovascular Surgery and Thoracic Transplantation, Heart Center of
theU niversityofLe ipzig, Leipzig, Germany

Mitsugi Nagashima, MD
Department of Surgery, Division of Cardiothoracic Surgery and Regenerative
Surgery, Ehime University School of Medicine, Stroke and Cardiovascular Center,
Shitsukawa,T oonc ity, Ehimepre fecture, Japan

Fábio NunesD ias
NiproM edicalLtda , Sorocaba SaoP aulo, Brazil

Harold Palevsky, MD
DepartmentofM edicine, PennsylvaniaH ospital, Philadelphia PA, USA
UniversityofPe nnsylvaniaSc hoolofM edicine, Philadelphia PA, USA
PennPre sbyterianM edicalC enter, Philadelphia PA, USA

Anthony L. Panos, MD
Division of Cardiothoracic Surgery, Miller School of Medicine,
UniversityofM iami,J acksonM emorialH ospital, Miami FL, USA

HelioP ennaGu imaraes, MD
IntensiveC areU nit,
FederalU niversityofSa oP aulo, SaoP aulo, Brazil

Si Pham, MD,F ACS,F AHA
UniversityofM iami, JacksonM emorialH ospital, Miami FL, USA

Tomas Pulido, MD
LaSa lleU niversity, MexicoC ity, Mexico
CardiopulmonaryD epartment, IgnacioC havezN ationalH eartI nstitute,
MexicoC ity, Mexico

Marco Ricci, MD
Department of Surgery, University of Miami Miller School of Medicine,
Miami FL, USA

Alain RiverosR ivera, MD,M Sc
Pontificia Universidad Javeriana, Universidad Militar "Nueva Granada",
BogotáD .C., Colombia

Maria M. Rodriguez, MD
DepartmentofP athology, Universityof M iami, MiamiFL , USA

Edwin RogerP arra, MD,PhD
Department of Pathology, University of Sao Paulo School of Medicine,
SaoP aulo, Brazil

Tomas Salerno, MD
Department of Surgery, University of Miami Miller School of Medicine,
Miami FL, USA

Stefano Salizzoni, MD
UniversityofPitts burghM edicalC enter, Pittsburgh PA, USA

Julio Sandoval, MD
Cardiopulmonary Department, Ignacio Chavez National Heart Institute,
MexicoC ity, Mexico

Leticia SandreV endrame, MD
FederalU niversityofSa oP aulo, SaoP aulo, Brazil

Luca Salvatore De Santo, MD
DepartmentofC ardiacS urgery, UniversityofF oggia, Foggia, Italy
Department of Cardiovascular Surgery and Transplant, V. Monaldi Hospital,
Naples, Italy

Christian Schlensak, MD
Department of Cardiovascular Surgery, University Medical Center, Freiburg, Germany

Toshiharu Shin'oka, MD,PhD
DepartmentofSur gery, YaleU niversitySc hoolofM edicine, NewH aven,C T, USA

Shirah Shore, MD
DepartmentofPe diatrics, Universityof Miami, Miami FL, USA

Salvatore Spagnolo, MD
DepartmentofC ardiacS urgery, PoliclinicodiM onza, Monza, Italy

Gustav Steinhoff, MD,PhD
DepartmentofC ardiacS urgery, UniversityofR ostock, Rostock, Germany

Maria R. Suarez, MD
Division of Cardiothoracic Surgery, University of Miami Miller School of Medicine andJ acksonM emorialH ospital, Miami Florida, USA

Takaaki Suzuki, MD
Department of Pediatric Cardiac Surgery, Saitama International Medical Center, Yamane Hidaka-City Saitama, Japan

Gilberto Szarf, MD,PhD
DepartmentofR adiology, FederalU niversityofSa oP aulo, SaoP aulo, Brazil
FleuryD iagnosticC enter, SaoP aulo, Brazil

Emmanuele Tafuri, MD
Abruzzos ection, ItalianSoc ietyforthe StudyofA therosclerosis, Chieti, Italy

Yoshiko Toyoda, MD
UniversityofPitts burghM edicalC enter, Pittsburgh PA, USA

Yoshiya Toyoda, MD,PhD
The Heart, Lung and Esophageal Surgery Institute, Division of Cardiac Surgery, UniversityofPitts burghM edicalC enter, Pittsburgh PA, USA

Cynara ViterboM ontoya
NiproM edicalLtda , Sorocaba SaoP aulo, Brazil

Wei Wang, MD,PhD
Department of Pediatric Thoracic and Cardiovascular Surgery, Shanghai Jiaotong University, School of Medicine, Shanghai Children's Medical Center, Shanghai, China

Yanmin Yang, MD,PhD
Department of Cardiovascular and Thoracic Surgery, Shanghai Children's Medical Center, School of Medicine, Shanghai Jiaotong University Shanghai, Shanghai, China

Qin Yang, MD,PhD
DepartmentofSur gery, TheC hineseU niversityofH ongK ong, HongK ong, China

Section

General Concepts

I

Anatomyo ft heL ungs

Colleen Gaughan and Anthony L. Panos

1.1 Introduction

Life and respiration are complementary. There is nothing living which does not breathe nor anything which breathing which does not live.

WilliamH arvey

Lectures on the Whole of Anatomy: An Annotated Translation of Prelectiones anatomiae universalis

Early descriptions of the lungs understood that breathing occurred in the lungs, which acted like a pair of bellows firing and cooling a furnace. Galen's description of the lung, for example, emphasized that it "has all the properties which make for easy evacuation; for it is very soft and warm and is kept in constant motion." From these early descriptions, it is evident that early concepts of respiration were influenced by humoral theories of the body, and that the lung was considered an organ for disposal of waste or "bad humors."[1,2]

Medieval and Renaissance physicians began to understand the connection between the lungs and respiration and between life and breath. The Galenic *pneuma* was a vitality, a life force, that was associated with the inhalation and exhalation of air.[3] Leonardo da Vinci described the process as follows in his unpublished notebooks of the late fifteenth century: "From the heart, impurities or 'sooty vapors' are carried back to the lung by way of the pulmonary artery, to be exhaled to the outer air."[4] Despite Leonardo's carefully drawn images of the anatomy of the lungs and the establishment of a five-lobe system of the

lungs, he did not yet understand the relationship between form and function in great detail. These careful anatomical studies of the human body conducted by Renaissance anatomists yielded a more precise physical description of the lungs. Thus, by the early seventeenth century, the new anatomy of the lung was in place.[5] William Harvey concurred with his Renaissance predecessors on the five-lobe structure of the lungs. Yet, he took their views several steps further in describing the significance of the lungs. In his treatise, *On the Circulation of the Blood* (1628), Harvey established a new physiology of the human body based on a different understanding of the relationship between arteries and veins – no longer separate circulatory systems within the body but a unified system. Harvey concluded that the lungs were the most important organs in the body and the place where respiration occurred, even though he could not see capillaries and did not understand the concept of gas exchange as his studies preceded the discovery of the microscope and oxygen. However, through a long series of dissections (from dogs and pigs down to slugs and oysters) and by a process of logical argument, Harvey was able to prove that the body contains only a single supply of blood, and that the heart is a muscle pumping the blood around a circuit.[4]

Scientists began to understand in the 1600s that there was a part of air that was necessary for life when John Mayow performed experiments demonstrating that some aspect of air necessary for life could be removed both by mouse respiration and by fire. He called the part of air that was necessary for respiration and for fire "ariel spirits." In 1774, Lavoisier repeated experiments performed by his contemporary Priestly, creating ariel spirits from the combustion of mercuric oxide, and confirmed the results, calling the air "eminently breathable air." Several years later, he coined the term *oxygen*.[1] The discovery of oxygen laid the groundwork for our current understanding of gas exchange and respiration.

A.L.P anos(✉)
Division of Cardiothoracic Surgery, Miller School of Medicine, University of Miami, Jackson Memorial Hospital, Miami, FL, USA
e-mail:a panos@med.miami.edu

E.A. Gabriel and T. Salerno (eds.), *Principles of Pulmonary Protection in Heart Surgery*, DOI: 10.1007/978-1-84996-308-4_1, © Springer-Verlag London Limited 2010

1.2 EmbryologyandL ungDevel opment

The process of lung development and maturation begins in the embryo with the emergence of lung buds from the ventral foregut and ends with the formation of gas-exchanging alveoli and an integrated capillary network.[6] A tube formed by endoderm arises in the ventral wall of the pharynx in the fourth week of development. By the sixth to seventh week of gestation, the right and left lung buds have become lobulated, forming three lobes on the right and two on the left. Although lung morphogenesis is a continuous process, developmental biologists have subdivided it, on the basis of histological features, into four successive stages: pseudoglandular, canalicular, saccular, and alveolar. Shortly after primary lung budding, the highly ordered sequence of events referred to as branching morphogenesis begins to generate the bronchial tree of the lung. By the 16th week of development, all of the conducting airways are formed, including the terminole bronchioles, concluding the pseudoglandular stage of development. In the canalicular phase, the canaliculi branch out of the terminal bronchioli. The canaliculi are composed of the part of the lung directly involved in respiration and gas exchange. The chief characteristic of this canalicular phase is the alteration of the epithelium and the surrounding mesenchyma, which is thinned, induced by the invasion of capillaries. In the last trimester, clusters of sacs form on the terminal bronchioli, which represent the last subdivision of the passages that supply air and are coated with type I and type II pneumocytes. It is difficult to define exactly when one phase of lung development ends and another begins, particularly the alveolar phase. By birth, approximately one third of alveoli have developed, starting cephalically and progressing caudally. Initially, the alveoli present are primitive in structure and are composed of saccules lined with pneumocytes, with primary septa separating these from the growing capillaries, and elastic fibers that form secondary septa between the capillary nets. In the first six postnatal months, the number of alveoli increases massively. This "alveolarization" and the formation of secondary septa continue up to the first year and a half of life. An important regulator of lung growth during the period of lung maturation is distension of the lung. Kitterman and colleagues created oligohydramnios in rats at 16 days of gestation to reduce fetal lung distension.[7] They observed in 21- to 22-day-old fetuses that the oligohydramnios reduced lung growth and impeded the formation of alveolar type I cells relative to type II cells.

Also developing in the sixth week of gestation is the main pulmonary artery, arising from the left sixth aortic arch. The pulmonary artery follows the branching of the bronchial tree, down to the level of the terminal bronchioles. The paired bronchiole and pulmonary artery establish a central location in the pulmonary lobule. The pulmonary veins develop as outgrowths of the cardiac atria, and small venules that develop in the periphery of the pulmonary lobule coalesce and receive tributaries from the pleura and the growing tips of the respiratory tree until they join to form intersegmental veins. These intersegmental veins then merge with the main pulmonary veins near the pulmonary hilum, accounting for the variability in the number of pulmonary veins that can be present.

1.3 Trachea

The trachea is a direct continuation of the larynx. The larynx functions to protect the airway, to prevent aspiration, and to allow phonation. The larynx marks the first space in the airway that is lined by ciliated respiratory epithelium. The trachea itself is, on average, 10–12 cm in length in the adult from the cricoid cartilage to the carina and 13–22 mm in width. There are 17–21 incomplete cartilaginous rings that run along its length and provide support for the fibromuscular tube. The cricoid cartilage can be palpated in the neck approximately 3 cm superior to the sternal notch, and the carina lies in the middle mediastinum at the level of the sternal angle of Louis (lower border of the fourth thoracic vertebra). Thus, approximately half of the trachea lies in the neck and half in the thorax. The trachea is attached to movable structures both proximally and distally and can move both superiorly and inferiorly; its diameter can change with the contraction of airway smooth muscle. In a young person, the airway can contract to one tenth of its normal diameter with coughing.

Due to its position in the superior mediastinum, the trachea has important anatomic relations. The posterior membranous trachea is adherent to the anterior muscular wall of the esophagus. Anteriorly, it is related to the thyroid gland in the neck, the innominate artery in the superior mediastinum, then the thymus, and continuing inferiorly the aorta and pulmonary artery. Laterally, the vagus nerves run in the tracheoesophageal groove in the neck. In the superior mediastinum, the brachiocephalic vein, superior vena cava, and azygous vein are on the right, while the left common carotid artery, aortic arch, and recurrent laryngeal nerve are on the left.

The trachea is lined with pseudostratified columnar ciliated epithelium, with goblet cells comprising about one third of epithelial cells. This epithelium rests on a basement membrane composed of a thick elastic lamina. The submucosa is comprised of glands, blood vessels, nerves, and a lymphatic plexus in a loose fibrous stroma and supported by the incomplete cartilaginous rings. In the posterior wall of the trachea, the cartilaginous rings are absent, and the submucosa lies directly on the muscular tube of the esophagus. In the remainder of the respiratory tree, the muscular tube runs longitudinally and helically along the bronchi, and the cartilaginous rings are complete. The posterior membranous portion of the trachea is a reflection of the embryologic formation of the trachea as an outpouching of the primitive foregut.

1.4 ConductingA irwayst oA lveoli

At the carina, the trachea bifurcates into the right and left main stem bronchi. The right main stem bronchi branches in a more direct line with the trachea than the left and passes behind the superior vena cava to reach the hilum of the lung. The right upper lobe bronchus originates from the right main stem bronchus very shortly after the takeoff from the carina and may even take off from the trachea itself, although this is rare. The left main stem bronchus is smaller (10–14 mm in diameter) than the right, but is longer (15–20 mm), and exits the trachea at a more oblique angle, passing below the aortic arch to reach the pulmonary hilum.

Jackson and Huber standardized the terminology for lung segment classification and the concept that each pulmonary segment is derived from its own segmental pulmonary bronchus[8] (Table 1.1). The right lung has three lobes and ten segments. The lower lobe is separated from the middle and upper lobes by the oblique or major fissure. The middle lobe is separated from the upper lobe by the horizontal or minor fissure. The horizontal fissure is complete in only about one third of the population and is completely absent is approximately 10% of the population. The left lung has two lobes and eight segments. The upper and lower lobes are separated

Table 1.1 Jackson–Huber pulmonary segmental classification

	Right	Left
Upper	Apical	Apical-posterior
	Posterior	
	Anterior	Anterior
Middle (left lingula)	Lateral	Superior
	Medial	Inferior
Lower	Superior	Superior
	Medialba sal	Anterior-medial basal
	Anteriorba sal	
	Lateralba sal	Lateralba sal
	Posteriorba sal	Posteriorba sal

by a major fissure. In 8% of the population, there is a horizontal fissure between the upper lobe and the lingular lobe on the left, but it is never complete.[9]

As the bronchi branch distally, each division results in an increase of bronchial surface area about 1.2 times greater than the parent branch. Structurally, the large conducting bronchi are similar to the trachea, except that the cartilaginous rings are complete, and the longitudinal muscle of the posterior membranous trachea runs longitudinally and helically around the bronchi. As the bronchi continue to branch into medium and smaller bronchi, the cartilage changes to plates of cartilage instead of rings, and the number of glands in the submucosa increases. A bronchiole is less than 1 mm in diameter and has no cartilaginous support. Bronchioles have the highest proportion of smooth muscle to diameter. The epithelium of the respiratory tract changes at the level of the bronchiole from pseudostratified columnar epithelium to ciliated columnar cells and goblet cells alone. As the bronchioles continue to branch and get smaller in diameter, this epithelium is replaced by columnar epithelium alone in the terminal bronchiole. The short columnar epithelium of the terminal bronchiole stops abruptly at the beginning of the alveolus, which is lined by type I and type II pneumocytes.

The pulmonary lobule, or secondary pulmonary nodule, is the smallest pulmonary division of the conducting airways and is visible on high-resolution computerized tomography. It is polyhedral in shape, contains less than a dozen acini, and is approximately 1–2.5 cm in diameter. It is surrounded by connective tissue septa and is cone shaped, with the base of the cone abutting the visceral pleura. The pulmonary arteriole and bronchus are centrally located with axial interstitium and parenchyma. Pulmonary veins and lymphatics are present peripherally within connective tissue septa. These septa coalesce into interlobar septa, which are continuous with the subpleural interstitium. The acinus is a functional unit of the lung at the end of a terminal bronchiole. It is 6–10 mm in diameter, and it is the largest unit in which all tissue participates in gas exchange. The final subdivision of the lung is the alveolus, the air sac directly involved in gas exchange. Alveoli are approximately 160 μm in size; there are approximately 300 million in two human lungs, encompassing a surface area of 140 m².

1.5 Pulmonary Vascular System

The anatomy of the pulmonary vascular tree and its relation to the bronchial tree is of obvious importance for pulmonary resection.[10] There is a dual arterial supply to the lung: the pulmonary circulation and the bronchial circulation. The pulmonary circulation returns deoxygenated blood to the lungs for gas exchange, while the bronchial circulation supplies oxygenated blood to the lung parenchyma itself.

The pulmonary artery and its branches have an intimate relationship with the bronchial tree but vary slightly on the right and left sides. The main pulmonary artery divides and the right pulmonary artery runs posterior to the aorta and the superior vena cava within the pericardial sac, emerging into the pleura lateral to the right atrium and slightly anterior to the right main stem bronchus. More than two thirds of the right pulmonary artery is within the pericardium; it forms the superior border of the transverse sinus, and as it passes out of the pericardium, it forms the superior border of the postcaval recess of Allison. The right upper lobe branches pass anteriorly to the right upper lobe bronchus. The interlobar right pulmonary artery continues in close approximation to the bronchus intermedius and becomes lateral to the bronchial tree as it supplies the middle and lower lobe segments. The arborization of the right pulmonary artery is highly variable, especially with reference to the right upper lobe, a fact that must be considered in right upper lobe pulmonary resections.[10] The first branch to the right upper lobe is the truncus anterior. The interlobar portion of the right pulmonary artery gives posterior ascending branches to the posterior segment of the right upper

lobe, and sometimes there is a common trunk that gives branches to both the posterior segment of the right upper lobe and the superior segment of the right lower lobe. The interlobar portion of the right pulmonary artery gives one or two branches to the middle lobe, then 1–2 cm distal there is a branch to the superior segment of the right lower lobe. In 80% of the population, this branch will be directly opposite the branch to the middle lobe. The interlobar portion then terminates in the segmental branches to the lower lobe.

The left pulmonary artery has a short course through the pericardium and passes anterior to the left main stem bronchus as it exits. Just distal to its origin, the left pulmonary artery is connected to the aorta by the ligamentum arteriosum. It courses posterior and laterally and wraps around the left upper lobe bronchus, ultimately becoming lateral to the left lower lobe bronchus. The left pulmonary artery is shorter than the right, but because the majority of its length is outside the pericardium, there is more length available for dissection during lung resections. The arborization of the left upper lobe pulmonary artery is even more variable than that of the right upper lobe.[10] The first branch of the left pulmonary artery is an anterior trunk that arises from the superior and lateral surface of the vessel about 1.5 cm distal to the ligamentum arteriosum. The left superior pulmonary vein is anterior and inferior to the left pulmonary artery as it exits the pericardium, making dissection of the anterior branches of the left pulmonary artery hazardous. A common variation in left pulmonary artery anatomy is that this first anterior branch will supply the lingula, rather than the supply branches to the apical-posterior and anterior segments. One or two branches divide posteriorly in the interlobar fissure beyond this. Two thirds of the population will have a single posterior branch that arises off the posterior and lateral aspect of the interlobar portion of the artery to supply the superior segment of the left lower lobe. The other one third of the population will have two branches to the superior segment of the lower lobe. Beyond these branches to the superior segment of the lower lobe, the artery terminates in branches to the segments of the lower lobe.

The vascular supply to the bronchial tree is derived from the systemic circulation and usually is comprised of short segmental branches either directly from the aorta or from the intercostal arteries.[11] On the right, a single artery from the posterior third intercostal artery to the right main stem bronchus is the most common arterial pattern. On the left, it is common that there are one or two branches coming directly from the descending aorta. These bronchial arteries form a peribronchial plexus and follow the bronchial tree deep into the lung parenchyma, supplying the visceral pleura and walls of the pulmonary artery as vasa vasorum.

Due to the embryologic formation of the venous drainage of the lung as a coalescence of venules in the developing pulmonary parenchyma merging with the cardiac atrium, the anatomy of the venous drainage of the lung is highly variable. As a rule, venous branches vary more than arterial branches, which vary more than the bronchi. Pulmonary veins do not travel with the bronchial tree but along interlobar septal planes and are attached to the lung parenchyma. There are some common anomalies of venous drainage that are worth mentioning. The superior and inferior lingular segments have separate draining veins, and the vein for the inferior segment may drain into the left inferior pulmonary vein. A right middle lobe vein may drain directly into the left atrium or, rarely, into the right inferior pulmonary vein. In 25% of the population, the superior and inferior pulmonary veins form a common trunk before entering the atrium. Venous drainage of the bronchi is through the azygous and hemiazygous veins. Some bronchial arteries also form anastomoses to pulmonary alveolar arterioles and drain via the pulmonary venous system. These communications, between the pulmonary and the bronchial arteries, constitute a physiological shunt.

1.6 Lymphatic Drainage of the Lung

The lungs are more extensively supplied by lymphatics than other more metabolically active organs.[12] There are two lymphatic drainage systems, the superficial and the deep. Both systems are connected at the beginning, the bronchioles, and the end, the bronchomediastinal trunk. Alveoli have no lymphatic drainage. Bronchi have lymphatic channels in the submucosa and around the bronchial periphery. The superficial plexus drains the visceral pleura and superficial lung. The two systems converge on the lymph nodes of the segmental bronchi and from the bronchomediastinal trunk at the hilum of the lung. At the hilum of the lung, the pulmonary lymphatics are thick walled and muscular and resemble the thoracic duct. Within the lung, there is communication at the periphery of the two systems such that obstruction of the deep system causes small peripheral channels to open to

allow lymph from the deep system to travel to the superficial. This can overwhelm the ability of the superficial to drain the lung and can result in pleural effusion as the lymphatic drainage leaks from the visceral pleura.

1.7 Innervation of the Lung

Both afferent and efferent nerve fibers follow the bronchial tree to the lungs. Parasympathetic innervation is derived from the bilateral vagus nerves in the neck, which send fibers to the anterior and posterior pulmonary plexuses. There are multiple ganglia along the vagus nerve branches to the lung, the cervical components are thought to contribute motor innervation, while the thoracic is thought to provide sensory innervation. Vagal afferent terminals are found in conducting airways, bronchioles, and alveoli. These terminals in the conducting airways are the afferent limb of the cough reflex. The vagus nerve also supplies secretomotor fibers to the pulmonary mucous glands and stretch receptors to the lung.

Sympathetic innervation to the lung is derived from the sympathetic ganglia at spinal levels T2–T4. The bronchial muscles receive bronchodilator fibers from the sympathetic system, which is also weakly vasoconstrictor to the bronchial vessels. Stimulation of the sympathetic innervation to the lungs thus improves oxygenation of the blood through bronchodilation and mild pulmonary vasoconstriction. A third system, the nonadrenergic, noncholinergic (NANC) system regulates airway smooth muscle contraction. One of the main mediators of this pathway is nitric oxide, and it may play a role in asthma and acute respiratory distress syndrome (ARDS).

References

1. Priestley J. *Considerations on the Doctrine of Phlogiston and the Decomposition of Water*. Philadelphia: Dobson; 1796.
2. Severinghaus JW. Priestley, the furious free thinker of the enlightenment, and Scheele, the taciturn apothecary of Uppsala. *Acta Anaesth Scand*.2002; 46:2-9.
3. Harvey W. Lectures on the whole of anatomy: an annotated translation of *Prelectiones anatomiae universalis*. In: O'Malley CD, Poynter FNL, Russell KF eds. and trans. Berkeley: University of California Press; 1961.
4. da Vinci L. *Leonardo da Vinci on the Human Body: The Anatomical, Physiological, and Embryological Drawings of Leonardo da Vinci*. In: Saunders J. B. de C. M, O'Malley CD eds. New York: Crown; 1982.

5. Cunningham A. *The anatomical Renaissance: The resurrection of the anatomical projects of the ancients.* Aldershot: Scolar;1997.

6. McMurtry IF. Introduction: pre- and postnatal lung development, maturation, and plasticity. *Am J Physiol Lung Cell Mol Physiol.*2002; 282:L341-L344.

7. Kitterman JA, Chapin CJ, Vanderbilt JN, et al. Effects of oligohydramnios on lung growth and maturation in the fetal rat. *Am J Physiol Lung Cell Mol Physiol.* 2002;282:L431-L439.

8. Jackson CL, Huber JF. Correlated applied anatomy of the bronchial tree and lungs with a system of nomenclature. *Chest.*1943;9:319- 326.

9. Webb WR. High-resolution computed tomography of the lung: normal and abnormal anatomy. *Semin Roentgenol.* 1991;26(2):110-117.

10. Smith FR. Segmental anatomy as applied to segmental resection. *Dis Chest.*1958; 34:602-606.

11. Ellis H, Feldman S, Harrop-Griffiths W. *Anatomy for anaesthetists.* 8th ed. Oxford: Blackwell; 2004.

12. Ellis H. Lungs: blood supply, lymphatic drainage and nerve supply. *Anaesth Intensive Care Med.*2008; 9(11):462-463.

RespiratoryPhys iology

Jesús Armando Sánchez-Godoy

2

2.1 Introduction

Organic evolution has been essentially linked to oxygen (O_2) since it was first introduced in the earth's atmosphere by photosynthesis of early cyanobacteria species some 2.5 billion years ago. In the steady state (i.e., normoxia), most of the oxygen consumed by a cell is used by mitochondria in the generation of adenosine triphosphate (ATP) via oxidative phosphorylation, providing eukaryotic cells with a highly sophisticated survival advantage. Whereas a total of 38 molecules of ATP are generated per molecule of glucose via oxidative phosphorylation, only 2 are produced via anaerobic metabolism. In fact, more than 90% of the oxygen consumption of the body is used for oxidative phosphorylation. Thus, since the chemical reduction of molecular oxygen is the primary source of metabolic energy for most eukaryotic cells, a constant oxygen supply is critical for continued cell function and survival.

Therefore, it is not surprising that dysoxia (i.e., inadequate supply of tissue oxygenation at levels impairing mitochondrial respiration)[1] and oxygen debt are major factors in the development and propagation of multiple-organ failures, especially in critically ill patients. Dysoxia is the result of an abnormal relationship between O_2 supply and O_2 demand. In mammals, the function of the lungs, heart, and vasculature must ensure a continuous and adequate supply of oxygen and nutrients to the tissues to maintain cellular integrity and function.

J.A.Sá nchez-Godoy
Departamento de Ciencias Fisiológicas, Pontificia Universidad Javeriana, Universidad Militar "Nueva Granada", Bogotá D.C., Colombia
e-mail:a rmandosanchezg@yahoo.com

The respiratory system allows gases to transfer by convective and diffusive processes between the atmospheric air and the blood. Furthermore, it also plays a central role in the maintenance of the acid–base balance and is related to other functions associated with the immune system and metabolism. This chapter focuses on the respiratory mechanisms that avoid tissue hypoxia by means of the analysis of the determinants of lung function.

2.2 OxygenDel ivery

The most important function of the respiratory and circulatory systems is the supply of oxygen to the cells of the body in adequate quantity and at satisfactory partial pressure.[2] On the one hand, the respiratory system allows appropriate partial oxygen pressure for the diffusion of gases through the alveolar-capillary barrier. On the other hand, the cardiovascular system favors an appropriate sanguineous flow to optimize the delivery, at the tissue level, of the oxygen already incorporated into the blood. The *oxygen delivery* $\left(\dot{D}_{O_2} \right)$ expresses this joint function of both systems. The quantity of oxygen made available to the body in 1 min is the product of the cardiac output (CO) and the *arterial oxygen content* $\left(CaO_2 \right)$:

$$\dot{D}_{O_2} = CO_{(1)} * Ca_{O_2} (dl / min) * 10 \qquad (2.1)$$

Under normal physiological conditions, the amount of oxygen delivered to the tissues is approximately 1,000 mL/min. Anaerobic metabolism occurs when $\dot{D}_{O_2}$ falls below about 3.03 ± 1.08 mL/kg/min (dysoxia), when oxygen demands exceed oxygen supply and tissue extraction to meet that need (e.g., beyond V_{O_2} max with severe exercise), or when the mitochondria are unable to utilize the oxygen. The essential feature of hypoxia is the cessation of oxidative phosphorylation when the mitochondrial P_{O_2} falls below a critical level. That is, hypoxia occurs when there is a reduction of $\dot{D}O_2$ due to hypoxemia (i.e., a reduced amount of oxygen being carried in the blood), to a restriction of the blood supply to the tissues, or to both.

Oxygen is carried by the blood in two forms: as solution (i.e., dissolved in the plasma) and as oxyhemoglobin. The quantity of hemoglobin (Hb) in solution in plasma at 37°C is defined by the capacitance coefficient, which is approximately 0.003 mL O_2/dL$_{blood}$×mmHg. The amount of oxygen that can be transported into the blood can be expressed by the equation describing CaO_2 :

$$Ca_{O_2} = [1.39(^{ml_{O_2}}/_{g_{Hb}}) \times Hb(^{g}/_{dl}) \times SaO_2] + \\ [Pa_{O_2}(mmHg) \times 0.0031(^{ml_{O_2}}/_{dl.mmHg})] \quad (2.2)$$

where 1.39 (Huffner's constant) is the amount of O_2 (mL) carried per gram of Hb at sea level. Therefore, CaO_2 could be impaired by a decrease in the Hb concentration or in the arterial oxygen pressure (Pa_{O_2}).

The function of the lung and its control system allows the maintenance of CaO_2 and avoids the hypoxia throughout four processes:

- The generation of a pressure gradient between the alveolar space and either the mouth or the airway opening, transairway pressure[3] to maintain an adequate alveolar oxygen pressure (PA_{O_2}) and alveolar pressure of carbon dioxide (PA_{CO_2}) by the cyclic ventilation of alveolar gas with atmospheric air.
- Gas exchange across the blood–air barrier. This requires a large, thin, moist exchange surface; a pump to move air; and a circulatory system to transport gases to the cells.
- Perfusion as the process by which deoxygenated blood passes through the lung and becomes reoxygenated, given an appropriate ventilation–perfusion ratio $\dot{V}A/\dot{Q}$.[1]
- The maintenance of a control system that allows permanent "sensing" of specific chemical and

physical conditions of the blood, especially gas pressures and acid–base status, which must follow the actual requirements of the body.

2.3 Pulmonary Ventilation

Ventilation is the process by which fresh gas moves in and out of the lung. *Minute ventilation* $(\dot{V}E)$ or total is the volume of air that enters or leaves the lung per minute and can be expressed by the equation

$$\dot{V}E = f \quad VT \quad (2.3)$$

where f is the number of breaths per minute, and V_T is the tidal volume or volume of air inspired (or exhaled) with each breath. Tidal volume varies with age, gender, body position, and metabolic activity. In an average-size adult, V_T is 500 mL (6–7 mL/kg). In children, the tidal volume is 3–5 mL/kg.[5] The initial portion of the tidal volume is directed into the alveoli to effect gas exchange. However, the last portion remains in the airway conducts and is commonly referred to as anatomical dead space ($V_{D(anat)}$). Therefore, the volume that enters the alveoli per breath V_A is

$$V_A = V_T - V_{D(anat)} \quad (2.4)$$

and the alveolar ventilation can be expressed as

$$\dot{V}_A = V_T \times f - V_{D(anat)} \times f \quad (2.5)$$

or

$$\dot{V}_A = f[V_T - V_D] \quad (2.6)$$

Thus, the alveolar ventilation depends on the breathing pattern and the volume of dead space. This dead space is called *anatomic dead space* because it represents the wasted ventilation of the airways that do not participate in gas exchange. The total volume of gas in each breath not participating in gas exchange is called the *physiological dead space* $V_{D(physiol)}$. Normally, $V_{D(physiol)}$ is approximately equal to $V_{D(anat)}$ and accounts for 25–30% of the V_T. It includes two separate components: (1) the anatomical dead space and (2) the dead space secondary to ventilated, but not perfused, alveoli or alveoli overventilated relative to the amount of perfusion. The physiological dead space may be determined by de Bohr's equation:

$$V_{D(physiol)}/V_T = (Pa_{CO2} - P\bar{E}_{CO_2})/Pa_{CO_2} \quad (2.7)$$

---

[1]The special symbols in respiratory physiology compiled by Pappenheimer et al.[4] are used throughout this chapter.

where $P\bar{E}_{CO_2}$ is the mixed expired P_{CO_2}. It is assumed that the P_{CO_2} of the exchanging (i.e., perfused) alveoli equals the P_{CO_2} of the arterial blood. As a consequence, a decrease in ventilation *out of proportion* to any decrease in metabolic V_{CO_2} (amount of CO_2 evolved from the body each minute) results in a high arterial P_{CO_2}. Hence, increase in dead space is a cause of hypercarbia.

At any given rate of metabolic CO_2 production, the steady-state value for PA_{CO_2} is therefore inversely related, in a hyperbolic fashion, to the rate of alveolar ventilation. The determinants of $\dot{V}A$ were expressed in (2.6).

2.3.1 Lung Volumes

The amount of gas in the lungs at different levels of inflation is represented as volumes (when they are single components) and capacities (when they are composed of two or more components). The balances between the elastic recoil properties of the lung and the properties of the chest wall and its muscles determine lung volumes. All lung volumes are subdivisions of the total lung capacity (TLC), and they are measured in liters. The static volumes of the lungs are shown in Fig. 2.1.[6]

The functional residual capacity (FRC) is the resting volume of the lung. It is determined by the balance between the lung elastic recoil pressure, which operates to decrease the lung volume, and the pressure generated by the chest wall to become larger. At FRC, the pressure difference across the respiratory system is zero, and it is approximately 50–60% of TLC (see the forces shown in Fig. 2.2 at resting volume). The interaction between elastic recoil forces of the chest wall, which pull the chest wall outward, and the elastic recoil forces of lung, which pull inward, creates a negative pressure in the intrapleural space with respect to atmosphericpre ssure(s ees ection2.3.2).

Vital capacity, tidal volume, inspiratory reserve, and expiratory reserve can all be measured with a simple spirometer. Total lung capacity, FRC, and residual volume (RV) all contain a fraction that cannot be measured by simple spirometry. However, RV and TLC can be measured using other methods: body plethysmography,[6,8,9] nitrogen washout,[10] or helium dilution[11] or using imaging techniques.[12] The methods more commonly used are nitrogen (N_2) washout (in its modern form, an open-circuit method) and helium (He) dilution (a closed-circuit method). The former method uses nitrogen washout by breathing 100% oxygen. Total quantity of nitrogen eliminated is measured as the product of the expired volume collected and the concentration of nitrogen. For example, if 4 L of nitrogen are collected and

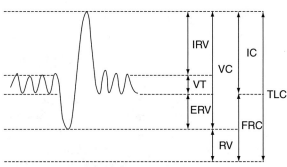

Volume and capacities	Typical ranges (liters)
IRV: Inspiratory reserve volume	1.9-2.5
VT: Tidal volume	0.4-0.5
ERV: Expiratory reserve volume	1.1-1.5
RV: Residual volume	1.5-1.9
TLC: Total lung capacity	4.9-6.4
IC: Inspiratory capacity	2.3-3.0
FRC: Functional Residual capacity	2.6-3.4
VC: Vital capacity	3.4-4.5

Fig. 2.1 Standard lung volumes and capacities. Typical values fora 70- kga dulta res hown

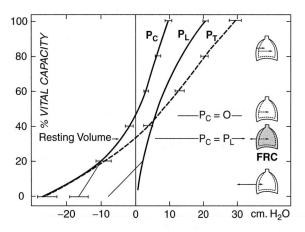

Fig. 2.2 Sitting pressure–volume curve of lung (P_L), thoracic cage (P_C), and the result of these two forces, the total respiratory system (P_T). Diagrams on the right side indicate direction and magnitude of forces for the two elastic systems of the chest at various lung volumes. *Dotted arrows* indicate lung tensions and *solid arrows* the thoracic-cage tension. Average vital capacity was 4,730 cm³ ATPS (Ambient temperature, ambient pressure, saturated with water vapor conditions of a volume of gas) at 26°C. Standard errors are indicated by brackets unless smaller than width of the line (From [7]w ithpe rmission)

the initial alveolar concentration was 80%, the estimated initial lung volume is 5 L. The latter method uses wash-in of a tracer gas such as helium (preferred for its low solubility in blood), which can be measured by katharometry. For example, if 50 mL of helium are introduced into the lungs and the helium concentration is then found to be 1%, the estimated lung volume is 5 L.

Measurements of lung volumes by radiographic, plethysmographic, gas dilution, or washout techniques produce on average similar results when normal subjects are tested. In contrast, the results of these techniques can differ significantly when ill patients are evaluated.[12]

2.3.2 Forces Involved in Breathing (Gradient Pressures)

Airflow in any system is directly proportional to the gradients of pressure and inversely related to the resistance to airflow, as expressed by Ohm's law:

$$\dot{Q} = \frac{P_1 - P_2}{R} \qquad (2.8)$$

where P_1 is the circuit initial pressure, P_2 is the pressure at the end, and R is the flow resistance. In the lung, the pressure gradient of concern is the difference between atmospheric (barometric) and alveolar pressure:

$$\dot{Q} = \frac{P_B - P_{alv}}{R_{aw}} \qquad (2.9)$$

where P_B is the barometric pressure, and P_{alv} is the alveolar pressure. Alternatively, it is described as the pressure gradient between the alveolar space and either the mouth (P_m) or the airway opening (P_{oa}), the transairway pressure.[3] R_{aw} represents the airway resistance. If the subject is breathing ambient air, atmospheric pressure (P_{atm}) does not change. This means that gas flow in the lungs results from changes in alveolar pressure; this is brought about by changes in the dimension of the thorax. *Inspirations* lead to expansion of the thorax, causing a fall in alveolar pressure sustained until the end of inspiration, when alveolar pressure equals atmospheric pressure. During *expiration*, the inspiration muscles relax, and the intrapleural pressure (P_{pl}) becomes less negative with respect to the atmospheric pressure. The elastic recoil of the lung then compresses the alveolar gas and raises its pressure above that of the mouth. If $P_{alv} > P_{atm}$, then, air flows out the lung

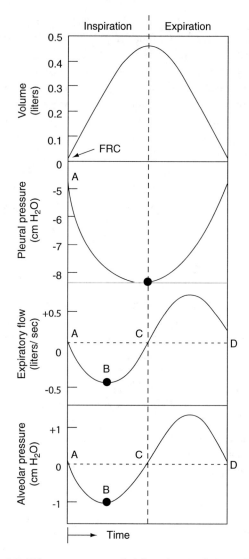

Fig. 2.3 Volume, pressure, and airflow changes during a single respiratory cycle

(Fig. 2.3). During quiet breathing in the supine position, the process occurs passively without much participation of the expiratory muscles because the energy required is provided by the elastic recoil of the lungs aided by the weight of the abdominal contents pushing the diaphragm in the cephalad direction. In the upright posture and during stimulated ventilation, the internal intercostal muscles and the abdominal wall muscles are active in returning the rib cage and diaphragm to the resting position.

Barometric pressure (P_B): Dalton's law (also called Dalton's law of partial pressures) states that the total pressure exerted by a gaseous mixture is equal to the sum of the partial pressures of each individual component in the mixture. This empirical law was observed by John Dalton in 1801 and is related to the ideal gas laws. Thus, the barometric pressure at a given location depends on the weight of the column of atmosphere directly over that point. Hence, places closer to sea level have "higher columns" of air above them and consequently greater "atmospheric" or "barometric" pressures. The air density and pressure decrease almost linearly with increasing altitude. It should be remembered that the atmospheric air is a mixture of gases, mostly nitrogen (78.09%), oxygen (20.95%), and small amounts of other gases. This remains largely unchanged around the globe. In other words, at high altitude the air contains the same percentage of oxygen as at sea level. However, since the air is less dense, a given volume of air contains fewer gas molecules, including oxygen. Thus, the partial pressure of oxygen (Po_2) is lower at high altitude due to the reduced barometric pressure.

Maximal inspiratory ($P_I mo,max$, MIP, or $P_{I'max}$) and expiratory pressure ($P_E mo,max$, MEP, or $P_{E'max}$) at the mouth. Both of these are simple indexes of ventilatory or respiratory muscle endurance. They are the most widely used measures of global inspiratory and expiratory muscle strength.[13–15] MIP decreases with age independent of gender. However, the decline is larger in men than in women.[16] The measurement is the maximal sustained pressure over 1 s, and the result is the maximal value of three measures. The result is compared with standardized values that take into account age, height, gender, and body mass. Typically, an MIP value that does not reach −80 cm H_2O is likely to be abnormal. Diaphragm contraction force can be estimated from the *transdiaphragmatic pressure* P_{di}, which is the difference between pressure above and below the diaphragm, measured as intragastric and intraesophageal pressure, respectively. Maximal contraction of the diaphragm is obtained by performing a maximal sniff maneuver or by phrenic nerve stimulation. Inspiratory muscle strength is often better reflected by esophageal pressure during a maximal sniff (sniff P_{oes}). Sniff P_{oes} is performed from FRC without a nose clip. In such a case, the volume increases about 500 mL, and diaphragm contraction is therefore relatively isometric. The normal mean sniff P_{oes} is 93 ± 20 cm H_2O, ranging between 74 and 135 cm H_2O.[17]

Alveolar pressure (P_{alv}): Boyle's law describes pressure–volume relationships of gases. Thus, in the alveolar space the pressure is determined for the size of the container (i.e., the alveolus). If the size of the container is reduced, the collisions between gas molecules and the walls become more frequent, and the pressure rises (i.e., at expiration, P_{alv} becomes greater than P_B, and the air flows out of the lungs). Therefore, the alveolar pressure depends on the alveolar volume, and the alveolar volume is determined by the relationship between forces involved in elastic lung and chest wall recoil. Hence, P_{alv} is simply the sum of the intrinsic recoil pressure (P_{recoil}) of the lung (at that volume) and the applied intrapleural pressure (P_{pl}). Therefore, to develop a change in P_{alv}, it is necessary to adjust the amount of P_{recoil}, P_{pl}, or both.

Causes of lung recoil: The lung tends to recoil to a lower volume even after a maximal volitional exhalation (i.e., at residual volume). Two basic factors account for this retractive, or recoil, force: elastic recoil and lungs urface tension.

1. *Elastic recoil*[18]: Elastic and collagen fibers are present in the alveolar walls and bronchial tree and, when distended, tend to return to equilibrium configuration. During inspiration, contraction of respiratory muscles stretches the elastic and collagen tissue network of the lungs and pleura, also overcoming the surface tension that is present at the interfaces between the air and alveoli, and the fluid lines alveolar walls. These features constitute an elastic hindrance to inspiration. At most lung volumes, the hindrance is mainly due to surface tension, but if lungs are nearly fully distended the recoil of the elastic and collagen fibers contributes as well. The work that is done in stretching the lung is not dissipated as heat. Instead, the energy is stored in the stretched structures and then spent in driving the subsequent expiration. This entails shrinking the lungs back to their previous volume. Hence, normal expiration is affected by the elastic recoil of the lung tissue. The energy applied to the lung in inspiration is not recovered in expiration. The property of dissipating energy is called *hysteresis*. Lung hysteresis can be quantified because it applies to the area between the ascending and descending portions of the pressure–volume curve and depends specifically on surface tension as discussed in item 2[19](s eea lsoFig. 2.4).

The network of fiber confers stability on the lungs because a local change in volume causes enlargement or shortening of collagen or elastic fibers in the immediate surrounding area. This is defined as *interdependence*.

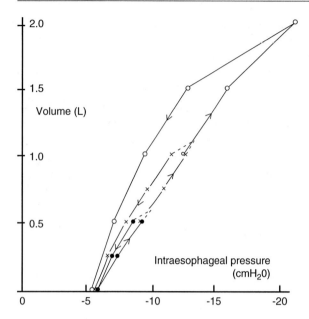

Fig. 2.4 The effect of tidal volume on hysteresis. Hysteresis is minimal at low tidal volumes but becomes larger as the tidal volume increases (From [20],w ithpe rmission.)

Interdependence mitigates the effect of local stress. The lung parenchyma, the airways, and the pulmonary and bronchial vascular systems are continuously subjected to a wide range of passive and active physical forces as a result of the dynamic nature of lung function. These forces include changes in *stress* (i.e., force per unit area) or *strain* (i.e., any forced change in length in relation to the initial length) and *shear stress* (i.e., the stress component parallel to a given surface).[21] The response to stress will be further analyzed in chapter numberfour .

2. *Lung surface tension*: In 1929, Kurt von Neergaard evacuated air from an isolated porcine lung, which he then filled with an isotonic gum solution to eliminate surface tension of the air tissue interfaces. Von Neergaard then obtained pressure–volume measurements and constructed curves based on the induced expansion of the lungs with air and liquid. From these experiments, he arrived at two main conclusions: (1) Surface tension is responsible for the greater part of total lung recoil compared to tissue elasticity. (2) A lower surface tension would be useful for the respiratory mechanism because without it pulmonary retraction might become too great, interfering with adequate expansion.[22,23] Surface tension is a measure of the force acting to pull a the surface

molecules of a liquid together at an air–liquid interface. Alveolar surface tension is similar to that existing in a spherical bubble. The surface tension created by the thin film of fluid is directed toward the center of the bubble and creates pressure in the interior. The law of Laplace is an expression of this pressure.

If the surface tension of the fluid was the same in the small and large alveoli, then small alveoli would have higher inwardly directed pressure than larger alveoli and consequently an increased resistance to stretch. As a result, more work would be needed to expand smaller alveoli. However, a *surfactant* reduces the surface tension, especially in the smaller alveoli, where higher concentrations are accumulated. Alveolar surfactant is well known for its ability to reduce minimal surface tension at the alveolar air–liquid interface to values below 5 mN/m. Hence, surfactant avoids collapse of the smaller alveoli. For this reason, alveoli with different diameters would have the same pressure (Fig. 2.5).

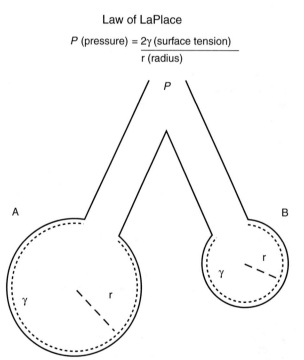

Fig. 2.5 According to Laplace's law, the surface tension in alveoli has to be dynamic. When the airway pressure is similar (pressure 1/4P) in alveoli of different sizes (difference in radius 1/4r), the surface tension (g) has to change accordingly. In this diagram, the surface tension in alveolus A will be higher than the surface tension in B to maintain alveolar stability. Pulmonary surfactant is able to dynamically reduce the surface tension (From [24],w ithpe rmission)

Production of surfactant is reduced when the lung parenchyma is damaged by breathing oxygen-enriched air, by severe shock, and by diversion of pulmonary blood flow through an extracorporeal circulation.

The surface tension also occurs in the airways. The airway surfactant existence reduces surface tension at the air–liquid interface of conducting airways.[25] This decreases the tendency of airway liquid to form bridges in the narrower airway lumen (film collapse). In addition, a low surface tension minimizes the amount of negative pressure in the airway wall and its adjacent liquid layer, which in turn decreases the tendency for airway wall (compliant) collapse. According to the law of Laplace, it becomes obvious that the smaller the airways, the higher the pressure would increase if surface-active material lowering the value of γ were absent. Surface tension in the conducting airways has been shown to be in the range between 25 and 30 mN/m.

Pleural (intrapleural) pressure (P_{pl}) depends on the elastic and chest wall recoil interaction forces. The recoil of the lung causes it to attempt to retract to its equilibrium volume (effectively that of a gas-free lung). The elastic properties of the chest wall cause it to expand to adopt its own equilibrium point (which is half the volume of the fully expanded state). Thus, at the same time elastic recoil of the lungs creates an inwardly directed force that tends to pull the lungs away from the chest wall. As a consequence, at the end of normal (passive) expiration (FRC), the combination of the outward pull of the thoracic cage and inward recoil

of the elastic lungs creates a subatmospheric intrapleural pressure of about −3 mmHg. When a person is in the upright position, the weight of the lungs pulls the lungs away from the chest wall at the top of the lungs and squeezes them against the chest wall at the base of the lungs. This means that intrapleural pressure is more negative at the top of the lungs and less negative at the bases. Consequently, the alveolar volume is different between apex and bases because the alveolar volume is determined by transpulmonary pressure ($P_{alv} - P_{pl}$). In any posture, the pleural fluid pressure with respect to atmospheric pressure is more negative at the top than at the bottom of the lung (Fig. 2.6).

The pleural space does not contain gas. This is because the sum of the tissue gas tensions is considerably less than atmospheric pressure, leading to the reabsorption of any gas in the pleural space. Also, the concentration of protein in the pleural fluid is low (1–2%), leading to a lower osmotic pressure than in the plasma. Therefore, the fluid is reabsorbed, and as a result the pleural space is relatively dry.

Respiratory muscles and P_{pl}: At FRC, neither the lung nor the chest wall are in equilibrium. However, the combined chest wall system adopts an equilibrium position due to the absence of volitional contraction of muscles of breathing applied to the chest wall. However, when respiratory muscles are contracted, the P_{pl} changes. The fall in P_{pl} obtained in response to a given stimulation of the phrenic nerves decreases rapidly as the lung volume is passively increased above

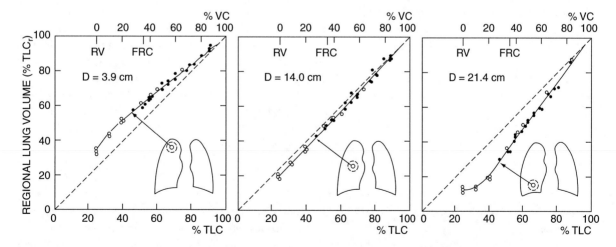

Fig. 2.6 Correlation between percentage total lung capacity (% TLC) and regional lung volume. Abscissa lower axis is the overall lung volume expressed as percentage TLC, and the upper axis is the overall lung volume expressed as percentage vital capacity (VC).

The *broken line* (line of identity) indicates percentile degree of expansion of the regions equal to that of the entire lungs. The vertical distance (*D*) from the top of the lungs (in centimeters) to the center of each counter is indicated (From [26], with permission).

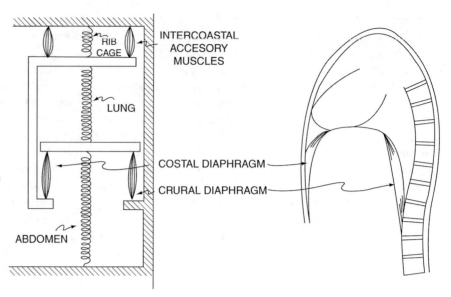

Fig.2.7 Mechanicalm odel of inspiratory musculature. Intercostal and accessory muscles are mechanically parallel with costal diaphragm. *Bar* into which crural and costal fibers insert represents central tendon. *Inverted L-shaped structure* represents rib cage, and *springs* attached to its upper surface indicate the elastic properties of the rib cage. The *hatched area* represents the rest of bony skeleton. *Right*: more anatomically realistic drawing of diaphragm illustrating separation of costal and crural parts (From [27], w ithpe rmission)

FRC, and muscle length is decreased. Inspiration is effected by three groups of muscles, diaphragm, external intercostals, and some accessory muscles (e.g., scalenes, sternocleidomastoids, and trapezius come into play at high rates of ventilation). When the diaphragm contracts, it loses its dome shape and drops down toward the abdomen. In quiet breathing, the diaphragm moves about 1.5 cm. This movement increases thoracic volume by flattening its floor. Contraction of the diaphragm causes between 60 and 75% of inspiratory volume change during normal breathing. Movement of the rib cage creates the remaining 25–40% of the volume change (Fig. 2.7). During inhalation in the upright position, the external intercostals and scalene muscles contract and pull the ribs upward andout.

Weakness of inspiratory or expiratory muscles reduces inspiratory capacity and expiratory reserve volume, respectively. That weakness can be caused by mechanical derangement, in association with critical or chronic illness and as a result of a neurological or muscular disorder. For this reason, on both accounts the vital capacity and TLC are reduced. If the reduction in vital capacity exceeds 50%, the hypoventilation is likely to occur with hypercapnia, and it can lead to hypoxemia.

Lung compliance (C) is the capability of the lungs to distend under pressure, as measured by pulmonary volume change per unit pressure change. The distending pressure across the lung is the difference in pressures between the inside and outside of the lung, that is, the transpulmonary pressure $(P_{alv} - P_{pl})$[2]:

$$C = \frac{\Delta V_{(ml)}}{\Delta P_{tp}} \Rightarrow C = \frac{\Delta V_{(ml)}}{\Delta(P_{alv} - P_{pl})_{(cmH_2O)}} \quad (2.10)$$

The measurement of lung *compliance* under conditions of no airflow (i.e., under *static conditions*) allows establishing the intrinsic elasticity or stiffness of the lungs without the confounding influence of needing additional pulmonary pressures to overcome the resistance to airflow. At the end of inspiration and expiration, P_{alv} must be exactly equal to P_{atm} because the airflow is zero. Thus, to measure *static lung compliance* only, the changes in the lung volume and intrapleural pressure are needed. The lung volume can be readily measured with a simple spirometer, and the pleural pressure is normally estimated by measuring the intraesophageal pressure. For normal adults, a change of P_{pl} from −4 to −6 cm H_2O would induce a volume change, a tidal volume, of approximately 600 mL. The compliance in this case would be 200 mL/cm H_2O. In a normal adult, it has a mean value of 240 mL/cm H_2O (Fig. 2.8). Recent studies have found that regular use of pressure–volume curves provides useful physiological data that help to optimize mechanical ventilation at the bedside and, more interestingly, to improve outcome.[28,29] In a normal subject on mechanical ventilation, compliance should

[2]A positive transpulmonary pressure is needed to increase the lung volume.

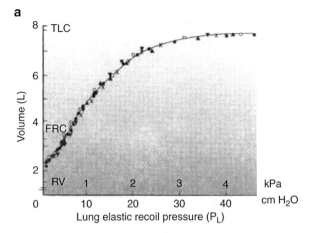

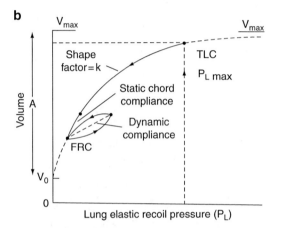

Fig. 2.8 (**a**) Static lung pressure–volume (PV) curve. Lung recoil pressure (P_L) plotted against absolute lung volume and total lung capacity (TLC), measured separately. Different symbols indicate measurements made during five separate interrupted expirations from TLC. At volumes below functional residual capacity (FRC), the slope of the PV curve becomes shallower. Note that maximum P_L in this healthy young individual is unusually high at approximately 50 cm H_2O. (**b**) Measurements from static lung PV curve and dynamic lung compliance. *Heavy line* is a diagrammatic static PV curve of lungs from TLC to FRC with extrapolation to V_{max} and V_0 (difference = A) to allow calculation of shape factor "k." In general, the greater the value of k, the more distensible the lungs (From [31], w ithpe rmission)

The specific compliance is usually reported for expiration at FRC; it then has a value in normal subjects of 0.08 cm H_2O (range 0.03–0.14 cm H_2O). Loss of compliance increases the work of breathing (WOB).

Measurements of transpulmonary pressure and volume also can be recorded continuously during tidal breathing. Then, the so-called dynamic compliance (C_{dyn}) can be obtained – usually on a plot of pressure vs. volume – by measuring the slope of a line crossing values of esophageal pressure and volume at end expiration and end inspiration as determined by zero airflow at the mouth. In normal subjects, dynamic compliance is only slightly less than static compliance. In patients with airway disease, redistribution of air continues through narrowed intrapulmonary airways even when flow at the mouth ceases. Consequently, some of the transpulmonary pressure apparently overcoming elastic forces is dissipated against resistive forces, and the apparent compliance is less than estimated statically. This effect goes along with increases in breathing frequency. Thus, in patients with even mild diffuse airway disease, the dynamic compliance falls as frequency increases.[31]

Compliance is different from *elastance* (elasticity). The fact that a lung stretches easily (high compliance) does not necessarily mean that it will return to its resting volume when the stretching force is released. For example, when destruction of elastin occurs, the lungs exhibit high compliance and stretch easily during inspiration. However, these lungs also have decreased elastance, so they do not recoil to their resting position during expiration. Thus, people with emphysema have more difficulty exhaling than inhaling.

Chest wall compliance is the relationship of the pressure change across the chest wall to thoracic volume. In normal subjects, it is on average 230 mL/cm H_2O. It can correlate negatively with age, disease of chondrovertebral joints, damage to thoracic vertebrae, scarring of the skin of the chest, large bosom, or central obesity.

Closing volume (CV) is the lung volume at which the dependent lung zones cease to ventilate, presumably as a result of airway closure (Fig. 2.9). At the point of maximal closure, the volume of gas remaining in the lungs is the residual volume. This volume is reached when the pleural pressure is greater than the airway pressure in the terminal bronchi (in normal subjects). Premature closure increases the residual volume; the most common cause is the loss of lung elasticity

be greater than 50–100 mL/cm H_2O.[30] Lower values are obtained in children and in women compared with men, mainly due to absolutely smaller lungs. However, when the lung volume is considered in relative terms (e.g., as a fraction of the TLC), no significant differences are found due to age and gender. This has the effect that the compliance per liter of lung volume, which is the *specific compliance* (sC), is effectively constant.

$$sC = C_{measured}/FCR \qquad (2.11)$$

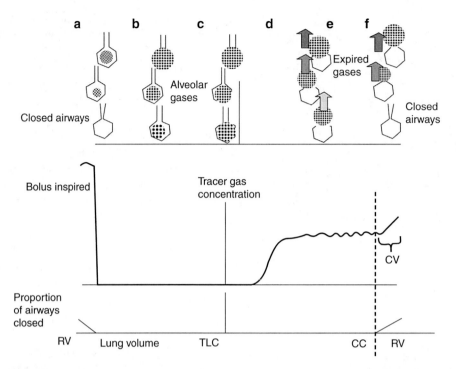

Fig. 2.9 The proposed mechanism for the closing volume (CV) maneuver with a tracer gas. *A* The lung is at residual volume (RV), and a bolus of tracer gas is inspired, passing into lung regions served by airways that remain open. Lung regions with closed airways do not receive any tracer gas. *B* The tracer gas bolus is followed by unlabeled air. As this unlabeled air is inspired, it dilutes the tracer gas according to the regional ventilation pattern of the lung. Regions previously closed are then open and receive air. *C* Total lung capacity (TLC) is reached. The alveoli that were open at RV contain tracer gas; the alveoli that were closed, and the airways, contain air only. *D* Expiration has started, and airway gas containing no tracer is exhaled; this is dead-space gas. *E* The "alveolar plateau" contains slightly varying contributions from different lung regions (partly because of cardiac movement). The exhaled concentration represents this variation in contributions from different regions. *F* As airway closure starts, the lung regions that contain less or no tracer gas cease to contribute to expired gas. Consequently, the tracer gas concentration in the expired gas increases as it is now only emerging from labeled lung regions. The lung volume at which airway closure starts is called the closing capacity (CC), and the difference between CC and RV is the CV (From [32],w ithpe rmission)

(increased compliance), which occurs with increasing age and with emphysema. Premature generalized closure can also occur as a consequence of narrowing of airways from other causes, including contraction of bronchial muscles and thickening of air walls.[32]

Several factors as well as the elastic recoil of the lungs and the chest wall must be overcome to move air into or out of the lungs. These factors include the inertia of the respiratory system and the frictional resistance of the airways to the flow of air. Inertial forces are of negligible magnitude except when a high-frequency oscillation is applied for mechanical ventilation or in experimental conditions. *Pulmonary tissue resistance* (R_{ti}) is caused by the friction encountered as the lung tissues move against each other during lung expansion. The R_{ti} itself is bigger in pulmonary fibrosis and other conditions in which the quantity of interstitial lung tissue is increased.

The *airways resistance* (R_{aw}) plus the pulmonary tissue resistance is often referred to as the *pulmonary resistance* (Rl). Pulmonary tissue resistance normally contributes about 10–20% of the pulmonary resistance, with airways resistance responsible for the rest. Pulmonary tissue resistance can be augmented in such conditions as pulmonary sarcoidosis and fibrosis. Since airways resistance is the major component of the total resistance, this chapter concentrates on airways resistance.

R_{aw}, as a part of pulmonary function testing, is the ratio of driving pressure to the rate of airflow. Three parameters contribute to resistance: the system's length L, the viscosity of the fluid (η), and the radius of the tubes in the system r. Poiseuille's law relates these factors to one another:

$$R \propto L\eta/r^4 \qquad (2.12)$$

In normal conditions, the length and viscosity are constant; then, the radius of the airways becomes the primary determinant of R_{aw}. However, the work needed by a normal subject to overcome resistance of the airways to airflow is much less than work needed to overcome the resistance of the lungs and thoracic cage to stretch.

Because the airways behave like a circuit in parallel, the resistance at each level of the airways depends on the cross-sectional area. For this reason, the resistance is greater in the proximal airway (e.g., trachea 2–2.5 cm²) than in the distal airway (5×10^3 cm²). The first eight airway generations are the major site of airway resistance. R_{aw} varies with lung volume because the airways diameter, as well as the alveoli, depends on the changes in the pleural pressure. The resistance is lower at large volumes when the airways are expanded; it rises during expiration as the airways diminish in size and becomes infinite at residual volume when some airways close.

The R_{aw} also depends on the pattern of flow. The airway resistance is the sum of its laminar and turbulent components. The determinants of this pattern were described by Reynolds:

$$\text{Re} = \dot{v}D\rho/\eta A \qquad (2.13)$$

where $\dot{v}$ is the bulk flow gas, A is the cross-sectional area, D is the diameter, ρ is the gas density, and η is the gas viscosity. Re numbers less than 100 and more than 4,000 are associated, respectively, with completely laminar and fully turbulent flow. With other values, Re would be intermediate. Thus, on the trachea it is intermediate, and in the bronchioles it is nearly laminar.

Work of breathing: The two main components of the WOB are the elastic recoil of the lungs and chest wall and the resistance to airflow. The inertia of the airway is also part of impedance, but its contribution is negligible in respiratory physiology. Impedance can be estimated through measurements of the WOB. In respiratory physiology, WOB describes the energy required as the flow begins to perform the task of ventilation. Breathing requires the use of respiratory muscles (diaphragm, intercostals, etc.), which expend energy. In general, the work performed during each respiratory cycle is mathematically expressed as $\text{WOB} = \int P \times V$ (i.e., the area on a pressure–volume diagram).[3] The *volume change* is

the volume of air moved into and out of the lung, the tidal volume. The *pressure change* is the change in transpulmonary pressure necessary to overcome the elastic WOB and the resistive WOB. *Impedance to airflow* includes the resistance to airflow as well as the force required to overcome the elasticity of the lungs and chest wall. The calculation of the WOB is usually associated with inspiratory effort because expiration is generally a passive process. However, in patients with air trapping or acute respiratory failure, expiration can be an active process and can require significant work.[33] Although ventilation normally requires 5% of total oxygen delivery,[34] this requirement increases during lung pathological states, such that the metabolic demand for oxygen may reach 25% of total oxygen delivery.

2.3.3 Alveolar Gas Pressures

The levels of oxygen and carbon dioxide in alveolar gas are determined by the altitude (P_B), the composition of the inspired air, the *alveolar ventilation volume* ($\dot{V}A$), the rate of *oxygen consumption* ($\dot{V}O_2$), and the *carbon dioxide production of the body* ($\dot{V}CO_2$).[35,36]

The partial pressure of oxygen changes as it flows through the airway. The partial pressure of oxygen in the ambient air is determined by P_B. Hence, the dry P_{O_2} can be calculated from the *fraction of oxygen* (F_{O_2}) in the gas mixture times the total or ambient (barometric) pressure. At sea level, that is,

$$\begin{aligned} P_{O_2} &= P_B \times F_{O_2} \Rightarrow P_{O_2} = 760\,mmHg \\ &\times 0.21 \Rightarrow P_{O_2} = 159.6\,mmHg \end{aligned} \qquad (2.14)$$

Evidently, P_{O_2} will be altered if the subject is at altitude or if using supplemental oxygen.

As inspiration begins, inspired gases become saturated with water vapor, which exerts a partial pressure (47 mmHg at normal body temperature). Because the total pressure remains constant at P_B, water vapor dilutes the total pressure of the other gases. Hence, in the conducting airways the partial pressure of oxygen may be calculated as

$$\begin{aligned} P_{I_{O_2}} &= F_{I_{O_2}} \times (P_B - P_{H_2O}) \xrightarrow{at\,sea\,level} P_{I_{O_2}} \\ &= 0.21 \times (760 - 47)_{mmHg} \end{aligned} \qquad (2.15)$$

At the end of inspiration or expiration, with the glottis open, the total alveolar pressure is equal to P_B. The gas

---

[3]In a healthy subject, the work per liter of ventilation (work per cycle divided by tidal volume) normal value is around 2.4 J/min, with 1 joule (J) the energy needed to move 1 L of gas through a 10-cm H_2O pressure gradient.

exchange decreases the P_{O_2} and increases the P_{CO_2}. Therefore, the *alveolar oxygen pressure* (PA_{O_2}) is slightly lower than PI_{O_2} and can be calculated by the alveolar gas equation:

$$PA_{O_2} = PI_{O_2} - \frac{PA_{CO_2}}{R} \Rightarrow PA_{O_2}$$
$$= FI_{O_2}(P_B - P_{H_2O}) - \frac{PA_{CO_2}}{R} \qquad (2.16)$$

The *respiratory exchange ratio* is the ratio of the rate at which carbon dioxide leaves the lung in expired gas ($\dot{V}_{CO_2}$) to the rate of oxygen consumption ($\dot{V}_{O_2}$). Under steady-state conditions, such a ratio is representative of the metabolism of the subject and is called the *respiratory quotient* (R). R varies between 0.7 and 1.0 when the metabolism is exclusively from fatty acid or when there is exclusive carbohydrate metabolism, respectively. R in a mixed diet is approximately 0.8.

The concentration of carbon dioxide in the alveolar gas is dependent on $\dot{V}A$ and on $\dot{V}CO_2$ (and its delivery to the lung in the mixed venous blood). The volume of carbon dioxide expired per unit of time ($\dot{V}E_{CO_2}$) is equal to $\dot{V}A$ times the alveolar fractional concentration of CO_2 (FA_{CO_2}). No carbon dioxide comes from the dead space. This relationship is defined by the alveolar carbon dioxide equation:

$$\dot{V}_{CO_2} = \dot{V}A \times FA_{CO_2} \qquad (2.17)$$

sincethe $PA_{CO_2}$is de fined by

$$PA_{CO_2} = FA_{CO_2} \times (P_B - P_{H_2O}) \qquad (2.18)$$

then,

$$PA_{CO_2} = \frac{\dot{V}_{CO_2} \times (P_B - P_{H_2O})}{\dot{V}A} \qquad (2.19)$$

Therefore, there is an inverse relationship between PA_{CO_2} and $\dot{V}A$. PA_{CO_2} is tightly regulated to remain constant around 40 mmHg at sea level via a ventilatory control system. In a normal subject, PA_{CO_2} is in equilibrium with arterial carbon dioxide pressure (Pa_{CO_2}). Thus, when $\dot{V}A$ decreases (hypoventilation), Pa_{CO_2} becomes greater, causing respiratory acidosis. Hyperventilation has the opposite effect (Fig. 2.10).

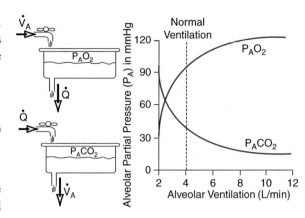

Fig. 2.10 PA_{O_2} and PA_{CO_2} are inversely related due the converse effects of ventilation. Hyperventilation (Pa_{CO2}<40 mmHg) results in increased Pa_{O_2} and decreased Pa_{CO_2}. Hypoventilation (Pa_{O_2}>40 mmHg) causes decreased PA_{O_2} and hypoxemia (From [37],w ithpe rmission)

When the alveolar oxygen equation and alveolar carbon dioxide equation are related to each other, it is possible to demonstrate that PaO_2 depends on the composition of the inspired air, $\dot{V}O_2$ (mL/min) and $\dot{V}A$(mL/min):

$$PA_{O_2} = PI_{O_2} - (P_B - 47)\frac{\dot{V}_{O_2}}{\dot{V}A} \qquad (2.20)$$

Distribution of ventilation: Studies performed on normal subjects seated upright have shown that alveoli in the lower regions of the lungs receive more ventilation per unit volume than those in the upper regions of the lung. As described previously, alveolar volume depends on transpulmonary pressure. Alveolar pressure is the same everywhere in the lungs, but because of these regional differences in P_{pl}, alveoli at the top of the lungs are at a larger volume (due to a more negative P_{pl}) than those at the base (less-negative P_{pl}).[4] Thus, at the beginning of a breath, some alveoli start at a larger volume than the other alveoli. As described, alveolar compliance depends on volume changes. At the beginning of a breath, intrapleural pressure decreases the same amount everywhere. However, because the alveoli at the top of the lungs start at a larger volume, they

---

[4]This is because the pleural pressure is lower at the apex than at the base because the weight of the lungs tends to pull it downward, away from the chest wall. If the pleural pressure is decreased, the transpulmonary pressure must be increased, and the alveolar volume increases in this area.

are less compliant and consequently change their volume less than alveoli of the bases despite the same fall in the P_{pl} (Fig. 2.6). Therefore, the weight of the lungs sets alveoli at different initial volumes, which affects how much their volume can be increased during a breath. Those at the base are ventilated more than those at the top of the lung.

In a theoretically constructed model of the lung, complete gas exchange equilibrium is reached between alveolar gas and pulmonary capillary blood, and partial pressures for CO_2 and O_2 in arterial blood are equal to those in alveolar gas. In fact, under basal conditions, most O_2 transfer across the alveolar–capillary membrane occurs within one third of the transit time for blood in the pulmonary capillaries.

In real lungs, partial pressure differences between alveolar gas and arterialized blood – an alveolar-to-arterial PO_2 difference ($AaDO_2$) and arterial-to-alveolar PCO_2 difference ($aADCO_2$) – are found. In the conventional model analysis of alveolar gas exchange, these differences are attributed to three mechanisms: (1) unequal distribution of alveolar ventilation to pulmonary blood flow; (2) shunt; and (3) diffusion limitation.

2.3.4 Unequal Distribution of Ventilation to Perfusion

Perfusion: The systemic and pulmonary circulations differ significantly with regard to blood flow and pressure–volume relationship. The pulmonary circulation is a low-pressure and low-resistance system with a driving pressure that is almost a 13th of the systemic circulation. This difference is partially caused by greater compliance of the pulmonary vessels than the systemic vessels. In contrast to systemic arterial vessels, the anatomical structure of pulmonary arteries is characterized by a thinner media and fewer smooth muscle cells surrounding precapillary resistance vessels. The pulmonary vessels are seven times more compliant than the systemic vessels. Hence, increased vascular distensibility causes decreased pulmonary vascular resistance (PVR) when compared with systemic vascular resistance despite an equal blood flow. This resistance is about ten times less than in the systemic circulation. Using an equation like Ohm's law, PVR can be calculated as the difference between mean pulmonary artery pressure (MPAP) and pressure of left atrium (PLA) divided by the cardiac output. PLA can be replaced with pulmonary artery wedge pressure (PAWP):

$$R_{pulmonary} = \frac{MPAP - PLA}{Cardiac\ output} \Rightarrow R_{pulmonary}$$
$$= \frac{MPAP - PAWP}{Cardiac\ output} \tag{2.21}$$

Lung volume can affect PVR through its influence on alveolar vessels, mainly on the capillaries. At the end of inspiration, the fully distended air-filled alveoli compress the alveolar capillaries and increase PVR. In contrast to the capillary beds in the systemic circulation, the capillary bed in the lung has a major influence on PVR, and it accounts for about 40% of the resistance. This stretching effect during inspiration has an opposite effect on larger extra-alveolar vessels, which increase in diameter due to radial traction by the connective tissue and alveolar septa holding the larger vessels in place in the lung (Fig. 2.11). The extra-alveolar vessels are not influenced by alveolar pressure changes, but they are affected by intrapleural and interstitial pressure changes. As lung volume is increased by making the intrapleural pressure more negative, the transmural pressure gradient of the larger arteries and veins increases, and they distend.[38]

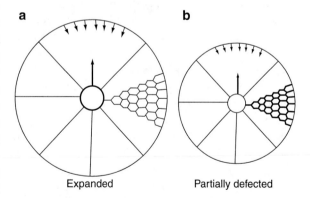

Fig. 2.11 The mechanism of radial traction on blood vessels. When the lungs are expanded (**a**) the capillaries in the alveolar walls are attenuated, and the volume of blood that they contain is less than when the lung is partially deflated. (**b**) By contrast, the alveolar corner vessels and the extra-alveolar vessels in the interstitial spaces are increased in size due to traction from surrounding structures (From [38], w ithpe rmission)

Fig.2.12 Recruitmenta nd
distentionof a lveolarv essels

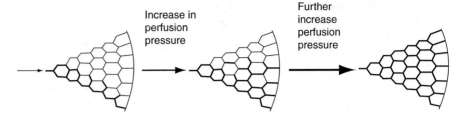

Increase in
perfusion
pressure

Further
increase
perfusion
pressure

PVR usually decreases with increases in pulmonary blood flow, pulmonary artery pressure, left atrial pressure, or pulmonary capillary blood volume because of distention of already open blood vessels, recruitment of previously unopened vessels, or both.[39] Therefore, recruitment of physiologically collapsed pulmonary vessels at rest provides constant PVR even in the presence of increased cardiac output during exercise[40] (Fig. 2.12). This effect is due to a decrease of the PVR occurring when the blood vessels are recruited and distended. Alveolar hypoxia (or hypercapnia) can cause constriction of precapillary pulmonary vessels, diverting blood flow away from poorly ventilated or unventilated alveoli. However, local hypoxia does not alter PVR. Approximately 20% of the vessels need to be hypoxic before a change in PVR can be measured. Low inspired oxygen levels due to exposure to high altitude will have a greater effect on PVR.

Regional perfusion changes because of gravity: In upright, resting subjects, blood flow increases linearly from the apex of the lung to the base of the lung, where the flow is the greatest. The marked effect of gravity on pulmonary circulation stems from the low arterial pulmonary pressure and the very different densities of blood and air. Because there is a hydrostatic gradient in blood but practically none in alveolar air, the transmural pressure in pulmonary vessels increases vertically from top to bottom, leading to distension of vessels and increased blood volume and blood flow in the lower (dependent) lung regions. The interplay of alveolar pressure, flow rate, and vascular resistance is best considered by dividing the lung field into four zones. Zone 1 represents the apex region, where blood does not flow under certain conditions. Under normal conditions, zone 1 does not exist; nevertheless, this state is reached during positive-pressure mechanical ventilation and conditions with severe decrease of the arterial pressure (Pa). In zone 2, which comprises the upper one third of the lung, Pa is greater than the PA, which is greater than

venous pressure (Pv). In zone 3, Pa is greater than Pv, which is greater than PA, and blood flow in this area parallels the pressure gradients.[41] In zone 4, in the most dependent part of the lung the intravascular hydrostatic pressure is relatively high. This can lead to fluid passing into the interstitial tissue. In normal circumstances, the quantity of fluid is small. It can increase dramatically if pulmonary venous pressure or the permeability of the pulmonary capillary membrane is increased or if the plasma osmotic pressure is reduced, thus causing alveolar interstitial edema (Fig. 2.13).

It has been known for many years that the distribution of ventilation–perfusion ratios ($\dot{V}_A/\dot{Q}$) is uneven in the lungs of normal subjects. The 1953 work of Martin, Cline, and Marshall[42] demonstrated interlobar differences in O_2 and CO_2 concentrations best explained by regional differences in ventilation and blood flow. On average, $\dot{V}_A/\dot{Q}$ is approximately 1. However, as described in previous sections, the effect of gravity produces differences in ventilation and perfusion from the top to the bottom of the lungs. Relative to the top of the lung, the base of the lung is ventilated (approximately 3 times) and perfused (18 times) better. However, because the change in ventilation from the top to the bottom of lungs is not as great as the change in blood flow, $\dot{V}_A/\dot{Q}$ decreases from the top to the bottom of the lungs (approximately five times). This means that the top of the lungs is overventilated relative to its blood flow, and the base of the lung is overperfused relative to its ventilation. In other words, $\dot{V}_A/\dot{Q}$ is high at the top of the lung and low at the base of the lung. This imbalance between alveolar ventilation and blood flow is also called $\dot{V}A - \dot{Q}$ *mismatch*.

Regional differences in $\dot{V}_A/\dot{Q}$ result in regional differences in gas exchanges from the top to the bottom of the normal lung. Thus, blood leaving the top of the lung has a higher P_{O_2} and a lower P_{CO_2} than the blood leaving the base of the lung.

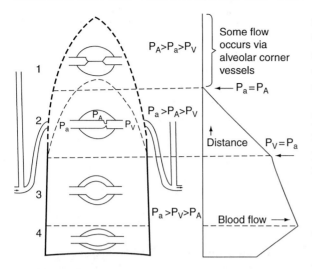

Fig. 2.13 Model to explain the effect of gravity on the vertical distribution of blood flow in lungs (Modified from [41], with permission)

Ventilation and perfusion must be matched on the alveolar–capillary level for optimal gas exchange. The alveolar–arterial P_{O_2} difference (AaD_{O_2}) due to $\dot{V}_A/\dot{Q}$ inequality may amount to 10–15 mmHg in normal individuals, the alveolar-arterial P_{CO_2} difference to 2–4 mmHg. The extreme cases are of particular interest. $\dot{V}_A/\dot{Q} = 0$ means lack of ventilation and therefore absence of gas exchange, its perfusion constituting *shunt* or *venous admixture*. $\dot{V}_A/\dot{Q} = \infty$, due to $\dot{Q} = 0$, designates the presence of ventilated but unperfused alveoli (Fig. 2.14). Again, there is no gas exchange, and the ventilation of such a compartment is functionally a dead space ventilation. It is called *parallel* or *alveolar dead space ventilation*, as distinguished from conducting airway ventilation, which is *series* or *anatomic dead space ventilation*. The sum of both is

equivalent to total ventilation not contributing to gas exchange. It is termed *physiologic dead space ventilation*. It can be calculated from Bohr's equation as described previously. Ventilation–perfusion ratios close to 1.0 result in alveolar PO_2s of approximately 100 mmHg and PCO_2s close to 40 mmHg (at sea level); ventilation–perfusion ratios greater than 1.0 increase the PO_2 and decrease the PCO_2; ventilation–perfusion ratios lower than 1.0 decrease the PO_2 and increase the PCO_2.

2.3.5 Shunt or Venous Admixture

A short circuit of blood passing gas-exchanging regions of the lungs leads to admixture of venous blood to arterialized blood and thus to a decrease of PO_2 and increase of PCO_2 in the arterial blood. *Shunt* refers to a condition in which $\dot{V}_A/\dot{Q}$ tends to zero because of no ventilation. The lack of ventilation may occur for two reasons: either the vasculature does not have access to alveoli or alveoli do not permit gas exchange because they are either physically plugged (not ventilated) or impermeable to gas. There are two types of shunts, anatomic and absolute. *Anatomic (extrapulmonary) shunt* refers to the amount of systemic venous blood that mixes with the pulmonary end-capillary blood on the arterial side of the circulation. In a normal healthy adult, about 2–5% of the cardiac output, including venous blood from the bronchial veins, the Thebesian veins, and the pleural veins, enters the left side of the circulation directly without passing through the pulmonary capillaries. In contrast, mixed venous blood perfusing pulmonary capillaries, associated with totally unventilated or collapsed alveoli, constitutes an

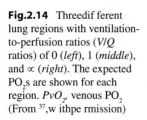

Fig.2.14 Three different lung regions with ventilation-to-perfusion ratios (*V/Q* ratios) of 0 (*left*), 1 (*middle*), and ∞ (*right*). The expected PO_2s are shown for each region. *PvO_2*, venous PO_2 (From [37], with permission)

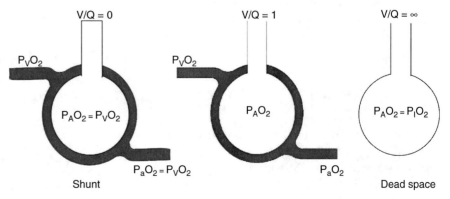

absolute shunt because no gas exchange occurs as the blood passes through thc lung. Absolute shunt is sometimes also referred to as *true shunt, alveolar shunt,* or *intrapulmonary shunt.* Alveolar–capillary units with low $\dot{V}_A/\dot{Q}$ also act to lower the arterial oxygen content because the blood draining these units has a lower PO_2 than blood from units with well-matched ventilation and perfusion. These are referred to as "shuntlike states." The combined effect of anatomical shunt, alveolar shunt, and "shuntlike" states is called *physiological shunt* and can be calculated by the shunt equation:

$$\frac{\dot{Q}s}{\dot{Q}t}(\%) = \frac{Cc'O_2 - CaO_2}{Cc'O_2 - C\bar{v}O_2} \times 100 \qquad (2.22)$$

where C is content of oxygen; c', a, and $\bar{v}$ refer, respectively, to the end-capillary, arterial, and mixed venous blood. In a healthy young adult at rest, 2% of cardiac output does not participate in gas exchange. At age 60, the average proportion is approximately 4%.[43] Among the intrapulmonary causes for an increased venous admixture effect, an enlarged anatomical shunt occurs in some cases of bronchiectasis, atelectasis, and pulmonary edema. Extrapulmonary causes include cyanotic congenital heart disease and portal cirrhosis.

According to experimental results, a substantial part of the $\dot{V}_A/\dot{Q}$ inequality appears not to be due to gravity but to anatomical heterogeneity of airways and blood vessels. The gravitational model of ventilation–perfusion distribution might fail to explain adequately several important observations regarding the distribution of ventilation and perfusion: heterogeneity at the same vertical level, postural inequality, and the persistence of heterogeneity in the absence of gravity. The underlying structure of the bronchial and pulmonary vascular anatomy with nonsymmetrical branching is now considered an important factor in causing heterogeneity in pulmonary perfusion and ventilation in both health and disease.[44]

2.3.6 Gas Diffusion

Diffusion is important for gas movement from the smaller airways to the alveoli and for gas movement across the alveoli into the blood and from the blood to the tissue and mitochondria (oxygen) and conversely from the tissue to blood, from the blood to the alveoli, and from alveoli to the smaller airways (carbon dioxide). Four factors determine the amount of gas diffusing through a sheet of tissue over time, but only one changes under normal conditions, the pressure gradient. Fick's law states that the rate of diffusion ($\dot{V}$) of a gas across a sheet of tissue is directly related to the surface area A of the tissue, the diffusion constant D of the specific gas, and the partial pressure difference $P_1 - P_2$ of each gas on each side of the tissue, and it is inversely related to the tissue thickness T. Thus ,

$$\dot{V}\text{gas} = \frac{(P_1 - P_2) \times A \times D}{T} \qquad (2.23)$$

Two properties of the gas contribute to the diffusing capacity of the lungs D_L: solubility S and molecular weight MW ($S/\sqrt{MW}$). First, the mobility of the gas should decrease as its molecular weight increases. Indeed, Graham's law states that the diffusion is inversely proportional to the square root of MW. Second, Fick's law states that the flow of the gas across the wet barrier is proportional to the concentration gradient of the gas dissolved in water. According to Henry's law, these concentrations are proportional to the respective partial pressures, and the proportionality constant is the solubility of gas. Therefore, poorly soluble gases like N_2 and helium diffuse poorly across the alveolar wall. The ratio $A \times D/T$ represents the conductance of a gas from alveolus to the blood. The physical properties of oxygen and carbon dioxide enable them to diffuse rapidly between the alveolar air and the blood. Therefore, the amount of these gases in the blood is not limited by diffusion. Nevertheless, the amount of these gases in the blood is limited by blood flow.[6] As carbon monoxide has a low solubility in the capillary membrane, it is limited by diffusion across the alveolar–capillary membrane. For this reason, CO is a useful gas for calculating D_L, also named the *transfer factor*, as follows:

$$DL = \frac{\dot{V}_{CO}}{P_{ACO}} \qquad (2.24)$$

---

[6] If the partial pressure of a gas in the plasma equilibrates with the alveolar partial pressure of the gas within the amount of time the blood is in the pulmonary capillary, its transfer is perfusion limited; if equilibration does not occur within the time the blood is in the capillary, its transfer is diffusion limited.

The *oxygen-diffusing capacity* of the lung (DL_{O_2}) is its conductance $(A \times D/T)$ when considered for the entire lung; thus, applying Fick's equation, the DL_{O_2} can be calculated (theoretically) as follows:

$$DL_{O_2} = \frac{\dot{V}_{O_2}}{PA_{O_2} - P\overline{c}_{O_2}} \qquad (2.25)$$

where $\dot{V}_{O_2}$ is the net diffusion of O_2, and $P\overline{c}_{O_2}$ is the mean pulmonary capillary P_{O_2}. But, as DL_{O_2} cannot be calculated directly, DL_{CO} is most frequently used in determinations of the diffusing capacity because the mean pulmonary capillary partial pressure of carbon monoxide is virtually zero when nonlethal alveolar partial pressures of carbon monoxide are used.

Although diffusion per se involves no expenditure of energy, the body must do work, in the form of ventilation and circulation, to create the concentration gradients under which O_2 and CO_2 diffuse as discussed.

References

1. Connett RJ, Honig CR, Gayeski TE, Brooks GA. Defining hypoxia: a systems view of VO₂, glycolysis, energetics, and intracellular PO₂. *J Appl Physiol*.1990; 68:833-842.
2. Nathan AT, Singer M. The oxygen trail: tissue oxygenation. *Br Med Bull*.1999; 55:96-108.
3. Wolfe DF, Sorbello JG. Comparison of published pressure gradient symbols and equations in mechanics of breathing. *Respir Care*.2006;51: 1450-1457.
4. Pappenheimer JR, Comroe JH, Cournand A, et al. Standardization of definitions and symbols in respiratory physiology. *Fed Proc*.1950; 9:602-605.
5. Berne RM, Levy M, Koeppen B, Stanton B. *Physiology*. St Louis: Mosby; 2004.
6. Wanger J, Clausen JL, Coates A, et al. Standardisation of the measurement of lung volumes. *Eur Respir J*. 2005;26:511-522.
7. Knowles JH, Hong SK, Rahn H. Possible errors using esophageal balloon in determination of pressure–volume characteristics of the lung and thoracic cage. *J Appl Physiol*. 1959;14:525-530.
8. Coates AL, Peslin R, Rodenstein D, Stocks J. Measurement of lung volumes by plethysmography. *Eur Respir J*. 1997;10:1415-1427.
9. Dubois AB, Botelho SY, Bedell GN, Marshall R, Comroe JH Jr. A rapid plethysmographic method for measuring thoracic gas volume: a comparison with a nitrogen washout method for measuring functional residual capacity in normal subjects. *J Clin Invest*.1956; 35:322-326.
10. Newth CJ, Enright P, Johnson RL. Multiple-breath nitrogen washout techniques: including measurements with patients on ventilators. *Eur Respir J*.1997; 10:2174-2185.
11. Meneely GR, Kaltreider NL. The volume of the lung determined by helium dilution. Description of the method and comparison with other procedures. *J Clin Invest*. 1949;28:129-139.
12. Clausen J. Measurement of absolute lung volumes by imaging techniques. *Eur Respir J*.1997; 10:2427-2431.
13. Rochester DF. Tests of respiratory muscle function. *Clin Chest Med*.1988; 9:249-261.
14. Syabbalo N. Assessment of respiratory muscle function and strength. *Postgrad Med J*.1998; 74:208-215.
15. Pacia EB, Aldrich TK. Assessment of diaphragm function. *Chest Surg Clin N Am*.1998; 8:225-236.
16. Harik-Khan RI, Wise RA, Fozard JL. Determinants of maximal inspiratory pressure. The Baltimore Longitudinal Study of Aging. *Am J Respir Crit Care Med*. 1998;158:1459-1464.
17. Koulouris N, Mulvey DA, Laroche CM, Sawicka EH, Green M, Moxham J. The measurement of inspiratory muscle strength by sniff esophageal, nasopharyngeal, and mouth pressures. *Am Rev Respir Dis*.1989; 139:641-646.
18. Cotes JE, Chinn DJ, Miller MR. *Lung function. Physiology, measurement and application in medicine*. Oxford: Blackwell;2006.
19. Escolar JD, Escolar A. Lung hysteresis: a morphological view. *Histol Histopathol*.2004; 19:159-166.
20. Mead J, Whittenberg JL, Radford EP Jr. Surface tension as a factor in pulmonary volume–pressure hysteresis. *J Appl Physiol*.1957; 10:191-196.
21. Garcia CS, Prota LF, Morales MM, Romero PV, Zin WA, Rocco PR. Understanding the mechanisms of lung mechanical stress. *Braz J Med Biol Res*.2006; 39:697-706.
22. Halliday HL. Surfactants: past, present and future. *J Perinatol*.2008; 28(suppl1) :S47-S56.
23. Neegaard KV. Neue auffassungen uber einen grundbegriff der atemmechanik. Die retraktionskraft der lunge, abhangig von der oberflachenspannung in den alveolen. *Gesund Wohlfahrt*.1948; 28:231-260.
24. Haitsma JJ. Physiology of mechanical ventilation. *Crit Care Clin*.2007; 23:117–134,vii
25. Bernhard W, Haagsman HP, Tschernig T, et al. Conductive airway surfactant: surface-tension function, biochemical composition, and possible alveolar origin. *Am J Respir Cell Mol Biol*.1997; 17:41-50.
26. Milic-Emili J, Henderson JA, Dolovich MB, Trop D, Kaneko K. Regional distribution of inspired gas in the lung. *J Appl Physiol*.1966; 21:749-759.
27. Macklem PT, Macklem DM, De TA. A model of inspiratory muscle mechanics. *J Appl Physiol*.1983; 55:547-557.
28. Albaiceta GM, Garcia E, Taboada F. Comparative study of four sigmoid models of pressure–volume curve in acute lung injury. *Biomed Eng Online*.2007; 6:7.
29. Albaiceta GM, Blanch L, Lucangelo U. Static pressure–volume curves of the respiratory system: were they just a passing fad? *Curr Opin Crit Care*.2008; 14:80-86.
30. MacIntyre NR. Evidence-based ventilator weaning and discontinuation. *Respir Care*.2004; 49:830-836.
31. Gibson GJ. Lung volumes and elasticity. *Clin Chest Med*. 2001;22:623–635,vii
32. Drummond GB, Milic-Emili J. Forty years of closing volume. *Br J Anaesth*.2007; 99:772-774.
33. Grinnan DC, Truwit JD. Clinical review: respiratory mechanics in spontaneous and assisted ventilation. *Crit Care*. 2005;9:472-484.

34. Roussos C, Macklem PT. The respiratory muscles. *N Engl J Med.*1982;307:7 86-797.
35. Fenn WO, Rahn H, Otis AB. A theoretical study of the composition of the alveolar air at altitude. *Am J Physiol.* 1946;146:637-653.
36. Curran-Everett D. A classic learning opportunity from Fenn, Rahn, and Otis (1946): the alveolar gas equation. *Adv Physiol Educ.*2006;30:58-6 2.
37. Glenny RW. Teaching ventilation/perfusion relationships in the lung. *Adv Physiol Educ.*2008; 32:192-195.
38. Howell JB, Permutt S, Proctor DF, Riley RL. Effect of inflation of the lung on different parts of pulmonary vascular bed. *J Appl Physiol.*1961; 16:71-76.
39. Levitzky MG. *Pulmonary Physiology*. New York: McGraw-Hill;2007.
40. Dembinski R, Henzler D, Rossaint R. Modulating the pulmonary circulation: an update. *Minerva Anestesiol.* 2004;70:239-243.
41. West JB, Dollery CT, Naimark A. Distribution of blood flow in isolated lung; relation to vascular and alveolar pressures. *J Appl Physiol.*1964; 19:713-724.
42. Martin CJ, Marshall H, Cline F Jr. Lobar alveolar gas concentrations; effect of body position. *J Clin Invest.* 1953;32:617-621.
43. Harris EA, Seelye ER, Whitlock RM. Gas exchange during exercise in healthy people II. Venous admixture. *Clin Sci Mol Med.*1976; 51:335-344.
44. Galvin I, Drummond GB, Nirmalan M. Distribution of blood flow and ventilation in the lung: gravity is not the only factor. *Br J Anaesth.*2007; 98:420-428.

3.1 HistologicalFe atrueso fL ungs in Cardiac Disease

The histological features of the lung are diverse when considering the processes that compromise the cardiac pump. The organic impairment of the heart can occur due to one of the following mechanisms: loss of blood; irregular heartbeat; flow obstruction; regurgitation; contractile impairment (systolic failure); or inadequate filling (diastolic failure).[1] Any of these causes, when sufficiently severe or advanced, can finally damage the heart function and render the heart incapable of maintaining enough blood outflow to meet the metabolic requirements of tissues, resulting in cardiac arrest and ischemia of different organs.[2,3]

The effects of the diastolic failure are manifested mainly as pulmonary effects. With the ongoing pooling of blood within the pulmonary circulation, the increased pressure of the pulmonary vessels promotes the capillary lesion and, subsequently, the lesion of alveolar-capillary membrane.[4,5] Although these alterations are reversible due to the highly reparative properties of the alveolar surface, when the alveolar-capillary membrane undergoes continuing damage, such as in chronic heart failure, its remodeling can occur.[6-8] These characteristics show that chronic heart failure leads to the organic impairment of the alveolar-capillary membrane, contributing to increased symptoms and, consequently, to the onset of pulmonary alterations and symptoms.[6-8] On the other hand, patients with chronic left ventricular failure can present all the symptoms of pulmonary disease and absence of typical symptoms of pulmonary vascular congestion, such as dyspnea and nocturnal paroxystic orthopnea. In addition, the pulmonary radiological results might not be coincident, with heart failure leading the physician to misdiagnosis.

Certainly, a combination of atypical clinical and radiological findings in the absence of cardiac signs and symptoms, such as galloping heart sounds, can prevent the clinician from attaining the correct diagnosis of chronic heart failure, and many of these findings can be considered prognostic factors that are independent from the clinical course of the heart disease. In this situation, the surgical pulmonary biopsy must be considered, especially if the noninvasive or minimally invasive procedures did not provide a specific diagnosis.

Ischemia is one of the main causes of tissue lesion, a condition in which there is an interruption in the oxygen and nutrient supply to a certain area, invariably leading to tissue dysfunction and posterior death. This lesion occurs at different time intervals, depending on the characteristics of the affected tissue, as well as of the capillary recruitment capacity of the microcirculation, the metabolic demand, the available oxygen stores, and the energy production capacity by the anaerobic metabolism.[9,10] Recent evidence has shown that the tissue lesion is not limited simply to the ischemic period, but that it can also extend to the reperfusion period.

Parks and Granger demonstrated that 3 h of continuous ischemia followed by 1 h of reperfusion determined a larger lesion in the intestinal mucosa than 4 h of ischemia.[11] Furthermore, Korthuis et al.[12] showed that the anoxic reperfusion of the ischemic tissues results in less damage than that occurring in the presence of oxygen. That suggests the participation of the oxygen supplied at the reperfusion among the mechanisms of tissue damage.

V.L.C apelozzi(✉)
Department of Pathology, University of Sao Paulo
School of Medicine, Av. Dr. Arnaldo 455, Room 1143
01296-903, SaoP aulo, SP,B razil
e-mail:vc apelozzi@lim05.fm.usp.br

E.A. Gabriel and T. Salerno (eds.), *Principles of Pulmonary Protection in Heart Surgery*,
DOI: 10.1007/978-1-84996-308-4_3, © Springer-Verlag London Limited 2010

The ischemia–reperfusion lesion, also called reperfusion lesion, can be defined as the damage that occurs in a certain tissue after the blood flow is restored after a period of ischemia.[13] Its identification is important so that the ischemia can be reverted, a crucial point for the maintenance of tissue viability, in a less-harmful way. The reperfusion can lead to the isolated lesion of the ischemic and then reperfused organ as it occurs in the myocardial reperfusion and organ transplantations.[14,15] However, the reperfusion damage can extend to distant organs due to the systemic inflammatory response, in which inflammatory mediators, toxic oxygen reactive species, metabolites of the arachidonic acid, and products of the complement are produced and released in the circulation, reaching different organs.

In the lungs, these inflammatory mediators can affect, the alveolar-capillary barrier, directly or indirectly or through the chemotaxis of polymorphonuclear cells, determining the onset of pulmonary edema, which can be present in situations of ischemia–reperfusion at a distance, such as the postoperative period of surgeries with temporary clamping of the aorta as well as circulatory shock or chronic heart failure.[16,17]

Recent studies have shown that there is a different degree of organic impairment of the alveolar-capillary membrane associated with alterations of heart failure. Similarly, the presence of different histological patterns associated with damage to the alveolar-capillary membrane have been described in open lung biopsies.[6,7]

One of the first histological patterns described is characterized by the prominent accumulation of edema in the alveolar spaces (Fig. 3.1a) in the perivascular and interstitial regions, particularly in the lobular septum region and inside the alveolar spaces (Fig. 3.1b).

Recent reports by Marenzi et al.[18] showed that this process is caused by the attempt to increase the intravenous volume and, consequently, the cardiac outflow to restore renal perfusion. In fact, with the progressive pooling of blood within the pulmonary circulation and the increased pressure of the pulmonary veins, the capillary congestion promotes the damage to the alveolar-capillary membrane, thus increasing the gas exchange resistance.[3]

The relevance of these pulmonary changes that led to alterations in gas exchange, mainly in the spaces distant from the airway point of origin, was emphasized by reports of De Pasquale[4] and Rasche,[5] who demonstrated under experimental circumstances that the pulmonary pressure or volume overload can affect the alveolar-capillary membrane. This can interrupt its anatomic

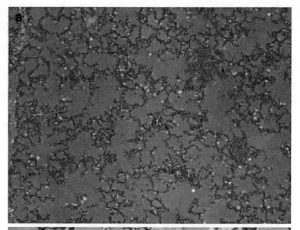
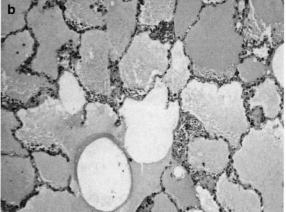

Fig. 3.1 Histological pattern of pulmonary edema; prominent accumulation of fluid in large pulmonary extensions can be observed (**a**) mainly in the region of the lobular septum and inside the alveolar spaces (**b**). Hematoxylin and eosin (**a** ×40; **b** ×400)

configuration, causing the loss of fluid regulation and affecting the conductibility of the alveolar gas; however, these alterations are reversible due to the reparative properties of the alveolar surface. Nevertheless, if the alveolar-capillary membrane is chronically affected, as it occurs in patients with chronic heart failure, the remodeling of the alveolar membrane can take place.[6]

Studies by De Pasquale et al.[4] showed that the cardiogenic acute pulmonary edema is associated with the damage to the alveolar-capillary membrane, demonstrated by the increased escape to circulation of specific pulmonary proteins, such as surfactant. On the other hand, it has been documented that the damage to the alveolar-capillary membrane is directly related to the time and adjustment of the inflammatory process in the pulmonary parenchyma; in fact, tumor necrosis factor (TNF) is increased in the circulation after acute cardiogenic pulmonary edema. Although the initial increase in proteins A and B of the surfactant might represent the hydrostatic failure of the alveolar-capillary membrane, the subsequent increase of TNF may represent the inflammation of the pulmonary parenchyma, which can further damage the alveolar-capillary membrane. This prolonged physiological defect of the alveolar-capillary membrane can clarify in part the vulnerability of these patients in accumulating pulmonary fluid.

Pulmonary congestion (Fig. 3.2a) is the second histological pattern described as associated with a slight remodeling of the extracellular matrix. Venous stasis, as well as alveolar veins and septa with a slight degree of thickening, often can be observed (Fig. 3.2b). An unspecific inflammatory infiltrate, dilation and distortion of the capillaries (Fig. 3.2c), as well as the accumulation of macrophages with hemosiderin inside the alveolar spaces (Fig. 3.2d) also encompass the described picture.

As reported by Marenzi et al.,[18] during cardiac arrest the compensatory mechanisms are incapable of increasing the blood outflow, resulting in increased water retention and posterior increased venous pressure, with the onset of pulmonary congestion. These anatomic changes produce important clinical manifestations, such as dyspnea and coughing. This retrograde hemodynamic effect exercises pressure, and the volume overload produces mechanical damage to the alveolar-capillary membrane. Matthay et al.[19] demonstrated that the process is acute and, consequently, reversible. However, when the alveolar-capillary membrane is chronically damaged by neurohumoral activation (angiotensin II, norepinephrine, cytotoxic stimulation, or genetic factors), the remodeling process of the membrane and alveolar capillaries becomes critical.[19,20] In this phase, the reversibility of the process is uncertain, considering that the extracellular matrix remodeling and the deterioration of the endothelial permeability are implicated in loss of fluid to the alveolar space and consequent damage to the gas exchange.[21]

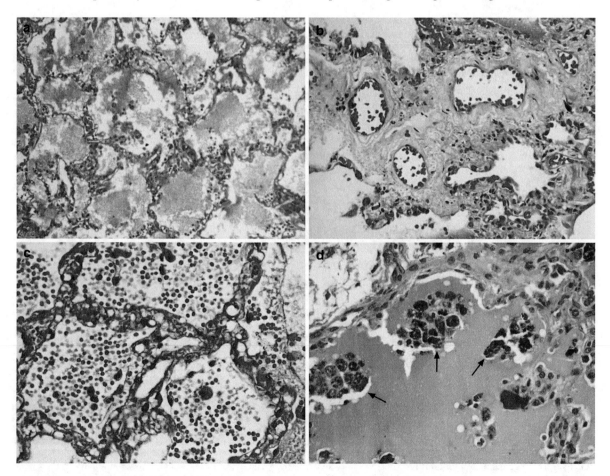

Fig. 3.2 Histological pattern of pulmonary congestion. Observe the significant vascular congestion present in the parenchyma (**a**), alveolar veins and septa with slight degree of thickening (**b**), dilation and distortion of the septal capillaries (**c**), and accumulation of macrophages with hemosiderin (*arrows*) in the alveolar spaces (**d**). Hematoxylin and eosin (**a** ×200; **b, c, d**× 400)

A third histological pattern of damage to the alveolar-capillary membrane is the presence of multiple foci of pulmonary lesions (Fig. 3.3a), observed mainly in patients with cardiac arrest. It is noteworthy that this pattern does not correspond to the classic pattern of diffuse alveolar damage, as observed in Hamman–Rich syndrome, characterized by the formation of hyaline membranes or pneumonia in organization with membrane remnants. The alterations found in patients with cardiac arrest are characterized by multiple foci of fibroblasts incorporated in septa of ducts and alveoli (Fig. 3.3b), as well as the presence of unspecific inflammatory infiltrate. In these cases, the interstitial edema and the chronic hypertension probably determine the damage to the alveolar-capillary membrane.[22]

The mechanism of hydrostatic pressure increase is gradual, as well as the increased lymphatic drainage that prevents the interstitial infiltration and the alveolar edema, at least up to the point when the transudate fluid oppresses the lymphatic system.[23-25] The chronic venous hypertension also encourages the formation of fibrin, which inhibits the passage of the edema to the intra-alveolar space and is often present in these lungs (Fig. 3.3c).

Compensatory measures such as the increase in the diastolic end phase, tachycardia, progressive hypertrophy of the ventricular wall, and increase in the adrenergic stimuli are somehow the compensatory mechanisms that attempt to counterbalance chronic left ventricular failure and the inadequate cardiac output that occur in chronic heart failure.

The sequelae of these compensatory measures are the increase in pulmonary venous pressure secondary to interstitial edema and dyspnea.[26] The pulmonary interstitial edema does not result in any abnormal sign on pulmonary auscultation in these cases, and the diagnosis is often based on the radiological alterations alone and clinical suspicion. These characteristics are important and can explain some symptoms in patients

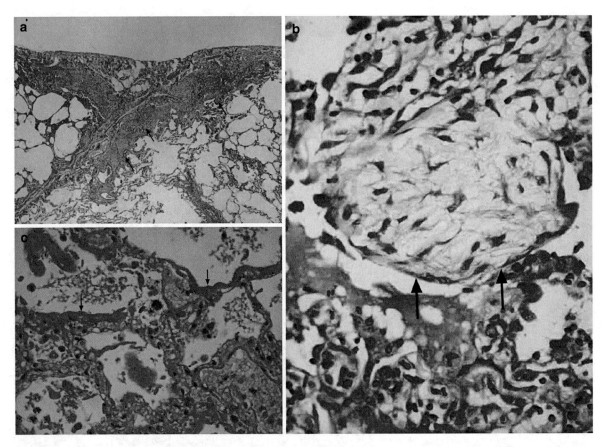

Fig. 3.3 Histological pattern of multifocal lesion of alveolar-capillary membrane characterized by multiple foci of fibroblasts (*arrows*) incorporated into the septa of ducts and alveoli (**a**), detail of proliferation of fibroblasts in the alveolar wall (**b**). Some regions can present foci of pulmonary lesions, characterized by the presence of hyaline membranes (*arrows*) (**c**). Hematoxylin and eosin (**a** ×200; **b, c** ×400)

with congestive cardiac arrest that present an initial picture of pulmonary disease. In this sense, Rosenow and Harrison[27] reported eight patients with congestive cardiac arrest who were diagnosed based on the pulmonary disease.

A histological pattern of acute pulmonary lesion can imitate very well a heart lesion. Rosenow and Harrison[27] reported that the response to cardiac arrest therapy can be the best way to differentiate primary pulmonary disease from a pulmonary lesion due to congestive cardiac arrest.

Our studies[28] have shown that the pulmonary changes resulting from cardiac arrest due to left heart impairment are a frequent cause of ischemic heart disease, aortic and mitral valve diseases (mainly calcified aortic stenosis and rheumatic heart disease), and myocardial diseases.

In brief, three different histological patterns can be found in patients with heart lesions; in fact, most of the examples of myocardial failure are a consequence of the progressive deterioration of the contractile function of the heart (organic systolic failure), which frequently occurs due to ischemic alterations, pressure or volume overload, or dilated cardiomyopathy.[29,30]

Ichihara et al.[20] showed that patients with characteristics of progressive pooling of the blood within the pulmonary circulation present a progressive increase in pulmonary venous pressure, which is transmitted, in a retrograde manner, to the capillaries. The cardiac arrest also determines the metabolic nutrition impairment of tissues caused by the ineffective arterial volume,[31] leading to the activation of the renin-angiotensin system, which causes sodium and water retention. The final result will be pulmonary congestion and edema.[21] Sometimes, the failure that results from the incapacity of the heart walls to expand adequately during diastole to accommodate adequate ventricular volume (organic diastolic failure) can also contribute to the pulmonary congestion process. This mechanism can be found in left ventricular hypertrophy, myocardial fibrosis, heart amyloidosis, or constrictive pericarditis.[29] Whatever the base, chronic heart failure is characterized by decreased blood outflow or by the retrograde pooling of blood in the venous system. Except for mitral valve obstruction or in processes that restrict the left ventricular size, this chamber is usually hypertrophic or dilated.[32] The secondary left ventricular dilation can frequently lead to ventricular fibrillation (i.e., the uncoordinated contraction of the ventricle). This fact can cause blood stasis and the consequent formation of thrombi.[33] Therefore, we can conclude that damage to the alveolar-capillary membrane due to acute overload or high-pressure volume overload can manifest with different histological patterns, and the identification of these patterns can influence prognosis and therapy.

The patients must be assessed for alveolar edema, for pulmonary congestion, and for alveolar damage. Concerning these patients, physicians must be aware of the possibility of congestive cardiac arrest, particularly if the patients are elderly or have a history of coronary,myoc ardial,or v alvulardis ease.

References

1. Gehlbach BK, BK GE. The pulmonary manifestations of left heart failure. *Chest*.2004; 125(2):669-682.
2. Ramadan MM, Okura Y, Ohno Y, et al. Comparative analysis of systolic and isolated diastolic dysfunction: Sado heart failure study. *Int Heart J*.2008; 49(4):459-469.
3. Vandiviere HM. Pulmonary hypertension and cor pulmonale. *South Med J*.1993; 86(10):2S7-2S10.
4. De Pasquale CG, Arnolda LF, Doyle IR, Grant RL, Aylward PE, Bersten AD. Prolonged alveolocapillary barrier damage after acute cardiogenic pulmonary edema. *Crit Care Med*. 2003;31(4):1060-1067.
5. Rasche K, Orth M, Duchna HW. Sequels of lung diseases on cardiac function. *Med Klin (Munich)*. 2006;101(suppl 1): 44-46(abstract).
6. West JB. Cellular responses to mechanical stress. *J Appl Physiol*.2000; 89(2):2483-2489.
7. Bhattacharya J. Pressure-induced capillary stress failure: is it regulated? *Am J Physiol Lung Cell Mol Physiol*. 2003; 284:L701-L702.
8. Han MK, McLaughlin VV, Criner GJ, Martinez FJ. Pulmonary diseases and the heart. *Circulation*. 2007;116(25):2992-3005.
9. Scannell G. Leukocyte responses to hypoxic/ischemic conditions. *New Horiz*.1996; 4:179-183.
10. Gutierrez G, Brown SD. Gastrointestinal tonometry: a monitor of regional dysoxia. *New Horiz*.1996; 4:413-419.
11. Parks DA, Granger DN. Contributions of ischemia and reperfusion to mucosal lesion formation. *Am J Physiol*. 1986;250:G749-G753.
12. Korthuis RJ, Smith JK, Carden DL. Hypoxic reperfusion attenuates postischemic microvascular injury. *Am J Physiol*. 1989;256:H315-H319.
13. Reily PM, Schiller HJ, Bulkley GB. Pharmacologic approach to tissue injury mediated by free radicals and other reactive oxygen metabolites. *Am J Surg*.1991; 161:488-503.
14. Becker LC, Ambrosio G. Myocardial consequences of reperfusion. *Prog Cardiovasc Dis*.1987; 30:23-44.
15. Horiguchi T, Harada Y. The effect of protease inhibitor on reperfusion injury after unilateral pulmonary ischemia. *Transplantation*.1993; 55:254-258.
16. Klausner JM, Paterson IS, Kobzik L, Valeri CR, Shepro D, Hechtman HB. Oxygen free radicals mediate ischemia-induced lung injury. *Surgery*.1989; 105:192-199.

17. Ar'rajab A, Dawidson I, Fabia R. Reperfusion injury. *New Horiz*.1996;4:224- 234.
18. Marenzi G, Agostoni P. Hemofiltration in heart failure. *Int J Artif Organs*.2004; 27(12):1070-1076.
19. Matthay MA, Fukuda N, Frank J, Kallet R, Daniel B, Sakuma T. Alveolar epithelial barrier. Role in lung fluid balance in clinical lung injury. *Clin Chest Med*. 2000;21(3):477-490.
20. Ichihara S, Senbonmatsu T, Price E Jr, Ichiki T, Gaffney FA, Inagami T. Angiotensin II type 2 receptor is essential for left ventricular hypertrophy and cardiac fibrosis in chronic angiotensin II-induced hypertension. *Circulation*. 2001; 104(3):346-351.
21. Zemans RL, Matthay MA. Bench-to-bedside review: the role of the alveolar epithelium in the resolution of pulmonary edema in acute lung injury. *Crit Care*. 2004;8(6):469-477.
22. Mutlu GM, Sznajder JI. Mechanisms of pulmonary edema clearance. *Am J Physiol Lung Cell Mol Physiol*. 2005;289(5): L685-L695.
23. Haddy FJ, Stephens G, Visscher MB. The physiology and pharmacology of lung edema. *Pharmacol Ver*. 1956;8(3): 389-434.
24. Uhley H, Leeds SE, Sampson JJ, Friedman M. Some observations on the role of the lymphatics in experimental acute pulmonary edema. *Circ Res*.1961; 9:688.
25. Grainger RU. Interstitial pulmonary oedema and its radiological diagnosis: a sign of pulmonary venous antecapillary hypertension. *Br J Radiol*.1958; 31(364):201.
26. Brown CC Jr, Fry DL, Ebert RV. The mechanics of pulmonary ventilation in patients with heart disease. *Am J Med*. 1954;17(4):438.
27. Rosenow EC III, Harrison CE Jr. Congestive heart failure masquerading as primary pulmonary disease. *Chest*. 1970;58(1):28-36.
28. de Castro Zampieri FM, Canzian M, Parra ER, Kairalla RA, Capelozzi VL. Alveolar-capillary membrane dysfunction in heart failure: histopathological changes. *Eur Resp J*. 2008; 661s,a bstract.
29. Mandinov L, Eberli FR, Seiler C, Hess OM. Diastolic heart failure. *Cardiovasc Res*.2000; 45(4):813-825.
30. Campbell FE. Cardiac effects of pulmonary disease. *Vet Clin N Am Small Anim Pract*.2007; 37(5):949-962.
31. Ravi K, Kappagoda CT. Left ventricular dysfunction and extravascular fluid in the lung: physiological basis for symptoms. *Indian J Chest Dis Allied Sci*.2008; 50(1):7-18.
32. Snow JB, Kitzis V, Norton CE, et al. Differential effects of chronic hypoxia and intermittent hypocapnic and eucapnic hypoxia on pulmonary vasoreactivity. *J Appl Physiol*. 2008;104(1):110-118.
33. Thiedemann KU, Ferrans VJ. Left atrial ultrastructure in mitral valvular disease. *Am J Pathol*.1977; 89(3):575-604.

Cellular and Molecular Aspects of Lung Function,i tsC ontrolandR egulation

4

Jesús Armando Sánchez Godoy and Alain Riveros Rivera

This chapter focuses on the molecular and cellular properties of the lung, and the mechanisms involved in the respiratory control throughout three integrative models:

- The defense mechanisms of the airways.
- The lung response to mechanical stress.
- Regulatory components of the respiratory regulation.

4.1 DefenseMec hanisms of the Respiratory System

The respiratory system is exposed to approximately 10,000 L of air per day and about 25 million particles per hour.[1] Thus, it is continuously at risk of exposure to noxious environmental agents (e.g., dust, soot, pollen, respiratory pathogens), which can be deposited all across the airways. The final location of these inhaled particles mainly depends on the particle size and density, which may determine the distance traveled across the tract. For example, larger and denser particles (>10 μm) are trapped in the nose and upper airways (above the cricoids ring) as result of inertial impaction. In addition to inertia, particle deposition may also depend on gravity (especially in small particles) and diffusion.[2]

In response to the risk exposure, the airway epithelium has developed diverse mechanisms that facilitate its clearance, aiming mainly to assure lung sterility. These mechanisms include cough, anatomical barriers,

aerodynamic changes and cellular mechanisms.[2,3] These mechanisms are related mainly with a mucociliary clearance and a specialized mucosal immune system, which constitute the focus of the first part of this chapter. In a second part, we will focus on the mechanisms of regulation of the respiratory system.

4.1.1 Mucociliary Clearance

Mucociliary clearance is a nonspecific mechanism that removes noxious particles from the lungs via ciliary and secretory activity. Thus, mucociliary clearance is based on the continuous transport of secretions from the peripheral airways towards the oropharynx. During its movement, the secretions act as a trap for particles, which are either swallowed or expectorated together with the secretion upon its arrival to the pharynx. Below, we briefly describe the mechanism of mucociliary clearance based on the production, composition and action of the viscoelastic mucus and the periciliary fluid.

Production and composition. The *viscoelastic mucus* is a fluid mainly composed of mucin glycoproteins, and produced in the bronchial tree by a wide diversity of specialized cells (goblet cells,[4] Clara cells, serous cells, and type II alveolar cells) located on the epithelium and the submucosal glands.[5] After its synthesis, mucus is stored in membrane-bound granules. As expected, production of mucous depends on the number of cells available for its secretion. Thus, areas with larger surface (and therefore more cells), such as the peripheral airways, produce greater amounts of mucus. On average, the total amount of mucus that reaches the trachea is ~10–20 mL/day.[6] However, during pathological conditions, levels of production can be globally elevated. Hence, some inflammatory airway diseases (e.g., asthma, chronic obstructive

J.A. Sánchez Godoy (✉)
Departamento de Ciencias Fisiológicas, Pontificia Universidad Javeriana, Universidad Militar "Nueva Granada",
Bogotá, DC, Colombia
e-mail:a rmandosanchezg@yahoo.com

E.A. Gabriel and T. Salerno (eds.), *Principles of Pulmonary Protection in Heart Surgery*,
DOI: 10.1007/978-1-84996-308-4_4, © Springer-Verlag London Limited 2010

pulmonary diseases, or cystic fibrosis) share common pathways of increased mucin protein genes (MUC genes) expression and goblet cell hyperplasia.[7,8] High levels of production, together with changes in physical properties of the mucus, may create favorable environments for pathogens' growth.[8-10] Physical properties of the mucus are determined by the expression of MUC genes, particularly MUC5AC and MUC5B.[7,10]

The second type of fluid, the *periciliary fluid,* is produced in the pseudoestratified and the columnar epithelium and contributes to facilitate cilia movement.[9] Airway surface fluid contains many components, including lysozyme, lactoferrin, secretory leukoprotease inhibitor (SLPI), glycoproteins, lipids, immunoglobuling A, and peroxidase, among others.[11] However, since the fluid is produced by active ion transport, its production creates a layer containing diverse ions. Thus, the periciliary fluid also contributes to modulate ionic gradients (see below).

Action and control of airway fluids Viscoelastic mucus has as its main function to be the "first line of defense," capturing particles that are later expulsed via the oropharynx. The mechanism of expulsion is based on the movement of the mucous layer, which is determined by the activity of ciliated cells. The cilia (~200 per cell) activate the movement by anchoring their apical claw-like projections to the mucous layer and then pushing it in the direction of the pharynx with beats of 8–15 Hz.[12] Thus, the viscoelastic mucus primarily acts as a physical barrier by capturing those particles that adhere to its surface.

Nevertheless, given the chemical composition of mucus, of the periciliary fluid and the components added by the ciliary cells (e.g., antimicrobial peptides (AMPs)), the two fluids act together as a truly chemical barrier during early stages of infection. Of particular relevance is the antimicrobial action of two main families of peptides, *Defensins* and *Cathelicidins,* secreted by epithelial cells constitutively or in response to the presence of noxious agents. The defensins are a family of peptides with antimicrobial action against bacteria (both Gram-negative and Gram-positive), fungi and viruses (enveloped viruses). In humans, β-defensins have other functions besides antimicrobial activity, including chemoattraction of macrophages and neutrophils, and modulation of tissue repair among others.[13]

On the other hand, cathelicidins are a family of cationic peptides with high structural diversity and broad taxonomic distribution. In humans, however, only have been described the cathelicidin hCAP-18/LL-37, which has broad antimicrobial activity and further contribute to the neutralization of microbial products with proinflammatory activity (e.g., lipopolysaccharide).[14] Additional functions of LL-37 include, among others: action as a chemotactic factor (for neutrophils, monocytes, mast cells and T cells), increase of gene expression during proinflammatory processes (e.g., in epithelial cells), epithelial proliferation and repair, and modulation of immunity.[13-15]

As mentioned before, periciliary fluids also contribute to the modulation of ionic gradients, which may, in turn, alter fluid secretion. Airway surface fluid is slightly hypotonic with 45% less Na^+ and Cl^- and 600% more K^+ than plasma.[16] Ionic gradients are regulated by intracellular cAMP, calcium ions, and ion-specific chloride channels across the epithelium. Active secretion of Cl^- into the airway lumen produces fluid secretion, whereas active Na^+ absorption accounts for the ability to absorb fluids. The balance between Cl^- secretion and Na^+ reabsorption regulates the depth of the periciliary fluid at 5–6 μm.

Although the secretion of fluids occurs in response to local exposure to foreign particles or pathogens (e.g., those leading to chronic inflammatory lung disease), it is also regulated centrally via the vagal nerve[17,18] and its mobilization can be affected by an individual's circadian rhythm[19,20]

4.1.2 Specialized Mucosal Immune System

Several types and subtypes of secondary lymphoid tissue form the specialized mucosal immune system. The mucosal associated lymphoid tissue (MALT) develops the immune response with the help of the local accessory cells (macrophages, dendritic cells, antigen presenting cells, and epithelial cells). A part of MALT, the bronchus-associated lymphoid tissue (BALT), is located in the bifurcation of the bronchus and formed by aggregates of lymph nodules throughout the conducting airways. Together with the nasal-associated lymphoid tissue (NALT), BALT is able to respond to inhaled antigens via T- and B-cells.[21] Indeed, most of the cells within BALT are B cells, which exhibit high expressions of surface IgA and IgM, acting as the primary immune response of BALT. Similarly to BALT, NALT is formed of B cells; however, NALT is also characterized by the presence of parafolicular T cells and its location on top of the soft palate and the bifurcation of the pharyngeal duct of the rodents.[21]

Alveolar macrophages (AM) play a major role in the innate immune response in the lung. AM ingest and remove inhaled particulate matter, microorganisms, and environmental toxins, as well as cellular debris from dead cells. AM are derived from myeloid progenitor cells in the bone marrow and then migrate to the lung. The response guided by AM includes the production of chemokines (e.g., monocyte chemoattractant protein-1, IL-8) and growth factors (e.g., macrophage colony-stimulating factor), which increase monocyte survival. Hence, AM may kill the foreign material rapidly, and without developing an inflammatory response.[22] However, if an inflammatory response is present, AM may contribute with the production of reactive oxygen and nitrogen species (ROS, RNS) and metalloproteases. Furthermore, AM also modulates the activity of the lung's immune system. Normally, resting, or quiescent, macrophages are anti-inflammatory, whereas activated macrophages are proinflammatory. A key regulatory molecule determining the AM's state of activation is a nuclear hormone receptor (peroxisome proliferator-activated receptor – PPAR-γ).[23] When the macrophage is activated, antigen presentation is facilitated, and release of proinflammatory mediators predominates. The Fc receptor of IgG (FcγR) are present in many components of the cellular immune response in the lung (including neutrophils, monocytes and macrophages) and are important to start the process of phagocytosis of viruses or bacteria.

4.2 Cellso ft heA lveoli

The alveolar epithelium is composed of cells type I and II. *Alveolar cells type I* are large and flat, with the basement membranes fused to the capillary endothelium and with extremely thin cytoplasm, which facilitate gas exchange. Alveolar cells cover ~95% of the alveolar surface, comprise ~8% of peripheral lung cells, and have a surface area of ~5,000 μm² per cell. Although alveolar cells have pumps and channels for sodium transport, it is unknown whether they participate in sodium absorption. However, alveolar cells lack of large numbers of mitochondria (a typical features of transporting epitheliums), which argues against its role in sodium transport. Furthermore, the absence of many mitochondria suggests the use of anaerobic glycolysis to generate ATP.

On the other hand, *type II cells* are small (apical surface area of ~250 μm²), cuboidal and characterized by the presence of apical microvilli. Type II cells comprise ~15% of the peripheral lung cells and cover ~2–5% of the alveolar surface area.[24] The main functions of the type II cells include:

- Synthesis and secretion of pulmonary surfactant proteins (SP), which, in the case of SP-B and SP-C, act together with saturated phosphatidylcholine, contributing to the decrease of surface tension on the alveolus to near 0 mN/m².[25-27]
- Serve as progenitor of alveolar epithelium after damage.
- Transcellular transport of sodium from the surface to the interstitium.
- Participation in innate immune responses, especially through the production of SP-A and SP-D.

4.3 Responset oPhys icalFo rces in the Lung

Diverse events of physical stress (e.g., strain, shear stress) may affect cells (Fig. 4.1). However, cell structure should be adapted to such conditions because innate cellular processes (e.g., growth, spreading, migration, etc.) involve mechanical stress.[28-31] In the case of lung cells, strain may be prominent in the epithelium and the alveolar wall during respiratory cycle, while shear forces

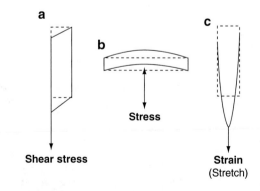

Fig. 4.1 Mechanical forces. When the stress is applied parallel or tangential to a face of a material is named "shear stress" (**a**) and is defined as a force per unit surface area in the direction of flow exerted at the fluid/surface interface. Otherwise, normal "stress" (**b**) is applied perpendicularly (force per unit area). Finally, "Strain" (**c**) is the geometrical measure of the change in length in relation to the initial length. The term "stretch" is interchangeablew ith" strain"

and hydrostatic pressure may have differential effects on the pulmonary vessels. Also, shear stress may affect other cells, including pleural mesothelial cells, whereas the fluid layer may affect alveolar epithelial cells.[32]

During the respiratory cycle, the alveolar epithelium contributes to the transduction of stimuli associated with inflation. In vitro, the responses of this epithelium to mechanical stress include: greater cell proliferation,[33] production of prostacyclin,[34] and synthesis and secretion of surfactants[35] (Fig. 4.2).

Cellular perception of mechanical stress involves many membrane components (e.g., membrane receptor kinases, integrins, G proteins, etc.) and the cytoskeleton. The mechanism of strain perception may involve increases of Ca^{2+} influx (via a mechanosensitive cation channel (Fig. 4.3)), the activation of Src (the proto-oncogene src (c-src) codes for a protein that is a member of the tyrosine kinase family), focal adhesion kinases (FAKs), and mitogen-activating protein kinases (MAP kinases). Remarkably, this mechanism may sense changes with

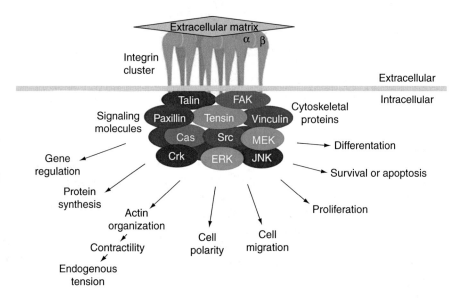

Fig.4.2 General mode lof cell–matrix adhesions and their downstream regulation. Cell-extracellular matrix adhesions containing clusters of integrins recruit cytoplasmic proteins, which in cooperation with other cell surface receptors control diverse cellular processes, functions, and phenotypes. (Reprinted with permission of John Wiley & Sons, Inc. J. Cell. Physiol. 213: 566, 2007. Copyright © 2007 Wiley-Liss, Inc. [36])

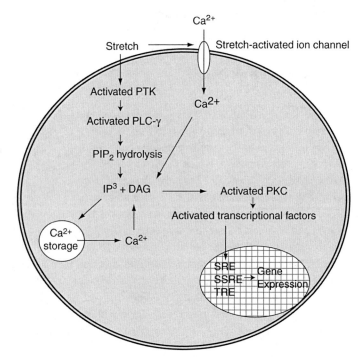

Fig.4.3 Mechanically activated ion channel pathway. Stretch induces Ca^{2+}i nflux via a stretch-activated ion channel. Mechanical stretch also activates protein tyrosine kinases (PTK) that activates phospholipase C-γ(PLC-γ) via its tyrosine phosphorylation. PLC-γ mediates the hydrolysis of phosphatidylinositol 4,5-bisphosphate (PIP2) to produce inositol 1,4,5-trisphosphate (IP3) and diacylglycerol (DAG). IP3 mobilizes Ca^{2+}f rom intracellular storage sites. DAG in the presence of intracellular and extracellular Ca^{2+} activates protein kinase C (PKC). PKC and other signals may activate transcriptional factors (c-*fos*) that bind to special response elements, such as stretch response elements (SRE), shear stress response elements (SSRE) and shear 12-*O*-tetradecanoylphorbol 13-acetate (TPA)-responsive element (TRE), boosting gene expression. (From [38],w ith permission)

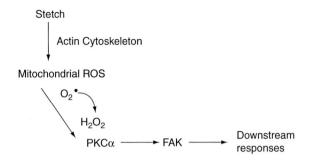

Fig. 4.4 Proposed pathway of mechanotransduction in bovine pulmonary artery endothelial cells. Cyclic stretch increases mitochondrial ROS production via the actin cytoskeleton. The mitochondrial ROS act as signaling molecules, activating PKC. PKC then phosphorylates FAK at Tyr397. This phosphorylation acts as the beginning of a wide variety of endothelial responses to mechanical stimuli. (Reprinted with permission of American Physiological Society. Copyright © 2006 by the American Physiological Society. [39])

intensities as low as 1 Pa. Consequences of stimulation include, but are not limited to, intracellular reorganization, extracellular remodeling and changes in protein expression. Similar responses to strain are observed in endothelial cells, suggesting the existence of a general mechanism of response to mechanical stress.[37]

In the case of shear stress, cell mechanoreception is linked to a series of signaling cascades leading to the production of ROS (which can act as secondary messenger), nitric oxide, and several transcription factors.[39] If adaptation is induced, new variations of the adapted "shear state" leads to the activation of the mechanisms of response. As a consequence of these events, diverse functional responses are elicited, including phosphorylation of focal adhesion kinase (FAK). As an alternative to this mechanism of perception, mechanical stress might be perceived at the level of the mitochondria if the strain is transmitted through the actin cytoskeleton. In this case, newly produced, or generated, superoxide or H_2O_2 to the cytosol acts as a signaling molecule to activate other cell responses. This mechanism has been associated with the increased inflammatory response and lung injury observed in patients ventilated with high tidal volumes (Fig. 4.4).

Another component of the cellular membrane associated with mechanoreception are the integrins (transmembrane proteins), which may play a major role in the airway smooth muscle (Fig. 4.5). If similar to nonmuscle cells, integrins in the airway smooth muscle might transduce mechanical information via a series of downstream pathways initiated by an increase in tyrosine phosphorylation[40] with the participation of actin and myosin filaments(Fig. 4.6).

This review has explored the molecular processes of local response. The next section will intend to explain the subcellular processes involved from local and systemic responses to integration.

4.4 ControlandR egulation of the Respiratory System

Like other control systems, the respiratory system has three levels of function:

- The *afferent (sensory) level* is responsible for sensing factors of the controlled system and sending information to the next level.
- The *level of analysis and command (controller)* receives and processes information from the sensory level in order to make decisions subsequently executed by the "effecter level."
- The *effecter level* executes a specific task based on the information processed by the controller level.

Each variable has a set point that allows the maintenance of homeostasis in the system. Such set point is likely to change according to circumstances in which the system is oscillating. To facilitate its comprehension, we will explore each of the three levels of control.

4.4.1 Afferents in Ventilatory Control

Just like the heart's, the lung's ventilatory pattern functions automatically, maintaining constant levels of activity. Nevertheless, this activity is susceptible of change according to modification in diverse variables. The sensors for the variables affecting the respiratory process are located virtually throughout the entire body because, as in the case of oxygen, many cells have specialized receptors, and are able to respond via changes in their function.[42] However, the aortic and carotid bodies, in the periphery, and chemoreceptors in the medulla oblongata, in the central nervous system, are some of the most relevant sites for acquisition of information on the respiratory pattern. Traditionally, the peripheral chemoreceptors are fundamentally associated with oxygen sensing, whereas the central chemoreceptors are associated with hydrons. This seems to be a rather crude approximation because, as we will see, others parameters can be considered.

Fig.4.5 (a)Sc hematic illustration of smooth muscle cellc ytoskeletalo rganization. Membrane adhesion junctions (box) connect the extracellular matrix surrounding the cells in smooth muscle tissues to actin filaments within the cell. Actin filaments are linked to integrin proteins at these adhesion junctions by structural proteins within macromolecular complexes that form around transmembrane integrin proteins. Actin that interacts with myosin generates tension and cell shortening. Additional actin not associated with myosin may regulate cell shape and structure. (**b**) Model of molecular organization of cytoskeletal/cell matrix membrane junctions in smooth muscle cells. (Reprinted with permission of Proceedings of the American Thoracic Society. Official Journal of American Thoracic Society. Copyright © 2009 by the American Thoracic Society. [41])

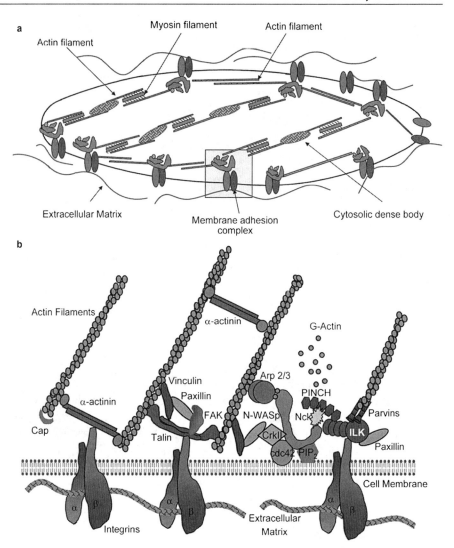

Peripheral chemoreceptors are better known as the carotid and aortic bodies, a cumulous of glomus cells with the machinery necessary to measure oxygen levels. Two main hypotheses aim to explain the mechanism of oxygen sensing. On the one hand, the "membrane hypothesis" proposes that glomus cells may rely on their membrane potential to sense oxygen changes. Similar to other cells, the glomus cells (GC) have a resting membrane potential with outward current of potassium, which keeps a relatively constant voltage.[43] However, if the potassium channels close, the accumulation of cations makes the membrane potential to become more positive, leading to the activation (depolarization) of GC. Under normal conditions, this closure

of potassium channels is inversely related with oxygen levels. Therefore, a decrease in oxygen levels is accompanied of depolarization. Simultaneously, this depolarization leads to the activation of voltage-gated calcium channels, thus increasing the levels of intracellular calcium. Inside the cell, calcium acts as a messenger, triggering processes to mobilize and release intercellular neurotransmitters (e.g., ATP, histamine, acetylcholine, dopamine, noradrenaline, adenosine) stored in the GC.[44,45]

An alternative to the "membrane hypothesis" is the so called "mitochondrial hypothesis." In contrast to the mechanism described above, the latter hypothesis suggests that mitochondrial oxidative phosphorylation is

Fig.4.6 Proposed cytoskeletal processes that occur during shortening and tension development in airway smooth muscle. (Reprinted with permission of Proceedings of the American Thoracic Society. Official Journal of American Thoracic Society. Copyright © 2009 by the American Thoracic Society.[41])

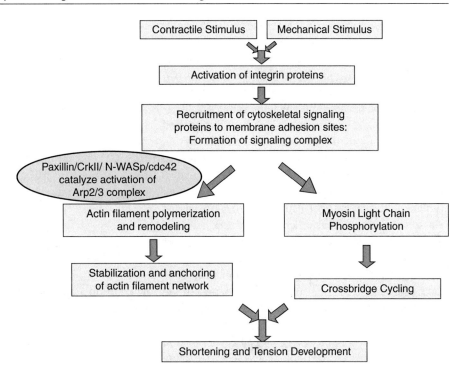

the fundamental process. Nevertheless, more recent research may lead to unify both hypotheses into a single model, centered on the role of protein kinase A (PKA). PKA is responsible for the phosphorylation of other molecules depending on the intracellular metabolic activity. Thus, PKA can radically alter the phenomena leading to the activation of GC.[46]

Of course, oxygen level is not the only parameter sensed by carotid bodies,[47] which may also acquire information on hydron concentration (i.e., pH) through channels of the families ASIC (acid-sensing ion channel) or TASK (tandem-p-domain, acid-sensitive K).[48,49] Even more interesting is the fact that the carotid body also senses temperature, osmolarity and glucose levels. Changes in all these variables may be triggered by glucopenia.[50,51]

In all cases, after the neurotransmitter release, the nerve terminals generate a signal that travels via Hering's nerve (a branch of the glosopharyngeal nerve transmitting information from the carotid bodies) and the vagus nerve (which transmits information from the aortic bodies). Information transmitted through both nerves (i.e., coming from carotid and aortic bodies) is received in the brainstem by the solitary tract, where it is processed to feed the next level, the "controller."

Interestingly, aortic bodies have more informative weight during childhood, whereas the carotid bodies are more important during adulthood.[52]

Central chemoreceptors are located in the locus ceruleus, midline raphe and medulla oblongata's ventrolateral quadrant and nucleus tractum solitarius.[53] In all cases, these structures are associated with CO_2 sensing, although the sensors seem to be more sensitive to hydrons.[54] Apparently, such stronger responses to hydrons are due to the conversion of CO_2 to HCO_3 plus H^+, a process catalyzed by carbonic anhydrase.[55] Importantly, it is not the plasma hydron what activates the neurons; rather the hydrons involved in the neuronal activation are a product of the catalyzed reaction. This is explained by the slow movement of the peripheral hydrons across the blood brain barrier, which is crossed faster by CO_2. Thus, CO_2 arrives first, and its conversion to HCO_3 produces hydrons that activate central chemoreceptors. Therefore, it is really the concentration of intracellular hydrons what generates the observed greater neuronal responses, leading, for example, to increases of up to 126% in firing rate in the locus ceruleus as a consequence of a slight decrease of only 0.43 pH units.[54] It is possible that CO_2 activates directly sensors, but the weight of its information is lower that hydron.[55] As in the carotid body, the pathways of activation involve potassium and calcium currents. However, there is growing evidence on the multiplicity of activation factors, involving at least two types of potassium channels, intra- and extracellular activation, and pH sensitive calcium channels.[56]

Peripheral mechanoreceptors include cells localized in the airway (both, the smooth muscle and the epithelium cells) or in the blood vessels. These cells have the potentiality to change the ventilatory pattern by stopping or starting a cycle if there is pulmonary distention (inflation or deflation).[57] This type of receptors can be classified as tonic or phasic, depending on the pattern of time response when the stimulus is present. If the sensor remains activated long after the stimulus begins, it is considered a slowly adapting receptor (or tonic, since the response is relatively permanent). In contrast, if the stimulus triggers a short lasting response, it is considered a rapidly adapting receptor (or phasic, since the response is present in the change of phase, either at the beginning or the end).[57] Traditionally, tonic receptors have been associated with static phenomena (e.g., muscle spindle in holding a position), while phasic receptors participate in dynamic phenomena (e.g., muscle spindle during changing position). If it is true in the ventilatory system, then the phasic receptors in the airway will be active when the inflation is active; if the ventilation stops, tonic receptors become highly active.[57]

Intracellular signaling events in mechanoreception have pointed to the involvement of membrane stress-dependent activity of Ca^{++} and Na^+ channels. For this to happen, inside of the channel, subunits are anchored to the cytoskeleton so that the inward current triggers an electrotonic potential. If several of these potentials coactivate the branches of a nerve, it is generated an action potential that travels through the vagus nerve towards the nodose ganglion, and later to nucleus tractus solitarii. Calculations over maximum firing rate in the vagus nerve (~150 Hz) consider a resolution in pressure change of 0.2 cmH_2O.[57]

Later on in here, we review the role of the integrative center in the control of ventilation. However, it is important to mention the effect that this may have on the inputs from the sensors. Traditionally, the sensory processing has been considered unidirectional, from sensors towards the controller, but not in the opposite direction. However, there is now sufficient evidence supporting the idea of a two-way process, where the controller also affects the signal input. Earlier research

in this field had already demonstrated the presence of efferents to the carotid bodies,[58] generating one of the first sources of debate. Nevertheless, it has been recently described a consensus model, which considers the importance of efferents in the inhibition of activities in the carotid bodies.[59] The neuromodulator is the nitric oxide, which acts on molecular targets in glomus cells promoting a state of hyperpolarization. In this state, the cells decrease the probability of activation by hypoxia, a process that can take part in the accommodation under long-term hypoxic conditions.[59]

4.4.2 Controller in Ventilatory Pattern

The information sent from chemoreceptors enters specific areas of the brainstem and may modify the ventilatory pattern. As already mentioned, there is an automatic and intrinsic pattern that makes the information received to change the frequency of ventilatory activation.

The automatic pattern (i.e., the ventilatory pacemaker) is generated in groups of neurons known as the pre-Bötzinger complex, located caudal to the facial nucleus and ventral to the ambiguus nucleus in brainstem of mammals.[60] Although initially described in rats, this ventilatory pacemaker recently has been studied in the human.[61] Similarly to the cardiac pacemaker, the pre-Bötzinger complex has a cyclic rhythm of electrical activity that depolarizes and repolarizes constantly.[60] Also similar to the process in the heart, the ventilatory pattern depends of slow sodium currents that keep the membrane potential more positive and with rhythmicity.[62,63]

This complex should be modified by opioids, which act preferentially in μ receptor.[61] In the pre-Bötzinger complex, μ receptors inhibit the intra-cellular cAMP pathway, which in part explains why the opioids behave as suppressors of ventilation. This effect is modified by activity of serotonin or dopamine which, behaving as antagonists of opioids, may represent a therapeutic alternative against ventilatory depression produced by opioids.[64]

Importantly, this "pacemaker hypothesis" is currently challenged by the apparent involvement of multiple nuclei (the retrotrapezoid nucleus and parafacial respiratory group) in the rhythmicity, which would be a process emerging from the interacting networks, rather than a property of cells.[65]

The dorsal group, in the medulla oblongata, is another neuronal group with a role in the inspiratory phase, and therefore, commanding the pathways associated with diaphragm's motoneurons.[65] A similar group of neurons in the medulla oblongata, the *ventral group*, can also start the expiratory phase or even the inspiratory phase, but mainly during forced ventilation.[65]

Furthermore, a group of neurons with pneumotaxic function (the Parabrachial nucleus and Kölliker-Fuse) has been described in the pons.[65-67] Those neurons have the potential to terminate the inspiratory activity; therefore, they are able to modify the frequency in the system: a higher fire rate lead to an increase in the ventilatory frequency.[65] Interestingly, these pneumotaxic neurons could lead to a learning process similar to the Hering–Breuer reflex.[60] Even more interesting is the finding of the cooperation between ventral and dorsal areas of the pons.[60]

In summary, the medulla oblongata and pons have neurons with the capacity to alter the ventilator activity. Increase o decrease of the ventilatory activity depends on the information received for chemoreceptors. Based on the subsequent process of "decision making" the controller sends commands to motoneurons, which activate the diaphragm and other muscles involved in respiration.

4.4.3 Effectors in Ventilatory Pattern

Once the controller has generated a command, this information is converted into a motor response executed by motor units of the inspiratory and expiratory muscles. Predominantly, the inspiratory activity is carried out by the diaphragm, a muscle whose motoneurons have their soma in C3–C5 segments of the spinal cord, and which generates 70% of tidal volume.[52] If it is necessary to strengthen the inspiratory response, other muscle groups work together, including the external intercostals, scalene, sternocleidomastoid and pectoralis muscles, among others.

This chapter analyzed how the study of the pulmonary function goes beyond the recognition of the parameters based on the respiratory mechanics and pulmonary hemodynamics. The analysis of the molecular and cellular aspects of the respiratory system has allowed recognizing the importance that these aspects have in the pulmonary performance, as much in physiological situations as in the disease.

References

1. Seaton A, MacNee W, Donaldson K, Godden D. Particulate air pollution and acute health effects. *Lancet*. 1995;345: 176-178.
2. Gerritsen J. Host defence mechanisms of the respiratory system. *Paediatr Respir Rev*.2000; 1:128-134.
3. Bals R, Hiemstra PS. Innate immunity in the lung: how epithelial cells fight against respiratory pathogens. *Eur Respir J*.2004; 23:327-333.
4. Davis CW, Dickey BF. Regulated airway goblet cell mucin secretion. *Annu Rev Physiol*.2008; 70:487-512.
5. Barton AD, Lourenco RV. Bronchial secretions and mucociliary clearance. Biochemical characteristics. *Arch Intern Med*.1973; 131:140-144.
6. Toremalm NG. The daily amoung of tracheo-bronchial secretions in man. A method for continuous tracheal aspiration in laryngectomized and tracheotomized patients. *Acta Otolaryngol Suppl*.1960; 158:43-53.
7. Rose MC, Voynow JA. Respiratory tract mucin genes and mucin glycoproteins in health and disease. *Physiol Rev*. 2006;86:245-278.
8. Williams OW, Sharafkhaneh A, Kim V, Dickey BF, Evans CM. Airway mucus: from production to secretion. *Am J Respir Cell Mol Biol*.2006; 34:527-536.
9. Chilvers MA, O'Callaghan C. Local mucociliary defence mechanisms. *Paediatr Respir Rev*.2000; 1:27-34.
10. Voynow JA, Rubin BK. Mucins, mucus, and sputum. *Chest*. 2009;135:505-512.
11. Travis SM, Conway BA, Zabner J, et al. Activity of abundant antimicrobials of the human airway. *Am J Respir Cell Mol Biol*.1999; 20:872-879.
12. Rutland J, Griffin WM, Cole PJ. Human ciliary beat frequency in epithelium from intrathoracic and extrathoracic airways. *Am Rev Respir Dis*.1982; 125:100-105.
13. Hiemstra PS. The role of epithelial beta-defensins and cathelicidins in host defense of the lung. *Exp Lung Res*. 2007;33:537-542.
14. Nijnik A, Hancock RE. The roles of cathelicidin LL-37 in immune defences and novel clinical applications. *Curr Opin Hematol*.2009; 16:41-47.
15. Zanetti M. Cathelicidins, multifunctional peptides of the innate immunity. *J Leukoc Biol*.2004; 75:39-48.
16. Joris L, Dab I, Quinton PM. Elemental composition of human airway surface fluid in healthy and diseased airways. *Am Rev Respir Dis*.1993; 148:1633-1637.
17. Baraniuk JN. Neural regulation of mucosal function. *Pulm Pharmacol Ther*.2008; 21:442-448.
18. Tai CF, Baraniuk JN. Upper airway neurogenic mechanisms. *Curr Opin Allergy Clin Immunol*.2002; 2:11-19.
19. Muers MF. Diurnal variation in asthma. *Arch Dis Child*. 1984;59:898-901.
20. Bateman JR, Pavia D, Clarke SW. The retention of lung secretions during the night in normal subjects. *Clin Sci Mol Med Suppl*.1978; 55:523-527.
21. Bienenstock J, McDermott MR. Bronchus- and nasal-associated lymphoid tissues. *Immunol Rev*. 2005;206:22-31.
22. Wu HM, Jin M, Marsh CB. Toward functional proteomics of alveolar macrophages. *Am J Physiol Lung Cell Mol Physiol*. 2005;288:L585-L595.

23. Reddy RC. Immunomodulatory role of PPAR-gamma in alveolar macrophages. *J Investig Med*.2008; 56:522-527.

24. Mason RJ. Biology of alveolar type II cells. *Respirology*. 2006;11(suppl):S12-S15.

25. Daniels CB, Orgeig S. Pulmonary surfactant: the key to the evolution of air breathing. *News Physiol Sci*. 2003;18: 151-157.

26. Ikegami M. Surfactant catabolism. *Respirology*. 2006; 11(suppl):S24-S27.

27. Perez-Gil J. Structure of pulmonary surfactant membranes and films: the role of proteins and lipid-protein interactions. *Biochim Biophys Acta*.2008; 1778:1676-1695.

28. Chicurel ME, Chen CS, Ingber DE. Cellular control lies in the balance of forces. *Curr Opin Cell Biol*. 1998;10: 232-239.

29. Ingber DE. Tensegrity: the architectural basis of cellular mechanotransduction. *Annu Rev Physiol*.1997; 59:575-599.

30. Janmey PA. The cytoskeleton and cell signaling: component localization and mechanical coupling. *Physiol Rev*. 1998; 78:763-781.

31. Janmey PA, McCulloch CA. Cell mechanics: integrating cell responses to mechanical stimuli. *Annu Rev Biomed Eng*. 2007;9:1-34.

32. Wirtz HR, Dobbs LG. The effects of mechanical forces on lung functions. *Respir Physiol*.2000; 119:1-17.

33. Liu M, Skinner SJ, Xu J, Han RN, Tanswell AK, Post M. Stimulation of fetal rat lung cell proliferation in vitro by mechanical stretch. *Am J Physiol*.1992; 263:L376-L383.

34. Skinner SJ, Somervell CE, Olson DM. The effects of mechanical stretching on fetal rat lung cell prostacyclin production. *Prostaglandins*.1992; 43:413-433.

35. Wirtz HR, Dobbs LG. Calcium mobilization and exocytosis after one mechanical stretch of lung epithelial cells. *Science*. 1990;250:1266-1269.

36. Berrier AL, Yamada KM. Cell-matrix adhesion. *J Cell Physiol*.2007;213:565- 573.

37. Fredberg JJ, Kamm RD. Stress transmission in the lung: pathways from organ to molecule. *Annu Rev Physiol*. 2006;68:507-541.

38. Garcia CS, Prota LF, Morales MM, Romero PV, Zin WA, Rocco PR. Understanding the mechanisms of lung mechanical stress. *Braz J Med Biol Res*.2006; 39:697-706.

39. Ali MH, Mungai PT, Schumacker PT. Stretch-induced phosphorylation of focal adhesion kinase in endothelial cells: role of mitochondrial oxidants. *Am J Physiol Lung Cell Mol Physiol*.2006;291: L38-L45.

40. Gunst SJ, Tang DD, Opazo SA. Cytoskeletal remodeling of the airway smooth muscle cell: a mechanism for adaptation to mechanical forces in the lung. *Respir Physiol Neurobiol*. 2003;137:151-168.

41. Zhang W, Gunst SJ. Interactions of airway smooth muscle cells with their tissue matrix: implications for contraction. *Proc Am Thorac Soc*.2008; 5:32-39.

42. Lahiri S, Roy A, Baby SM, Hoshi T, Semenza GL, Prabhakar NR. Oxygen sensing in the body. *Prog Biophys Mol Biol*. 2006;91:249-286.

43. Gonzalez C, Rocher A, Zapata P. Arterial chemoreceptors: cellular and molecular mechanisms in the adaptative and homeostatic function of the carotid body. *Rev Neurol*. 2003;36:239-254.

44. Koerner P, Hesslinger C, Schaefermeyer A, Prinz C, Gratzl M. Evidence for histamine as a transmitter in rat carotid body sensor cells. *J Neurochem*.2004; 91:493-500.

45. Lazarov NE, Reindl S, Fischer F, Gratzl M. Histaminergic and dopaminergic traits in the human carotid body. *Respir Physiol Neurobiol*.2009; 165:131-136.

46. Wyatt CN, Evans AM. AMP-activated protein kinase and chemotransduction in the carotid body. *Respir Physiol Neurobiol*.2007; 157:22-29.

47. Zapata P, Larrain C. How the carotid body works: different strategies and preparations to solve different problems. *Biol Res*.2005; 38:315-328.

48. Tan ZY, Lu Y, Whiteis CA, Benson CJ, Chapleau MW, Abboud FM. Acid-sensing ion channels contribute to transduction of extracellular acidosis in rat carotid body glomus cells. *Circ Res*.2007; 101:1009-1019.

49. Trapp S, Aller MI, Wisden W, Gourine AV. A role for TASK-1 (KCNK3) channels in the chemosensory control of breathing. *J Neurosci*.2008; 28:8844-8850.

50. Garcia-Fernandez M, Ortega-Saenz P, Castellano A, Lopez-Barneo J. Mechanisms of low-glucose sensitivity in carotid body glomus cells. *Diabetes*.2007; 56:2893-2900.

51. Kumar P, Bin-Jaliah I. Adequate stimuli of the carotid body: more than an oxygen sensor? *Respir Physiol Neurobiol*. 2007;157:12-21.

52. Benditt JO. The neuromuscular respiratory system: physiology, pathophysiology, and a respiratory care approach to patients. *Respir Care*.2006; 51:829-837.

53. Coates EL, Li A, Nattie EE. Widespread sites of brain stem ventilatory chemoreceptors. *J Appl Physiol*.1993; 75:5-14.

54. Filosa JA, Dean JB, Putnam RW. Role of intracellular and extracellular pH in the chemosensitive response of rat locus coeruleus neurones. *J Physiol*.2002; 541:493-509.

55. Nattie E. CO2, brainstem chemoreceptors and breathing. *Prog Neurobiol*.1999; 59:299-331.

56. Filosa JA, Putnam RW. Multiple targets of chemosensitive signaling in locus coeruleus neurons: role of K+ and Ca2+ channels. *Am J Physiol Cell Physiol*. 2003;284: C145-C155.

57. Yu J. Airway mechanosensors. *Respir Physiol Neurobiol*. 2005;148:217-243.

58. Biscoe TJ, Stehbens WE. Ultrastructure of the denervated carotid body. *Q J Exp Physiol Cogn Med Sci*. 1967;52: 31-36.

59. Campanucci VA, Nurse CA. Autonomic innervation of the carotid body: role in efferent inhibition. *Respir Physiol Neurobiol*.2007; 157:83-92.

60. Smith JC, Ellenberger HH, Ballanyi K, Richter DW, Feldman JL. Pre-Botzinger complex: a brainstem region that may generate respiratory rhythm in mammals. *Science*. 1991; 254:726-729.

61. Lavezzi AM, Matturri L. Functional neuroanatomy of the human pre-Botzinger complex with particular reference to sudden unexplained perinatal and infant death. *Neuropathology*. 2008;28:10-16.

62. Chevalier M, Ben-Mabrouk F, Tryba AK. Background sodium current underlying respiratory rhythm regularity. *Eur J Neurosci*.2008; 28:2423-2433.

63. Ptak K, Zummo GG, Alheid GF, Tkatch T, Surmeier DJ, McCrimmon DR. Sodium currents in medullary neurons

isolated from the pre-Botzinger complex region. *J Neurosci.* 2005;25:5159-5170.

64. Pattinson KT. Opioids and the control of respiration. *Br J Anaesth*.2008;100: 747-758.

65. Feldman JL, McCrimmon DR. Neural control of breathing. In: Squire LR, Berg D, Bloom FE, du Lac S, Ghosh A, Spitzer NC, eds. *Fundamental Neuroscience*. Oxford: Elsevier;2008: 855-872.

66. Alheid GF, McCrimmon DR. The chemical neuroanatomy of breathing. *Respir Physiol Neurobiol*.2008; 164:3-11.

67. Lumsden T. Observations on the respiratory centres in the cat. *J Physiol*.1923; 57:153-160.

ImagingEval uationo ft heT horax

5

Gilberto Szarf and Henrique M. Lederman

Different imaging techniques are available for thoracic evaluation. Depending on the clinical scenario, the assistant physician can choose among them, focusing on the indication and prioritizing imaging of the thoracic wall, pleural space, mediastinum or lungs. We briefly review the most available noninvasive imaging methods for the evaluation of the thorax.

5.1 ChestR adiography

Chest radiography is the most commonly performed imaging procedure in most radiology practices. Usually, the postero-anterior (PA) and the left lateral projection are used for routine evaluation. Oblique radiographs can be performed to confirm the presence of focal lesions. The lateral decubitus can help to evaluate pleural effusions; expiratory radiographs can help to detect pneumothoraces.

The thoracic bone structures can be examined for the presence of lesions. Metastases usually are characterized by lytic lesions with bone erosion.

Pulmonary parenchymal alterations include areas of increased density, which can be seen in different clinical settings, like infection (consolidation) and neoplasms (lung nodule or mass). The first one usually presents with a pattern of confluent opacification, frequently with air bronchograms. Such opacification may be multifocal and involve multiple lobes. Pulmonary neoplasms can present as a nodule, usually with speculated and ill-defined borders or as a mass. Those lesions can be peripheral or central, sometimes with involvement of the central airways with obstruction.

It is possible to evaluate the pulmonary vasculature with chest radiographs based on the size of the pulmonary arteries. Signs of pulmonary artery hypertension (PAH) include enlargement of the main and hilar pulmonary arteries associated with small peripheral vessels. On PA erect radiographs, a right interlobar artery more than 16 mm in diameter is considered to be hilar vessel enlargement. Right ventricular enlargement maybe pre sent (Fig. 5.1).

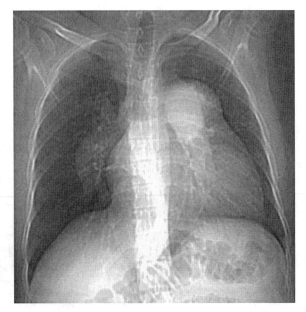

Fig. 5.1 Chest radiography demonstrating enlargement of the pulmonarya rterya ndi tsbr anches

G.S zarf(✉)
Department of Radiology, Federal University of Sao Paulo, Sao Paulo, Brazil

FleuryD iagnosticC enter, SaoP aulo, Brazil
e-mail:gs zarf@yaoo.com.br

E.A. Gabriel and T. Salerno (eds.), *Principles of Pulmonary Protection in Heart Surgery*,
DOI: 10.1007/978-1-84996-308-4_5, © Springer-Verlag London Limited 2010

An increased caliber of the upper lobe vessels is also a sign of pulmonary hypertension. In normal individuals, the caliber of the lower lobe vessels is bigger due to gravity. In PAH, there can be a reversal of this appearance secondary to a diversion of blood flow to the upper lobes.

Pulmonary edema due to congestive heart failure and elevated pulmonary microvascular pressure (cardiogenic edema) occurs secondary to elevated pulmonary venous pressure secondary to heart failure. Initially, there is edema with thickening of the interlobular septa, known as Kerley lines. Fluid accumulation in the peribronchovascular sheath can result in peribronchial cuffing. Fluid can also accumulate in the subpleural space, resulting in thickening of the interlobar fissures on chest radiograph. More severe cases can present also with extension of fluid into the alveolar spaces, which are identified on chest radiograph as poorly defined nodular opacities that can coalesce and produce consolidation. This condition usually has a rapid onset and quick resolution in response to adequate therapy.

Mediastinal contours and lines can be used to diagnose lesions in this compartment. Using this approach, generally it is possible to narrow the differential diagnosis based on lesion locations in the different mediastinalc ompartments(Fig. 5.2).

5.2 Fluoroscopy

With the widespread application of computed tomography (CT), fluoroscopy became restricted to the evaluation of diaphragmatic motion, for which both diaphragms should be visualized simultaneously and both inspiratory and expiratory maneuvers should be performed.

5.3 ComputedT omography

CT usually is used following abnormal chest radiography, to examine the tracheal and bronchial tree, for the assessment of focal or diffuse pulmonary lesions, and for staging of lung cancer. It is also used in the evaluation of mediastinal, hilar, or pleural abnormalities and to investigate chest wall lesions.

An understanding of the normal anatomy of the airways allows for the detection of abnormalities, including bronchiectasis, which is defined as abnormal and irreversible dilatation of the bronchial tree (Figs. 5.3 and 5.4).[1-4]

Air trapping, which is usually found in large airway obstruction and in small airway disease, can be seen on expiratory images as areas of lower density (Fig. 5.5).[5]

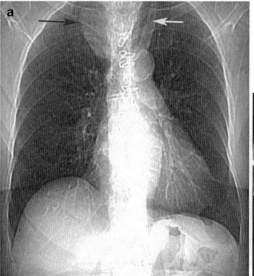
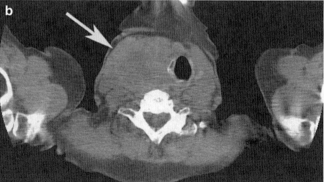

Fig. 5.2 (**a**) Superior mediastinal widening on thoracic radiography as shown between the white and the black arrows. (**b**) This lesion corresponds to an enlarged thyroid gland observed in the cervical computed tomography (*white arrow*).

Fig.5.3 (**a**) Trachea (*black asterisk*), (**b**) right upper lobe bronchus (*black arrow*), (**c**) middle lobe bronchus (*black arrowhead*) and left upper lobe bronchus (*white arrowhead*), (**d**) bronchi to thel owerl obes

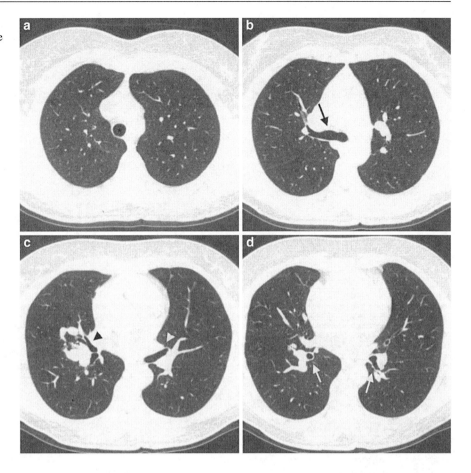

Pulmonary parenchymal alterations can be classified as lesions with increased density (including consolidation, linear opacities, nodular opacities, and ground glass attenuation) or decreased attenuation (including emphysema, cysts, cavities, and areas of decreased perfusion) (Figs. 5.6–5.8).[6-15]

On the vascular side, the pulmonary vasculature is readily accessible on CT. A main pulmonary artery diameter of more the 2.9 cm is considered abnormal and can suggest pulmonary hypertension. The upper limit of normal diameters for the proximal left and right pulmonary arteries are 2.8 and 2.4 cm, respectively.[16,17]

Contrast-enhanced images allow for the diagnosis of pulmonary thromboembolism, with the thrombus visualized in the pulmonary artery or in one of its branches.[18]

It is also possible to diagnose pulmonary infarction in this setting; it appears as a peripheral area of

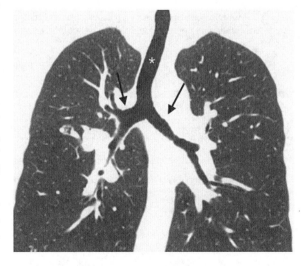

Fig. 5.4 Coronal reconstruction showing the trachea (*asterisk*), right and left main bronchi (*black arrows*)

Fig.5.5 (**a**) Inspiratory and (**b**) expiratory images at the level of the lower lobes. Air trapping is seen as areas of lower density, best identified duringe xpiration

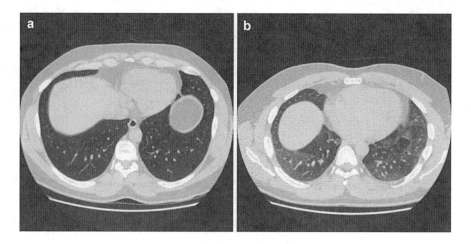

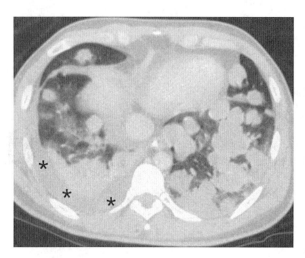

Fig. 5.6 Multiple round pulmonary opacities corresponding to metastatic pulmonary nodules. There is also right plural effusion (*asterisk*)

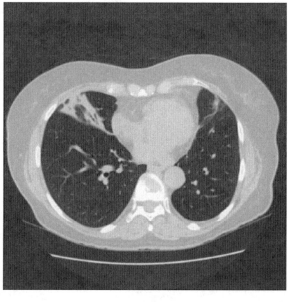

Fig. 5.7 Area of consolidation with air bronchograms in the middlel obe

consolidation, which can have diminished perfusion (Fig. 5.9).

Contrast-enhanced CT (angio CT) can also provide useful information about the aorta, including evaluation for aneurysms (Figs. 5.10 and 5.11).[19]

CT is the preferred imaging modality for evaluation of mediastinal masses. It provides information concerning location and relationship to adjacent structures. It can also determine whether a mass is cystic or solid or if it contains fat or calcium (which can be used to narrow the differential diagnosis). It also can evaluate the relation of lesions with the mediastinal adjacent structures(Fig. 5.12).

Pleural space alterations include effusions that can be seen as crescent-shaped opacities in the most dependent part of the thorax. Loculated effusions are seen as lenticular opacities in fixed position. Pleural plaques are irregular areas of pleural thickening that can involve the parietal pleura and the fissures. Pleural tumors appear as round or lobulated pleural masses.[20,21]

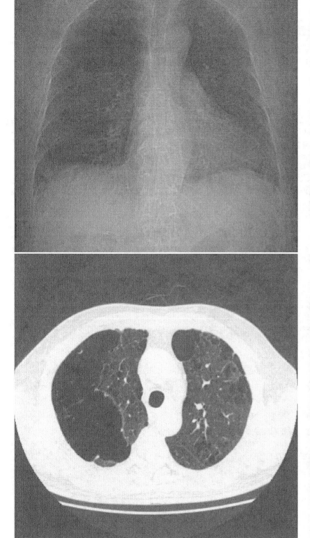

Fig. 5.8 Areas of lower density, more pronounced on the upper lobes, w ithoutd istinctw alls,c ompatiblew ithe mphysema

5.4 Ventilation-PerfusionSc an

The ventilation-perfusion scan is a nuclear medicine study that is performed by administering an inhaled ventilation agent (usually xenon-133) and an intravenously injected perfusion agent (technetium-99m-macroaggregated human albumin). This kind of scan permits visualization of alterations in the lung ventilation and perfusion patterns.

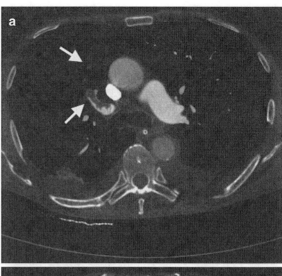
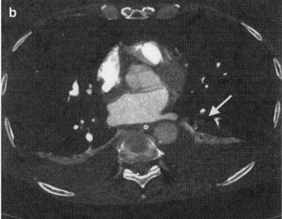
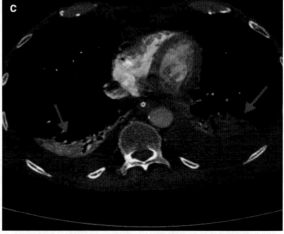

Fig. 5.9 (**a**, **b**) Contrast-enhanced computed tomographic image demonstrating thrombus in pulmonary artery branches (*white arrows*). (**c**) Hypoperfusion of the infarcted lower left lobe (*blue arrow*). Compare with the right atelectatic right lower lobe that is normally perfused (*red arrow*)

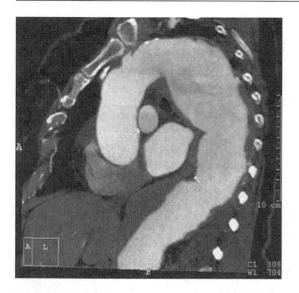

Fig. 5.10 Postcontrast thoracic computed tomographic image with sagittal oblique reformation shows diffuse dilation of the thoracica orta

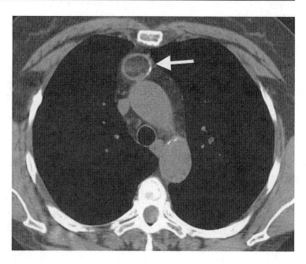

Fig. 5.12 Anterior mediastinal lesion with fat density inside corresponding to a teratoma (*white arrow*).

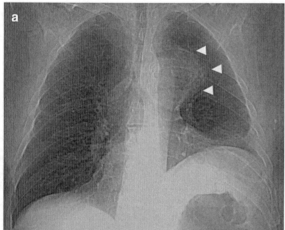

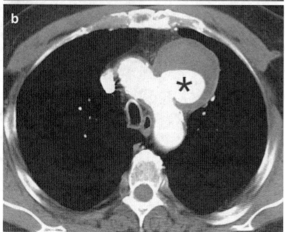

Fig. 5.11 (**a**) Mediastinal widening adjacent to the descending aorta (*white arrowheads*) corresponding to a (**b**) saccular aneurysm partially filled with thrombus (*black asterisk*)

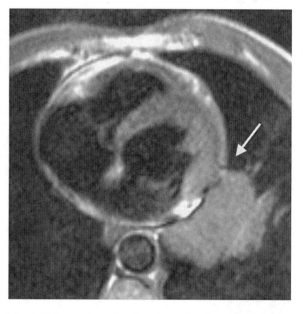

Fig. 5.13 Lung tumor invading the pericardium, which can be seen as a *dark line* interrupted by the tumor (*white arrow*)

5.5 MagneticR esonancel maging

Magnetic resonance imaging (MRI) provides excellent images of the chest wall, including the superior sulcus. The mediastinum, including the heart and great vessels, is also well visualized with this imaging modality (Fig. 5.13).

Fig.5.14 Magnetic resonance (MR) black
blood images and MR angiography of the
thoracic aorta demonstrating an area of
coarctation

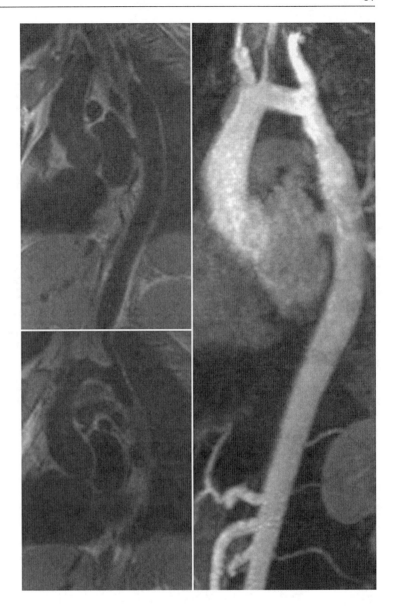

Magnetic resonance (MR) angiography, with the
intravenous injection of paramagnetic contrast material
(gadolinium), can provide high-quality images of the
thoracic vascular structures. It is also possible to access
the pulmonary vasculature and perfusion, acquiring
images in multiple phases after contrast injection
(Fig. 5.14).

The normal lung does not produce a MR signal
because of its low proton density and magnetic susceptibility effects. In the literature we can find studies
using polarized helium, which is an inert gas, to study
pulmonaryv entilation.

5.6 Conclusion

Multiple thoracic imaging methods are available. The
choice of which to use depends on which structure is to
bevis ualized.

References

1. Perhomaa M, Lahde S, Rossi O, Suramo I. Helical CT in
   evaluation of the bronchial tree. *Acta Radiol.* 1997;38(1):
   83-91.

2. Naidich DP, Gruden JF, McGuinness G, McCauley DI, Bhalla M. Volumetric (helical/spiral) CT (VCT) of the airways. *J Thorac Imaging*.1997; 12(1):11-28.

3. Gamsu G, Webb WR. Computed tomography of the trachea: normal and abnormal. *AJR Am J Roentgenol*. 1982;139(2): 321-326.

4. Naidich DP, Terry PB, Stitik FP, Siegelman SS. Computed tomography of the bronchi: 1. Normal anatomy. *J Comput Assist Tomogr*.1980; 4(6):746-753.

5. Stern EJ, Frank MS. Small-airway diseases of the lungs: findings at expiratory CT. *AJR Am J Roentgenol*. 1994;163(1): 37-41.

6. Bessis L, Callard P, Gotheil C, Biaggi A, Grenier P. High-resolution CT of parenchymal lung disease: precise correlation with histologic findings. *Radiographics*. 1992;12(1):45-58.

7. Leung AN, Miller RR, Muller NL. Parenchymal opacification in chronic infiltrative lung diseases: CT-pathologic correlation. *Radiology*.1993; 188(1):209-214.

8. Storto ML, Kee ST, Golden JA, Webb WR. Hydrostatic pulmonary edema: high-resolution CT findings. *AJR Am J Roentgenol*.1995;1 65(4):817-820.

9. Stein MG, Mayo J, Muller N, Aberle DR, Webb WR, Gamsu G. Pulmonary lymphangitic spread of carcinoma: appearance on CT scans. *Radiology*. 1987;162(2):371-375.

10. Akira M, Kita N, Higashihara T, Sakatani M, Kozuka T. Summer-type hypersensitivity pneumonitis: comparison of high-resolution CT and plain radiographic findings. *AJR Am J Roentgenol*.1992; 158(6):1223-1228.

11. Murata K, Takahashi M, Mori M, et al. Pulmonary metastatic nodules: CT-pathologic correlation. *Radiology*. 1992;182(2):331-335.

12. Remy-Jardin M, Giraud F, Remy J, Copin MC, Gosselin B, Duhamel A. Importance of ground-glass attenuation in chronic diffuse infiltrative lung disease: pathologic-CT correlation. *Radiology*.1993; 189(3):693-698.

13. Thurlbeck WM, Muller NL. Emphysema: definition, imaging, and quantification. *AJR Am J Roentgenol*. 1994;163(5): 1017-1025.

14. Aberle DR, Hansell DM, Brown K, Tashkin DP. Lymphangiomyomatosis: CT, chest radiographic, and functional correlations. *Radiology*.1990; 176(2):381-387.

15. Worthy SA, Muller NL, Hartman TE, Swensen SJ, Padley SP, Hansell DM. Mosaic attenuation pattern on thin-section CT scans of the lung: differentiation among infiltrative lung, airway, and vascular diseases as a cause. *Radiology*. 1997;205(2): 465-470.

16. Guthaner DF, Wexler L, Harell G. CT demonstration of cardiac structures. *AJR Am J Roentgenol*.1979; 133(1):75-81.

17. Kuriyama K, Gamsu G, Stern RG, Cann CE, Herfkens RJ, Brundage BH. CT-determined pulmonary artery diameters in predicting pulmonary hypertension. *Invest Radiol*. 1984; 19(1):16-22.

18. Garg K, Welsh CH, Feyerabend AJ, et al. Pulmonary embolism: diagnosis with spiral CT and ventilation-perfusion scanning–correlation with pulmonary angiographic results or clinical outcome. *Radiology*.1998; 208(1):201-208.

19. Rubin GD. Helical CT angiography of the thoracic aorta. *J Thorac Imaging*.1997; 12(2):128-149.

20. Shin MS, Ho KJ. Computed tomographic characteristics of pleural empyema. *J Comput Tomogr*.1983; 7(2):179-182.

21. Lee KS, Im JG, Choe KO, Kim CJ, Lee BH. CT findings in benign fibrous mesothelioma of the pleura: pathologic correlation in nine patients. *AJR Am J Roentgenol*. 1992;158(5): 983-986.

Endothelial Protection During Heart Surgery and Lung Transplantation

Qin Yang and Guo-Wei He

6

The endothelium in the cardiovascular system is crucial in the regulation of systemic and pulmonary blood circulation. A growing body of evidence demonstrates the occurrence of coronary endothelial dysfunction in cardiopulmonary bypass surgery. In addition, hypothermic circulatory arrest may cause pulmonary dysfunction that is manifested by increased pulmonary vascular resistance and decreased response to acetylcholine.[1,2] As a consequence, postoperative organ performance may be jeopardized by the compromised coronary or pulmonary blood circulation.

The cause of endothelial dysfunction during heart and lung surgery is multifold. To better understand the change of endothelial function under this situation, the alteration of individual relaxing factors (endothelium-derived relaxing factors [EDRFs]) nitric oxide (NO) and prostacyclin (PGI_2) and endothelium-derived hyperpolarizing factor (EDHF)[3-5] released from endothelial cells during heart and lung surgery should be addressed. In this chapter, we discuss these issues in detail by covering the strategy of endothelial protection, which still remains a challenge in cardiopulmonary bypass surgery as well as in heart or lung transplantation and therefore deserves continuous effort.

Q.Yang (✉)
Department of Surgery, The Chinese University of Hong Kong, HongKong, China
e-mail:qyang@surgery.cuhk.edu.hk

6.1 Endothelium Damage in Heart and Lung Surgery: Possible Mechanisms

The alteration of endothelial function in heart and lung surgery is a combined effect of several factors, including the following:

1. Ischemia-reperfusion injury. In cardiac surgery, acute ischemia due to cardiac arrest leads to damage of the myocardium. In the case of heart or lung transplantation, cardioplegia or organ preservation solutions are used to preserve the donor organ. The donor organ is therefore inevitably subjected to ischemia during preservation and the transplantation. When the heart or lung starts to function, it is subjected to reperfusion injury. The ischemia-reperfusion injury is a key point in cardiac surgery and heart or lung transplantation that may involve both myocytes or lung parenchymal cells and coronary or pulmonary endothelium-smooth muscle.

2. Direct action of the cardioplegic and organ preservation solutions due to their intrinsic characteristics (the components of the solution, such as hyperkalemia). Cardioplegic and organ preservation solutions were originally developed to protect the heart or lung by controlling the risk factors involved in cardiac surgery and heart or lung transplantation. The strategy includes reducing oxygen demand, Ca^{2+} overload, and edema as well as substrate supply. However, due to the differences between the cardiac myocytes or lung parenchymal cells and vascular (endothelial and smooth muscle) cells in structure and function, these solutions have been unfavorable to the function of

E.A. Gabriel and T. Salerno (eds.), *Principles of Pulmonary Protection in Heart Surgery*,
DOI: 10.1007/978-1-84996-308-4_6, © Springer-Verlag London Limited 2010

coronary or pulmonary endothelium,[6-8] as indicated by reduced ability of endothelial cell replication and attenuated endothelium-dependent relaxation. However, in most of the studies, the so-called effect of solutions on the endothelium was often mixed with the injury of ischemia-reperfusion. With the exclusion of the effect of ischemia, we have demonstrated the impact of hyperkalemic cardioplegia on endothelial function, particularly the EDHF-mediated endothelial function in coronary circulation,[9-12] which is discussed further in the next section.

3. Adjuncts to the cardioplegic procedure, such as hypothermia or the infusion pressure or duration, act both as independent factors and through their interaction with cardioplegic solutions.[13]

6.2 EndothelialDys functionU nder Ischemia-Reperfusion

Due to the simultaneous use of cardioplegia in cardiac surgery or preservation solutions in heart or lung transplantation, it is difficult to isolate the impact of ischemia-reperfusion in the clinical setting. However, experimental studies provided solid evidence regarding the detrimental effect of ischemia-reperfusion on the function of coronary or pulmonary endothelium. In isolated rabbit hearts, after 30 min of ischemic arrest and reperfusion, although coronary artery smooth muscle function was comparable, the endothelium-dependent increments of coronary flow to serotonin were significantly impaired,[14] which was consistent with the study conducted in rat and dog hearts.[15,16] Such vascular endothelial dysfunction plays a role in myocardial dysfunction that is marked by morphologic changes and creatine phosphokinase rise in coronary effluent.[15] Further studies on individual relaxing factors released by endothelium after ischemia-reperfusion suggested decreased PGI_2 synthesis[14] and the dominant target of ischemia-reperfusion injury: the NO transduction pathway.[17-19] This point was supported by the improved endothelial and myocardial function with supplementation of NO precursor or NO donor during the process of ischemia-reperfusion.[18,20,21] Regarding EDHF, the blunted response has been shown in porcine coronary arteries and veins after hypoxia-reoxygenation.[22-24] In dog coronary arteries exposed to 1-h ischemia followed by 2-h reperfusion, EDHF-mediated response was enhanced,[25] suggesting the backup role of EDHF in vasodilation when the function of NO is compromised.

Although the mechanism of ischemia-reperfusion injury is not fully understood yet, the oxidative stress-induced endothelial cell activation is recognized as the key component of the detrimental effect of ischemia-reperfusion. With expression of a set of proinflammatory, procoagulant, and vasoactive genes, a series of steps in protein production process is promoted in endothelial cells that causes intravascular microthrombosis, reduced blood flow, and activation of inflammatory cells. Among these proteins, the production of E-selectin, P-selectin, and intercellular adhesion molecules (ICAMs) leads to neutrophil recruitment, and neutrophils have been recognized as the principal effector cells of ischemia-reperfusion injury.[26] Leukocyte-endothelium adherence was indeed observed following cardioplegic arrest and reperfusion.[27] The cellular mechanism underlying the endothelial activation has been revealed with the study of nuclear factor kappa-B (NF-κB). Oxidative stress activates the tyrosine phosphorylation of IκBα, an inhibitor of NF-κB that binds to NF-κB in the cytoplasm, and such phosphorylation dissociates IkappaBalpha (IκBα)from NF-κB. The translocation of functional NF-κB to the nucleus with binding to the target genes results in transcriptional activation of these genes.[28] In patients undergoing cardiopulmonary bypass with cardioplegic arrest, NF-κB increased dramatically after reperfusion compared with before cardioplegia.[29] Therefore, targeting of the signaling pathway of endothelial cell activation may ameliorate cardioplegic arrest- and reperfusion-induced endothelium impairment. Better recovery of the coronary vascular response to serotonin and bradykinin in porcine coronary vessels[30] and to acetylcholine in the neonatal lamb heart[31] was obtained by adding deferoxamine or manganese superoxide dismutase to the cardioplegic solution to reduce the oxygen-derived free radicals[30] or by preischemic administration of leukocyte molecule CD18 (ligand for ICAM-1) antibody to the heart prior cardioplegic arrest.[31] Moreover, transfection of NF-κB decoy oligonucleotides into isolated heart blocked ICAM-1 upregulation and inhibited increase in neutrophil adhesion.[32] A study on peroxynitrite (ONOO⁻) suggested the inhibitory effect of this radical on K_{Ca} channel activity on the cellular membrane of human coronary arteriolar smooth muscle with reduced hyperpolarization-mediated vasodilation.[33] This mechanism may contribute to impaired EDHF-mediated dilation in conditions such as ischemia-reperfusion, in which an elevated level of ONOO⁻ is expected in the presence of excess of O_2^-.

6.3 EndothelialDys function Caused by Cardioplegic and Organ Preservation Solutions

As illustrated, the authentic effect of the solutions on the endothelium should be carefully distinguished from other factors to identify the possible damaging effect due to the intrinsic characteristics of the solutions. The solution-related impact on the endothelial function, particularly on individual EDRFs, is addressed next.

6.3.1 Effect of Cardioplegic and Organ Preservation Solutions on Individual EDRFs

6.3.1.1 Effecto nPG I$_2$

The increased release of PGI_2 during myocardial ischemia with/without cardioplegic arrest has been demonstrated.[34,35] Gene expression of COX (cyclooxygenase) 1 and PGI_2 synthase was not altered after cardioplegia, but the COX-1 protein level was significantly reduced, accompanied by increased expression of COX-2.[36] However, the combined effect of ischemia-reperfusion was not excluded. It is also unknown how long this increase would be maintained for under hypoxic conditions.

6.3.1.2 Effecto nN O

Studies have suggested impaired NO-related endothelial function during heart and lung surgery. By measuring the end products of NO (nitrite and nitrate), NO release decreased significantly at approximately 70 min of crystalloid cardioplegic arrest in human coronary vasculature, and it was further reduced after reperfusion.[37] Similarly, the inability of the endothelium to release NO associated with reduced endothelium-

dependent vasodilation after infusion with University of Wisconsin solution[38] or loss of NO production after cardioplegia-reperfusion associated with decreased protein level of constitutive NO synthase[36] was demonstrated. The NO loss after cold (4°C) ischemic storage with crystalloid cardioplegia was recovered by chronic oral administration of L-arginine, the physiological substrate of NO.[39] In an experimental lung transplantation model, both NO and cGMP (cyclic guanosine monophosphate) levels decreased markedly at the onset of reperfusion after preservation[40] and supplementation of a cGMP analog in Euro-Collin solution decreased pulmonary vascular resistance and improved recipient survival.[41] Furthermore, the attenuation of endothelium-dependent relaxation was observed in pulmonary arteries after several hours of cold storage in lung preservation solutions, such as University of Wisconsin solution or Euro-Collin solution.[8] However, the combined ischemia-reperfusion injury was probably the main cause of the NO-related endothelial dysfunction in these and other studies.[18,42]

We have demonstrated that, when the effect of ischemia-reperfusion is excluded, the NO-related, endothelium-dependent vasorelaxation after exposure to oxygenated crystalloid hyperkalemic cardioplegia to acetylcholine or substance P is well preserved in either porcine epicardial coronary arteries[43] or neonatal rabbit aorta.[44] Although in these studies the indomethacin-resistant relaxation was actually mediated by both NO and EDHF, the unchanged endothelium-dependent response and the susceptibility of EDHF to cardioplegic solution[9,10,45] provide convincing evidence for the minimal impact of hyperkalemic cardioplegic solution on the NO-related function after exposure for a certain period (1 or 2 h).

6.3.1.3 Effecto nEDHF

Our research group has conducted a series of experiments to investigate the effect of cardioplegic solution and organ preservation solutions on EDHF-mediated function. With exclusion of the effect of ischemia-reperfusion and elimination of the effect of PGI_2 and NO, we have demonstrated that hyperkalemia,[9,10] St. Thomas's Hospital cardioplegia[45] and University of Wisconsin solution[46] impair EDHF-related function in either porcine or human coronary arteries.[9,10] Decreased membrane hyperpolarization and associated vasorelaxation mediated by EDHF were also observed in pulmonary vasculature after exposure to organ preservation solutions, such as University of Wisconsin and Euro-Collins solutions.[47,48] The mechanism is due to the opposite effect of EDHF and hyperkalemia. Hyperkalemia depolarizes, whereas EDHF hyperpolarizes, the smooth muscle membrane. The persistent depolarizing effect of hyperkalemia even after washout of cardioplegic solution restricts the hyperpolarizing effect of EDHF.[10,46,49] Use of hyperpolarizing cardioplegia composed of potassium channel openers may overcome this shortage of hyperkalemic cardioplegia.[50]

6.3.2 Effect of Individual Components in Cardioplegic and Organ Preservation Solutions on Endothelial Function

6.3.2.1 Effect of K⁺

K^+ is the key component in cardioplegic and organ preservation solutions. The concentration of K^+ varies in different solutions. In University of Wisconsin solution, it is as high as 125 mM, whereas it is only 20 mM in St. Thomas's Hospital cardioplegia and 10 mM in histidine-tryptophan-ketoglutarate (HTK) solution. The importance of K^+ concentration with regard to coronary endothelial impairment was revealed. K^+ at 30 mmol/L but not at 20 mmol/L, abolished the endothelium-dependent, 5-hydroxytryptamine-induced vasodilation.[51]

In contrast, our studies and those by others[52] have demonstrated that hyperkalemia per se does not significantly alter the endothelium-dependent relaxation as a whole to acetylcholine or substance P in porcine coronary arteries (to K^+ 50 mmol/L)[43] and neonatal rabbit aorta (to K^+ 100 mmol/L).[44] These contradictory results stimulate further investigations regarding the effect of hyperkalemia on individual relaxing factors derived from endothelial cells. To date, there is a little evidence showing that the reduction of the production of NO is due to hyperkalemia. Rather, it is most likely due to the combined ischemia-reperfusion injury. When the capability of the endothelium to release NO is preserved or there is no presence of specific NO

inhibitors, the endothelium is tolerant to hyperkalemia as far as the endothelium-dependent relaxation is concerned, as discussed here.[43,44,52] With measurement of NO by a NO-specific electrode, we provided direct evidence for the first time that NO release is not affected by 1-h exposure to 20 mM K^+.[53]

On the other hand, in contrast to NO, susceptibility of EDHF to a high concentration of K^+ has been demonstrated in accumulating studies. When the effect of PGI_2 and NO is inhibited by indomethacin and N^G-nitro-L-arginine (L-NNA), the endothelium-dependent relaxation/hyperpolarization (mediated by EDHF) to a number of EDRF stimuli is impaired by incubation with K^+, ranging from 20 to 125 mM in porcine and human coronary arteries.[9,10,49] Realizing that L-NNA cannot abolish the production of NO, we further added oxyhemoglobin, a scavenger of NO, to abolish the effect of residual NO and demonstrated again the detrimental effect of hyperkalemia on the EDHF-mediated relaxation and hyperpolarization in porcine coronary microarteries[11] as well as in pulmonary arteries.[47]

The mechanism of the reduced EDHF-mediated relaxation in hyperkalemic solutions is twofold. First, hyperkalemia depolarizes the vascular smooth muscle membrane, and the prolonged depolarization increases the difficulty for subsequent hyperpolarization. Second, EDHF hyperpolarizes the vascular smooth muscle cell through opening K^+ channels, In contrast, as a natural K^+ channel blocker, high concentration of K^+ may block K^+c hannels.[10,49]

6.3.2.2 Effect of Mg²⁺

The introduction of Mg^{2+} into cardioplegia helps to achieve immediate heart arrest during cardiac surgery, and the enrichment of Mg^{2+} may counteract the unfavorable effect of hypocalcemia on sarcolemmal membrane by preventing calcium influx and thus obtain better membrane stabilization.[54] In addition to the protective effect on myocardium,[55,56] Mg^{2+} has been proven to be a potent vasodilator through both endothelium-dependent and -independent mechanisms.[57,58] The fact that Mg^{2+} infusion improves methacholine-induced vasorelaxation demonstrated the importance of endothelium in the effect of Mg^{2+} in human forearm vessels.[59] Pretreatment with NO synthase inhibitor L-NAME/L-NMMA reduces Mg^{2+}-mediated vasodilation and NO donor sodium nitroprusside or a cGMP analog, 3-guanosine monophosphate, restores the response to Mg^{2+}, indicating the role of the NO-cGMP pathway in the action of Mg^{2+} [57,58] Moreover, the involvement of the COX system with the production of PGI_2 has also been suggested in Mg^{2+}-induced relaxation.[58,60] Tofukuji and associates reported that hyper-Mg^{2+} cardioplegia (25 mM Mg^{2+}) was superior to hyper-K^+ cardioplegia in terms of preserving beta-adrenoceptor-mediated and endothelium-dependent regulation of the coronary microcirculation in pigs undergoing cardiopulmonary bypass.[61] Further, the inhibitory effect of hypomagnesemia was observed on endothelium-dependent vasodilation induced by acetylcholine or adenosine diphosphate, and such impairment of endothelial function was proposed to be due to the decreased release of NO.[62]

In addition, a study by our laboratory demonstrated that, in porcine coronary arteries, Mg^{2+} preserved the EDHF-mediated relaxation and hyperpolarization and restored the EDHF function impaired by hyperkalemia.[11]

6.3.2.3 Effecto fP rocaine

Similar to Mg^{2+}, the local anesthetic procaine is added to cardioplegia to induce asystole and obtain membrane stabilization.[54] Procaine is recognized as a vasodilator.[63,64] At 1 mM, procaine relaxes vascular smooth muscle in not only an endothelium-independent but also an endothelium-dependent manner that is closely related to NO but not PGI_2.[64] We further showed that procaine does not affect EDHF function in the coronary circulation[65] despite the fact that it depolarizes the membrane of vascular smooth muscle cells by reducing K^+c onductance.[66]

6.4 EndothelialPr otectioni nHear t Surgery and Lung Transplantation

6.4.1 Preconditioning

The concept of ischemic preconditioning was introduced in myocardial protection two decades ago. After brief episodes of ischemia, the heart becomes more

tolerant to prolonged periods of ischemic injury, suggesting a cardioadaptive response to stress.[67] Further studies on preconditioning revealed that the protection is not restricted only to myocardium, but also applies to coronary endothelium.[68] In an in vitro study mimicking the clinical setting, we demonstrated that hypoxic preconditioning restored EDHF-mediated responses impaired by hypoxia in porcine coronary arteries.[24,69] Similar protection of ischemic preconditioning was also observed in lung transplantation.[70,71] Repetitive periods of transient ischemia prior to pulmonary preservation can significantly reduce edema in the lung graft on reperfusion and improve oxygenation capacity. Further studies suggested that ischemic preconditioning of the lung prevented the decrease in the vasodilator responses to histamine and acetylcholine in the rat pulmonary vascular bed, and the protective effect may be mediated by NO and K_{ATP}c hannels.[72,73]

6.4.2 Postconditioning

Although ischemic preconditioning once raised great hope in the field of myocardial protection, due to the fact that in patients with acute myocardial infarction the coronary artery is already occluded at the time of hospital admission, ischemic preconditioning is therefore somehow not feasible in clinical practice. This fact led to the attempt at postconditioning. Since interventions are implemented at the time of predictable reperfusion, postconditioning showed greater clinical potential than preconditioning in ischemic myocardial protection. Studies of postconditioning so far have been focused on its efficacy in limiting myocardial infarction,[74-77] with its effect on vascular endothelium rarely explored. However, evidence derived from limited studies does suggest the potential of postconditioning in endothelial protection. Postconditioning protected endothelium from ischemia-reperfusion injury in the human forearm,[78] and the blunted endothelium-dependent vasodilation to acetylcholine in postischemic epicardial macrovessels in dogs was reversed by both preconditioning and postconditioning.[79] The protective effect of postconditioning on coronary endothelial function was further observed in patients with acute myocardial infarction.[80]

6.4.3 Additives to Cardioplegic or Organ Preservation Solutions

The additives aimed at protecting endothelial function may be categorized as follows.

1. *NO substrates or donors.* The benefit of the supplementation of NO precursor L-arginine or NO donors such as nitroglycerin in cardioplegia on postischemic ventricular performance and endothelial function has been well established, and thus it is considered as an effective replacement therapy in cardiac surgery.[81-83] In lung transplantation, supplementation of L-arginine in University of Wisconsin solution ameliorates impaired endothelium-dependent relaxation in pulmonary arteries following prolonged lung preservation,[84] and the use of nitroglycerin-supplemented Perfadex solution further enhances functional outcome of Perfadex-preserved lungs with improved pulmonary vascular resistance.[85]

2. *PGI$_2$ analogs.* PGI$_2$ analogs such as iloprost and OP-41483, added to crystalloid cardioplegia and lung preservation solutions, result in a significant amelioration of ischemia-reperfusion injury and improved preservation of cardiac and pulmonary graft function.[86-88]

3. *EDHF analogs.* Addition of epoxyeicosatrienoic 11, 12 (EET11, 12), the possible analog of EDHF, to a hyperkalemic solution may partially restore the bradykinin-induced, EDHF-mediated endothelial function in porcine coronary arteries.[89] Further, the benefit of EET11, 12 supplementation in St. Thomas's Hospital cardioplegia was shown under moderate hypothermia.[90]

4. *K$^+$ channel openers (KCOs).* When added to hyperkalemic cardioplegia, aprikalim reduces the Na$^+$–Ca^{2+} exchange outward current elevated by hyperkalemia and thus may attenuate the [Ca^{2+}]$_i$ elevation, leading to improved contractile function after cardioplegia in the ventricular myocyte.[91] In addition, supplementation with aprikalim in traditional hyperkalemic solutions preserves EDHF-mediated coronary relaxation, indicating its protective effect on endothelial function.[92] Other KCOs, such as KRN4884, have been demonstrated to have a preconditioning effect on the EDHF-mediated relaxation and may be beneficial if added to cardioplegic solutions.[24] The importance of intermediate- and small-conductance K$_{Ca}$ in endothelial function renders these channels potential targets in endothelial protection, which has been demonstrated in our recent studies.[93]

5. *Scavengers of oxygen-derived free radicals.* Supplementation of crystalloid cardioplegic solution with free radical scavengers, such as ascorbate and deferoxamine, reduces postreperfusion myocardial injury[94] and preserves the endothelium-dependent vasodilation in coronary microvessels.[30]

6. *Sodium-hydrogen ion exchange (NHE) inhibitors.* The cardioprotective effect of NHE inhibitors not only is observed with perioperative administration to patients undergoing bypass surgery[95] but also is demonstrated when added to blood cardioplegia.[96] The decreased accumulation of intracellular Na$^+$ and subsequently decreased Ca^{2+} overload contribute to the reduced postischemic infarct size and tissue edema due to the supplementation of selective NHE type 1 isoform inhibitor cariporide. In isolated postischemic left anterior descending coronary artery rings, maximal relaxation in response to acetylcholine was significantly greater in the cariporide group than in the vehicle group, indicating the preservation effect of cariporide on endothelium.[96]

7. *Other substances.* Adenosine has been shown to partially attenuate the microcirculatory injury by cardioplegia,[97] but the effect is controversial.[98] Adding phosphodiesterase III inhibitor (E-1020) to Bretschneider's HTK cardioplegic solution has been shown to improve myocardial functional recovery.[99] The finding that 17β-estradiol prevented intracellular Ca^{2+} loading or hypercontracture of ventricular cardiomyocytes in high K$^+$ exposure,[100] together with its direct favorable effects on vascular endothelial function,[101] raises the possibility of 17β-estradiol as a cardioprotective adjunct in hyperkalemic cardioplegia. The effect of prevention of Ca^{2+} overloading by Ca^{2+} antagonists highlights the cardiovascular protective effect of Ca^{2+} antagonist-supplemented cardioplegic solutions.[102,103] In addition to these strategies, solutions enriched with metabolic substrate (i.e., glutamate, aspartate, fumarate, etc.) have been clinically used for a long time for better myocardial protection.[104] However, little is known regarding the consequence of such enrichment on endothelial performance.

Figure 6.1 is a scheme of the contents in this chapter.

In conclusion, ischemia-reperfusion injury in cardiopulmonary bypass surgery and heart and lung

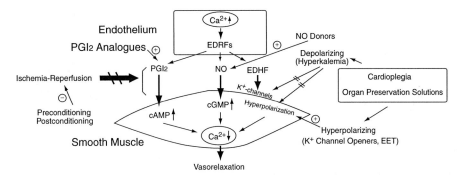

Fig. 6.1 Endothelium-smooth muscle interaction is altered during heart surgery and lung transplantation. In addition to ischemia-reperfusion, direct action of cardioplegic or organ preservation solutions due to their intrinsic characteristics (the components of the solution, such as hyperkalemic content) is another important cause of endothelial dysfunction. Several strategies have been proposed to protect endothelium, including the alleviation of ischemia-reperfusion injury by preconditioning or postconditioning and the improvement of cardioplegia or organ preservation solutions with additives targeting on different pathways of endothelium-dependent vasorelaxation. Ca^{2+} intracellular calcium; $cAMP$ cyclic 3′, 5′-adenosine monophosphate; $cGMP$ cyclic 3′, 5′-guanosine monophosphate; $EDRFs$ endothelium-derived relaxing factors; $EDHF$ endothelium-derived hyperpolarizing factor; EET epoxyeicosatrienoic acid; NO nitric oxide; PGI_2 prostacyclin; K^+ channel potassium channel

transplantation is a key factor that causes impairment to both myocytes or lung parenchymal cells and coronary or pulmonary endothelium. Due to the differences between the cardiac myocytes or lung parenchymal cells and vascular (endothelial and smooth muscle) cells in structure and function, the cardioplegic or organ preservation solutions primarily designed to protect the myocardium or lung parenchymal cells may have a detrimental effect on coronary or pulmonary vascular endothelial cells. One must be aware that under either experimental or clinical settings, the reported effect of the solutions on endothelium is often mixed, with many other factors, such as ischemia-reperfusion injury, temperature, and perfusion pressure and duration, not just the components of the solutions per se. In evaluation of a clinically used solution and in the development of a new solution, these factors should be carefully distinguished from the effect of the solution. The key component of the cardioplegic and heart or lung preservation solutions – high concentrations of potassium ion (hyperkalemia) – is the major component that has been studied regarding the endothelial function. The primary contributor of the endothelium-dependent relaxation, the NO pathway, is mainly impaired due to ischemia-reperfusion injury. Its resistance to the moderately increased potassium concentrations used for cardioplegia (~20 mEq/L) explains the excellent clinical results by using either crystalloid or blood cardioplegia. On the other hand, the second endothelium-dependent relaxation pathway – the EDHF

pathway, which is usually a "backup" of the NO pathway – is significantly altered (damaged) by hyperkalemia even at the moderately high concentration of potassium. This is because hyperkalemia inhibits potassium channels in the endothelium and smooth muscle that are related to either the release of EDHF from the endothelium or the target of the action of EDHF. Magnesium has a protective effect on this pathway because it hyperpolarizes the coronary smooth muscle membrane and therefore has a "synergetic" effect with EDHF. When combined with ischemia-reperfusion and other factors that significantly impair the NO pathway, the effect of hyperkalemia on the EDHF pathway becomes an important issue in the protection of endothelium. In short, endothelial protection is an important aspect that cannot be neglected in cardiopulmonary bypass surgery and heart or lung transplantation. Maximally limiting ischemia-reperfusion injury and optimizing the formula of cardioplegic and preservation solutions are the future directions in surgery-related coronary and pulmonary endothelial protection.

Acknowledgment This work was supported by Hong Kong GRF grant (CUHK4651/07M and CUHK 4789/09M), CUHK direct grants 2041561 2041457 Providence St. Vincent Medical Foundation, Portland, Oregon, USA, and China National Ministry of Science and Technology Grands 2009 DFB 30560 and 2010 CB 529502 (973), Tianjin Municipal Science and Technology Commission great 09ZCZDSF04200.

References

1. Cooper WA, Duarte IG, Thourani VH, Nakamura M, Wang NP, Brown WM III, Gott JP, Vinten-Johansen J, Guyton RA. Hypothermic circulatory arrest causes multisystem vascular endothelial dysfunction and apoptosis. *Ann Thorac Surg.* 2000;69:696-702; discussion 703.
2. Skaryak LA, Lodge AJ, Kirshbom PM, et al. Low-flow cardiopulmonary bypass produces greater pulmonary dysfunction than circulatory arrest. *Ann Thorac Surg.* 1996;62:1284-1288.
3. Ignarro LJ, Buga GM, Wood KS, Byrns RE, Chaudhuri G. Endothelium-derived relaxing factor produced and released from artery and vein is nitric oxide. *Proc Natl Acad Sci U S A.*1987;84:9265-9 269.
4. Moncada S, Gryglewski R, Bunting S, Vane JR. An enzyme isolated from arteries transforms prostagland in endoperoxides to an unstable substance that inhibits platelet aggregation. *Nature.*1976 ;263:663-665.
5. Feletou M, Vanhoutte PM. Endothelium-dependent hyperpolarization of canine coronary smooth muscle. *Br J Pharmacol.* 1988;93:515-524.
6. Follet DM, Buckberg GD, Mulder DG, Fonkalsrud EW. Deleterious effects of crystalloid hyperkalemic cardioplegic solutions on arterial endothelial cells. *Surg Forum.* 1980;31:253.
7. Nilsson FN, Miller VM, Johnson CM, Tazelaar H, McGregor CG. Cardioplegia alters porcine coronary endothelial cell growth and responses to aggregating platelets. *J Vasc Res.* 1993;30:43-52.
8. Strüber M, Ehlers KA, Nilsson FN, Miller VM, McGregor CG, Haverich A. Effects of lung preservation with Euro-Collins and University of Wisconsin solutions on endothelium-dependent relaxations. *Ann Thorac Surg.* 1997;63:1428-1435.
9. He GW. Hyperkalemia exposure impairs EDHF-mediated endothelial function in the human coronary artery. *Ann Thorac Surg.*1997 ;63:84-87.
10. He GW, Yang CQ, Yang JA. Depolarizing cardiac arrest and endothelium-derived hyperpolarizing factor-mediated hyperpolarization and relaxation in coronary arteries: the effect and mechanism. *J Thorac Cardiovasc Surg.* 1997; 113:932-941.
11. Yang Q, Liu YC, Zou W, Yim AP, He GW. Protective effect of magnesium on the endothelial function mediated by endothelium-derived hyperpolarizing factor in coronary arteries during cardioplegic arrest in a porcine model. *J Thorac Cardiovasc Surg.* 2002;124:361-370.
12. Yang Q, He GW. Effect of cardioplegic and organ preservation solutions and their components on coronary endothelium-derived relaxing factors. *Ann Thorac Surg.* 2005; 80:757;El–E13.
13. Parolari A, Rubini P, Cannata A, et al. Endothelial damage during myocardial preservation and storage. *Ann Thorac Surg.*2002;73:682 -690.
14. Hashimoto K, Pearson PJ, Schaff HV, Cartier R. Endothelial cell dysfunction after ischemic arrest and reperfusion: a possible mechanism of myocardial injury during reflow. *J Thorac Cardiovasc Surg.*1991; 102:688-694.
15. Qi XL, Nguyen TL, Andries L, Sys SU, Rouleau JL. Vascular endothelial dysfunction contributes to myocardial depression in ischemia-reperfusion in the rat. *Can J Physiol Pharmacol.*1998; 76:35-45.
16. Jorge PA, Osaki MR, de Almeida E, Dalva M, Credidio Neto L. Endothelium-dependent coronary flow in ischemia reperfusion. *Exp Toxicol Pathol.*1997; 49:147-151.
17. Seccombe JF, Schaff HV. Coronary artery endothelial function after myocardial ischemia and reperfusion. *Ann Thorac Surg.* 1995;60:778-788.
18. Engelman DT, Watanabe M, Engelman RM, et al. Constitutive nitric oxide release is impaired after ischemia and reperfusion. *J Thorac Cardiovasc Surg.* 1995;110:1047-1053.
19. Tiefenbacher CP, Chilian WM, Mitchell M, DeFily DV. Restoration of endothelium-dependent vasodilation after reperfusion injury by tetrahydrobiopterin. *Circulation.* 1996;94:1423-1429.
20. Vinten-Johansen J, Sato H, Zhao ZQ. The role of nitric oxide and NO-donor agents in myocardial protection from surgical ischemic-reperfusion injury. *Int J Cardiol.* 1995;50:273-281.
21. Gourine AV, Bulhak AA, Gonon AT, Pernow J, Sjöquist PO. Cardioprotective effect induced by brief exposure to nitric oxide before myocardial ischemia-reperfusion in vivo. *Nitric Oxide.* 2002;7:210-216.
22. Dong YY, Wu M, Yim AP, He GW. Hypoxia-reoxygenation, St. Thomas cardioplegic solution, and nicorandil on endothelium-derived hyperpolarizing factor in coronary microarteries. *Ann Thorac Surg.* 2005;80:1803-1811.
23. Dong YY, Wu M, Yim AP, He GW. Effect of hypoxia-reoxygenation on endothelial function in porcine cardiac microveins. *Ann Thorac Surg.* 2006;81:1708-1714.
24. Ren Z, Yang Q, Floten HS, Furnary AP, Yim AP, He GW. ATP-sensitive potassium channel openers may mimic the effects of hypoxic preconditioning on the coronary artery. *Ann Thorac Surg.*2001; 71:642-647.
25. Chan EC, Woodman OL. Enhanced role for the opening of potassium channels in relaxant responses to acetylcholine after myocardial ischaemia and reperfusion in dog coronary arteries. *Br J Pharmacol.*1999; 126:925-932.
26. Winn RK, Ramamoorthy C, Vedder NB, Sharar SR, Harlan JM. Leukocyte-endothelial cell interactions in ische-mia-reperfusion injury. *Ann N Y Acad Sci.* 1997;832:311-321.
27. Sellke FW, Friedman M, Dai HB, et al. Mechanisms causing coronary microvascular dysfunction following crystalloid cardioplegia and reperfusion. *Cardiovasc Res.* 1993;27:1925-1932.
28. Boyle EM Jr, Canty TG Jr, Morgan EN, Yun W, Pohlman TH, Verrier ED. Treating myocardial ischemia-re-perfusion injury by targeting endothelial cell transcription. *Ann Thorac Surg.* 1999;68:1949-1953.
29. Valen G, Paulsson G, Vaage J. Induction of inflammatory mediators during reperfusion of the human heart. *Ann Thorac Surg.*2001; 71:226-232.
30. Sellke FW, Shafique T, Ely DL, Weintraub RM. Coronary endothelial injury after cardiopulmonary bypass and ischemic cardioplegia is mediated by oxygen-derived free radicals. *Circulation.*1993; 88:II395-II400.

31. Kawata H, Aoki M, Hickey PR, Mayer JE Jr. Effect of antibody to leukocyte adhesion molecule CD18 on recovery of neonatal lamb hearts after 2 hours of cold ischemia. *Circulation.*1992; 86:II364-II370.

32. Kupatt C, Habazettl H, Goedecke A, et al. Tumor necrosis factor-alpha contributes to ischemiaand reperfusion-induced endothelial activation in isolated hearts. *Circ Res.* 1999;84:392-400.

33. Liu Y, Terata K, Chai Q, Li H, Kleinman LH, Gutterman DD. Peroxynitrite Inhibits Ca^{2+}-activated K^+ channel activity in smooth muscle of human coronary arterioles. *Circ Res.* 2002;91:1070-1076.

34. Wennmalm A, Pham-Huu-Chanh, Junstad S. Hypoxia causes prostaglandin release from perfused rabbit hearts. *Acta Physiol Scand.*1974; 91:133-135.

35. Nomura F, Matsuda H, Hirose H, et al. Assessment of prostacyclin and thromboxane A2 release during reperfusion after global ischemia induced by crystalloid cardioplegia – comparison between warm and cold ischemia. *Eur Surg Res.*1988;20:110- 119.

36. Metais C, Li J, Simons M, Sellke FW. Serotonin-in-duced coronary contraction increases after blood cardioplegia-reperfusion: role of COX-2 expression. *Circulation.* 1999; 100(Suppl):II328-II334.

37. Gohra H, Fujimura Y, Hamano K, et al. Nitric oxide release from coronary vasculature before, during, and following cardioplegic arrest. *World J Surg.*1999; 23:1249-1253.

38. Pearl JM, Laks H, Drinkwater DC, et al. Loss of endothelium-dependent vasodilatation and nitric oxide release after myocardial protection with University of Wisconsin solution. *J Thorac Cardiovasc Surg.* 1994; 107:257-264.

39. Nakamura K, Schmidt I, Gray CC, et al. The effect of chronic L-arginine administration on vascular recovery following cold cardioplegic arrest in rats. *Eur J Cardiothorac Surg.*2002;21:753- 759.

40. Pinsky DJ, Naka Y, Chowdhury NC, et al. The nitric oxide/cyclic GMP pathway in organ transplantation: critical role in successful lung preservation. *Proc Natl Acad Sci U S A.* 1994;91:12086-12090.

41. Naka Y, Roy DK, Smerling AJ, Michler RE, Smith CR, Stern DM, Oz MC, Pinsky DJ. Inhaled nitric oxide fails to confer the pulmonary protection provided by distal stimulation of the nitric oxide pathway at the level of cyclic guanosine monophosphate. *J Thorac Cardiovasc Surg.* 1995;110:1434-1440; discussion 1440-1441.

42. Dignan RJ, Dyke CM, Abd-Elfattah AS, et al. Coronary artery endothelial cell and smooth muscle dysfunction after global myocardial ischemia. *Ann Thorac Surg.* 1992;53: 311-317.

43. He GW, Yang CQ, Wilson GJ, Rebeyka IM. Tolerance of epicardial coronary endothelium and smooth muscle to hyperkalemia. *Ann Thorac Surg.*1994; 57:682-688.

44. He GW, Yang CQ, Rebeyka IM, Wilson GJ. Effects of hyperkalemia on neonatal endothelium and smooth muscle. *J Heart Lung Transplant.*1995; 14:92-101.

45. Ge ZD, He GW. Altered endothelium-derived hyperpolarizing factor-mediated endothelial function in coronary microarteries by St Thomas' Hospital solution. *J Thorac Cardiovasc Surg.*1999; 118:173-180.

46. Ge ZD, He GW. Comparison of University of Wisconsin and St Thomas' Hospital solutions on endotheli-um-derived hyperpolarizing factor-mediated function in coronary micro-arteries. *Transplantation.*2000; 70:22-31.

47. Zou W, Yang Q, Yim AP, He GW. Impaired endothelium-derived hyperpolarizing factor-mediated relaxation in porcine pulmonary microarteries after cold storage with Euro-Collins and University of Wisconsin solutions. *J Thorac Cardiovasc Surg.*2003; 126:208-215.

48. Zhang RZ, Yang Q, Yim AP, He GW. Alteration of cellular electrophysiologic properties in porcine pulmonary microcirculation after preservation with University of Wisconsin and Euro-Collins solutions. *Ann Thorac Surg.* 2004;77: 1944-1950.

49. He GW, Yang CQ, Graier WF, Yang JA. Hyperkalemia alters EDHF-mediated hyperpolarization and relaxation in coronary arteries. *Am J Physiol.*1996; 271:H760-H767.

50. He GW, Yang CQ. Superiority of hyperpolarizing to depolarizing cardioplegia in protection of coronary endothelial function. *J Thorac Cardiovasc Surg.*1997; 114:643-650.

51. Mankad PS, Chester AH, Yacoub MH. Role of potassium concentration in cardioplegic solutions in mediating endothelial damage. *Ann Thorac Surg.*1991; 51:89-93.

52. Evora PR, Pearson PJ, Schaff HV. Crystalloid cardioplegia and hypothermia do not impair endothelium-dependent relaxation or damage vascular smooth muscle of epicardial coronary arteries. *J Thorac Cardiovasc Surg.* 1992;104:365-1374.

53. Yang Q, Zhang RZ, Yim AP, He GW. Release of nitric oxide and endothelium-derived hyperpolarizing factor (EDHF) in porcine coronary arteries exposed to hyperkalemia: effect of nicorandil. *Ann Thorac Surg.* 2005;79: 2065-2071.

54. Vinten-Johansen J, Hammon JW. Myocardial protection during cardiac surgery. In: Gravlee GP et al., eds. *Cardiopulmonary Bypass: Principles and Practice.* Baltimore: Williams & Wilkins; 1993:155-206.

55. Hearse DJ, Stewart DA, Braimbridge MV. Myocardial protection during ischemia cardiac arrest: the importance of magnesium in cardioplegic infusates. *J Thorac Cardiovasc Surg.*1978; 75:877-885.

56. Shakerinia T, Ali IM, Sullivan JA. Magnesium in cardioplegia: is it necessary? *Can J Surg.*1996; 39:397-400.

57. Yang ZW, Gebrewold A, Nowakowski M, Altura BT, Altura BM. Mg(2+)-induced endothelium-dependent relaxation of blood vessels and blood pressure lowering: role of NO. *Am J Physiol.*2000; 278:R628-R639.

58. Longo M, Jain V, Vedernikov YP, Facchinetti F, Saade GR, Garfield RE. Endothelium dependence and gestational regulation of inhibition of vascular tone by magnesium sulfate in rat aorta. *Am J Obstet Gynecol.*2001; 184:971-978.

59. Haenni A, Johansson K, Lind L, Lithell H. Magnesium infusion improves endothelium-dependent vasodilation in the human forearm. *Am J Hypertens.*2002; 15:5-10.

60. Laurant P, Berthelot A. Influence of endothelium in the vitro vasorelaxant effect of magnesium on aortic basal tension in DOCA-salt hypertensive rat. *Magnes Res.* 1992;5:255-260.

61. Tofukuji M, Stamler A, Li J, et al. Effects of magnesium cardioplegia on regulation of the porcine coronary circulation. *J Surg Res.*1997; 69:233-239.

62. Pearson PJ, Evora PR, Seccombe JF, Schaff HV. Hypomagnesemia inhibits nitric oxide release from coronary endothelium: protective role of magnesium infusion after cardiac operations. *Ann Thorac Surg*. 1998;65:967-972.

63. Ahn HY, Karaki H. Inhibitory effects of procaine on contraction and movement in vascular and intestinal smooth muscles. *Br J Pharmacol*.1988; 94:789-796.

64. Huang Y, Lau CW, Chan FL, Yao XQ. Contribution of nitric oxide and K^+channel activation to vasorelaxation of isolated rat aorta induced by procaine. *Eur J Pharmacol*. 1999;367:231-237.

65. Yang Q, Liu YC, Zou W, Yim AP, He GW. Procaine in cardioplegia: the effect on EDHF-mediated function in porcine coronary arteries. *J Card Surg*.2002; 17:470-475.

66. Itoh T, Kuriyama H, Suzuki H. Excitation-contraction coupling in smooth muscle cells of the guinea pig mesenteric artery. *J Physiol*.1 981;321:513-535.

67. Murry CE, Jennings RB, Reimer KA. Preconditioning with ischemia: a delay of lethal cell injury in ischemic myocardium. *Circulation*.1986; 74:1124-1136.

68. Rubino A, Yellon DM. Ischaemic preconditioning of the vasculature: an overlooked phenomenon for protecting the heart? *Trends Pharmacol Sci*.2000; 21:225-230.

69. Ren Z, Yang Q, Floten HS, He GW. Hypoxic preconditioning in coronary microarteries: role of EDHF and K^+ channel openers. *Ann Thorac Surg*.2002; 74:143-148.

70. Gasparri RI, Jannis NC, Flameng WJ, Lerut TE, Van Raemdonck DE. Ischemic preconditioning enhances donor lung preservation in the rabbit. *Eur J Cardiothorac Surg*. 1999;16:639-646.

71. Li G, Chen S, Lou W, Lu E. Protective effects of ischemic preconditioning on donor lung in canine lung transplantation. *Chest*.1998;113: 1356-1359.

72. Kandilci HB, Gumusel B, Topaloglu E, et al. Effects of ischemic preconditioning on rat lung: role of nitric oxide. *Exp Lung Res*.200 6;32:287-303.

73. Kandilci HB, Gümüşel B, Demiryürek AT, Lippton H. Preconditioning modulates pulmonary endothelial dysfunction following ischemia-reperfusion injury in the rat lung: role of potassium channels. *Life Sci*. 2006;79: 2172-2178.

74. Argaud L, Gateau-Roesch O, Raisky O, Loufouat J, Robert D, Ovize M. Postconditioning inhibits mitochondrial permeability transition. *Circulation*. 2005;111:194-197.

75. Crisostomo PR, Wairiuko GM, Wang M, Tsai BM, Morrell ED, Meldrum DR. Preconditioning versus postconditioning: mechanisms and therapeutic potentials. *J Am Coll Surg*.2006;202:79 7-812.

76. Staat P, Rioufol G, Piot C, et al. Postconditioning the human heart. *Circulation*.2005; 112:2143-2148.

77. Vinten-Johansen J, Zhao ZQ, Zatta AJ, Kin H, Halkos ME, Kerendi F. Postconditioning–a new link in nature's armor against myocardial ischemia-reperfusion injury. *Basic Res Cardiol*.2005;100 :295-310.

78. Loukogeorgakis SP, Panagiotidou AT, Yellon DM, Deanfield JE, MacAllister RJ. Postconditioning protects against endothelial ischemia-reperfusion injury in the human forearm. *Circulation*.2006; 113:1015-1019.

79. Zhao ZQ, Corvera JS, Halkos ME, et al. Inhibition of myocardial injury by ischemic postconditioning during reperfusion: comparison with ischemic preconditioning. *Am J Physiol*.2003; 285:H579-H588.

80. Ma X, Zhang X, Li C, Luo M. Effect of postconditioning on coronary blood flow velocity and endothelial function and LV recovery after myocardial infarction. *J Interv Cardiol*.2006; 19:367-375.

81. Sato H, Zhao ZQ, McGee DS, Williams MW, Hammon JW Jr, Vinten-Johansen J. Supplemental L-arginine during cardioplegic arrest and reperfusion avoids regional postischemic injury. *J Thorac Cardiovasc Surg*. 1995;110: 302-314.

82. Lefer AM. Attenuation of myocardial ischemia-re-perfusion injury with nitric oxide replacement therapy. *Ann Thorac Surg*.1995; 60:847-851.

83. McKeown PP, McClelland JS, Bone DK, et al. Nitroglycerin as an adjunct to hypothermic hyperkalemic cardioplegia. *Circulation*.1983; 68:II107-II111.

84. Chu Y, Wu YC, Chou YC, et al. Endothelium-dependent relaxation of canine pulmonary artery after prolonged lung graft preservation in University of Wisconsin solution: role of L-arginine supplementation. *J Heart Lung Transplant*. 2004;23:592-598.

85. Wittwer T, Albes JM, Fehrenbach A, et al. Experimental lung preservation with Perfadex: effect of the NO-donor nitroglycerin on postischemic outcome. *J Thorac Cardiovasc Surg*.2003; 125:1208-1216.

86. Feng J, Wu G, Tang S, Chahine R, Lamontagne D. Beneficial effects of iloprost cardioplegia in ischemic arrest in isolated working rat heart. *Prostaglandins Leukot Essent Fatty Acids*.1996; 54:279-283.

87. Nomura F, Matsuda H, Shirakura R, et al. Experimental evaluation of myocardial protective effect of prostacyclin analog (OP41483) as an adjunct to cardioplegic solution. *J Thorac Cardiovasc Surg*.1991; 101:860-865.

88. Gohrbandt B, Sommer SP, Fischer S, et al. Iloprost to improve surfactant function in porcine pulmonary grafts stored for twenty-four hours in low-potassium dextran solution. *J Thorac Cardiovasc Surg*.2005; 129:80-86.

89. Zou W, Yang Q, Yim AP, He GW. Epoxyeicosatrienoic acids (EET(11, 12)) may partially restore endothelium-derived hyperpolarizing factor-mediated function in coronary microarteries. *Ann Thorac Surg*.2001; 72:1970-1976.

90. Yang Q, Zhang RZ, Yim AP, He GW. Effect of 11, 12 epoxyeicosatrienoic acid (EET11, 12) as additive to St. Thomas' cardioplegia or University of Wisconsin solution on endothelium-derived hyperpolarizing factor-mediated function in coronary microarteries: influence of temperature and time. *Ann Thorac Surg*.2003; 76:1623-1630.

91. Li HY, Wu S, He GW, Wong TM. Aprikalim reduces the Na^+-Ca^{2+} exchange outward current enhanced by hyperkalemia in rat ventricular myocytes. *Ann Thorac Surg*. 2002;73:1253-1259; discussion 1259-1260.

92. He GW. Potassium channel opener in cardioplegia may restore coronary endothelial function. *Ann Thorac Surg*. 1998;66:1318-1322.

93. Yang Q, Huang JH, Dong YY, Underwood MJ, He GW. New strategy to protect coronary endothelium from ischemia-reperfusion injury by using Ca^{2+}-activated K^+ channel activators: functional and cellular electrophysiological studies (abstract). *Circ J*.2009; 73(SuppII):397.

94. Chambers DJ, Astras G, Takahashi A, Manning AS, Braimbridge MV, Hearse DJ. Free radicals and cardioplegia: organic antioxidants as additives to the St Thomas' Hospital cardioplegic solution. *Cardiovasc Res*. 1989;23: 351-358.

95. Theroux P, Chaitman BR, Danchin N, et al. Inhibition of the sodium-hydrogen exchanger with cariporide to prevent myocardial infarction in high-risk ischemic situations. Main results of the GUARDIAN trial. Guard during ischemia against necrosis (GUARDIAN) Investigators. *Circulation*.2000;102: 3032-3038.

96. Muraki S, Morris CD, Budde JM, Zhao ZQ, Guyton RA, Vinten-Johansen J. Blood cardioplegia supplementation with the sodium-hydrogen ion exchange inhibitor cariporide to attenuate infarct size and coronary artery endothelial dysfunction after severe regional ischemia in a canine model. *J Thorac Cardiovasc Surg*.2003; 125:155-164.

97. Keller MW, Geddes L, Spotnitz W, Kaul S, Duling BR. Microcirculatory dysfunction following perfusion with hyperkalemic, hypothermic, cardioplegic solutions and blood reperfusion. Effects of adenosine. *Circulation*. 1991;84:2485-2494.

98. Sellke FW, Friedman M, Wang SY, Piana RN, Dai HB, Johnson RG. Adenosine and AICA-riboside fail to enhance microvascular endothelial preservation. *Ann Thorac Surg*. 1994;58:200-206.

99. Wang Y, Sunamori M, Suzuki A. Effect of phosphodiesterase III-inhibitor (E-1020) adjunct to Bretschnei-der's HTK cardioplegic solution on myocardial preservation in rabbit heart. *Thorac Cardiovasc Surg*.1996; 44:167-172.

100. Jovanovic S, Jovanovic A, Shen WK, Terzic A. Protective action of 17beta-estradiol in cardiac cells: implications for hyperkalemic cardioplegia. *Ann Thorac Surg*. 1998;66: 1658-1661.

101. Rubanyi GM, Johns A, Kauser K. Effect of estrogen on endothelial function and angiogenesis. *Vascul Pharmacol*. 2002;38:89-98.

102. Standeven JW, Jellinek M, Menz LJ, Kolata RJ, Barner HB. Cold blood potassium diltiazem cardioplegia. *J Thorac Cardiovasc Surg*.1984; 87:201-212.

103. Trubel W, Zwoelfer W, Moritz A, Laczkovics A, Haider W. Cardioprotection by nifedipine cardioplegia during coronary artery surgery. *Eur J Anaesthesiol*.1994; 11:101-106.

104. Rosenkranz ER. Substrate enhancement of cardioplegic solution: experimental studies and clinical evaluation. *Ann Thorac Surg*.1995; 60:797-800.

Vascular Endothelial Growth Factor andPul monaryl njury

7

Vineet Bhandari

7.1 Introduction

Vascular endothelial growth factor (VEGF) is a pluripotent growth factor that is essential for lung development[1,2] and has significant regulatory roles in angiogenesis and vascular permeability.[3] This chapter briefly discusses the biology of VEGF[3,4] and the role of VEGF in the varied forms of pulmonary injury.[5-8]

7.2 VEGF:B iology,R eceptors, and Regulation

VEGF is a widely expressed dimeric glycoprotein, but the highest level of expression in normal tissues is in the lung.[6,8,9] The VEGF family has many members, including VEGF-A to -E and placental growth factor (PlGF).[3-5] Alternative exon splicing of the VEGF genes results in various isoforms that have biological and functional specificity. VEGF-A is the best studied of all and is referred to as VEGF from this point in the discussion. VEGF is a 34- to 46-kDa dimeric glycoprotein produced by alternative splicing of the eight-exon VEGF gene located at p12–21 on chromosome 6 in humans.[9] In normal human tissues, the VEGF gene is expressed as proteins of 206, 189, 183, 165, 145, and 121 amino acids.[4,5,9] $VEGF_{165}$ is the predominant isoform.

The biological activity of VEGF is dependent on its interaction with specific transmembrane receptor

tyrosine kinase (RTK) receptors; the two well-defined ones are VEGF receptor-1/fms-like tyrosine kinase-1 (VEGFR-1/Flk-1) and VEGF receptor-2/kinase insert domain receptor/fetal liver kinase-1 (VEGFR-2/KDR/Flk-1).[10] VEGFR-3/Flt-4 is a member of the same family, but binds to VEGF-C/D.[4,5,7] Neuropilin 1 (NRP-1), a receptor for semaphorins in the nervous system, also binds VEGF (and PlGF).[4,5,7] It has been suggested that NRP-1 presents $VEGF_{165}$ to VEGFR-2, which enhances the latter's signal transduction.[7] A wide variety of cells expresses VEGF receptors in the lung, including activated macrophages, neutrophils, vascular endothelial cells, and alveolar type II pneumocytes (TIIPs).[10] VEGF is thus potentially capable of having effects on alveolar epithelial cells and endothelial cells.[10,11]

VEGF is known to be influenced by various factors, including hypoxia, cytokines, and other inflammatory mediators.[5,7] Hypoxic exposure to the lung led to increased VEGF messenger RNA (mRNA), mostly in the alveolar epithelium.[5] This is said to be mediated by binding of the hypoxia-inducible factor 1 (HIF-1) to a site located in the VEGF promoter and the stabilization of VEGF mRNA.[7] Various inflammatory cytokines and growth factors known to increase VEGF levels include tumor necrosis factor-alpha (TNF-α), interleukin 6 (IL-6), interferon-gamma (IFN-γ), endothelin 1 (ET-1), epidermal growth factor (EGF), transforming growth factor-beta (TGF-β), keratinocyte growth factor (KGF), and insulin-like growth factor (IGF).[5,7] The paracrine or autocrine release of these factors influences the release, and hence the biological effects, of VEGF in the pulmonary microenvironment.[7]

The major effects of VEGF are the critical roles in angiogenesis, endothelial cell survival, cell proliferation, activation and recruitment of inflammatory cells, and potent vascular-permeability enhancing effects.[2,3,5,12]

V.B handari
Department of Pediatrics, Yale University
Schoolof M edicine, NewH aven, CT, USA
e-mail:vi neet.bhandari@yale.edu

E.A. Gabriel and T. Salerno (eds.), *Principles of Pulmonary Protection in Heart Surgery*,
DOI: 10.1007/978-1-84996-308-4_7, © Springer-Verlag London Limited 2010

67

7.3 VEGF and the Lung

VEGF is expressed in the developing mouse lung by the early third trimester of murine fetal development at embryonic (E) day 14 and E17.[13] In normal lung development in the mouse, VEGF and VEGFR-2 mRNAs undergo coordinate, threefold increases in expression during the canalicular and saccular stages of lung development between E13 and E18, and a further two- to threefold increase by 2 weeks following delivery.[14] VEGF mRNA expression appears localized primarily to the alveolar epithelium from E18 onward, with specific expression in TIIP by postnatal day 8 in mice[15,16] and rabbits.[17] VEGF protein immunostaining is more diffuse, with protein detected in epithelial, mesenchymal, and vascular smooth muscle cells.[14] VEGF is said to play a role not only in the formation of the pulmonary vasculature, but also in the epithelial-endothelial interactions that are critical for normal lung development.[7,18] In addition, VEGF has been shown to stimulate surfactant production and pulmonary maturation.[1,19]

In healthy humans, VEGF protein levels are compartmentalized to the alveolar epithelium, with the levels 500 times that of plasma.[20] Under normal circumstances, this physiological reservoir exerts its biological functions, which may get exaggerated under conditions of stress, leading to the manifestations of lung injury.[5,20] In injured lungs, alveolar macrophages and migrating neutrophils and monocytes are mobilized to the lung.[5] These cells are additional sources of intrapulmonary VEGF.[5]

7.4 VEGF and Pulmonary Injury

In the early phase of lung injury, the high local concentrations of VEGF that are released from TIIP and inflammatory cells may disrupt the junctional integrity of endothelial cells, leading to vascular leakage and pulmonary edema. During the next phase, the damaged alveolar epithelium and release of proteases from neutrophils decrease the VEGF levels in the alveolar compartment. Simultaneously, the serum levels of VEGF are increased as a result of the loss of compartmentalization and release of VEGF from other organs and circulating inflammatory cells.[5] We speculate that the initial increase in VEGF levels could potentially contribute to lung injury or pulmonary edema, leading to cellular damage or death, which in turn results in decreased VEGF levels. Subsequently, there is a surge

in VEGF levels associated with lung repair.[1] This phasic pattern of VEGF release has been shown to occur during acute myocardial infarction in human adults,[21] lung injury in adult animals,[5,22] and hyperoxia-induced lung injury in newborn animals[23] and humans.[1]

7.5 VEGF and Hyperoxia-Induced Lung Injury

Adult Sprague-Dawley rats exposed to 95% O_2 had a reduction in VEGF mRNA at 24 h, which decreased to less than 50% of control values by 48 h.[24] Adult rabbits exposed to 100% O_2 for 64 h have a marked decrease in VEGF mRNA.[25] In contrast, secreted VEGF protein measured in the bronchoalveolar lavage (BAL) fluid of hyperoxia-exposed adult rabbits increased during a 64-h exposure, then decreased, followed by a dramatic increase during recovery in room air.[26] In adult mice exposed to 95% O_2 for 72 h, there was a significant increase in BAL VEGF protein levels.[27]

Using our transgenic system, we overexpressed VEGF$_{165}$ in the murine adult lung.[28] There was significantly increased survival on hyperoxia exposure compared to controls.[29] Furthermore, this protection was in part mediated via an A1-dependent mechanism.[29]

On gene expression profiling with confirmation by real-time reverse-transcriptase polymerase chain reaction (RT-PCR), premature rat lungs exposed to prolonged hyperoxia (10 days) had a downregulation of VEGFR-2.[30] In newborn rabbits, the amount of VEGF protein in the BAL fluid increased twofold on exposure to 95% O_2, dropped to barely detectable levels at the 50% lethal dose time point, and increased eightfold compared with control levels during the first 5 days of recovery (in 60% O_2).[26] By 2 weeks of recovery, VEGF levels had reached normal values.[26] Interestingly, exposure of neonatal rats to hyperoxia for 12 days impaired alveolarization and vessel density that persisted despite recovery in room air at day 22.[31] Recombinant human VEGF treatment, started at day 14 during the recovery period, enhanced vessel growth and alveolarization in infant rats.[31]

In summary, the data would suggest that exposure to hyperoxia (in the adult and developing lung) has a phasic response. Initially, there is an increased amount of VEGF release that could account for lung injury by causing vascular permeability alterations, followed by a decrease in VEGF. If adequate recovery is to occur, there is a tremendous surge in VEGF levels, allowing for angiogenesis and alveolarization that underlie the process of lung healing and repair. However, in the clinical arena, under most circumstances, exposure to hyperoxia is combined with mechanical ventilation. Hence, it would be important to assess the effects on VEGF under these circumstances.

7.6 VEGFandV entilation and Hyperoxia-Induced Lung Injury

In a rabbit model, VEGF mRNA levels were not changed after high lung inflation (positive end expiratory pressure) and room air for 4 h.[32] VEGF BAL fluid concentrations were increased in adult rats ventilated with high tidal volumes (35 mL/kg) and 45% O_2.[33] However, in an acid-aspiration model ventilated with high tidal volumes (17 mL/kg) with 100% O_2, pulmonary injury was associated with increased lung levels of IL-6 and VEGFR-2 but not VEGF.[34]

In 4- to 6-day-old newborn mice mechanically ventilated with 40% O_2 for 24 h, there was reduced lung protein abundance of VEGF and VEGFR-2.[35] Similarly, in a preterm lamb model, VEGF mRNA was decreased by 40% after 4 h of mechanical ventilation with 100% O_2.[36]

VEGF levels were measured in lung epithelial lining fluid (ELF) collected from adult patients with acute lung injury (ALI).[37] On days 0, 5, 7, and 10, the VEGF levels in ELF were significantly greater in survivors than in nonsurvivors, but did not differ on days 1 and 3. There was no significant difference in ELF VEGF levels between control subjects and patients with ALI at any time point. Lung injury score was inversely correlated with VEGF concentration in ELF. In patients with ALI, elevated VEGF levels in ELF may predict a better outcome. Increased production of VEGF in the injured lung may contribute to resolution of inflammation in the lung.[37]

In the premature fetal baboon delivered at 125 days (term is 140 days) and treated with oxygen and mechanical ventilation as needed for 14 days, overall expression of VEGF mRNA and protein was markedly decreased; expression of VEGFR-1 was decreased by 30–40%, while VEGFR2 mRNA expression was unchanged.[38] Other investigators, using the same preterm baboon model, have found increased[39] or decreased[40] VEGF but consistently decreased VEGFR-1 and VEGFR-2.[39,40]

Studies done in intubated premature neonates revealed an increase by at least three- to fourfold over the first 3–10 days after birth.[15] The discrepancy with the fetal baboon studies could be due to different concentrations of isoforms of VEGF being secreted in the BAL fluid or other variables, like chorioamnionitis or corticosteroid administration in humans.[1515] However, the subset of human infants who recover without bronchopulmonary dysplasia (BPD), a form of chronic lung disease in neonates secondary to lung injury contributed, in part, by mechanical ventilation and hyperoxia,[41] has a trend toward increasing VEGF levels over time, while babies who did develop BPD appeared to have decreased VEGF levels.[15] In our study of neonates exposed to hyperoxia, VEGF was readily apparent in tracheal aspirates (TAs). A subset of neonatal patients with respiratory distress syndrome (RDS) develops lung injury and pulmonary edema, subsequently leading to BPD and even death. Interestingly, the levels of TA VEGF measured in the first 12 h of life were significantly higher in babies who subsequently developed BPD or died. Subsequent measurements of VEGF revealed a significant decrease at days 3–5 (compared to patients with no BPD) followed by significantly increased levels by days 21–28. These studies demonstrated that VEGF levels appear to follow a specific pattern in conditions characterized by exposure to high concentrations of oxygen and ALI in neonatal patients.[1] Others[42] have not found such an association. However, this could be due to the variable timing or measurement technique utilized or the different characteristics of the patient population studied. These data appear to conform to the neonatal animal studies as enumerated in this chapter.

7.7 VEGFandL ipopolysaccharide- and Sepsis-Induced Lung Injury

In two adult murine (C57Bl/6 and 129/J) models of ALI induced by aerosolized lipopolysaccharide (LPS), increased BAL protein leak and inflammation correlated with time-dependent increase in lung tissue VEGF.[43] In contrast, in another study using C57Bl/6 mice, VEGF was shown to be protective of LPS-induced lung injury.[44] Interestingly, in a different strain (imprinting control region or ICR) of mice, pulmonary expression of VEGF and its receptors declined with age and was further downregulated by intratracheal LPS administration.[45] Again, differences in methodology, including timing of measurement or intervention, are important variables to take into consideration when analyzing these results.

In an ovine sepsis model, lung edema formation was the result of marked increases in both pulmonary microvascular permeability and pressure.[46] Pulmonary vascular hyperpermeability peaked 12 h postinjury and was related to VEGF overexpression. Early myocardial failure was a potential contributor to the constant increase in pulmonary capillary pressure.[46]

7.8 VEGFandI schemia-Reperfusion-Induced Lung Injury

Enhanced VEGF cell signaling has been shown to also mediate ischemia-reperfusion (I/R) injury in rat lungs.[47] On the other hand, decreased VEGF levels have been associated with increased alveolar epithelial damage in a rat model of I/R injury.[48] In a model of ALI secondary to intestinal I/R, VEGF was increased in the BAL, but VEGF and VEGFR-1 were significantly reduced in the lung tissues.[22] Significant negative correlations were noted with the number of VEGF- and VEGFR-1-positive cells and epithelial cells undergoing cell death.[22] Besides the differences in the modeling systems, the timing of measurement can potentially explain these discrepant results.[22,48]

In terms of the mechanism, which can potentially suggest therapeutic targets, activation of the zinc-finger transcription factor early growth response (Egr) 1 has been considered a major regulator of pulmonary I/R injury. Among other mediators, VEGF transcripts and protein were increased in wild-type adult mice subjected to pulmonary I/R but not in Egr-1 null mutant mice.[49] Integrin $\alpha v\beta 5$ has also been implicated as a regulator of pulmonary vascular permeability in I/R injury.[50] Since VEGF is known to have acted through nitric oxide (NO),[1,51] blockade of NO signaling attenuated lung injury secondary to aortic I/R.[52]

7.9 CardiacC onditions and Pulmonary VEGF

In a piglet model, the left pulmonary artery (PA) was ligated to induce lung ischemia then reimplanted into the main PA to reperfuse the lung. Animals sacrificed 5 weeks after ligation, 2 days after reperfusion, or 5 weeks after reperfusion were compared to a sham-operated group.[53] While VEGF levels were unchanged, chronic lung ischemia led to overexpression of other proapoptotic factors and a dramatic transient increase in endothelial cell death.[53]

In an experimental murine model of cardiac arrest, endothelial-specific molecules were assessed as biomarkers to predict lung injury due to warm ischemia. There were no changes in VEGF expression over 4 h.[54] Serum VEGF levels were increased after coronary artery bypass graft (CABG) surgery.[55] Interestingly, in post-CABG pleural effusions, local production of VEGF in the pleural space correlated with markers of inflammation and vascular permeability,[56] suggesting a possible deleterious role of VEGF.

Pulmonary VEGF has been shown to be upregulated after cavopulmonary anastomosis in lamb[57] and rat[58] models as well as in human children.[59] Children with cyanotic heart disease had increased serum VEGF levels, but these did not correlate with the presence of abnormal vessel proliferation (which included pulmonary collaterals and arteriovenous malformations).[60] However, another study found a positive correlation with pulmonary VEGF staining and advanced pulmonary plexogenic arteriopathy.[61] Serum VEGF levels were significantly increased in patients with cyanotic heart disease and those who underwent the Fontan procedure, compared to controls.[62] Aortopulmonary collaterals increased after the Fontan procedure, and the serum VEGF levels correlated with the development of these collaterals.[62] Transbronchial VEGF gene transfer led to pulmonary angiogenesis and proximal pulmonary arterial growth in a fetal lamb model.[63]

7.10 Conclusions

It is apparent that there is an obvious duality of the role of VEGF in lung injury. This is exemplified by reviews highlighting this issue.[6-8] While there are significant methodological differences in the animal models and human studies looking at VEGF and its signaling process, there does appear to be a pattern that can explain this biological phenomenon. Given the large stores of VEGF in the lung, an early increase (release) of VEGF may enhance pulmonary vascular permeability in response to an instigating event (e.g., ischemia), followed by decreased VEGF (and VEGF

Fig. 7.1 Proposedpha sic role of vascular endothelial growth factor (VEGF) during pulmonary injury. Various lung injury stimuli result in the *early phase* of VEGF release from the type II pneumocytes, which attracts inflammatory cells (monocytes-macrophages and neutrophils), which in turn also increase VEGF locally in the lung. This results in disruption of the alveolar-capillary barriers, causing pulmonary edema and endothelial and epithelial cell death. This is followed by the *intermediate phase,* during which there is a decrease in VEGF levels in the lung. Subsequent recovery of the pulmonary epithelium results in the *late phase* of increased VEGF production, which promotes angiogenesisa ndc ells urvival

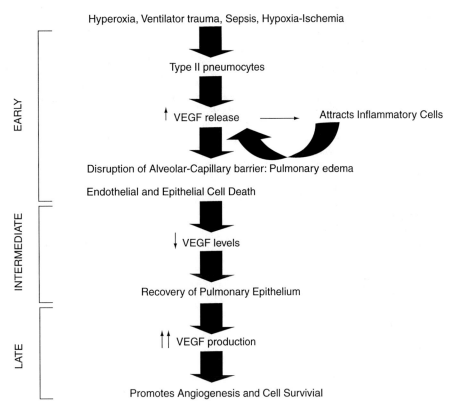

receptors) tissue levels, which may contribute to cell death. This aggravates pulmonary injury. What follows is a surge in VEGF levels secondary to an attempt at lung repair. This is illustrated in Fig. 7.1. There are supportive data suggesting such a phasic response.[1,5,22,23] Cardiac conditions that promote ischemia or hypoxia upregulate pulmonary VEGF levels and can have deleterious consequences. On the other hand, VEGF can be beneficial under specific circumstances.

Thus, not surprisingly, VEGF-enhancing[19,64-66] as well anti-VEGF[67,68] approaches have been proposed to attenuate lung injury. This reflects the need for better characterization of the modeling systems used and translation into human disease, especially in terms of timing. Developmental regulation is an additional confounding variable that needs to be taken into consideration.[1] Hence, an improved understanding of the pathobiology of VEGF and its signaling pathways is critical in terms of the translational potential of the utilization of VEGF-enhancing or anti-VEGF approaches as therapeutic approaches to ameliorate the various forms of pulmonary injury.[69]

Acknowledgments   VB was supported by grants from NHLBI K08 HL 074195, AHA 0755843T, ATS 07-005.

References

1. Bhandari V, Choo-Wing R, Lee CG, et al. Developmental regulation of NO-mediated VEGF-induced effects in the lung. *Am J Respir Cell Mol Biol*.2008; 39:420-430.
2. Voelkel NF, Vandivier RW, Tuder RM. Vascular endothelial growth factor in the lung. *Am J Physiol Lung Cell Mol Physiol*.2006; 290:L209-L221.
3. Ferrara N. Vascular endothelial growth factor: basic science and clinical progress. *Endocr Rev*.2004; 25:581-611.
4. Ferrara N, Gerber HP, LeCouter J. The biology of VEGF and its receptors. *Nat Med*.2003; 9:669-676.
5. Mura M, dos Santos CC, Stewart D, Liu M. Vascular endothelial growth factor and related molecules in acute lung injury. *J Appl Physiol*.2004; 97:1605-1617.
6. Medford AR, Millar AB. Vascular endothelial growth factor (VEGF) in acute lung injury (ALI) and acute respiratory distress syndrome (ARDS): paradox or paradigm? *Thorax*. 2006;61:621-626.
7. Papaioannou AI, Kostikas K, Kollia P, Gourgoulianis KI. Clinical implications for vascular endothelial growth factor in the lung: friend or foe? *Respir Res*.2006; 7:128.

8. Tuder RM, Yun JH. Vascular endothelial growth factor of the lung: friend or foe. *Curr Opin Pharmacol*. 2008;8:255-260.

9. Kaner RJ, Ladetto JV, Singh R, Fukuda N, Matthay MA, Crystal RG. Lung overexpression of the vascular endothelial growth factor gene induces pulmonary edema. *Am J Respir Cell Mol Biol*.2000; 22:657-664.

10. Thickett DR, Armstrong L, Christie SJ, Millar AB. Vascular endothelial growth factor may contribute to increased vascular permeability in acute respiratory distress syndrome. *Am J Respir Crit Care Med*.2001; 164:1601-1605.

11. Gebb SA, Shannon JM. Tissue interactions mediate early events in pulmonary vasculogenesis. *Dev Dyn*. 2000;217:159-169.

12. Suarez S, Ballmer-Hofer K. VEGF transiently disrupts gap junctional communication in endothelial cells. *J Cell Sci*. 2001;114:1229-1235.

13. Lagercrantz J, Farnebo F, Larsson C, Tvrdik T, Weber G, Piehl F. A comparative study of the expression patterns for vegf, vegf-b/vrf and vegf-c in the developing and adult mouse. *Biochim Biophys Acta*.1998; 1398:157-163.

14. Bhatt AJ, Amin SB, Chess PR, Watkins RH, Maniscalco WM. Expression of vascular endothelial growth factor and Flk-1 in developing and glucocorticoid-treated mouse lung. *Pediatr Res*. 2000;47:606-613.

15. D'Angio CT, Maniscalco WM. The role of vascular growth factors in hyperoxia-induced injury to the developing lung. *Front Biosci*.2002; 7:d1609-d1623.

16. Ng YS, Rohan R, Sunday ME, Demello DE, D'Amore PA. Differential expression of VEGF isoforms in mouse during development and in the adult. *Dev Dyn*. 2001;220:112-121.

17. Maniscalco WM, Watkins RH, D'Angio CT, Ryan RM. Hyperoxic injury decreases alveolar epithelial cell expression of vascular endothelial growth factor (VEGF) in neonatal rabbit lung. *Am J Respir Cell Mol Biol*. 1997;16:557-567.

18. Maeda S, Suzuki S, Suzuki T, et al. Analysis of intrapulmonary vessels and epithelial-endothelial interactions in the human developing lung. *Lab Invest*.2002; 82:293-301.

19. Compernolle V, Brusselmans K, Acker T, et al. Loss of HIF-2alpha and inhibition of VEGF impair fetal lung maturation, whereas treatment with VEGF prevents fatal respiratory distress in premature mice. *Nat Med*.2002; 8:702-710.

20. Kaner RJ, Crystal RG. Compartmentalization of vascular endothelial growth factor to the epithelial surface of the human lung. *Mol Med*.2001; 7:240-246.

21. Pannitteri G, Petrucci E, Testa U. Coordinate release of angiogenic growth factors after acute myocardial infarction: evidence of a two-wave production. *J Cardiovasc Med (Hagerstown)*.2006 ;7:872-879.

22. Mura M, Han B, Andrade CF, et al. The early responses of VEGF and its receptors during acute lung injury: implication of VEGF in alveolar epithelial cell survival. *Crit Care*. 2006;10:R130.

23. Hosford GE, Olson DM. Effects of hyperoxia on VEGF, its receptors, and HIF-2alpha in the newborn rat lung. *Am J Physiol Lung Cell Mol Physiol*.2003; 285:L161-L168.

24. Klekamp JG, Jarzecka K, Perkett EA. Exposure to hyperoxia decreases the expression of vascular endothelial growth factor and its receptors in adult rat lungs. *Am J Pathol*. 1999;154:823-831.

25. Maniscalco WM, Watkins RH, Finkelstein JN, Campbell MH. Vascular endothelial growth factor mRNA increases in alveolar epithelial cells during recovery from oxygen injury. *Am J Respir Cell Mol Biol*. 1995;13:377-386.

26. Watkins RH, D'Angio CT, Ryan RM, Patel A, Maniscalco WM. Differential expression of VEGF mRNA splice variants in newborn and adult hyperoxic lung injury. *Am J Physiol*. 1999; 276:L858-L867.

27. Corne J, Chupp G, Lee CG, et al. IL-13 stimulates vascular endothelial cell growth factor and protects against hyperoxic acute lung injury. *J Clin Invest*.2000; 106:783-791.

28. Lee CG, Link H, Baluk P, et al. Vascular endothelial growth factor (VEGF) induces remodeling and enhances TH2-mediated sensitization and inflammation in the lung. *Nat Med*.2004; 10:1095-1103.

29. He CH, Waxman AB, Lee CG, et al. Bcl-2-related protein A1 is an endogenous and cytokine-stimulated mediator of cytoprotection in hyperoxic acute lung injury. *J Clin Invest*. 2005;115:1039-1048.

30. Wagenaar GT, ter Horst SA, van Gastelen MA, et al. Gene expression profile and histopathology of experimental bronchopulmonary dysplasia induced by prolonged oxidative stress. *Free Radic Biol Med*.2004; 36:782-801.

31. Kunig AM, Balasubramaniam V, Markham NE, et al. Recombinant human VEGF treatment enhances alveolarization after hyperoxic lung injury in neonatal rats. *Am J Physiol Lung Cell Mol Physiol*2005; 289:L529–L535.

32. Berg JT, Fu Z, Breen EC, Tran HC, Mathieu-Costello O, West JB. High lung inflation increases mRNA levels of ECM components and growth factors in lung parenchyma. *J Appl Physiol*.1997; 83:120-128.

33. Nin N, Lorente JA, de Paula M, et al. Rats surviving injurious mechanical ventilation show reversible pulmonary, vascular and inflammatory changes. *Intensive Care Med*. 2008; 34:948-956.

34. Gurkan OU, O'Donnell C, Brower R, Ruckdeschel E, Becker PM. Differential effects of mechanical ventilatory strategy on lung injury and systemic organ inflammation in mice. *Am J Physiol Lung Cell Mol Physiol*.2003; 285:L710-L718.

35. Bland RD, Mokres LM, Ertsey R, et al. Mechanical ventilation with 40% oxygen reduces pulmonary expression of genes that regulate lung development and impairs alveolar septation in newborn mice. *Am J Physiol Lung Cell Mol Physiol*.2007; 293:L1099-L1110.

36. Grover TR, Asikainen TM, Kinsella JP, Abman SH, White CW. Hypoxia-inducible factors HIF-1alpha and HIF-2alpha are decreased in an experimental model of severe respiratory distress syndrome in preterm lambs. *Am J Physiol Lung Cell Mol Physiol*.2007; 292:L1345-L1351.

37. Koh H, Tasaka S, Hasegawa N, et al. Vascular endothelial growth factor in epithelial lining fluid of patients with acute respiratory distress syndrome. *Respirology*. 2008;13:281-284.

38. Maniscalco WM, Watkins RH, Pryhuber GS, Bhatt A, Shea C, Huyck H. Angiogenic factors and alveolar vasculature: development and alterations by injury in very premature baboons. *Am J Physiol Lung Cell Mol Physiol*. 2002;282:L811-L823.

39. Asikainen TM, Ahmad A, Schneider BK, White CW. Effect of preterm birth on hypoxia-inducible factors and vascular endothelial growth factor in primate lungs. *Pediatr Pulmonol*. 2005;40:538-546.

40. Tambunting F, Beharry KD, Waltzman J, Modanlou HD. Impaired lung vascular endothelial growth factor in extremely premature baboons developing bronchopulmonary dysplasia/chronic lung disease. *J Investig Med.* 2005; 53:253-262.
41. Bhandari A, Bhandari V. Bronchopulmonary dysplasia: an update. *Indian J Pediatr.*2007; 74:73-77.
42. Ambalavanan N, Novak ZE. Peptide growth factors in tracheal aspirates of mechanically ventilated preterm neonates. *Pediatr Res.*2003;53: 240-244.
43. Karmpaliotis D, Kosmidou I, Ingenito EP, et al. Angiogenic growth factors in the pathophysiology of a murine model of acute lung injury. *Am J Physiol Lung Cell Mol Physiol.* 2002;283:L585-L595.
44. Koh H, Tasaka S, Hasegawa N, et al. Protective role of vascular endothelial growth factor in endotoxin-induced acute lung injury in mice. *Respir Res.*2007; 8:60.
45. Ito Y, Betsuyaku T, Nagai K, Nasuhara Y, Nishimura M. Expression of pulmonary VEGF family declines with age and is further down-regulated in lipopolysaccharide (LPS)-induced lung injury. *Exp Gerontol.*2005; 40:315-323.
46. Lange M, Hamahata A, Enkhbaatar P, et al. Assessment of vascular permeability in an ovine model of acute lung injury and pneumonia-induced Pseudomonas aeruginosa sepsis. *Crit Care Med.*2008; 36:1284-1289.
47. Godzich M, Hodnett M, Frank JA, et al. Activation of the stress protein response prevents the development of pulmonary edema by inhibiting VEGF cell signaling in a model of lung ischemia-reperfusion injury in rats. *FASEB J.* 2006;20: 1519-1521.
48. Fehrenbach A, Pufe T, Wittwer T, et al. Reduced vascular endothelial growth factor correlates with alveolar epithelial damage after experimental ischemia and reperfusion. *J Heart Lung Transplant.* 2003;22:967-978.
49. Yan SF, Fujita T, Lu J, et al. Egr-1, a master switch coordinating upregulation of divergent gene families underlying ischemic stress. *Nat Med.*2000; 6:1355-1361.
50. Su G, Hodnett M, Wu N, et al. Integrin alphavbeta5 regulates lung vascular permeability and pulmonary endothelial barrier function. *Am J Respir Cell Mol Biol.* 2007;36:377-386.
51. Bhandari V, Choo-Wing R, Chapoval SP, et al. Essential role of nitric oxide in VEGF-induced, asthma-like angiogenic, inflammatory, mucus, and physiologic responses in the lung. *Proc Natl Acad Sci U S A.*2006; 103:11021-11026.
52. Okutan H, Kiris I, Adiloglu AK, et al. The effect of Nomega-nitro-L-arginine methyl ester and L-arginine on lung injury induced by abdominal aortic occlusion-reperfusion. *Surg Today.*2008;38:30- 37.
53. Sage E, Mercier O, Van den Eyden F, et al. Endothelial cell apoptosis in chronically obstructed and reperfused pulmonary artery. *Respir Res.*2008; 9:19.
54. Chen F, Kondo N, Sonobe M, Fujinaga T, Wada H, Bando T. Expression of endothelial cell-specific adhesion molecules in lungs after cardiac arrest. *Interact Cardiovasc Thorac Surg.*2008;7:437-440.
55. Burton PB, Owen VJ, Hafizi S, et al. Vascular endothelial growth factor release following coronary artery bypass surgery: extracorporeal circulation versus "beating heart" surgery. *Eur Heart J.*2000; 21:1708-1713.
56. Kalomenidis I, Stathopoulos GT, Barnette R, et al. Vascular endothelial growth factor levels in post-CABG pleural effusions are associated with pleural inflammation and permeability. *Respir Med.*2007; 101:223-229.
57. Malhotra SP, Reddy VM, Thelitz S, et al. The role of oxidative stress in the development of pulmonary arteriovenous malformations after cavopulmonary anastomosis. *J Thorac Cardiovasc Surg.*2002; 124:479-485.
58. Mumtaz MA, Fraga CH, Nicholls CM, et al. Increased expression of vascular endothelial growth factor messenger RNA in lungs of rats after cavopulmonary anastomosis. *J Thorac Cardiovasc Surg.*2005; 129:209-210.
59. Starnes SL, Duncan BW, Kneebone JM, et al. Angiogenic proteins in the lungs of children after cavopulmonary anastomosis. *J Thorac Cardiovasc Surg.*2001; 122:518-523.
60. Ootaki Y, Yamaguchi M, Yoshimura N, Oka S, Yoshida M, Hasegawa T. Vascular endothelial growth factor in children with congenital heart disease. *Ann Thorac Surg.* 2003;75: 1523-1526.
61. Geiger R, Berger RM, Hess J, Bogers AJ, Sharma HS, Mooi WJ. Enhanced expression of vascular endothelial growth factor in pulmonary plexogenic arteriopathy due to congenital heart disease. *J Pathol.*2000; 191:202-207.
62. Mori Y, Shoji M, Nakanishi T, Fujii T, Nakazawa M. Elevated vascular endothelial growth factor levels are associated with aortopulmonary collateral vessels in patients before and after the Fontan procedure. *Am Heart J.* 2007;153:987-994.
63. Lambert V, Michel R, Mazmanian GM, et al. Induction of pulmonary angiogenesis by adenoviral-mediated gene transfer of vascular endothelial growth factor. *Ann Thorac Surg* 2004;77:458–463; discussion 463.
64. Kunig AM, Balasubramaniam V, Markham NE, et al. Recombinant human VEGF treatment enhances alveolarization after hyperoxic lung injury in neonatal rats. *Am J Physiol Lung Cell Mol Physiol.*2005; 289:L529-L535.
65. Kunig AM, Balasubramaniam V, Markham NE, Seedorf G, Gien J, Abman SH. Recombinant human VEGF treatment transiently increases lung edema but enhances lung structure after neonatal hyperoxia. *Am J Physiol Lung Cell Mol Physiol.*2006; 291:L1068-L1078.
66. Thebaud B, Ladha F, Michelakis ED, et al. Vascular endothelial growth factor gene therapy increases survival, promotes lung angiogenesis, and prevents alveolar damage in hyperoxia-induced lung injury: evidence that angiogenesis participates in alveolarization. *Circulation.*2005; 112:2477-2486.
67. Rossiter HB, Scadeng M, Tang K, Wagner PD, Breen EC. Doxycycline treatment prevents alveolar destruction in VEGF-deficient mouse lung. *J Cell Biochem.* 2008;104:525-535.
68. Hamada N, Kuwano K, Yamada M, et al. Anti-vascular endothelial growth factor gene therapy attenuates lung injury and fibrosis in mice. *J Immunol.*2005; 175:1224-1231.
69. Lahm T, Crisostomo PR, Markel TA, Wang M, Lillemoe KD, Meldrum DR. The critical role of vascular endothelial growth factor in pulmonary vascular remodeling after lung injury. *Shock.* 2007;28:4-14.

Aprotinin Decreases Lung Reperfusion Injury and Dys function

8

Hartmuth B. Bittner, Peter S. Dahlberg, Cynthia S. Herrington, and Friedrich W. Mohr

8.1 Introduction

Reduced lung perfusion and subsequent pulmonary ischemia can cause increased pulmonary vascular resistance, decreased oxygenation capacity, worsened compliance, and edema formation. The initial ischemic insult to the lung correlates with the production of cytokines and increased expression of adhesion molecules by hypoxic parenchymal and endothelial cells. Once reperfusion is reestablished, the injury cascade is mediated in large part by neutrophil–endothelial adherence and subsequent neutrophil-mediated organ injury. Applying leukocyte depletion strategy already reduces pulmonary microvascular pressure and improves pulmonary status in patients undergoing cardiopulmonary bypass-supported coronary artery bypass surgery.[1] Cardiopulmonary bypass can trigger the systemic inflammatory response syndrome (SIRS), which can cause severe pulmonary dysfunction, necessitating prolonged mechanical ventilation and intensive care treatment.[2] By avoiding cardiopulmonary bypass in patients at high respiratory risk (forced expiratory volume in the first second of expiration [FEV_1]<65%, predicted) who then undergo off-pump coronary artery bypass (OPCABG) grafting, lower A-a gradients and significantly shorter postoperative mechanical ventilation time can be achieved.[3] However, these results are discussed controversially since physiological differences in terms of pulmonary gas exchange indices were not consistently observed when comparing on-pump with off-pump coronary artery bypass surgery in nonselected patients.[4,5] Staton et al. investigated pulmonary outcomes of off-pump coronary artery bypass vs. OPCABG surgery in a randomized trial in which OPCABG surgery yielded better gas exchange and earlier extubation.[6] There were no differences in morbidity or mortality observed.

In limited studies, the potential protective effect of aprotinin against lung damage was investigated in patients undergoing on-pump coronary artery bypass grafting (CABG). Aprotinin (Trasylol®, Bayer Pharmaceutical), a monomeric 58-amino acid polypeptide, inhibits several serine proteases, including plasmin and kallikrein. Although it has been primarily used as a blood conservation drug during cardiopulmonary bypass procedures, it also has multiple anti-inflammatory effects on leukocyte activation and cytotoxic mediator release.[7,8]

In a prospective randomized trial, Rahman et al. showed that by adding two million units of aprotinin to the prime solution of the cardiopulmonary bypass circuit patients following CABG had reduced lung reperfusion injury compared to controls.[9] In a similar study, aprotinin was directly administered into the pulmonary artery during cardiopulmonary bypass. Aprotinin had a protective effect against lung damage after open-heart surgery, which was reflected by significantly improved postoperative lung function and FEV_1 testing.[10]

Even in 391 consecutive patients undergoing off-pump CABG who received aprotinin intraoperatively, shorter intensive care unit (ICU) stays and mechanical ventilation times were demonstrated. This suggests less lung injury in the aprotinin-treated group compared to 370 control OPCABG patients managed without aprotinin bolus therapy.[11]

H.B.B ittner (✉)
Division of Cardiovascular Surgery and Thoracic Transplantation, Heart Center of the University of Leipzig, Leipzig, Germany
e-mail:H eartbeatgermany@aol.com

E.A. Gabriel and T. Salerno (eds.), *Principles of Pulmonary Protection in Heart Surgery*,
DOI: 10.1007/978-1-84996-308-4_8, © Springer-Verlag London Limited 2010

The indirect pulmonary protective effects may result from its extraordinarily well-documented ability to decrease bleeding and reduce the rate of blood product transfusion in on-pump cardiac surgery. Transfusion-related lung injury is a thoroughly described phenomenon and clinically similar to the adult respiratory distress syndrome.[12] It has been linked to the transfusion of leukocyte antibodies in blood components. There are several potential mechanisms by which massive transfusion might predispose to direct lung injury and have an impact on the immune system: cognate antigen–antibody interactions, activation of nonspecific immunity through soluble mediators present in transfused blood, an increased risk of infection through transfusion-associated immunomodulation leading to infection and sepsis, and volume overload in the face of increased permeability of the alveolar capillary membrane.[13]

However, in all the described procedures the occurrence of severe lung reperfusion injury is questionable since lung ischemia has not really been observed. On cardiopulmonary bypass and during the required heart manipulations in off-pump cardiac surgery, pulmonary artery perfusion is only reduced, and the blood flow through the bronchial arteries is definitely maintained, indicating that ischemia of the lungs does not exist. The observed decline in lung function might rather be associated with different fluid management regimens, variable quantities of cardiopulmonary bypass prime solutions, and the application of various volume restriction protocols.

The prevalence of severe pulmonary reperfusion injury following controlled ischemia and hypothermic organ preservation is well documented in lung transplantation surgery. Many hours of ischemic organ preservation are required for lung graft procurement and donor organ transport to distant lung transplantation centers, where the recipient with end-stage lung disease is prepared for single- or double-lung transplantation. Lung transplantation is now carried out on a routine basis with low operative mortality. The immediate success of lung transplantation is directly related to the incidence of primary graft dysfunction (PGD), which is a primary cause for early morbidity and mortality.[14] Pulmonary ischemia and the subsequently developing reperfusion injury are considered to be the principal mechanisms leading to early graft dysfunction. Ischemia-reperfusion injury-associated PGD is one of many terms used to describe poor pulmonary function following lung transplantation. The syndrome is characterized by hypoxia, increased pulmonary vascular permeability, and infiltrates on chest X-ray. In 2004, an International Society for Heart and Lung Transplant (ISHLT) working group developed definitions of PGD. They proposed severity grading from I to III, which is based on the P/F ratio of arterial PO_2 to the FIO_2 (fraction of inspired oxygen) and measured within the initial 48 h following lung transplantation. Patients with grade I severity have infiltrates on chest X-ray. For patients with grade II severity, the P/F ratio falls between 200 and 300. For grade III severity, the least-favorable grade, the ratio becomes less than 200. Of all lung transplants, 57–97% showed some degree of perihilar infiltrates or reperfusion edema on chest X-ray examinations after implantation.[15] Approximately 20–40% of lung transplant recipients will experience a clinically significant degree of reperfusion injury, which has an associated mortality rate of 40%.[16,17] A therapy effective in preventing PGD might improve both short- and long-term rates of survival as well as the quality of life for patients following the procedure.

Key Cellular Mechanisms

Identifying key cellular events mediating the phenomenon of ischemia-reperfusion injury has been an important goal of lung transplantation research in the past few years. It is now widely accepted that lung transplant ischemia-reperfusion injury involves pulmonary macrophages and circulating leukocytes in a biphasic response.[18] The early phase is mediated by donor pulmonary macrophages, followed by a late injury, which is induced by recipient circulating leukocytes. The specific reperfusion component of the injury cascade is mediated in large part by neutrophil-endothelial adherence and subsequent extravasation into surrounding tissue, causing neutrophil-mediated organ injury.[17,19] In fact, as soon as the neutrophils are activated by their adherence to the endothelium, they start secreting reactive oxygen species and proteolytic enzymes. This initiates pulmonary vascular endothelial dysfunction, leading to profound lung parenchymal destruction. Inflammatory substances and interleukins (ILs) are released; especially, IL-8 seems to be upregulated. High levels of IL-8 were found to correlate with the incidence of primary graft failure after reperfusion.[20] The mechanism by which reperfusion injury develops in these patients is thought to be through mechanical disruption of the pulmonary vascular endothelium and production of IL-8 and platelet-activating factor.[21] As described, this results in a profound structural and functional breakdown of delicate lung parenchyma, causing capillary leaks with subsequent interstitial fluid accumulation, which leads to pronounced pulmonary edema with associated lung transplant dysfunction and finally to the SIRS.

Asmiakopoulos et al. thoroughly demonstrated in vivo and in vitro that aprotinin inhibits neutrophil extravasation and secretion of myeloperoxidase from neutrophils.[19] In addition to the attenuation of neutrophil activation, aprotinin decreased IL-8 concentration and leukocyte adhesion molecule expression.[22,23]

Aprotinin and Lung Transplantation Surgery

By adding aprotinin to organ preservation solution, lung reperfusion-injury decreased in experimental studies.[24] It also significantly improved pulmonary function during reperfusion in an isolated, whole-blood perfused rabbit lung model.[25] Adding aprotinin to Low-potassium dextrane (LPD) single-flush pulmonary solution in an in situ normothermic ischemic lung model prevented lung ischemia-reperfusion injury and maintained the morphological, functional, and biochemical integrity of the lungs.[26] The Groningen Lung Transplant Group showed that the administration of aprotinin is safe, and that clotting and fibrinolytic disturbances were reduced in clinical lung transplantation.[27]

We used the high-dose regimen of aprotinin (2 million Kallikrein inhibiting units (KIU) loading dose, 500,000 KIU/h during surgery, 2 million KIU supplemented to the pump prime when cardiopulmonary bypass was used), which was applied for 59 patients who underwent single and bilateral sequential lung transplantation for similar end-stage lung disease as the 112 patients of the control group without treatment with the aprotinin regimen. Using the ISHLT lung transplant injury grade III, defined by a FIO_2/PaO_2 (partial pressure of oxygen, arterial) ratio of less than 200 mmHg measured within the initial 48 h after transplantation, we identified 20 patients (18%) with severe posttransplant ischemia-reperfusion injury and acute graft failure in the control group. Eight patients died within 90 days (mortality rate of 40%). Early ECMO (extracorporeal

membrane oxygenation) was used in five patients. Three patients were successfully weaned off ECMO support. The factors significantly correlating with reperfusion injury were older donor age and markedly increased pulmonary artery pressure in the recipient. The use of cardiopulmonary bypass, the procedure itself, or the ischemic times could not be attributed to the occurrence of reperfusion injury.[28] A significant reduction of ischemia-reperfusion injury and of primary graft failure were observed in the aprotinin-treated lung transplant patients, which resulted in a markedly decreased mortality rate. Adverse effects were not documented in association with aprotinin administration. Based on these results, aprotinin became an important part of the management protocol for lung transplantation patients in many centers.

In 2003, we initiated a prospective, randomized, single-center, nonblinded clinical trial to study the effect of aprotinin in reducing PGD following lung transplantation.[29] There were 48 patients randomized, with diagnosis and bypass use inconsistent among groups. Although not reaching the level of significance, patients at higher risk of developing severe lung reperfusion injury were included in the aprotinin group. Compared to the placebo group, there were more patients with idiopathic pulmonary fibrosis and fewer patients with chronic obstructive pulmonary disease (COPD) in the aprotinin group. In our study, the primary end point was the occurrence of grade III PGD during the first 48 h following transplantation (T_{0-48}). The 90-day rate of death and early survival were also secondary end points of the study. For the entire study population, the 90-day death rate was 2% (one death), and the actual 1-year survival for the study cohort was 94%. No significant differences were measured between groups. There were trends regarding early incidence of PGD favoring the use of aprotinin. The study was prematurely stopped at the interim point because of published concerns about renal toxicity associated with aprotinin administration in cardiac surgery.

A report was published that described a doubling in the risk of renal failure requiring dialysis among patients undergoing complex coronary artery surgery.[30,31] Therefore, post hoc we analyzed trends in renal function among patients enrolled in the study. Although there were no significant differences attributable to aprotinin administration at any of the time points measured (0, 12, 24, 48, 72 h; 7 and 30 days), enrollment of new patients into the study was suspended, and the study, as described, was stopped prematurely.

At the Heart Center Leipzig, Germany, we successfully used aprotinin in lung transplantation surgery, incorporating the compassionate application guidelines, until it was withdrawn from the market in 2007.

Lung transplantation is a complex undertaking that is fraught with many possible complications, among which ischemia-reperfusion injury is the most important cause of early death following the procedure. Despite improvements in patient selection, preservation solutions, and postoperative management, the most severe forms of acute lung injury still have an impact on 15–25% of all patients.[32] Progress in preventing or treating ischemia-reperfusion injury has been hampered by the challenges of performing clinical trials. The number of patients transplanted at any one center is small, and until recently, standardized and validated end points that occur with sufficient frequency and predictive poor outcomes have not been able to be utilized in trial design.

Because the transplanted lung is highly susceptible to the deleterious effects of ischemia-reperfusion injury, an agent that may combat this process is much sought after in clinical and investigative lung transplantation.

References

1. Olivencia-Yurvati AH, Ferrara CA, Tierney N, Wallace N, Mallet RT. Strategic leukocyte depletion reduces pulmonary microvascular pressure and improves pulmonary status postcardiopulmonary bypass. *Perfusion*.2003; 18:23-31.
2. Asimakopoulos G, Smith PLC, Ratnatunga CP, Taylor KM. Lung injury and acute respiratory distress syndrome after cardiopulmonary bypass. *Ann Thorac Surg*. 1999;68:1107-1115.
3. Reddy SL, Grayson AD, Oo AY, Pullan MD, Poonacha T, Fabri BM. Does off-pump surgery offer benefit in high respiratory risk patients? A respiratory risk stratified analysis in a propensity-matched cohort. *Eur J Cardiothorac Surg*. 2006; 30(1):126-131.
4. Montes FR, Maldonado JD, Paez S, Ariza F. Off-pump versus on-pump coronary artery bypass surgery and postoperative pulmonary dysfunction. *J Cardiothorac Vasc Anesth*. 2004;18(6):698-703.
5. Syed A, Fawzy H, Farag A, Nemlander A. Comparison of pulmonary gas exchange in OPCABG versus conventional CABG. *Heart Lung Circ*.2004; 13(2):168-172.
6. Staton GW, Williams WH, Mahoney EM, et al. Pulmonary outcomes of off-pump versus on-pump coronary artery bypass surgery in a randomized trial. *Chest*. 2005;127(3):892-901.
7. Landis RC, Asimakopoulos G, Poullis M, Haskard DO, Taylor KM. The antithrombotic and anti-inflammatory mechanisms of action of aprotinin. *Ann Thorac Surg*. 2001;72(6):2169-2175.
8. Royston D, Bidstrup BP, Taylor KM, Sapford RN. Effect of aprotinin on need for blood transfusions after repeat open heart surgery. *Lancet*.1987; 2:1289-1291.
9. Rahman A, Ustünda B, Burma O, Ozercan IH, Cekirdekçi A, Bayar MK. Does aprotinin reduce lung reperfusion damage after cardiopulmonary bypass? *Eur J Cardiothorac Surg*. 2000;18(5):583-588.
10. Erdogan M, Kalaycioglu S, Iriz E. Protective effect of aprotinin against lung damage in patients undergoing CABG surgery. *Acta Cardiol*.2005; 60(4):367-372.
11. Bittner HB, Lemke J, Lange M, Rastan A, Mohr FW. The impact of aprotinin on blood loss and blood transfusion in off-pump coronary artery bypass grafting. *Ann Thorac Surg*. 2008;85(5):1662-1668.
12. Silliman CC, Paterson AJ, Dickey WO, et al. The association of biologically active lipids with the development of transfusion-related acute lung injury: a retrospective study. *Transfusion*.1997; 37:719-726.
13. Nathens AB. Massive transfusion as a risk factor for acute lung injury: association or causation? *Crit Care Med*. 2006; 34(5s uppl):144-150.
14. Cooper JD, Patterson GA, Trulock EP; Washington University Lung Transplant Group. Results of 131 consecutive single and bilateral lung transplant recipients. *J Thorac Cardiovasc Surg*1994; 107(2):460-471.
15. Khan SU, Salloum J, O'Donovan PB, et al. Acute pulmonary edema after lung transplantation. *Chest*. 1999;116:187-194.
16. Burdine J, Hertz MI, Snover DC, Bolman RM. Heart-lung and lung transplantation: perioperative pulmonary dysfunction. *Transplant Proc*.1991; 23:1176-1177.
17. Novick RJ, Gehman KE, Ali IS, Lee J. Lung preservation: the importance of endothelial and alveolar type II cell integrity. *Ann Thorac Surg*.1996; 62:302-314.
18. Fiser SM, Tribble CG, Long SM, et al. Lung transplant reperfusion injury involves pulmonary macrophages and circulating leukocytes in a biphasic response. *J Thorac Cardiovasc Surg*.2001; 121:1069-1075.
19. Asimakopoulos G, Thompson R, Nourshargh S, et al. An anti-inflammatory property of aprotinin detected at the level of leukocyte extravasation. *J Thorac Cardiovasc Surg*. 2000; 120:361-369.
20. de Perrot M, Sekine Y, Fischer S, et al. Interleukin-8 release during early reperfusion predicts graft function in human lung transplantation. *Am J Respir Crit Care Med*. 2002;165: 211-215.
21. Jorens PG, Van Damme J, De Backer W, et al. Interleukin-8 in the bronchoalveolar lavage fluid from patients with the adult respiratory distress syndrome (ARDS) and patients at risk for ARDS. *Cytokine*.1992; 4:592-597.
22. Hill GE, Pohorecki R, Alonso A, Rennard SI, Robbins RA. Aprotinin reduces interleukin-8 production and lung neutrophil accumulation after cardiopulmonary bypass. *Anesth Analg*.1996; 83:696-700.
23. Gilliland HE, Armstrong MA, Uprichard S, Clarke G, McMurray TJ. The effect of aprotinin on interleukin-8 concentration and leukocyte adhesion molecule expression in an isolated cardiopulmonary bypass system. *Anaesthesia*. 1999;54:427-433.

24. Roberts RF, Nishanian GP, Carey JN, et al. Addition of apro-tinin to organ preservation solutions decreases lung reperfusion injury. *Ann Thorac Surg*.1998; 66:225-230.

25. Mathias MA, Tribble CG, Dietz JF, et al. Aprotinin improves pulmonary function during reperfusion in an isolated lung model. *Ann Thorac Surg*.2000; 70:1671-1674.

26. Eren S, Esme H, Balci AE, et al. The effect of aprotinin on ischemia-reperfusion injury in an in situ normothermic ischemic lung model. *Eur J Cardiothorac Surg*.2003; 23:60-65.

27. Gu YJ, De Vries AJ, Vos P, Boonstra PW, Oeveren WV. Leukocyte depletion during cardiac operation: a new approach through the venous bypass circuit. *Ann Thorac Surg*.1999;67:604-609.

28. Bittner HB, Richter M, Kuntze T, et al. Aprotinin decreases reperfusion injury and allograft dysfunction in clinical lung transplantation. *Eur J Cardiothorac Surg*. 2006;29(2):210-215.

29. Herrington CS, Prekker ME, Hertz MI, Studenski LL, Radosevich DM, Shumway SJ, Kelly RF, Arrington AK, Susanto D, Baltzell JW, Bittner HB, Dahlberg PS. A randomized, placebo controlled trial of aprotinin to reduce primary graft dysfunction following lung transplantation. *J Transplant* 2009 [accepted].

30. Mangano DT, Tudor IC, Detzel C. The risk associated with aprotinin in cardiac surgery. *N Engl J Med*. 2006;354(4): 353-365.

31. Mangano DT, Miao Y, Vuylsteke A, Tudor IC, Juneja R, Filipescu D, Hoeft A, Fontes ML, Hillel Z, Ott E, Titov T, Dietzel C, Levin J; Investigators of the Multicenter Study of Perioperative Ischemia Research Group; Ischemia Research and Education Foundation. Mortality associated with aprotinin during 5 years following coronary artery bypass graft surgery. *JAMA*2007; 297(5):471–479.

32. King RC, Binns OAR, Rodriguez F, et al. Reperfusion injury significantly impacts clinical outcome after pulmonary transplantation. *Ann Thorac Surg*.2000; 69:1681-1685.

Effects of Prostaglandin E1 and Nitroglycerin on Lung Preservation

9

Stefano Salizzoni, Yoshiko Toyoda, and Yoshiya Toyoda

9.1 Introduction

The term *lung preservation* usually refers to protection of the lungs from ischemia-reperfusion injury (IRI). The most extreme situation in which IRI can be observed is in lung transplantation as the ischemic time can be more than 10 h. Adequate preservation of the lungs is critical to achieve a good outcome following lung transplantation.

Since 1973 much of the experimental work on lung preservation has focused on optimizing methods to reduce the impact of IRI on posttransplant lung function, and since the 1980s, when the number of lung transplantations performed increased exponentially, the research has focused on new techniques that might prolong the acceptable graft ischemic time. However, despite continuous improvements in lung preservation and operative technique, injury from ischemia-reperfusion leads to primary graft dysfunction and remains a significant cause of morbidity and mortality. The primary graft dysfunction typically occurs within 3 days after transplantation, and it is characterized by nonspecific alveolar damage, lung edema, and hypoxemia.

Based on the results of the studies by the Toronto group, which in 1986 reported the first two successful midterm (at 26 and 14 months) outcomes after lung transplantation, the pulmonary flush technique for lung procurement, with different preservation solutions, has

been adopted by the vast majority of lung transplantation centers worldwide.[1]

Other techniques, such as simple hypothermic atelectatic immersion, ex vivo normothermic heart-lung autoperfusion, and donor core cooling, were abandoned in favor of pulmonary artery flush, which allowed longer ischemic times.[2-4]

The aim of this chapter is to describe how prostaglandins, nitric oxide (NO), and nitroglycerin, the most commonly used NO donor, had a central role in the development and improvement in lung preservation and consequently in lung transplantation. To better understand the importance of prostaglandins and nitroglycerin, a description of the mechanism of IRI and of the evolution of the preservation solutions and its additives is necessary.

9.2 Mechanism of Ischemia-Reperfusion Injury

When a tissue is subjected to ischemia, a sequence of chemical reactions is initiated, which may ultimately lead to cellular dysfunction and necrosis. Although no single process can be identified as the critical event in ischemia-induced tissue injury, most studies indicated that depletion of cellular energy stores and accumulation of toxic metabolites may contribute to cell death. Several terms, such as reperfusion injury or early acute respiratory distress, have been used to describe this syndrome, but IRI is most commonly used.

IRI still remains one of the major problems associated with lung transplantation in the early postoperative course. Up to 97% of transplanted lungs will have some degree of peripheral edema during the immediate postoperative period, and it is estimated that IRI

Y. Toyoda (✉)
The Heart, Lung and Esophageal Surgery Institute,
Division of Cardiac Surgery, University of Pittsburgh
Medical Center, Pittsburgh, PA, USA

E.A. Gabriel and T. Salerno (eds.), *Principles of Pulmonary Protection in Heart Surgery*,
DOI: 10.1007/978-1-84996-308-4_9, © Springer-Verlag London Limited 2010

81

occurs in 15–20% of lung transplant recipients.[5-7] Originally, IRI was thought to be due to either inadequate preservation or prolonged graft ischemia before implantation. Several studies demonstrated that IRI is not dependent on the duration of donor ischemia[7-9], while other reports have confirmed an increased incidence of clinical IRI in recipients with preoperative pulmonary hypertension.[7]

Clinical manifestations of early IRI are similar to those of hydrostatic pulmonary edema, with interstitial or patchy infiltrates, nonspecific alveolar damage, decreased compliance, and impaired gas exchange that occurs within 72 h after lung transplantation.[10] One of the most important modulators of IRI is the interaction between leukocytes and pulmonary endothelial cells.[11] The first event in the cycle is the migration of circulating pulmonary leukocytes from pulmonary capillaries into the lung parenchyma. The first step in this process is the "rolling" of leukocytes along the endothelial surface, and it is mediated by selectines.[12] Another important role performed by the sodium (Na^+/K^+-ATPase [adenosine triphosphatase]) pump is to preserve the proper intracellular electrolyte concentration and to maintain adequate clearance of the alveolar fluid. Hypothermia results in the loss of function of the sodium pump and leads to accumulation of sodium in the cell, resulting in cell swelling. Even if it is clear that prolonged ischemia leads to IRI, it has also been demonstrated that a rapid reoxygenation of hypoxic tissues can lead to a sequence of events that produce the same consequences of prolonged hypoxia.[13] This happens because of the formation of reactive oxygen metabolites, such as superoxide, hydrogen peroxide, and the hydroxyl radical, which has been shown to be clearly involved in mechanisms of IRI.[14] The consequence of oxygen radical formation is a series of biochemical events (lipid peroxidation, sulfhydryl oxidation, protein degradation, hemoprotein and cytochrome inactivation, formation of inflammatory mediators) that results in the damage of the cell membrane and death of the cell.[15] The most important studies to prevent IRI are focused on understanding the role of NO, which is discussed further in this chapter. Other strategies to reduce IRI are the use of exogenous surfactant[16]; leukocyte filtering to deplete cells before reperfusion[17]; endobronchial gene transfer using adenovirus that encodes human interleukin (IL) 10[18]; and the administration of melatonin, a radical scavenger and antioxidant.[19]

9.3 Flush Solution for Lung Preservation

Two types of preservation solutions, intracellular and extracellular, have been developed to counteract the decreased activity of the Na^+/K^+-ATPase pump during the period of organ ischemia and the increased permeability of the plasma membrane during hypothermia. Table 9.1 shows the composition of the various most important intracellular and extracellular solutions.

The most commonly used intracellular solutions for lung preservation are Euro-Collins solution and the University of Wisconsin solution, also known as Viaspan. The Euro-Collins® (Fresenius Biotech, Bad Homburgh, DE) was originally developed for kidney preservation.[20] It is a crystalloid solution with a high concentration of K^+ and low concentration of Na^+. Euro-Collins solution is normally modified by addition of magnesium sulfate and 50% dextrose.[21] The University of Wisconsin® (Fresenius Hemocare, Emmer-Compascuum, NE) solution was initially developed by Folkert Belzer for pancreas and liver preservation in the late 1980s.[22] It consists of several components, including magnesium, glutathione, allopurinol, phosphate, lactobionate, raffinose, hydroxyethyl starch, adenosine phosphate, and a high concentration of K^+.[23]

Extracellular solutions commonly used in lung transplantation are Wallwork, Perfadex, and Celsior. The Wallwork solution is based on third-party, cold donor blood modified by the addition of substrates such as epoprostenol (prostacyclin), buffers, and human proteins.[24] Perfadex® (Vitrolife, Gothenburg, Sweden) is a low-potassium, 5% dextran-based solution that has been specifically developed for lung preservation.[25] Celsior® (SangStat Medical Corporation, Fremont, CA) is a low-viscosity preservation solution that was developed for heart preservation.[26]

The concept of using a modified extracellular fluid solution for lung preservation was developed by Fujimura in 1987.[27] Fujimura demonstrated that a modified extracellular solution was better than an intracellular solution for prolonged lung preservation. Following Fujimura's experiments, other authors demonstrated that the high potassium concentration of the intracellular solution can cause severe pulmonary vasoconstriction followed by the formation of edema. Therefore, the use of intracellular solutions was gradually abandoned in lung transplantation.[28] In particular, the beneficial effects of preservation with Perfadex are due to the combination of a low potassium concentration and the presence of dextran.[29] Low

Table 9.1 Composition of preservations olutions

Composition	Intracellulars olutions		Extracellulars olutions	
	Euro-Collins	University of Wisconsin	Perfadex	Celsior
Na^+ (mmol/L)	10	28–30	138	100
K^+ (mmol/L)	115	125	6	15
Cl^- (mmol/L)	15	–	142	41.5
Mg^{2++} (mmol/L)	–	0–5	0.8	13
SO_4^{2-} (mmol/L)	–	4–5	0.8	–
HPO_4^{2-} (mmol/L)	42.5	25	0.8	–
Ca^{2+} (mmol/L)	–	–	0.3	0.26
HCO^{3-} (mmol/L)	10	5	1	–
Dextran40 (g/L)	–	–	50	–
Glucose (g/L)	194	–	0.91	–
Raffinose (mmol/L)	3.5	30	–	–
Lactobionate (mmol/L)	–	100	–	80
Glutathione (mmol/L)	–	3	–	3
Adenosine (mmol/L)	–	5	–	–
Allopurinol (mmol/L)	–	1	–	–
Pentafraction (g/L)	–	50	–	–
Glutamate (mmol/L)	–	–	–	20
Histidine (mmol/L)	–	–	–	30
Mannitol (mmol/L)	–	–	–	60
pH	6.8–7.8	7.4	7.45	7.2–7.4
Osmolarity (mO sm/L)	370	320–327	280–325	320–360

potassium concentrations cause less damage to the integrity of the endothelial cells, which may decrease the release of pulmonary vasoconstrictors and the production of oxidants. Dextran coats endothelial surfaces and platelets. It prevents erythrocyte aggregation, improves erythrocyte deformability, induces disaggregation of already aggregated cells, and has antithrombotic effects. Together, these effects improve pulmonary microcirculation and preserve the endothelial-epithelial barrier, which may prevent the no-reflow phenomenon (inadequate perfusion without evident obstruction) and the reflow paradox (activation of leukocytes following reperfusion-reoxygenation following ischemia) and reduce the degree of water and protein extravasation at the time of reperfusion.[30,31]

Despite the benefits that these solutions provide, it is controversial whether any solution is superior to another, partially due to the fact that the exact composition of each solution may change from institution to institution.[32-37] However, there is growing evidence suggesting that Perfadex may be better than other solutions for lung preservation. Wu et al. demonstrated that Perfadex preserves endothelium-dependent smooth muscle relaxation and hyperpolarization better than Celsior at cellular and vascular levels using in vitro analysis of the electrophysiologic and mechanical proprieties.[38] Moreover, Oto et al. demonstrated that Perfadex prevents moderate-to-severe primary graft dysfunction better than Euro-Collins can.[39] Bertolotti et al. demonstrated that Perfadex affords good lung preservation by reducing early graft injury, as indicated by decreased levels of IL-8 (a marker that predicts early graft failure[40]) and reduced myeloperoxidase activity, tissue injury, and polymorphonuclear neutrophil accumulation in pulmonary tissue as compared with the Euro-Collins solution.[41] Wittwer et al.[42] demonstrated that Perfadex is superior to Celsior in an experiment testing the ability of the solutions to provide 27 h of protection against cold ischemia.

9.4 Prostaglandinsi nL ungPr eservation

A variety of pharmacologic additives have been investigated in animal models of lung preservation and transplantation, and several studies demonstrated that the addition of prostaglandins or nitroglycerin to the preservation solution improved organ preservation.[43-53]

The prostaglandins are members of a group of lipid compounds that are derived enzymatically from fatty acids. Every prostaglandin contains 20 carbon atoms, including a 5-carbon ring. They are mediator molecules and have a variety of strong physiological effects. Although they are technically hormones, they are rarely classified as such. They are produced by all nucleated cells except lymphocytes. The most important prostaglandins are prostaglandin E1 (PGE1), prostacyclin (PGI_2), prostaglandin F2 alpha, and prostaglandin A2. Basically, PGE1 and PGI_2 are the two prostaglandins used for lung preservation because their vasodilatory effects counteract vasoconstriction, which normally occurs in cold preservation solution, allowing better distribution of perfusion.[43] Moreover, PGE1 is also beneficial to the lung because it promotes pulmonary protection by stimulating cyclic $3',5'$-adenosine monophosphate (c-GMP)-dependent protein kinase during cold ischemic time. This decreases neutrophil infiltration, vascular permeability, and platelet deposition.[44] In 2001, De Perrot et al. used a rat single-lung transplantation model to show that PGE1 administered during the reperfusion period reduces IRI and improves lung function through a mechanism that is likely mediated by a shift between pro- and anti-inflammatory cytokine releases.[45] Evidence of increased levels of IL-10 and reduced levels of the proinflammatory cytokines IL-12, tumor necrosis factor-alpha, and interferon-gamma were observed in transplanted lung tissue. Gohrbandt et al. showed, in a porcine left single-lung transplantation model, that iloprost, a PGI_2 analog, resulted in a significant amelioration of IRI and improved preservation of surfactant function in transplanted lungs.[46] PGE1, PGI_2, and their analogs may be administered during donor lung procurement via antegrade or retrograde flush or by aerosolization directly into the alveolar compartment to avoid the side effects of systemic application, especially systemic hypotension and increasing intrapulmonary shunt.[54-56] Aerosolization of iloprost causes marked pulmonary vasodilation with maintenance of pulmonary gas exchange and systemic arterial pressure.[57] Evidence exists that aerosolized PGI_2 exerts its beneficial actions directly rather than via secondary release of endogenous NO.[58]

In 2008, Toyoda et al. published an article on lung transplantation for idiopathic pulmonary arterial hypertension (IPAH) that demonstrated that short- and long-term outcomes after lung and heart-lung transplantation for IPAH benefited from upgrading the pulmonary protection donor protocols.[59] In particular, the patients benefited from the addition of PGE1 before cross clamping and the addition of PGE1 and nitroglycerine to the first bag of Perfadex. IPAH is a pathology that clearly demonstrates the effects of improving lung preservation techniques. Data from the International Society of Heart and Lung Transplantation Registry from January 1994 to June 2004 indicated that recipients with IPAH had the lowest survival rate at 1 year among all the major diagnostic categories of lung transplant recipients, and that the actuarial survival after lung transplantation for IPAH was 66% at 1 year, 47% at 5 years, and 27% at 10 years.[60] At the University of Pittsburgh Medical Center (UPMC), the cardiothoracic transplant program experienced similar results, with 58% survival at 1 year, 39% at 5 years, and 27% at 10 years from 1982 to 1993. However, the UMPC outcomes improved significantly to 86% at 1 year, 75% at 5 years, and 66% at 10 years from 1994 to 2006 because of the introduction of PGE1 (indicated by multivariate analysis).[59]

9.5 Nitroglycerini nL ungPr eservation

Several studies have demonstrated that lung ischemia-reperfusion leads to an apparent deficit of endogenous NO.[61,62] The role of endothelial nitric oxide synthase (eNOS), which produces NO from the terminal nitrogen atom of L-arginine in the presence of NADPH (Nicotinamide adenine dinucleotide phosphate) and dioxygen (O_2), is not clearly defined. However, eNOS does seem to have an important role during the ischemia and reperfusion process, and a better understanding of changes in NO and NO metabolism will provide more information at the molecular level regarding IRI of the lung.[63-66]

NO is a key modulator of normal pulmonary vascular physiology.[67,68] It prevents neutrophil adherence to the endothelium, maintains endothelial barrier properties, and inhibits platelet aggregation and has an important role in modulating pulmonary vascular tone.[69-71] Moreover, NO can be identified in exhaled air and is thought to regulate basal pulmonary vascular resistance in humans.[72,73] Reactive oxygen intermediates are formed and are especially abundant in the pulmonary reperfusion microenvironment.[74,75] Therefore, endothelium-dependent vascular homeostatic properties might be perturbed by the lack of available NO during IRI, and pulmonary preservation might be enhanced by nitroglycerin, which produces antineutrophil and antiplatelet effects, as well as harvest vasodilation.[47]

However, NO can react with superoxide anion and form peroxynitrous acid, especially in the presence of a high concentration oxygen. Peroxynitrous acid can induce the release of endothelin 1 (a potent vasoconstrictor[10]), damage alveolar type II cells even after a short period of ischemic time, and cause structural and functional alteration of surfactant proteins.[76] Therefore, this reaction may explain why some have shown that NO administered during ischemia or early reperfusion may be ineffective or even harmful, particularly when it is given with a high fraction of inspired oxygen immediately after reperfusion.[77,78]

Exogenous NO can be administered directly by inhalation, by infusion, or by a NO donor, such as nitroglycerine, FK409, nitroprusside, glyceryl nitrate, or 3-morpholinosydnonimine (SIN-1). Addition of nitroglycerin has been shown to maintain pulmonary vascular homeostatic properties, reduce neutrophil and platelet accumulation, modulate vasomotor tone, and enhance the protective effects of Perfadex.[47,48] Therefore, nitroglycerin is now commonly added to preservation solutions in many centers around the world. Moreover, other strategies have been developed to increase the activity of eNOS by addition one of its cofactors, such as tetrahydrobiopterin, to the preservation solutions or by transfecting the donor with an adenovirus containing eNOS before lung retrieval.[64,65] Clearly, nitroglycerin and other NO donors are simple

and effective additives that improve lung preservation fortra nsplantation.

9.6 "Pulmonoplegia" and Other Additives

Our group at UPMC demonstrated that "pulmonoplegia" significantly improves lung transplant outcomes.[59] One of the senior surgeons at the University of Pittsburgh, the late Brack G. Hattler (1935–2008) (Fig. 9.1), developed a pulmonoplegia for lung preservation, similar to cardioplegia for heart protection. The pulmonoplegia, named the "Hattler solution," is given as cold (4–6°C) blood solution intermittently between the bronchial and pulmonary arterial anastomoses and as terminal warm (34–36°C) blood solution right before perfusing the new

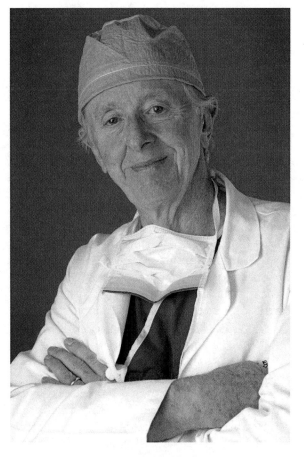

Fig. 9.1 BrackG .H attler(1935–2008)

Table 9.2 Composition of pne umoplegia

Composition	
Dextrose (50%)	5g/ L
Insulin(regular)	20uni ts/L
Glutamate/aspartate	0.92M
Lidocaine	100m g/L
Adenosine	3m g/L
Nitroglycerin	2.5m g/L
Verapamil	2.5m g/L
Deferoxamine	125m g/L
Ascorbica cid	250m g/L
Hematocrit	20±5%

lungs to protect the lungs from IRI. This pulmonoplegia contains glucose, insulin, glutamate, aspartate, lidocaine, adenosine, nitroglycerin, verapamil, deferoxamine, and vitamin C with blood (hematocrit 20±5%) (Table 9.2).

The efficacy of glutamate/aspartate for cardioprotection was well documented by Rosenkranz et al., who showed that glutamate/aspartate improves metabolic and functional recovery of cardiac myocytes and decreases the incidence of lung IRI by improving oxidative metabolism during cardioplegic infusion and during postischemic work.[79] Lidocaine is also reported to reduce reperfusion injury in lung allografts by inhibiting neutrophil adhesion and migration to the lung allograft.[80] Previously, it has been shown that adenosine enhances cardioprotection through antistunning, anti-infarct, and antiapoptotic effects against IRI via adenosine receptors and adenosine triphosphate (ATP)-sensitive potassium channels.[81-83] Adenosine also reduced inflammation and preserved pulmonary function in an in vivo model of lung transplantation through adenosine A_{2A} receptor activation.[84] Verapamil, a calcium antagonist, prevents Ca^{2+} overload and reduces myocardial infarct size via the prostacyclin pathway.[85] Iron chelation with deferoxamine, an oxygen free radical scavenger, has been shown to improve lung preservation, resulting in increased oxygenation and decreased pulmonary vascular resistance.[86]

8-Bromo-cyclic guanosine monophosphate (8-bromo-cGMP) is another additive that has been shown to improve pulmonary function when added to a preservation solution. 8-Bromo-cGMP is a membrane-permeable cGMP analog and is a potent second messenger for the NO pathway in the pulmonary vasculature.[87,88]

9.7 Summary

An overview of the current status of lung preservation has been presented. Evident progress has been made in lung preservation over the past decades, especially with modifying preservation solutions and sampling new additives. An important role of prostaglandins and NO and its donor, nitroglycerin, and their effects and mechanisms in lung preservation were described. A better understanding of the roles of NO and NO metabolism could provide clues on how to better use exogenous NO in lung transplantation to improve the outcomes.

References

1. Toronto Lung Transplant Group. Unilateral lung transplantation for pulmonary fibrosis. *N Engl J Med*. 1986;314: 1140-1145.
2. Baldwin JC, Frist WH, Starkey TD, et al. Distant graft procurement for combined heart and lung transplantation using pulmonary artery flush and simple topical hypothermia for graft preservation. *Ann Thorac Surg*.1987; 43:670-673.
3. Cooper JD, Pearson FG, Patterson GA, et al. Technique of successful lung transplantation in humans. *J Thorac Cardiovasc Surg*.1987; 93:173-181.
4. Patterson GA, Cooper JD, Dark JH, Jones MT. Experimental and clinical double lung transplantation. *J Thorac Cardiovasc Surg*.1988; 95:70-74.
5. Anderson DC, Glazer HS, Semenkovich JW, et al. Lung transplant edema: chest radiography after lung transplantation – the first 10 days. *Radiology*.1995; 195:275-281.
6. Christie JD, Bavaria JE, Palevsky HI, et al. Primary graft failure following lung transplantation. *Chest*. 1998;114: 51-60.
7. King RC, Binns OA, Rodriguez F, et al. Reperfusion injury significantly impacts clinical outcome after pulmonary transplantation. *Ann Thorac Surg*.2000; 69:1681-1685.
8. Lee KH, Martich GD, Boujoukos AJ, Keenan RJ, Griffith BP. Predicting ICU length of stay following single lung transplantation. *Chest*. 1996;110:1014-1017.
9. Novick RJ, Bennett LE, Meyer DM, Hosenpud JD. Influence of graft ischemic time and donor age on survival after lung transplantation. *J Heart Lung Transplant*. 1999;18:425-431.
10. de Perrot M, Liu M, Waddell TK, Keshavjee S. Ischemia-reperfusion-induced lung injury. *Am J Respir Crit Care Med*. 2003;167:490-511.
11. Novick RJ, Gehman KE, Ali IS, Lee J. Lung preservation: the importance of endothelial and alveolar type II cell integrity. *Ann Thorac Surg*.1996; 62:302-314.
12. McEver RP. Selectins: novel receptors that mediate leukocyte adhesion during inflammation. *Thromb Haemost*. 1991; 65:223-228.
13. Parks DA, Granger DN. Contributions of ischemia and reperfusion to mucosal lesion formation. *Am J Physiol*. 1986; 250(6 pt 1):G749-G753.

14. Jurmann MJ, Dammenhayn L, Schaefers HJ, Haverich A. Pulmonary reperfusion injury: evidence for oxygen-derived free radical mediated damage and effects of different free radical scavengers. *Eur J Cardiothorac Surg.* 1990;4:665-670.
15. Zimmerman BJ, Granger DN. Mechanisms of reperfusion injury. *Am J Med Sci.*1994; 307:284-392.
16. van Putte BP, Cobelens PM, van der Kaaij N, et al. Exogenous surfactant attenuation of ischemia-reperfusion injury in the lung through alteration of inflammatory and apoptotic factors. *J Thorac Cardiovasc Surg.*2009; 137:824-828.
17. Levine AJ, Parkes K, Rooney S, Bonser RS. Reduction of endothelial injury after hypothermic lung preservation by initial leukocyte-depleted reperfusion. *J Thorac Cardiovasc Surg.*2000;120:47- 54.
18. Tagawa T, Suda T, Daddi N, et al. Low-dose endobronchial gene transfer to ameliorate lung graft ischemia-reperfusion injury. *J Thorac Cardiovasc Surg.*2002; 123:795-802.
19. Inci I, Inci D, Dutly A, Boehler A, Weder W. Melatonin attenuates posttransplant lung ischemia-reperfusion injury. *Ann Thorac Surg.*2002; 73:220-225.
20. Squifflet JP, Pirson Y, Gianello P, Van Cangh P, Alexandre GP. Safe preservation of human renal cadaver transplants by Euro-Collins solution up to 50 hours. *Transplant Proc.* 1981; 13(1 pt 2):693-966.
21. Konertz WF, Saka B, Berhard A. Euro-Collins solution for heart preservation: experimental and clinical experience. *Transplant Proc.*1988; 20:984-986.
22. Belzer FO, Ashby BS, Dunphy JE. 24- and 72-hour preservation of canine kidneys. *Lancet.*1967; 2:536-538.
23. Jeevanandam V, Barr ML, Auteri JS, et al. University of Wisconsin solution versus crystalloid cardioplegia for human donor heart preservation. A randomized blinded prospective clinical trial. *J Thorac Cardiovasc Surg.* 1992;103:194-199.
24. Wallwork J, Jones K, Cavarocchi N, Hakim M, Higenbottam T. Distant procurement of organs for clinical heart-lung transplantation using a single flush technique. *Transplantation.* 1987;44: 654-658.
25. Yamazaki F, Yokomise H, Keshavjee SH, et al. The superiority of an extracellular fluid solution over Euro-Collins' solution for pulmonary preservation. *Transplantation.* 1990; 49:690-694.
26. Wittwer T, Wahlers T, Cornelius JF, Elki S, Haverich A. Celsior solution for improvement of currently used clinical standards of lung preservation in an ex vivo rat model. *Eur J Cardiothorac Surg.*1999; 15:667-671.
27. Fujimura S, Handa M, Kondo T, Ichinose T, Shiraishi Y, Nakada T. Successful 48-hour simple hypothermic preservation of canine lung transplants. *Transplant Proc.* 1987;19(1 pt2):1334-1336.
28. Kimblad PA, Sjöberg T, Massa G, Solem JO, Steen S. High potassium contents in organ preservation solutions causes strong pulmonary vasoconstriction. *Ann Thorac Surg.* 1991;52:523-528.
29. Keshavjee SH, Yamazaki F, Yokomise H, Cardoso PF, Slutsky AS, Patterson GA. The role of dextran 40 and potassium in extended hypothermic lung preservation for transplantation. *J Thorac Cardiovasc Surg.*1992; 103:314-325.
30. Rezkalla SH, Kloner RA. No-reflow phenomenon. *Circulation.*2002;105: 656-662.
31. Menger MD. Microcirculatory disturbances secondary to ischemia-reperfusion. *Transplant Proc.* 1995;27:2863-2865.
32. Rabanal JM, Ibañez AM, Mons R, et al. Influence of preservation solution on early lung function (Euro-Collins vs Perfadex). *Transplant Proc.*2003; 35:1938-1939.
33. Wittwer T, Fehrenbach A, Meyer D, et al. Retrograde flush perfusion with low-potassium solutions for improvement of experimental pulmonary preservation.*J Heart Lung Transplant.* 2000;19:976-983.
34. Müller C, Fürst H, Reichenspurner H, Briegel J, Groh J, Reichart B; Munich Lung Transplant Group. Lung procurement by low-potassium dextran and the effect on preservation injury. *Transplantation*1999; 68:1139–1143.
35. Albes JM, Brandes H, Heinemann MK, Scheule A, Wahlers T. Potassium-reduced lung preservation solutions: a screening study. *Eur Surg Res.* 1997;29:327-338.
36. Liu CC, Hsu PK, Huang WC, Huang MH, Hsu HS. Two-layer method (UW solution/perfluorochemical plus O_2) for lung preservation in rat lung transplantation. *Transplant Proc.* 2007;39:3019-3023.
37. Aziz TM, Pillay TM, Corris PA, et al. Perfadex for clinical lung procurement: is it an advance? *Ann Thorac Surg.* 2003;75: 990-995.
38. Wu M, Yang Q, Yim AP, Underwood MJ, He GW. Cellular electrophysiologic and mechanical evidence of superior vascular protection in pulmonary microcirculation by Perfadex compared with Celsior. *J Thorac Cardiovasc Surg.* 2009; 13:492-498.
39. Oto T, Griffiths AP, Rosenfeldt F, Levvey BJ, Williams TJ, Snell GI. Early outcomes comparing Perfadex, Euro-Collins, and Papworth solutions in lung transplantation. *Ann Thorac Surg.*2006; 82:1842-1848.
40. De Perrot M, Sekine Y, Fischer S, et al. Interleukin-8 release during early reperfusion predicts graft function in human lung transplantation. *Am J Respir Crit Care Med.* 2002;165: 211-215.
41. Bertolotti A, Gómez C, Lascano E, et al. Effect of preservation solution on graft viability in single-lung transplantation from heart-beating donors in pigs. *Transplant Proc.* 2007;39: 355-357.
42. Wittwer T, Franke UF, Fehrenbach A, et al. Experimental lung transplantation: impact of preservation solution and route of delivery. *J Heart Lung Transplant.* 2005;24: 1081-1090.
43. Puskas JD, Cardoso PF, Mayer E, Shi S, Slutsky AS, Patterson GA. Equivalent eighteen-hour lung preservation with low-potassium dextran or Euro-Collins solution after prostaglandin E1 infusion. *J Thorac Cardiovasc Surg.* 1992; 104:83-89.
44. Naka Y, Roy DK, Liao H, et al. cAMP-mediated vascular protection in an orthotopic rat lung transplant model. Insights into the mechanism of action of prostaglandin E1 to improve lung preservation. *Circ Res.*1996; 79:773-783.
45. de Perrot M, Fischer S, Liu M, et al. Prostaglandin E1 protects lung transplants from ischemia-reperfusion injury: a shift from pro- to anti-inflammatory cytokines. *Transplantation.* 2001;72:1505-1512.
46. Gohrbandt B, Sommer SP, Fischer S, et al. Iloprost to improve surfactant function in porcine pulmonary grafts stored for twenty-four hours in low-potassium dextran solution. *J Thorac Cardiovasc Surg.*2005; 129:80-86.
47. Naka Y, Chowdhury NC, Liao H, et al. Enhanced preservation of orthotopically transplanted rat lungs by nitroglycerin but

not hydralazine. Requirement for graft vascular homeostasis beyond harvest vasodilation. *Circ Res.* 1995;76:900-906.

48. Wittwer T, Albes JM, Fehrenbach A, et al. Experimental lung preservation with Perfadex: effect of the NO-donor nitroglycerin on postischemic outcome. *J Thorac Cardiovasc Surg.*2003;125:1208- 1216.

49. Dandel M, Lehmkuhl HB, Mulahasanovic S, et al. Survival of patients with idiopathic pulmonary arterial hypertension after listing for transplantation: impact of iloprost and bosentan treatment. *J Heart Lung Transplant.*2007; 26:898-906.

50. Santillan-Doherty P, Sotres-Vega A, Jasso-Victoria R, Olmos-Zuñiga R, Arreola-Ramirez JL, Cedillo-Ley I. Effect of prostaglandin E2 on the tracheobronchial distribution of lung preservation perfusate. *J Invest Surg.* 1998;11:259-265.

51. Chiang CH, Wu K, Yu CP, Yan HC, Perng WC, Wu CP. Hypothermia and prostaglandin E(1) produce synergistic attenuation of ischemia-reperfusion lung injury. *Am J Respir Crit Care Med.*199 9;160:1319-1323.

52. Wittwer T, Wahlers T, Fehrenbach A, et al. Combined use of prostacyclin and higher perfusate temperatures further enhances the superior lung preservation by Celsior solution in the isolated rat lung. *J Heart Lung Transplant.* 1999; 18:684-692.

53. Sasaki S, Yasuda K, McCully JD, LoCicero J III. Does PGE1 attenuate potassium-induced vasoconstriction in initial pulmonary artery flush on lung preservation? *J Heart Lung Transplant.*1999;18: 139-142.

54. Löckinger A, Schütte H, Walmrath D, Seeger W, Grimminger F. Protection against gas exchange abnormalities by preaerosolized PGE1, iloprost, and nitroprusside in lung ischemia-reperfusion. *Transplantation.*2001; 71:185-193.

55. Fiser SM, Cope JT, Kron IL, et al. Aerosolized prostacyclin (Epoprostenol) as an alternative to inhaled nitric oxide for patients with reperfusion injury after lung transplantation. *J Thorac Cardiovasc Surg.*2001; 121:981-982.

56. Schütte H, Löckinger A, Seeger W, Grimminger F. Aerosolized PGE1, PGI2 and nitroprusside protect against vascular leakage in lung ischemia-reperfusion. *Eur Respir J.*2001;18:15-22.

57. Olschewski H, Ghofrani HA, Walmrath D, et al. Inhaled prostacyclin and iloprost in severe pulmonary hypertension secondary to lung fibrosis. *Am J Respir Crit Care Med.* 1999;160:600-607.

58. Ikeda S, Shirai M, Shimouchi A, et al. Pulmonary microvascular responses to inhaled prostacyclin, nitric oxide and their combination in anesthetized cats. *Jpn J Physiol.* 1999;49:89-98.

59. Toyoda Y, Thacker J, Santos R, et al. Long-term outcome of lung and heart-lung transplantation for idiopathic pulmonary arterial hypertension. *Ann Thorac Surg.* 2008;86:1116-1122.

60. Trulock EP, Christie JD, Edwards LB, et al. Registry of the International Society for Heart and Lung Transplantation: twenty-third official adult lung and heart–lung transplantation report – 2007. *J Heart Lung Transplant.* 2007;26:782-795.

61. Pinsky DJ, Naka Y, Chowdhury NC, et al. The nitric oxide/cyclic GMP pathway in organ transplantation: critical role in successful lung preservation. *Proc Natl Acad Sci U S A.* 1994;91:12086-12090.

62. Marczin N, Riedel B, Gal J, Polak J, Yacoub M. Exhaled nitric oxide during lung transplantation. *Lancet.* 1997;350: 1681-1682.

63. Liu M, Tremblay L, Cassivi SD, et al. Alterations of nitric oxide synthase expression and activity during rat lung transplantation. *Am J Physiol Lung Cell Mol Physiol.* 2000; 278:L1071-L1081.

64. Schmid RA, Hillinger S, Walter R, et al. The nitric oxide synthase cofactor tetrahydrobiopterin reduces allograft ischemia-reperfusion injury after lung transplantation. *J Thorac Cardiovasc Surg.*1999; 118:726-732.

65. Suda T, Mora BN, D'Ovidio F, et al. In vivo adenovirus-mediated endothelial nitric oxide synthase gene transfer ameliorates lung allograft ischemia-reperfusion injury. *J Thorac Cardiovasc Surg.*2000; 119:297-304.

66. Cardella JA, Keshavjee SH, Bai XH, et al. Increased expression of nitric oxide synthase in human lung transplants after nitric oxide inhalation. *Transplantation.*2004; 77:886-890.

67. Cremona G, Dinh Xuan AT, Higenbottam TW. Endothelium-derived relaxing factor and the pulmonary circulation. *Lung.* 1991;169:185-202.

68. Feelisch M, te Poel M, Zamora R, Deussen A, Moncada S. Understanding the controversy over the identity of EDRF. *Nature.*1994; 368:62-65.

69. Kubes P, Suzuki M, Granger DN. Nitric oxide: an endogenous modulator of leukocyte adhesion. *Proc Natl Acad Sci U S A.*1991; 88:4651-4655.

70. Kubes P, Granger DN. Nitric oxide modulates microvascular permeability. *Am J Physiol.*1992; 262:H611-H615.

71. Pinsky DJ, Oz MC, Koga S, et al. Cardiac preservation is enhanced in a heterotopic rat transplant model by supplementing the nitric oxide pathway. *J Clin Invest.* 1994;93: 2291-2297.

72. Gustafsson LE, Leone AM, Person MG, Wiklung NP, Moncada S. Endogenous nitric oxide is present in the exhaled air of rabbits, guinea pigs, and humans. *Biochem Biophys Res Commun.*1991; 181:852-857.

73. Stamler JS, Loh E, Roddy M-A, Currie KE, Creager MA. Nitric oxide regulates basal and systemic pulmonary vascular resistance in healthy humans. *Circulation.* 1994;89: 2035-2040.

74. Adkins WK, Taylor AE. Role of xanthine oxidase and neutrophils in ischemia-reperfusion injury in rabbit lung. *J Appl Physiol.*1990; 69:2012-2018.

75. Kirk AJ, Colguhoun IW, Dark JH. Lung preservation: a review of current practice and future directions. *Ann Thorac Surg.*1993; 56:990-1000.

76. de Perrot M, Keshavjee S. Lung preservation. *Semin Thorac Cardiovasc Surg.*2004; 16:300-308.

77. Naka Y, Roy DK, Smerling AJ, et al. Inhaled nitric oxide fails to confer the pulmonary protection provided by distal stimulation of the nitric oxide pathway at the level of cyclic guanosine monophosphate. *J Thorac Cardiovasc Surg.* 1995;110:1434-1441.

78. Eppinger MJ, Ward PA, Jones ML, Bolling SF, Deeb GM. Disparate effects of nitric oxide on lung ischemia-reperfusion injury. *Ann Thorac Surg.* 1995;60:1169-1176.

79. Rosenkranz ER, Okamoto F, Buckberg GD, Vinten-Johansen J, Robertson JM, Buqyi H. Safety of prolonged aortic clamping with blood cardioplegia. III. Aspartate enrichment of glutamate-blood cardioplegia in energy-depleted hearts after ischemia and reperfusion injury. *J Thorac Cardiovasc Surg.* 1986;91:428-435.

80. Schmid RA, Yamashita M, Ando K, Tanaka Y, Cooper JD, Patterson GA. Lidocaine reduces reperfusion injury and neutrophil migration in canine lung allografts. *Ann Thorac Surg*.1996;61:949- 955.

81. Toyoda Y, Di Gregorio V, Parker RA, Levitsky S, McCully JD. Anti-stunning and anti-infarct effects of adenosine-enhanced ischemic preconditioning. *Circulation*. 2000;102: III326-III331.

82. Stadler B, Phillips J, Toyoda Y, Federman M, Levitsky S, McCully JD. Adenosine-enhanced ischemic preconditioning modulates necrosis and apoptosis: effects of stunning and ischemia-reperfusion. *Ann Thorac Surg*. 2001;72:555-563.

83. Toyoda Y, Friehs I, Parker RA, Levitsky S, McCully JD. Differential role of sarcolemmal and mitochondrial K(ATP) channels in adenosine-enhanced ischemic preconditioning. *Am J Physiol Heart Circ Physiol*.2000; 279:H2694-H2703.

84. Reece TB, Ellman PI, Maxey TS, et al. Adenosine A_{2A} receptor activation reduces inflammation and preserves pulmonary function in an in vivo model of lung transplantation. *J Thorac Cardiovasc Surg*.2005; 129:1137-1143.

85. Sullivan AT, Baker DJ, Drew GM. Effect of calcium channel blocking agents on infarct size after ischemia-reperfusion in anaesthetized pigs: relationship between cardioprotection and cardiodepression. *J Cardiovasc Pharmacol*. 1991;17: 707-717.

86. Conte JV Jr, Katz NM, Foegh ML, Wallace RB, Ramwell PW. Iron chelation therapy and lung transplantation. Effects of deferoxamine on lung preservation in canine single lung transplantation. *J Thorac Cardiovasc Surg*. 1991;101: 1024-1029.

87. King RC, Laubach VE, Kanithanon RC, et al. Preservation with 8-bromo-cyclic GMP improves pulmonary function after prolonged ischemia. *Ann Thorac Surg*. 1998;66:1732-1738.

88. Hillinger S, Schmid RA, Sandera P, et al. 8-Br-cGMP is superior to prostaglandin E1 for lung preservation. *Ann Thorac Surg*.1999; 68:1138-1143.

Endothelin and Ischemia-Reperfusion Injury

10

Matthias Gorenflo

10.1 Introduction

The lung vasculature is subject to the net effect of various vasoactive stimuli that influence pulmonary vascular tone.[1] Among these are gaseous factors (e.g., oxygen), the effect of autonomic innervation (e.g., alpha adrenergic innervation) and mediators from endothelial or inflammatory cells that act in concert to influence the pulmonary vascular tone (Fig. 10.1). Endothelin (ET) was discovered in 1988 by Yanagisawa et al.[2] It was originally derived from cultured endothelial cells. ET-1 belongs to a family of closely related 21-amino acid peptides which are designated ET-1, ET-2 and ET-3 (Fig. 10.2) characterized by two disulfide bridges and six conserved amino acid residues at the COOH-terminus. Among the three isoforms ET-1 is responsible for most of the physiological and pathophysiological actions in human lung and vascular tissue.[3]

The ET-1 peptide is encoded by a distinct gene, mapped on chromosome 6 in humans. This gene codes for a precursor peptide (pre-proendothelin-1) that is cleaved to a 38-aminoacid intermediate form called big-ET-1 or pro-ET-1 (Fig. 10.3). This pro-ET-1 is then rapidly converted to form the mature ET-1 by cleavage by a specific enzyme called endothelin-converting enzyme-1 (ECE-1). ECE-1 is a type II integral membrane protein belonging to the family of membrane bound metalloproteases, inhibited by phosphoramidone.

The expression of ET-1 is regulated genetically by different factors.[4] Proinflammatory cytokines such as tumor necrosis factor-α (TNF-α), transforming growth factor-β (TGF-β) and interleukin (IL)-1β are able to increase the expression of ET-1. ETs are stored within the cell and are synthesized by activation within the cell. Secretion of ETs is regulated at the level of peptide synthesis. ET-1 is released from endothelial cells via two pathways: (1) the peptide is continuously transported in and released from secretory vesicles by the constitutive pathway.[5] By this it contributes to intense constriction of the underlying smooth muscle cell and to basal vascular tone. (2) ET-1 is stored in Weibel-Palade bodies and released from these intracellular storage granules by the regulated pathway in response to a stimulus (physiological or pathological) and may thus produce further vasoconstriction.[6,7] The terminal half-life of ET-1 has been reported to be 455 ± 59 min,[8] and the kinetics of clearance is best described by using a three-compartment model. The pharmacological responses to ET-1 are mediated by at least two subtypes of receptors. These are designated ET_A and ET_B receptor. In the human, ET_A receptor predominantely is to find on vascular smooth muscle cells, whereas the ET_B receptor is located on the luminal site of the endothelial cell. ET-1 related vasoconstriction of smooth muscle cells in human pulmonary artery is mediated by the ET_A receptor, whereas ET-1 coupling to the ET_B receptor will result in consecutive NO mediated vasodilation (Fig. 10.4). The ET_B receptor plays an important role by clearing circulating ET-1 from the circulation and may primarily serve to keep tissue ET-1 concentrations low.[9]

The effects of ET-1 are mediated by several signal transduction pathways utilizing intracellular second messengers. These include inositol 1,4,5-triphosphate (IP3), 1,2 diacylglycerol (DAG), calcium, cAMP, protein kinase C and phospholipase A2.[10] The biological effects of ET-1 are summarized in Table 10.1: there are effects on vascular tone as well as mitogenic activities and interactions with other mediators.

M.G orenflo
Department of Paediatric Cardiology, UZ Leuven Campus
Gasthuisberg,H erestraat49 , B-3000Le uven, Belgie
e-mail:ma tthias.gorenflo@uz.kuleuven.ac.be

E.A. Gabriel and T. Salerno (eds.), *Principles of Pulmonary Protection in Heart Surgery*,
DOI: 10.1007/978-1-84996-308-4_10, © Springer-Verlag London Limited 2010

Fig.10.1 Theinfl uence of different factors on the balance of pulmonary vascular tone. The *boxes* represent the specific receptors which are located on the endothelial or smooth muscle cells. The effect of different gaseous factors, hormones and neural innervations is mediated by these receptors. *paO₂* pa rtial pressure of oxygen; *5-HT* serotonin; *ANP* a trial atriuretic peptide; *PGI₂* prostacyclin

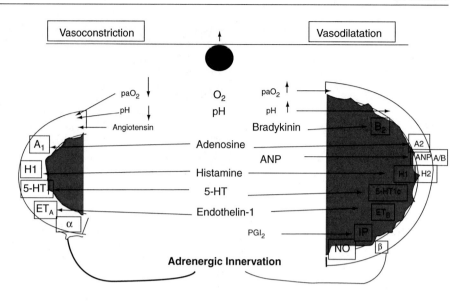

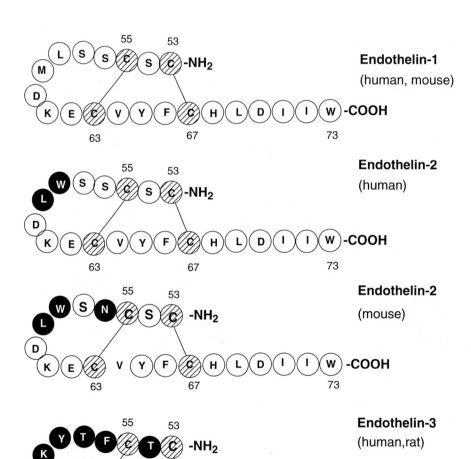

Fig.10.2 Structureof endothelins (ETs) in different species. Differences in amino acids compared to ET-1 are marked in *black*

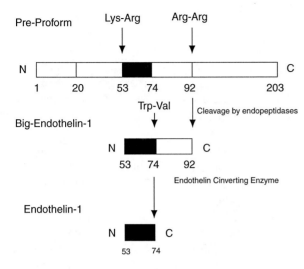

Fig.10.3 Processofs ynthesisof ET -1bypr otein-cleavage

10.2 ET-1i nI schemia/Reperfusion Injury of the Lung

It is well known that cardiopulmonary bypass surgery and major surgical procedures are associated with a systemic inflammatory response and impaired peripheral circulation. This has been shown to be associated with an increase in ET-1 plasma levels.[11,12] Patients with left-to-right shunt show increased ET-1 immunoreactivity and an increase in ETA receptor density in the vessel wall of pulmonary artery resistance vessels[13] (Fig. 10.5). Children undergoing intracardiac repair for left-to-right shunt show an increase in plasma ET-1[14] and decreased L-arginine plasma levels.[15] At present it is unsettled whether the combination of an increase in (vasoconstrictive) ET-1 with a decrease in plasma

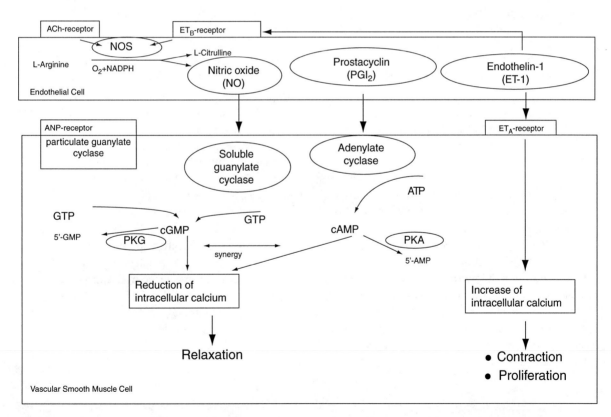

Fig. 10.4 Different actions of ET-1: vasodilatation is mediated by coupling to the ET$_B$ receptor on endothelial cells with subsequent generation of nitric oxide (NO). Vasoconstriction is mediated by coupling to the ET$_A$ receptor on the vascular smooth muscle cell. *cAMP* cyclic adenosine monophosphate; *ATP* adenosine triphosphate; *cGMP* cyclic guanosine monophosphate; *GTP* guanosine triphosphate; *PKA* protein kinase A; *PKG* proteinki naseG

Table 10.1 Biological effects of ET-1 and interaction with other mediators important in ischemia / reperfusion (adapted from Göttmann et al[27])

Effects of ET-1
Vasoconstriction
Release of NO
Increased oxidant stress
Infiltration of polymorphnuclear leucocytes
Release of GM-CSF, IL-5, IL-6, IL-8
Production of bFGF, VEGF, PAF
Proliferation of vascular smooth muscle cells
Production of collagen and fibronectin
Increase of ET-1 production in response to
Ischemia
Hypoxia
Reduced extracellular pH
IGF-1,TG F-β,TN F-α
IL-1α,IL-1 β, IL-2, IL-6
Thromboxane A2, PDGF, thrombin

bFGF basic fibroblast growth factor; *GM-CSF* granulocyte-macrophage colony-stimulating factor; *IGF-1* insulin-like growth factor I; *IL* interleukin; *PAF* platelet activating factor; *PDGF* platelet derived growth factor; *TGF-β* transforming growth factor beta, *TNF-α* transforming growth factor alpha; *VEGF* vascular endothelial growth factor

L-Arginine (as substrate for eNOS) will render these patients more vulnerable to postoperative pulmonary hypertensive crises.

The endothelium is clearly one of the key players in the pathophysiology of lung injury in response to ischemia-reperfusion: Pulmonary ischemia studied with the isolated murine lung or flow adapted pulmonary microvascular endothelial cells in vitro results in endothelial generation of reactive oxygen species (ROS) and NO. These mediators generated in response to oxidative stress, can promote vasodilation and angiogenesis which may be seen in compensation for decreased tissue perfusion.[16] In a rat model of lung injury induced by abdominal aortic ischemia-reperfusion Kiris et al[17] demonstrated an increase in lung tissue levels of mediators associated with increased oxidative stress (malondialdehyde, catalase and myeloperoxidase). Treatment of these animals with tezosentan, a dual ET receptor antagonist attenuated as well the histological findings associated with lung injury as well as plasma levels of mediators associated with oxidative stress.

In a dog model an elevation of ET-1 levels early after lung transplantation was found, indicating that ET-1 may play an important role in early high pulmonary vascular resistance and temporary graft dysfunction[18] and studies in human lung transplant recipients confirm these observations.[19] In a rabbit model of lung transplantation the treatment with the dual ET receptor antagonist SB209670 resulted in a significant decrease in mean pulmonary artery pressure, PVR, and pulmonary edema, and improvement in pulmonary compliance and paO$_2$.[20]

There is evidence that the ischemia-reperfusion injury mainly is mediated by the ET$_A$ receptor: Both, a dual ET receptor antagonists (PD-156707-0015) and a selective ET$_A$ receptor antagonists (BQ-610) have been found to effectively reduce the ischemia-reperfusion injury in experimental models of lung transplantation.[21] In contrast the severity of ischemia-reperfusion injury was not influenced by an ET$_B$ receptor *agonist* (IRL-1620) and treatment with a selective ET$_B$ receptor *antagonist* (IRL-1038) did not ameliorate the ischemia-reperfusion injury.[21] In a rat model of lung transplantation the combined treatment with a platelet activating factor (PAF) antagonist (TCV-309) and a ET receptor antagonist (TAK-044) resulted in superior posttransplant graft function 24 h after reperfusion, suggesting a synergistic role of ET-1 and PAF in the mediation of reperfusion injury in this model. Single treatment with either of the antagonists revealed only a slight improvement compared to untreated controls in this study.[22]

In the human undergoing lung transplantation an increase in plasma ET-1 levels was found and associated with detrimental effect during the postoperative course early after transplantation.[19] Taken together there is considerable evidence from experimental models as well as from studies in the human that ET-1 plays an important role in the pathophysiology of ischemia-reperfusion injury of the lung.

10.3 ETR eceptorA ntagonistT reatment of Ischemia-Reperfusion in the Human

Treatment with sitaxsentan – a selective ET$_A$ receptor antagonist – in patients undergoing cardiopulmonary bypass for coronary artery bypass surgery has shown to

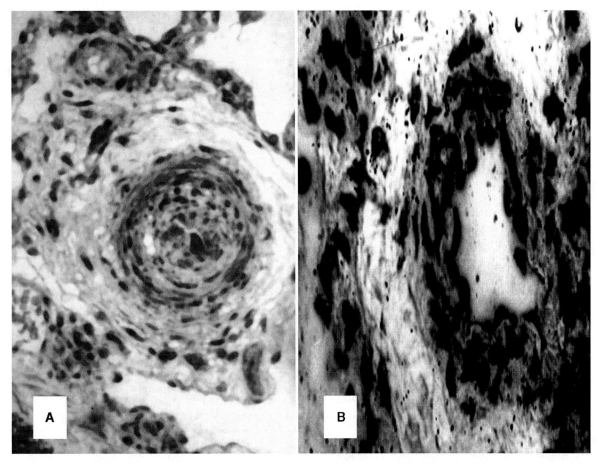

Fig. 10.5 ET immunoreactivity as demonstrated by *red* colorization of ET in intima and smooth muscle cells in a pulmonary resistance artery (**a**; 40×). Autoradiography of ET_A receptor (*black dots*) on vascular smooth muscle cells within the tunica media (**b**)

have a beneficial effect with respect to systemic and pulmonary vascular resistance after weaning from cardiopulmonary bypass.[23] A second study by the same group has demonstrated that plasma levels of TNF-α and TNF receptor 2 were reduced in sitaxsentan treated patients undergoing cardiopulmonary bypass.[24] This demonstrates that ET_A receptor antagonists may effectively reduce ischemia-reperfusion injury. However treatment with ET receptor antagonists in the human after cardiopulmonary bypass is not without risks: Prendergast et al[25] have found that treatment with the ET_A receptor antagonist BQ-123 in infants with postoperative pulmonary hypertension after corrective surgery for congenital heart disease was well associated with a significant improvement in pulmonary hemodynamic indices. However, these benefits were associated with reductions in systemic blood pressure and arterial oxygen saturation, the

latter consistent with a ventilation-perfusion mismatch. More clinical studies that analyze the effect of treatment with ET receptor antagonists on lung injury after ischemia-reperfusion in different disease entities are clearly needed before the potential benefit of these substances can be ascertained. Given the fact that ET-1 has a major role in maintaining a normal blood pressure in the human,[9] potential deleterious effects of treatment with ET receptor antagonists in the setting of postoperative care after cardiopulmonary bypass are easy to explain. It remains to be established whether treatment with substances leading to decreased ET-1 *production* (rather than *antagonizing* its actions) may have a potential role in preventing ischemia-reperfusion injury. A pharmacological candidate for such an approach is e.g., estrogen: Estrogen leads to increased levels of prostacyclin and NO as well as decreased levels of ET-1 and may thus be a potential therapeutic agent for future experimental and clinical studies.[26]

In summary, ET-1 contributes considerably to the pathophysiology of lung injury after ischemia-reperfusion. Treatment with ET receptor antagonists has been effective in some disease entities, but their precise role needs to be clarified by further studies. Future research may well be directed to substances thatprima rilyre duceET-1produc tion.

References

1. Barns PJ, Liu SF. Regulation of pulmonary vascular tone. *Pharmacol Rev*.1995; 47:87-131.
2. Yanagisawa M, Kurihara H, Kimure S, et al. A novel potent vasoconstrictor peptide produced by vascular endothelial cells. *Nature Lond*.1988; 332:411-415.
3. Barnes PJ. Endothelins and pulmonary diseases. *J Appl Physiol*.1994;77:1051- 1059.
4. Masaki T, Yanagisawa M, Goto K. Physiology and pharmacology of endothelins. *Med Res Rev*.1992; 12:391-421.
5. Russell FD, Skepper JN, Davenport AP. Evidence using electron microscopy for regulated and constitutive pathways in the transport and release of endothelin. *J Cardiovasc Pharmacol*.1998;31: 424-430.
6. Ozaka T, Doi Y, Kayashima K, Fujimoto S. Weibel-Palade bodies as a storage site of calcitonin gene related peptide and endothelin-1 in blood vessels of the rat carotid body. *Anat Rec*.1997;247:388- 394.
7. Kayashima K, Doi Y, Kudo HKiyonaga H, Fujimoto S. Effects of endothelin-1 on vasoreactivity and its synthesis, storage, and acting sites in the rat superior mesenteric vasculature: an ultrastructural and immuncytochemical study. *Med Electron Microsc*.1999; 32:36-42.
8. Parker JD, Thiessen JJ, Reilly R, Tong JH, Stewart DJ, Pandey AS. Human endothelin-1 clearance kinetics revealed by a radiotracer technique. *J Pharmacol Exp Ther*. 1999; 289:261-265.
9. Brunner F, Brás-Silva C, Cerdeira AS, Leite-Moreira AF. Cardiovascular endothelins: essential regulators of cardiovascular homeostasis. *Pharmacol Ther*.2006; 111:508-531.
10. Miller RC, Pelton JT, Huggins JP. Endothelins – from receptors to medicine. *Trends Pharmacol Sci*.1993; 14:54-60.
11. Komai H, Adatia IT, Elliott MJ, de Leval MR, Haworth SG. Increased plasma levels of endothelin-1 after cardiopulmonary bypass in patients with pulmonary hypertension and congenital heart disease. *J Thorac Cardiovasc Surg*. 1993; 106:473-478.
12. Shirakami G, Magaribuchi T, Shingu K, et al. Effects of anesthesia and surgery on plasma endothelin levels. *Anesth Analg*.1995;80:449- 453.
13. Lutz J, Gorenflo M, Habighorst M, Vogel M, Lange PE, Hocher B. Endothelin-1 and endothelin-receptors in lung biopsies of patients with pulmonary hypertension due to congenital heart disease. *Clin Chem Lab Med*. 1999;37:423-428.
14. Loukanov T, Arnold R, Gross J, et al. Endothelin-1 and asymmetric dimethylarginine in children with left-to-right shunt after intracardiac repair. *Clin Res Cardiol*. 2008;97: 383-388.
15. Gorenflo M, Ullmann MV, Eitel K, et al. Plasma L-arginine and metabolites of nitric oxide synthase in patients with left-to-right shunt after intracardiac repair. *Chest*. 2005;127:1184-1189.
16. Chatterjee S, Chapman KE, Fisher AB. Lung ischemia: a model for endothelial mechanotransduction. *Cell Biochem Biophys*.2008; 52:125-138.
17. Kiri I, Narin C, Gülmen S, Yılmaz N, Sütçü R, Kapucuo lu N. Endothelin receptor antagonism by tezosentan attenuates lung injury induced by aortic ischemia-reperfusion. *Ann Vasc Surg*. 2009;23(3):382-91.
18. Shennib H, Serrick C, Saleh D, Adoumie R, Stewart DJ, Giaid A. Alterations in bronchoalveolar lavage and plasma endothelin-1 levels early after lung transplantation. *Transplantation*.1995; 59:994-998.
19. Shennib H, Serrick C, Saleh D, Reis A, Stewart DJ, Giaid A. Plasma endothelin-1 levels in human lung transplant recipients. *J Cardiovasc Pharmacol*. 1995;26(suppl 3):S516-S518.
20. Shennib H, Kuang JQ, Ohlstein EH, Giaid A. Endothelin receptor antagonist improves pulmonary hemodynamics during lung ischemia/reperfusion injury. *Transplantation*. 1998;66:917-937.
21. Khimenko PL, Moore TM, Taylor AE. Blocked ETA receptors prevent ischemia and reperfusion injury in rat lungs. *J Appl Physiol*.1996; 80:203-207.
22. Stammberger U, Carboni GL, Hillinger S, Schneiter D, Weder W, Schmid RA. Combined treatment with endothelin- and PAF-antagonists reduces posttransplant lung ischemia/reperfusion injury. *J Heart Lung Transplant*. 1999;18: 862-868.
23. Ikonomidis JS, Hilton EJ, Payne K, Harrell A, Finklea L, Clark L, Reeves S, Stroud RE, Leonardi A, Crawford FA Jr, Spinale FG. Selective endothelin-A receptor inhibition after cardiac surgery: a safety and feasibility study. *Ann Thorac Surg*. 2007;83:2153-2160; discussion 2161.
24. Ford RL, Mains IM, Hilton EJ, et al. Endothelin-A receptor inhibition after cardiopulmonary bypass: cytokines and receptor activation. *Ann Thorac Surg*.2008; 86:1576-1583.
25. Prendergast B, Newby DE, Wilson LE, Webb DJ, Mankad PS. Early therapeutic experience with the endothelin antagonist BQ-123 in pulmonary hypertension after congenital heart surgery. *Heart*.1999; 82:505-508.
26. Lahm T, Crisostomo PR, Markel TA, et al. The effects of estrogen on pulmonary artery vasoreactivity and hypoxic pulmonary vasoconstriction: potential new clinical implications for an old hormone. *Crit Care Med*. 2008;36:2174-2183.
27. Göttmann U, van der Woude FJ, Braun C. Endothelin receptor antagonists: a new therapeutic option for improving the outcome after solid organ transplantation? *Curr Vasc Pharmacol*.2003; 1:281-299.

L-Arginine and Ischemia-ReperfusionI njury

Yanmin Yang and Jiming Cai

11

11.1 Introduction

Despite continuous optimization of lung preservation strategies, the lung remains extremely vulnerable to ischemia-reperfusion (I/R) injury.[1] It is generally known that I/R-induced lung injury is characterized by (1) increased microvascular permeability and edema, (2) dysfunction of the pulmonary endothelium, (3) aggregation of neutrophils and platelets, and (4) sometimes hemorrhage.

In 1987, a new metabolic pathway was proposed, the products of which include L-citrulline as well as the highly reactive and unstable nitric oxide (NO).[2] The enzyme responsible for the production of NO has been named nitric oxide synthase (NOS). In the presence of reduced nicotinamide adenine dinucleotide phosphate (NADPH) and O_2, NOS produces NO by catalyzing a five-electron oxidation of a guanidino nitrogen of L-arginine. Two moles of O_2 and 1.5 moles of NADPH are consumed per mole of NO formed. Soon, it became clear that this newly identified pathway actually exists in various eukaryotic cells, including pulmonary arterial endothelial cells (PAECs). Also, three isoforms of NOS were distinguished based on such varied properties as encoding genes, intracellular localization, regulation of activity, catalytic features, and inhibitor sensitivity. In human beings, there exists about 50%

homology among the three isoforms. These isoforms are usually referred to by the most common nomenclature: nNOS (also known as type I, NOS-I, and NOS-1) was the isoform first found (and predominating) in neuronal tissue, iNOS (also known as type II, NOS-II, and NOS-2) the isoform inducible in a wide range of cells and tissues; and eNOS (also known as type III, NOS-III, and NOS-3), the isoform first found in vascular endothelial cells.[3] In the past, these isoforms also have been differentiated on the basis of their constitutive (eNOS and nNOS) vs. inducible (iNOS) expression, and their calcium dependence (eNOS and nNOS) vs. independence (iNOS).

Because NO contains an unpaired electron, it can rapidly react with superoxide anion (O_2^-) to form peroxynitrite anion (ONOO⁻). During the decomposition of peroxynitrite, the highly reactive oxygen species, hydroxyl radical (HO) is formed. It has been observed that HOs destroy tissue by oxidation of proteins as well as peroxidation of membrane lipids and nucleic acids. Due to these observations in other tissue and because reperfusion of ischemic tissue causes superoxide generation, suspicion that NO production in postischemic lung tissues is a major factor causing I/R injury due to peroxynitrite formation is proposed. However, studies showing that use of exogenous NO to reperfuse lung tissues, when superoxide production is elevated, prevents leukocyte adherence and emigration as well as attenuates the I/R-induced microvascular dysfunction cast doubt on such suspicion. Furthermore, it has been shown that acute oxidative lung injury indeed can be attenuated by NO ventilation. As a result, the exact role of L-arginine and its product NO on normal lung and those subjected to I/R insult deserves to be discussed in detail.

Y.Y ang(✉)
Institute for Biodiagnostics, National Research Council of Canada, Winnipeg, MB, Canadaa nd
Department of Cardiovascular and Thoracic Surgery, Shanghai Children's Medical Center, School of Medicine, ShanghaiJ iaoT ongU niversity, Shanghai, China
e-mail:vi ctor.yang@nrc-cnrc.gc.ca

E.A. Gabriel and T. Salerno (eds.), *Principles of Pulmonary Protection in Heart Surgery*,
DOI: 10.1007/978-1-84996-308-4_11, © Springer-Verlag London Limited 2010

11.2 Role of L-Arginine/NO Pathway in the Regulation of Normal Lung Physiology

NO production depends on intracellular L-arginine content, a nutritionally nonessential amino acid and an exclusive biosynthetic precursor. Consistent transport of extracellular L-arginine is a prerequisite for its continuous synthesis. Under physiological conditions, L-arginine transport into endothelium is mediated by system y+, which is a sodium-independent plasmalemmal transport system accounting for about 60% of its transport, and system b0, +, a sodium-dependent system that accounts for about 40% of its transport. Low levels of NO are produced under normal physiologic conditions. NO is a highly reactive and unstable substance with a short half-life. Considerable evidence has emerged suggesting that the effects of NO in some physiological processes are mediated through the activation of guanylate cyclase, resulting in an increased level of cyclic guanosine monophosphate (cGMP) in the target cell.

11.2.1 Maintenance of Normal Lung Vascular Resistance

NO regulates pulmonary vascular resistance (PVR) via relaxing vascular smooth muscle. NO, diffusing from neighboring PAECs, increases the conversion of guanosine triphosphate (GTP) to cGMP by activating guanylate cyclase in vascular smooth muscle cells. Increasing the intracellular cGMP level (1) decreases the Ca^{2+} sensitivity of contraction of smooth muscle by activating cGMP-dependent protein kinase, which stimulates myosin light chain phosphatase; (2) inhibits Ca^{2+} entry into the cell; and (3) activates K^+ channels, which leads to hyperpolarization. These actions lead to endothelium-dependent vasodilation and resultant increment of pulmonary blood flow. This is supported by the finding that N^G-nitro-L-arginine methyl ester (L-NAME), a competitive inhibitor of NOS, results in an increased PVR in isolated, perfused pig and human lungs. It is generally believed that under normal physiological conditions L-arginine is in excess as the half-maximal effective concentration (EC50) for activation of eNOS is 1–10 µM, yet the intracellular concentration of L-arginine in the endothelial cell is significantly

higher than 100 µM and sufficient to maximally activate the enzyme.[4] Classical endothelium-dependent vasodilators such as acetylcholine and bradykinin execute their function via activation of eNOS. However, their efficiency is not directly dependent on extracellular L-arginine concentration. Rather, release of Ca^{2+} from intracellular stores is the initiating factor for activation of eNOS by these agents, which is then maintained by a sustained phase of Ca^{2+} entry across the membrane.[5] A high proportion of eNOS is known to be located in plasmalemmal caveolae, which contain structural proteins called caveolins. The increase in Ca^{2+} results in Ca^{2+}-calmodulin binding and subsequent dissociation of eNOS from caveolin 1, allowing activation of the enzyme.[6] In this way, the activated eNOS has access to the high concentration of L-arginine in the cytosol of the endothelial cell.

Of course, there also exists an alternative NO-dependent pathway of pulmonary artery relaxation, which is a Ca^{2+}-independent eNOS activation and acetylcholine independent. It functions as a physiological response to the presence of isoprenaline (a nonselective β-receptor agonist) in the pulmonary circulation. It is mediated by cyclic adenosine monophosphate (cAMP) and exclusively associated with extracellular L-arginine content and its direct entry into the pulmonary vascular endothelium. The concentration of extracellular L-arginine delivered to the eNOS is a rate-limiting step for NO production via this pathway. When eNOS is activated by a rise in cAMP, it only has access to L-arginine that enters across the cell membrane. In PAECs, the proteins for eNOS, caveolin 1, and CAT-1 (cationic amino acid transporter associated with system y+) all collocate, and eNOS and CAT1 form a complex within the caveolae. This allows directed delivery of extracellular L-arginine to the eNOS,[7] which explains the critical dependence of cAMP-induced, NO-mediated relaxation on extracellular L-arginine.

11.2.2 Maintenance of Normal Microvascular Endothelial Function

Functional and anatomical integrity of the microvascular endothelium is critical for control of the movement of water and solutes between the vascular lumen and the interstitial space. Under normal conditions, the pulmonary microvascular endothelial barrier regulates the passage of macromolecules and circulating cells from blood to the lung. L-Arginine-derived NO, again, is a key factor in maintaining microvascular endothelial normal function, the result of which is an integral microvascular permeability and balanced fluids movement. It has been observed that reduction of intrinsic NO production (induced by L-NAME) may reduce cGMP levels and cause endothelial cell contraction, which would produce larger interendothelial junctions, an event that results in increased microvascular permeability.[8]

11.2.3 Inhibition of Neutrophil Adhesion to Endothelium and Transmigration into Interstitium

Normally, a limited amount of unstimulated neutrophils in the blood will adhere to and transmigrate across the microvascular endothelial barrier. During inflammation, stimulants such as cytokines will activate neutrophils, the result of which is an increased tendency for adhesion and transmigration.[9] It has been proved that, during acute inflammation, expression of iNOS increased significantly in stimulated inflammatory cells.[10,11] It seems that the acutely formed iNOS plays a key role in limiting adhesion of neutrophils with endothelium and subsequent transmigration. For example, with iNOS knockout mice as an animal model, transmigration across microvascular endothelium significantly increased when compared with wild-type mice.[12] Similar results were also found between the interaction of human neutrophils and pulmonary microvascular endothelial cells when expressed iNOS was chemically inhibited.[9] As a ubiquitous signaling pathway, the increased NO level in activated neutrophils translates to an enhanced cGMP level.[13] Studies have shown that high concentrations of cGMP can inhibit host neutrophil rolling, adhesion, transmigration, and deformability[14] by blunting adhesion molecule expression.[15,16]

11.2.4 Inhibition of Platelet Aggregation and Thrombosis Formation

Thrombosis is the most commonly encountered obstructive process in pulmonary arteries, leading to pulmonary hypertension with significant morbidity and mortality. It has been observed that inhibition of NOS by L-NAME significantly potentiated and the administration of L-arginine significantly reduced the accumulation of ^{111}In-labeled platelets in the pulmonary vasculature of rabbits induced by intravenous collagen plus epinephrine.[17] What is more, inhalation of exogenous NO can significantly reduce ex vivo collagen-induced and in vivo massive pulmonary embolism-induced platelet aggregation.[18,19] As a result, it is clear that L-arginine-derived NO, during platelet activation, plays an important role in preventing their subsequent massive aggregation in respective organs such as the lung. It has been proved that the amount of NO available for the regulation of platelet function depends mainly on vascular endothelium. However, platelets also contain NOS, with eNOS as a predominant isoform, and increase NO production during activation. Although it is true that stimuli that increase intracellular Ca^{2+} such as ADP (adenosine diphosphate) and thrombin activate platelet eNOS and induce NO generation, many other stimuli have been identified as capable of activating the enzyme with no detectable effect on intracellular Ca^{2+}.[20] The amount of NO produced by platelets is relatively lower than produced by endothelial cells,[21] but this NO acts as a negative feedback mechanism in regulating platelet activation. It appears that, compared with endothelium-generated NO diffusing into adjacent cells to exert its action in a paracrine manner, platelet-derived NO exerts its effects within the same cell in an autocrine manner.

The NO in platelets derived from both endothelium and itself stimulates intracellular guanylate cyclase, causing an increase in cGMP and hence activation of cGMP-dependent protein kinase (PKG). This in turn causes inhibition of platelet activation through various pathways. First, PKG promotes sarcoplasmic reticulum ATPase-dependent refilling of intraplatelet Ca^{2+} stores, thereby inhibiting influx of Ca^{2+} and other cations and decreasing intracellular Ca^{2+} levels. Second, it also inhibits inositol-1,4,5-triphosphate-stimulated Ca^{2+} release from the sarcoplasmic reticulum, which also contributes to decreasing cytosolic Ca^{2+}. It has been further proved that cGMP can inhibit platelet aggregation via other pathways. For example, cGMP inhibits the activation of phosphoinositide 3 kinase, which in turn causes activation of platelet glycoprotein IIb/IIIa fibrinogen receptors, facilitating its interaction with fibrinogen. Platelet aggregation that occurs at this stage is called primary aggregation, which is still reversible. The primarily aggregated platelets then initiate the second stage of aggregation, which is irreversible, by recruitment of more activated platelet via releasing their dense granules (containing ADP or ATP, Ca^{2+}, and serotonin) and α-granules (containing platelet factor 4, platelet-derived growth factor [PDGF], fibronectin, β-thromboglobulin, von Willebrand factor [vWF], fibrinogen, and coagulation factors V and XIII).

11.3 Disturbanceo f L-Arginine/NO Pathway Due to Lung I/R Insult

During cardiovascular surgery requiring the use of cardiopulmonary bypass (CPB) for a period of heart arrest, the lung also has to experience transient significant reduction of blood flow. It has been observed that such insult can increase pulmonary microvascular endothelium permeability, causing increased lung water retention and albumin leakage. Meanwhile, such insult also promotes neutrophil adhesion to endothelium and transmigration into lung interstitial and alveolar space, causing tissue inflammation. Consequently, lung function characterized by gas exchange is impaired, and the clinical features of acute lung injury result. In addition, endothelial dysfunction, manifested as decreased reactivity in the pulmonary circulation to infusions of acetylcholine, has been reported in both children[22] and adults[23,24] after heart surgery with CPB. As such, PVR often is increased in these patients after cardiac surgery. As it was also noted that the L-arginine concentration decreased significantly after surgery compared to the preoperative values,[24] a clear explanation for the change in the L-arginine/NO pathway and its relationship with impaired pulmonary function is desired.

11.3.1 Rapid Depletion of L-Arginine Pool During CPB

It had been found in patients with congenital heart disease that the plasma level of L-arginine dropped significantly after surgical correction with the use of CPB. The reasons for that decrease are not only associated with hemodilution by priming fluids but also related to reduced synthesis and increased metabolism due to CPB-induced systemic inflammation. It has been shown that employment of CPB would induce the systemic inflammatory response syndrome (SIRS) due to direct contact of leukocytes with the CPB circuit, therefore causing massive induction of iNOS.[25] Unlike nNOS and eNOS, the activity of iNOS is independent of intracellular Ca^{2+} level as calmodulin almost has no regulatory effects on it. As a result, sudden increment of L-arginine metabolism due to SIRS will inevitably subject all organs, including the lung, to a reduced L-arginine substrate pool. In addition, the massively activated acute inflammatory cells, including macrophages and neutrophils, during CPB will further exhaust the L-arginine pool via not only the NOS[26] but also the arginase pathway, the product of which is L-ornithine and urea. It has been indicated that whole-body inflammation induced by burn injuries can cause reduced de novo synthesis of L-arginine[27,28] and increased rate of L-arginine disposal, as reflected by equivalent increases in L-ornithine turnover and oxidation,[29] which suggests that this amino acid may become a conditionally indispensable amino acid if large-scale systemic inflammation occurs abruptly. For example, Schapira et al. found that lung inflammatory cells increased L-arginine uptake and its metabolism via both NOS and arginase pathways following in vivo silica exposure, which plays a significant role in the fast depletion of extracellular L-arginine content in the lung.[30] Another study further indicated that, when PAECs encounter circulating proinflammatory cytokines such as interleukin (IL) 1β, IL-6, and tumor necrosis factor alpha (TNF-α), they can increase iNOS and arginase expression, which is mediated by the Src family tyrosine kinase signaling pathway.[31]

11.3.2 Change of NOS Catalyzing Property Due to L-Arginine Shortage

The known NOS enzymes are usually referred to as "dimeric" in their active form, containing both reductase and oxygenase domains. In the presence of sufficient L-arginine, NADPH, and O_2, they catalyze the reaction to form NO, L-citrulline, and Nicotinamide adenine dinucleotide phosphate (NADP). During the reaction, electrons are donated by NADPH to the reductase

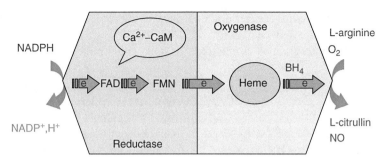

Fig. 11.1 Nitric oxide synthases (NOSs) exhibit a bidomain structure in which an N-terminal oxygenase domain containing binding sites for heme, BH_4 (tetrahydrobiopterin), and L-arginine is linked by a calmodulin (CaM) recognition site to a C-terminal reductase domain that contains binding sites for flavin adenine dinucleotide (FAD), flavin mononucleotide (FMN), and nicotinamide adenine dinucleotide phosphate (NADPH). NADPH donates electrons to the reductase domain and these electrons proceed via FAD and FMN to the oxygenase domain. Then, they interact with the heme iron and BH_4 to catalyze the reaction between oxygen and L-arginine, generating L-citrulline andni tricoxi de(NO)

domain of the enzyme and proceed via flavin adenine dinucleotide (FAD) and flavin mononucleotide (FMN) in sequence to the oxygenase domain. Then, they interact with the heme iron and tetrahydrobiopterin to catalyze the reaction of O_2 with L-arginine, generating L-citrulline and NO as products (Fig. 11.1).

When L-arginine tends to be inadequate (e.g., during CPB), NOS can catalyze an "uncoupled" NADPH oxidation (uncoupled with NO formation), forming superoxide. All three isoforms can make such a shift, although the respective inclinations toward it vary. It appears that nNOS has a particular propensity to catalyze this uncoupled reaction at a subsaturating level of L-arginine (i.e., below the K_m). In contrast, eNOS appears to have the least penchant. Because of the rapid reaction of superoxide with NO, synthesis of both species by the same enzyme is likely to result in peroxynitrite formation under such circumstances.

11.3.3 Lung Ischemia Followed by Reperfusion: A Further Nightmare for Endangered L-Arginine/NO Pathway

During lung ischemia, consistent provision of L-arginine is not available. Moreover, local hypoxia resulting from both ischemia and termination of ventilation further impairs the transport of L-arginine across the cell membrane. It has been shown that, when oxygen concentration is lowered below 5%, cultured PAECs experience significantly reduced transportation of extracellular L-arginine[4] due to hypoxia-induced decreasing membrane potential, a driving force for transport via system y+.[32] Meanwhile, during the ischemic period, there exists severe metabolic derangement, including hypoxia-anoxia, acidosis, and depletion of high-energy phosphates.

At the initial stage of lung reperfusion, refill of the depleted extracellular and intracellular L-arginine pool for various cells, including PAECs and entrapped inflammatory cells, requires a relatively long period. In contrast, refueling of tissue O_2 content is instantaneous due to its significantly higher transmembrane diffusion rate. As a result, NOS, including those newly formed NOS during CPB (especially iNOS), begins to catalyze the "uncoupled" NADPH oxidation, forming superoxide. In turn, the newly formed superoxide acts like an in situ scavenger of NO, which is gradually synthesized during the process of replenishment of the L-arginine pool in the cytosol, to form a powerful oxidant, that is, peroxynitrite. When biological systems are exposed to peroxynitrite, a multitude of adverse effects proceeds subsequently with potential risk to the viability and function of cells.[33] It can impair the function of endothelial cells by modifying actin[34] and increasing adhesion molecule expression,[35] the result of which includes increased albumin leakage from the blood into the lung[36] and pulmonary fluid accumulation.[37] They can increase stimulated neutrophils to adhere to endothelium and transmigrate into interstitial tissue.[9] In the mean time, the tissue NO level remains low, the result of which is further deterioration of the microvascular endothelium, reduced control of neutrophil adhesion and transmigration, as well as plateleta ggregation.

11.4 Effectso fExo genous L-Arginine on Lung Experiencing I/R Injury

As evidence-based research has gradually revealed that disturbance of the L-arginine/NO pathway plays a major role in the development of lung I/R injury, it seems reasonable to test the effects of exogenous L-arginine. So far, the majority of research indicated that administration of L-arginine is beneficial in reducing lung I/R injury.

11.4.1 Reduced Deterioration of Microvascular Permeability and PVR After Lung I/R Injury

In a groundbreaking study by Moore et al., it was proved that NO played a key role in reducing microvascular damage.[38] With isolated buffer-perfused rat lung as the I/R model, they found that its microvascular permeability K_f significantly increased after 45 min of ischemia followed by 30 min of reperfusion. Lung that was pretreated with NOS inhibitors showed even worse increases in K_f after I/R. In contrast, use of NO donors such as spermine-NO and *S*-nitroso-*N*-acetylpenacillamine could prevent such increase. Similar results were also reported by other groups when L-arginine was used as the NO donor. For instance, with isolated rabbit lung as the I/R model, Yoshida et al. found that 2 h of warm ischemia followed by reperfusion incurred double increment of K_f. In contrast, attenuated deterioration of K_f and PVR could be achieved when L-arginine was added into the perfusate. As a further proof of L-arginine/NO pathway involvement, simultaneous use of L-NAME with L-arginine or addition of D-arginine alone all significantly reduced the beneficial effects of L-arginine.[39]

A potential mechanism by which NO prevents I/R-induced increase in microvascular permeability may be related to the maintenance of the intracellular cGMP level in endothelium as it was found that use of dibutyryl-cGMP (a membrane permeant cGMP analog), also provided protective effects. As a result, L-arginine-mediated lung protection against I/R injury possibly is via increased endothelial NO production and resultant increment of endothelial cGMP content. Another potential explanation is that L-arginine-derived NO inhibits the activation of inflammatory cells (neutrophils, mast cells, and macrophages), which further inhibits neutrophil adhesion and transmigration.[40]

11.4.2 Mitigated Lung Inflammatory Injury

Of course, the beneficial effect with the use of L-arginine is also related to its inhibiting effects on SIRS. It has been established that the activated neutrophils, once having transmigrated into the lung interstitium, will damage the lung tissue by producing oxygen metabolites and releasing lysosomal enzymes. As L-arginine-derived NO has been proposed to be capable of reducing neutrophil chemotaxis, activation, and adherence to endothelial cells, effects of exogenous L-arginine on lung inflammatory injury have been studied. Sheridan et al. found that L-arginine could reduce endotoxin-induced neutrophil accumulation in the lung by more than 50%.[41] The results from our most recent study also supported this notion that L-arginine could reduce the extent of neutrophil infiltration in the lung tissue.[42]

This inhibitory effect of L-arginine is related to the attenuation of chemokine production, which is mediated by nuclear factor kappa B (NF-κB), an inducible transcription factor under the control of inhibitory factor kappa B (IκB), from the lung. For instance, Calkins et al.[43] examined the effect of L-arginine on the relationship of chemokine production with NF-κB DNA binding in the lung after systemic lipopolysaccharide-induced inflammation. They found that use of L-arginine could attenuate increased expression of chemokines, prevent reduction of intracellular IκB levels, and inhibited NF-κB DNA binding. Inhibition of NOS abolished the effects of L-arginine on all measured variables. As such, it could be inferred that L-arginine-derived NO could abrogate chemokine production during systemic inflammation. Reduced pulmonary retention of leukocytes further contributes to reduced lung water retention and improved pulmonary oxygenation. Also, the beneficial effects of exogenous L-arginine during acute lung injury may be partly attributable to decreased alveolar macrophage proinflammatory cytokine production, such as TNF-α and IL-1β.[44]

11.4.3 Improved Lung Surfactant Integrity After I/R Injury

The initial evidence indicating an interaction of pulmonary surfactant and L-arginine came from research focusing on understanding the relationship between NO and surfactant metabolism. Sun et al.[45] examined the effects of NO on lung surfactant secretion. They found that administration of L-NAME through the pulmonary circulation led to significantly decreased surfactant secretion. Further tests revealed that such inhibition mainly involved specific blockage of eNOS. Their subsequent investigation focusing on the NO signaling pathway revealed that NO-mediated surfactant secretion was related to cGMP and PKG within the alveolar type II cells. As a result, lack of sufficient NO production would inevitably lead to disturbed metabolism of surfactant and lung function.

Pulmonary vascular endothelium is a major source of NO production, and its impairment would inevitably impair surfactant production and secretion. Of course, leakage of serum proteins into the alveoli due to increased filtration could further aggravate surfactant dysfunction due to direct inhibition.[46]

11.5 PracticalC onsideration When Administration of L-Arginine Is Planned

11.5.1 Timing for L-Arginine Use

As reduced bioavailability of L-arginine within the lung tissue usually begins at the initial stage of CPB due to hemodilution and inflammation-induced exhaustion, the optimal timing for administration of L-arginine aimed at prevention of lung I/R injury is therefore at the beginning of CPB, which is well before the onset of lung ischemia. For example, it was proved that, during inflammation, proinflammatory cytokines and endotoxin quickly stimulate the expression of iNOS in endothelial cells, smooth muscle cells, macrophages, neutrophils, and other cell types,[47,48] whereas early administration of exogenous L-arginine can prevent endotoxin-induced neutrophil accumulation in the lung and attenuate associated impairment of endothelium-dependent cGMP-mediated pulmonary vascular smooth muscle relaxation.[41] What is more, even without preceding hemodilution and CPB-induced SIRS, L-arginine within the lung tissue was immediately depleted when the lung experienced microembolism-induced ischemia.[49] It is speculated that increased superoxide generation during ischemia leads to eNOS uncoupling through increased oxidative stress-induced oxidation and depletion of tetrahydrobiopterin, a cofactor required for NO synthesis.[50] As described in the previous section, administration of L-arginine after ischemia may further increase superoxide/peroxynitrite formation, thus interfering with its protective potential.

As a result, early administration of L-arginine may be a better option to ensure optimal protective effects in reducing lung I/R injury, whereas its delayed use may be simply too late.[49] Giving further support to this argument, an early pilot clinical study for patients undergoing cardiac surgery showed that delayed use of L-arginine had no influence on increased postoperative PVR. In that study, 20 adult patients, with ischemic or valvular cardiac disease and presenting significant reduction of PVR during acetylcholine administration before surgery, were randomized to receive L-arginine or placebo. The dose of L-arginine was 30 mg·kg^{-1} administered as a bolus 5 min before declamping of the aorta, followed by a continuous infusion of 300 mg·kg^{-1}·h^{-1} until 2 h after CPB. In the placebo group, saline was given in the same volumes (bolus and infusion). In contrast, to test if a lower concentration would also be effective in humans, a much smaller dose was given to a few pilot patients. These patients received a bolus dose of 1 mg·kg^{-1} followed by an infusion of 10 mg·kg^{-1}·h^{-1}, the administration of which was started before surgery. The results from those pilot patients revealed a better-maintained reactivity to acetylcholine. Of course, if L-arginine cannot be used before the onset of ischemia, its delayed use might still be beneficial. For example, Schulze-Neick et al. found that intravenous infusion of 15 mg·kg^{-1}·min^{-1} L-arginine even at 2 h after CPB could reduce PVR by about 15% for young patients with congenital heart diseases,[51] which indicated that lack of sufficient substrate pool played a significant role in the escalation of postoperative PVR. As such, it seems that dysfunction of pulmonary artery endothelium due to a short period of I/R injury with the use CPB remains controllable.

11.5.2 Additional Exclusive Perfusion with L-Arginine During Lung Ischemia

Based on pathophysiology of lung I/R injury during cardiac operation involving the use of CPB, depletion of L-arginine and other important nutrients indeed occurs during heart arrest. During this period, pulmonary blood flow from systemic circulation is completely terminated, which becomes a key rationale for the recommendation of continuous pulmonary replenishment of L-arginine. Our most recent research indicated that continuous infusion of L-arginine into the pulmonary circulation during this stage could provide protection against lung injury. With piglets as an animal model, we initially decreased body temperature through hypothermic CPB to 18°C followed by circulatory arrest for 90 min. During this period, antegrade infusion of L-arginine was provided via a cannula secured inside the main pulmonary artery. At 4 h after rewarming, L-arginine significantly mitigated the deterioration of pulmonary static compliance, pulmonary oxygenation index, PVR, and pulmonary surfactant. In addition, water retention and neutrophil sequestration were significantly reduced.[42] As a result, it appears that continuous provision of substrate in lung is beneficial during its ischemic period. Of course, its clinical efficiency remains to be further determined.

11.5.3 Inhibition of iNOS: A New Strategy in Adjusting L-Arginine/NO Pathway

Exclusive administration of exogenous L-arginine may not be enough to maximally reduce the extent of lung I/R injury when CPB is applied. Although newly expressed iNOS inside inflammatory cells such as neutrophils has been indicated to be beneficial in limiting its lung sequestration, its massive expression in both inflammatory cells and other cell types still easily jeopardizes the L-arginine pool. As a result, identification of selective inhibitors of iNOS has been proposed as a goal for both academic and pharmaceutical researchers. The observation of very high structural homology between the heme domains of iNOS and eNOS[52] initially led to pessimism regarding the potential to identify specific inhibitors of iNOS. Fortunately, identification of several inhibitors with more than 100-fold selectivity for iNOS vs. eNOS translates to a renewed optimism. Among all these selective inhibitors, 1,400 W appears to have the greatest potential for its clinical translation as it is not only highly selective as an iNOS inhibitor vs. both eNOS and nNOS but also can enter different cell types.[53]

11.6 Summary

Although many other components of pulmonary I/R injury have been studied in the past, one important research branch of contemporary studies is the L-arginine/NO pathway, which arguably is the most clinically important system for vasodilation and inflammatory syndrome. Furthermore, abnormalities of this pathway probably reflect an early stage of acute lung injury, preceding irreversible, histological changes. Defining the function of the L-arginine/NO pathway should pave the way to a better understanding and ultimately a more focused treatment of lung I/R injury.

References

1. Carvalho EM, Gabriel EA, Salerno TA. Pulmonary protection during cardiac surgery: systematic literature review. *Asian Cardiovasc Thorac Ann*.2008; 16(6):503-507.
2. Palmer RM, Ferrige AG, Moncada S. Nitric oxide release accounts for the biological activity of endothelium-derived relaxing factor. *Nature*.1987; 327(6122):524-526.
3. Alderton WK, Cooper CE, Knowles RG. Nitric oxide synthases: structure, function and inhibition. *Biochem J.* 2001;357(pt3) :593-615.
4. Block ER, Herrera H, Couch M. Hypoxia inhibits L-arginine uptake by pulmonary artery endothelial cells. *Am J Physiol*. 1995;269(5 pt 1):L574-L580.
5. Zheng XF, Kwan CY, Daniel EE. Role of intracellular Ca2+ in EDRF release in rat aorta. *J Vasc Res*.1994; 31(1):18-24.
6. Feron O, Saldana F, Michel JB, Michel T. The endothelial nitric-oxide synthase-caveolin regulatory cycle. *J Biol Chem*. 1998;273(6):3125-3128.
7. McDonald KK, Zharikov S, Block ER, Kilberg MS. A caveolar complex between the cationic amino acid transporter 1 and endothelial nitric-oxide synthase may explain the "arginine paradox". *J Biol Chem*.1997; 272(50):31213-31216.

8. Mundy AL, Dorrington KL. Inhibition of nitric oxide synthesis augments pulmonary oedema in isolated perfused rabbit lung. *Br J Anaesth*.2000; 85(4):570-576.

9. Shelton JL, Wang L, Cepinskas G, Inculet R, Mehta S. Human neutrophil-pulmonary microvascular endothelial cell interactions in vitro: differential effects of nitric oxide vs. peroxynitrite. *Microvasc Res*.2008; 76(2):80-88.

10. Farley KS, Wang LF, Razavi HM, et al. Effects of macrophage inducible nitric oxide synthase in murine septic lung injury. *Am J Physiol Lung Cell Mol Physiol*. 2006;290(6):L1164-L1172.

11. Sittipunt C, Steinberg KP, Ruzinski JT, et al. Nitric oxide and nitrotyrosine in the lungs of patients with acute respiratory distress syndrome. *Am J Respir Crit Care Med*. 2001;163(2):503-510.

12. Razavi HM, Wang IF, Weicker S, et al. Pulmonary neutrophil infiltration in murine sepsis: role of inducible nitric oxide synthase. *Am J Respir Crit Care Med*. 2004;170(3):227-233.

13. Schmidt HH, Lohmann SM, Walter U. The nitric oxide and cGMP signal transduction system: regulation and mechanism of action. *Biochim Biophys Acta*. 1993;1178(2):153-175.

14. Dal SD, Paron JA, de Oliveira SH, Ferreira SH, Silva JS, Cunha FQ. Neutrophil migration in inflammation: nitric oxide inhibits rolling, adhesion and induces apoptosis. *Nitric Oxide*.2003;9(3):153- 164.

15. Dal SD, Moreira AP, Freitas A, et al. Nitric oxide inhibits neutrophil migration by a mechanism dependent on ICAM-1: role of soluble guanylate cyclase. *Nitric Oxide*. 2006; 15(1):77-86.

16. Rios-Santos F, ves Filho JC, Souto FO, et al. Downregulation of CXCR2 on neutrophils in severe sepsis is mediated by inducible nitric oxide synthase-derived nitric oxide. *Am J Respir Crit Care Med*.2007; 175(5):490-497.

17. Emerson M, Momi S, Paul W, Alberti PF, Page C, Gresele P. Endogenous nitric oxide acts as a natural antithrombotic agent in vivo by inhibiting platelet aggregation in the pulmonary vasculature. *Thromb Haemost*.1999; 81(6):961-966.

18. Nong Z, Hoylaerts M, Van PN, Collen D, Janssens S. Nitric oxide inhalation inhibits platelet aggregation and platelet-mediated pulmonary thrombosis in rats. *Circ Res*. 1997;81(5):865-869.

19. Gries A, Bottiger BW, Dorsam J, et al. Inhaled nitric oxide inhibits platelet aggregation after pulmonary embolism in pigs. *Anesthesiology*.1997; 86(2):387-393.

20. Gkaliagkousi E, Ritter J, Ferro A. Platelet-derived nitric oxide signaling and regulation. *Circ Res*. 2007;101(7):654-662.

21. Radomski MW, Palmer RM, Moncada S. Characterization of the L-arginine:nitric oxide pathway in human platelets. *Br J Pharmacol*.1990 ;101(2):325-328.

22. Wessel DL, Adatia I, Giglia TM, Thompson JE, Kulik TJ. Use of inhaled nitric oxide and acetylcholine in the evaluation of pulmonary hypertension and endothelial function after cardiopulmonary bypass. *Circulation*. 1993;88(5 pt 1):2128-2138.

23. Angdin M, Settergren G, Astudillo R, Liska J. Altered reactivity to acetylcholine in the pulmonary circulation after cardiopulmonary bypass is part of reperfusion injury. *J Clin Anesth*.1998;10(2) :126-132.

24. Angdin M, Settergren G. Acetylcholine reactivity in the pulmonary artery during cardiac surgery in patients with ischemic or valvular heart disease. *J Cardiothorac Vasc Anesth*.1997;11(4) :458-462.

25. Hayashi Y, Sawa Y, Fukuyama N, Nakazawa H, Matsuda H. Inducible nitric oxide production is an adaptation to cardiopulmonary bypass-induced inflammatory response. *Ann Thorac Surg*.2001; 72(1):149-155.

26. Yuen IS, Hartsky MA, Snajdr SI, Warheit DB. Time course of chemotactic factor generation and neutrophil recruitment in the lungs of dust-exposed rats. *Am J Respir Cell Mol Biol*. 1996;15(2):268-274.

27. Yu YM, Ryan CM, Burke JF, Tompkins RG, Young VR. Relations among arginine, citrulline, ornithine, and leucine kinetics in adult burn patients. *Am J Clin Nutr*. 1995;62(5): 960-968.

28. Yu YM, Sheridan RL, Burke JF, Chapman TE, Tompkins RG, Young VR. Kinetics of plasma arginine and leucine in pediatric burn patients. *Am J Clin Nutr*.1996; 64(1):60-66.

29. Yu YM, Ryan CM, Castillo L, et al. Arginine and ornithine kinetics in severely burned patients: increased rate of arginine disposal. *Am J Physiol Endocrinol Metab*. 2001; 280(3):E509-E517.

30. Schapira RM, Wiessner JH, Morrisey JF, Almagro UA, Nelin LD. L-arginine uptake and metabolism by lung macrophages and neutrophils following intratracheal instillation of silica in vivo. *Am J Respir Cell Mol Biol*. 1998;19(2):308-315.

31. Chang R, Chicoine LG, Cui H, et al. Cytokine-induced arginase activity in pulmonary endothelial cells is dependent on Src family tyrosine kinase activity. *Am J Physiol Lung Cell Mol Physiol*.2008; 295(4):L688-L697.

32. Zharikov SI, Herrera H, Block ER. Role of membrane potential in hypoxic inhibition of L-arginine uptake by lung endothelial cells. *Am J Physiol*. 1997;272(1 pt 1): L78-L84.

33. Szabo C, Ischiropoulos H, Radi R. Peroxynitrite: biochemistry, pathophysiology and development of therapeutics. *Nat Rev Drug Discov*.2007; 6(8):662-680.

34. Gao J, Zhao WX, Zhou LJ, et al. Protective effects of propofol on lipopolysaccharide-activated endothelial cell barrier dysfunction. *Inflamm Res*.2006; 55(9):385-392.

35. Mazzon E, De SA, Caputi AP, Cuzzocrea S. Role of tight junction derangement in the endothelial dysfunction elicited by exogenous and endogenous peroxynitrite and poly(ADP-ribose) synthetase. *Shock*.2002; 18(5):434-439.

36. Shelton JL, Wang L, Cepinskas G, et al. Inducible NO synthase (iNOS) in human neutrophils but not pulmonary microvascular endothelial cells (PMVEC) mediates septic protein leak in vitro. *Microvasc Res*.2007; 74(1):23-31.

37. Beckman DL, Mehta P, Hanks V, Rowan WH, Liu L. Effects of peroxynitrite on pulmonary edema and the oxidative state. *Exp Lung Res*.2000; 26(5):349-359.

38. Moore TM, Khimenko PL, Wilson PS, Taylor AE. Role of nitric oxide in lung ischemia and reperfusion injury. *Am J Physiol*. 1996;271(5 pt 2):H1970-H1977.

39. Yoshida K, Yoshimura K, Haniuda M. L-arginine inhibits ischemia-reperfusion lung injury in rabbits. *J Surg Res*. 1999;85(1):9-16.

40. Kubes P, Suzuki M, Granger DN. Nitric oxide: an endogenous modulator of leukocyte adhesion. *Proc Natl Acad Sci U S A*.1991; 88(11):4651-4655.

41. Sheridan BC, McIntyre RC Jr, Meldrum DR, Fullerton DA. L-arginine prevents lung neutrophil accumulation and preserves pulmonary endothelial function after endotoxin. *Am J Physiol*. 1998;274(3 pt 1):L337-L342.

42. Yang Y, Su Z, Cai J, et al. Continuous pulmonary infusion of L-arginine during deep hypothermia and circulatory arrest improves pulmonary surfactant integrity in piglets. *Ann Thorac Surg*.2008;86(2):429-435.

43. Calkins CM, Bensard DD, Heimbach JK, et al. L-arginine attenuates lipopolysaccharide-induced lung chemokine production. *Am J Physiol Lung Cell Mol Physiol*. 2001;280(3):L400-L408.

44. Meldrum DR, McIntyre RC, Sheridan BC, Cleveland JC Jr, Fullerton DA, Harken AH. L-arginine decreases alveolar macrophage proinflammatory monokine production during acute lung injury by a nitric oxide synthase-dependent mechanism. *J Trauma*.1997; 43(6):888-893.

45. Sun P, Wang J, Mehta P, Beckman DL, Liu L. Effect of nitric oxide on lung surfactant secretion. *Exp Lung Res*. 2003;29(5):303-314.

46. Bruni R, Fan BR, David-Cu R, Taeusch HW, Walther FJ. Inactivation of surfactant in rat lungs. *Pediatr Res*. 1996;39(2):236-240.

47. Liaudet L, Soriano FG, Szabo C. Biology of nitric oxide signaling. *Crit Care Med*.2000; 28(4s uppl):N37-N52.

48. Aktan F. iNOS-mediated nitric oxide production and its regulation. *Life Sci*.2004; 75(6):639-653.

49. Souza-Costa DC, Zerbini T, Metzger IF, Rocha JB, Gerlach RF, Tanus-Santos JE. l-Arginine attenuates acute pulmonary embolism-induced oxidative stress and pulmonary hypertension. *Nitric Oxide*.2005; 12(1):9-14.

50. Li H, Wallerath T, Munzel T, Forstermann U. Regulation of endothelial-type NO synthase expression in pathophysiology and in response to drugs. *Nitric Oxide*. 2002;7(3):149-164.

51. Schulze-Neick I, Penny DJ, Rigby ML, et al. L-arginine and substance P reverse the pulmonary endothelial dysfunction caused by congenital heart surgery. *Circulation*. 1999;100(7):749-755.

52. Fischmann TO, Hruza A, Niu XD, et al. Structural characterization of nitric oxide synthase isoforms reveals striking active-site conservation. *Nat Struct Biol*. 1999;6(3):233-242.

53. Garvey EP, Oplinger JA, Furfine ES, et al. 1400W is a slow, tight binding, and highly selective inhibitor of inducible nitric-oxide synthase in vitro and in vivo. *J Biol Chem*. 1997;272(8):4959-4963.

The Role of Nitric Oxide in Pulmonary Ischemia-Reperfusion Injury

12

Peter Donndorf, Alexander Kaminski, and Gustav Steinhoff

Impaired pulmonary function remains a major clinical problem in a variety of settings, such as shock, lung transplantation, and cardiac surgery with cardiopulmonary bypass or circulatory arrest. Pulmonary damage in this context is often associated with ischemia-reperfusion injury, leading to endothelial dysfunction, capillary leakage, and an intense neutrophilic inflammatory response. Clinically, this is recognized as a progressive deterioration in gas exchange, opacification of the chest X-ray, and increased pulmonary vascular resistance.[1]

Nitric oxide (NO) is well known as a potent vasodilator and is mainly involved in the vasomotor regulation after ischemia-reperfusion. Furthermore, NO is believed to modulate postischemic tissue damage, exhibiting both pro- and anti-inflammatory actions, and may therefore significantly modulate ischemia-reperfusion injury.[2,3]

12.1 Nitric Oxide and Nitric Oxide-Producing Enzymes

NO is produced by nitric oxide synthase (NOS), a heme-containing enzyme that is linked to Nictotinamide dinucleotide phospphate (NADPH)-derived electron transport by flavin adenine dinucleotide and flavin mononucleotide. There are three isoforms of NOS. All these isoforms produce NO via oxidation of its precursor arginine.[4] Endothelial NOS (eNOS) is constitutively expressed by vascular endothelial cells. It has a calcium-dependent activity and generates relatively low levels of NO. The NO produced by eNOS mediates a variety of physiological functions in vivo, including regulation of blood vessel tone, neovascularization and stem cell recruitment, platelet aggregation, vascular permeability, and leukocyte-endothelial interaction.[5,6]

By contrast, inducible NOS (iNOS) is transcriptionally regulated by inflammatory cytokines and other stimuli; it is calcium independent and generates higher levels of NO than eNOS, which can induce cytostatic or toxic effects. Finally, neuronal NOS (nNOS) mediates the transmission of neuronal signals.[6] Pathways by with NO may mediate cytotoxic effects include the ability to form peroxynitrate and thereby the impairment of mitochondrial function, the inhibition of Na^+/K^+ ATPase (adenosine triphosphatase) activity and other oxidative protein modifications.[7] On the other hand, NO is believed to prevent vascular remodeling and to protect against ischemia-reperfusion injury via its scavenging capacity for reactive oxygen species and inhibition of leukocyte adhesion to the microvascular endothelium.[8]

In this chapter, we focus on the role of NO and NOS in modulating ischemia-reperfusion injury.

12.2 Protective Role of Endothelial Nitric Oxide Synthase in Pulmonary Ischemia-Reperfusion Injury

The eNOS isoform has been identified as the predominant isoform upregulated during pulmonary ischemia-reperfusion.[9] Kaminski et al. were able to show that postischemic upregulation of eNOS limits the local inflammatory cell infiltration in the mouse lung

P.D onndorf (✉)
Department of Cardiac Surgery, University of Rostock, Rostock, Germany
e-mail: pe ter.donndorf@med.uni-rostock.de

E.A. Gabriel and T. Salerno (eds.), *Principles of Pulmonary Protection in Heart Surgery*,
DOI: 10.1007/978-1-84996-308-4_12, © Springer-Verlag London Limited 2010

107

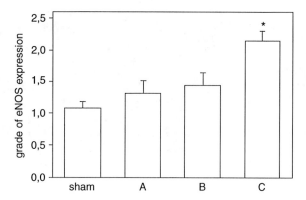

Fig. 12.1 Average immunohistochemical expression of pulmonary endothelial nitric oxide synthase (eNOS) protein is displayed in sham-operated control lungs (*sham*) and left lungs exposed to 1 h of ischemia, followed by 0.5 h of reperfusion (*group A*), 5 h of reperfusion (*group B*), or 24 h of reperfusion (*group C*). Experiments were performed in wild-type (WT) animals. Mean± standard deviation; $*p < 0.05$v ersuss ham

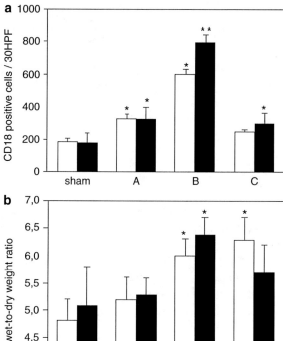

Fig. 12.2 (**a**) Quantitative assessment of the number of CD18-positive cells in alveolar interstitium of pulmonary tissue from sham-operated lungs (*sham*)and left lungs exposed to 1 h of ischemia followed by 0.5 h of reperfusion (*group A*), 5 h of reperfusion (*group B*), or 24 h of reperfusion (*group C*). *Open bars* indicate data from wild-type (WT) mice, while *filled bars* indicate data from endothelial nitric oxide synthase knockout (eNOS-KO) mice. Mean±standard deviation; $*p < 0.05$ versus sham, $\# p < 0.05$ versus WT mice. (**b**) Quantitative assessment of wet-to-dry weight ratio of pulmonary tissue from sham-operated lungs (*sham*) and left lungs exposed to 1 h of ischemia, followed by 0.5 h of reperfusion (*group A*), 5 h of reperfusion (*group B*), or 24 h of reperfusion (*group C*). *Open bars* indicate data from WT mice, while *filled bars* indicate data from eNOS-KO mice. Mean ± standard deviation; $*p < 0.05$v ersuss ham

(Fig. 12.1). Animals lacking the gene for the eNOS (eNOS knockout) showed increased leukocyte infiltration of lung tissue after a pulmonary ischemia-reperfusion maneuver. Furthermore, eNOS knockout animals revealed higher lung tissue water content and an increased postoperative mortality after pulmonary ischemia-reperfusion (Fig. 12.2). The mechanism linking eNOS expression and postischemic leukocyte infiltration seems to involve endothelial vascular cell adhesion molecule (VCAM) transcription, as evidenced by higher messenger RNA (mRNA) and protein levels in postischemic eNOS knockout animals (Fig. 12.3). It has been well established that activation and migration of polymorphonuclear leukocytes into lung tissue contributes to inflammatory tissue injury and pathological remodeling of tissue architecture.[10]

The view that eNOS is the key isoform in the non-septic pulmonary stress response was further supported by the findings of Fagan et al., who demonstrated a predominant upregulation of eNOS in a mouse model of chronic severe hypoxia.[11] The hypothesis that eNOS upregulation might be a protective response to pulmonary ischemia is also supported by the increased susceptibility of eNOS knockout mice for postischemic reperfusion injury. These animals die more often than similar treated wild-type animals, presenting severe symptoms of pulmonary edema, indicating a disruption of the endothelial-alveolar barrier with acute fluid extravasation. Although parameters of lung injury have been found more modest in surviving animals, it is still reasonable to speculate that eNOS deficiency is responsible for aggravation of local inflammation, as indicated by significantly higher postischemic leukocyte infiltration in eNOS knockout animals versus wild-type animals. Taken together, there is strong evidence that endogenous upregulation of eNOS is a protective mechanism against inflammatory pulmonary tissue damage following ischemia-reperfusion. For this reason, therapeutic strategies to augment eNOS expression may help to improve postischemic pulmonary function in clinical settings.

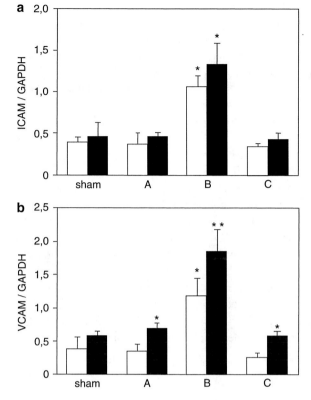

Fig. 12.3 Densitometric assessment of pulmonary (**a**) intercellular adhesion molecule 1 (ICAM-1) to Glyceraldehyde 3 phosphate dehydrogenase (GAPDH) transcript ratio and (**b**) vascular cell adhesion molecule (VCAM) to GAPDH transcript ratio in sham-operated control lungs (*sham*) and left lungs exposed to 1 h of ischemia followed by 0.5 h of reperfusion (*group A*), 5 h of reperfusion (*group B*), or 24 h of reperfusion (*group C*). *Open bars* indicate data from wild-type (WT) mice, while *filled bars* indicate data from endothelial nitric oxide synthase knockout (eNOS-KO) mice. Mean ± standard deviation; *$p < 0.05$ versus sham, # $p < 0.05$ versuss ham

12.3 Importanceo fN itricOxi def or Hypothermic Protection Against Ischemia-Reperfusion Injury

Injury of the endothelium is a frequent consequence of an ischemic insult. During reperfusion, release of oxygen radicals and proinflammatory cytokines can also harm endothelial function.[12] Several experimental and clinical studies have shown the protective action of hypothermia against postischemic inflammatory and endothelial function.[13] In accordance with these reports, Zhang et al. were able to show that intraischemic mild hypothermia dramatically attenuates lung injury and abolishes mortality during the reperfusion period in mice. Moreover, they found that the beneficial effect of mild hypothermia during lung ischemia is dependent on the presence of eNOS and even is associated with eNOS overexpression as mild hypothermia significantly reduced endothelial disturbance after ischemia-reperfusion in wild-type mice but not in mice lacking the gene for eNOS.[14] Several studies have investigated the role of NO during ischemia-reperfusion injury in brain and mesenteric tissue. It was found that the protective effect of intraischemic hypothermia is associated with suppression of iNOS/nNOS expression and NO release during reperfusion. In contrast to these findings, an *augmentation* of the expression of the eNOS seems to play a substantial role in hypothermia-induced protection of lungs. The importance of the eNOS in this regard was demonstrated by two lines of evidence: First, hypothermia-induced protection against ischemia-reperfusion injury is completely abolished in eNOS knockout mice. Second, hypothermia is associated with postischemic upregulation of eNOS.[14] Liu et al.[16] demonstrated a marked increase of eNOS expression in rat lungs after hypothermic ischemia within 2 h of reperfusion.[15] How hypothermia may affect the eNOS expression is still unclear. The eNOS expression is a function of balance between protein synthesis and degradation. Regulation of this process is complex, and the exact analysis of the mechanisms involved in hypothermia-induced upregulation of eNOS still needs to be done.

12.4 EndothelialN itricOxi de Synthase and Hypoxic Preconditioning in Lungs

The protective effects of hypoxic treatment before ischemia-reperfusion injury have been noted. For several organs, it has been shown that hypoxic preconditioning improves tolerance to an ischemic injury. Oxidant radicals are thought to mediate protection by hypoxic preconditioning in the heart,[16] and activation of the transcription factor hypoxia-inducible factor 1 by hypoxic and oxidative stress seems to induce a specific target gene expression pattern.[15] One of these target genes, eNOS, is known to be upregulated following hypoxia in the heart and to induce an increase in ischemic tolerance after ischemic preconditioning in the rat liver[17] and in cultured human coronary artery endothelial cells.

For the lung, our group was able to show that the absence of eNOS expression reverses the protective effects of hypoxic preconditioning, suggesting that eNOS does play an active role in pulmonary protection against ischemia-reperfusion injury by hypoxic preconditioning.[18] In this context, the altered functional performance of endothelial cells during local NO-mediated relaxation with preservation of endothelial barrier function might be just as important as eNOS-related changes in adhesion molecule expression pattern and modified leukocyte migration behavior. The differential effect of eNOS on both preservation of endothelial barrier function and neutrophil cell migration in the lungs has not been clearly explained until recently, but, for example, Blais and coworkers have suggested eNOS-derived NO as an endogenous inhibitor of tumor necrosis factor alpha (TNF-α)-induced nuclear factor kappa B (NF-κB) activation and cyclooxygenase 2 (COX-2) transcription.[19]

All in all, eNOS seems to be particularly relevant for preservation of endothelial permeability and attenuation of leukocyte infiltration achieved by hypoxia-based preconditioning protocols.

12.5 Inhaled Nitric Oxide and Ischemia-Reperfusion Injury

From the experimental results discussed, one can conclude that NO might be a promising therapeutic agent in cardiothoracic surgery to modulate ischemia-reperfusion injury occurring during cardiopulmonary bypass. One way of taking advantage of the possible beneficial effects of NO is the use of NO inhalation before and during cardiothoracic operations. Inhaled NO has been shown to preserve cardiac function after ischemia-reperfusion in rats. Geury and colleagues found that breathing air with NO for 4 h before coronary artery occlusion and reperfusion led to improved systolic and diastolic function.[20] In line with these results, Hataishi et al. were able to show that breathing NO decreased myocardial infarction size in mice subjected to different times of cardiac ischemia followed by reperfusion. In clinical use, inhaled NO has been shown to reduce pulmonary vascular resistance, pulmonary hypertension of the newborn, and severe

pulmonary hypertension in adults.[21] These same effects can also be seen in cardiac surgery patients, including children with congenital cardiopathy during hemodynamic diagnostic investigations after pediatric and adult surgical corrections.[1] Furthermore, a number of uncontrolled clinical studies have demonstrated that inhalation of NO (20–40 ppm) effectively decreases pulmonary artery pressure (PAP) when coronary artery bypass grafting or surgery of valvular heart disease is complicated by perioperative pulmonary hypertension.[22] As the pulmonary vasodilator effects of NO are transient when the gas is discontinued, it must be administered continuously with careful monitoring of NO and NO^2 concentrations. Commercially available equipment permits the safe delivery of NO gas in intubated and nonintubated patients. In the presence of severe left ventricular failure, administration of NO to relieve pulmonary vasoconstriction may augment left ventricular filling and raise the pulmonary capillary wedge pressure. Therefore, caution should be exercised when patients with severe left ventricular failure are treated with NO.[23] Regarding the treatment of ischemia-reperfusion injury, some small uncontrolled clinical trials have been performed. While two studies suggested that inhaled NO might be protective in patients who develop lung ischemia-reperfusion injury,[24,25] a small, randomized, placebo-controlled trial demonstrated that inhaling NO (20 ppm) commencing 20 min after reperfusion did not affect the clinical or physiological outcome of patients after lung transplantation.[26] Additional studies will be required to define the therapeutic role of inhaled NO in cardiothoracic surgery and its possible impact on preventing ischemia-reperfusion injury in the lung.

12.6 Exhaled Nitric Oxide as a Diagnostic Parameter in Cardiac Surgery

As discussed, one major consequence of ischemia-reperfusion injury is endothelial damage and dysfunction, which may affect the release of NO. Endothelial dysfunction in the lung with consecutive attenuated pulmonary vasodilation has been demonstrated both in children and in adults. However, detecting this endothelial dysfunction requires invasive pulmonary artery catheterization. A less-invasive technique could be to quantify changes in mediators responsible for vasodilation. One way could be the detection of NO in the exhaled air. Törnberg and colleagues performed a study of exhaled NO as a marker of pulmonary endothelial dysfunction after ischemia-reperfusion injury occurring during open heart surgery with cardiopulmonary bypass. They found that, in patients with open-heart surgery, pulmonary vascular dysfunction after cardiopulmonary bypass was accompanied by lower levels of basal exhaled NO and a reduction of exhaled NO response to nitroglycerin.[27] In line with these results, in a study performed on children undergoing closure of an atrial septal defect either by a surgical approach using cardiopulmonary bypass or by closure in the catheter laboratory, the authors found a decrease of exhaled NO levels in patients undergoing surgical closure with cardiopulmonary bypass. In contrast, exhaled NO levels increased after catheter-based closure.[28] Exhaled NO levels and dynamics after pharmacological stimulation may reflect endothelial dysfunction after cardiopulmonary bypass with consecutive ischemia-reperfusion injury.

Taken together, there is growing experimental evidence suggesting that NO is a key regulator of the amount of endothelial damage occurring after ischemia-reperfusion injury in the lung. Especially, NO produced by the endothelial isoform of the NO synthesizing enzymes seems to be particularly relevant. Whether this role of NO can be used successfully as a therapeutic or diagnostic tool in the clinical setting of cardiothoracic surgery will need further studies in randomizedc linicaltri als.

References

1. Della Rocca G, Coccia C. Nitric oxide in thoracic surgery. *Minerva Anestesiol.*2005; 71:313-318.
2. Vinten-Johansen J, Zhao ZQ, Nakamura M, et al. Nitric oxide and the vascular endothelium in myocardial ischemia-reperfusion injury. *Ann N Y Acad Sci.*1999; 874:354-370.
3. Hickey MJ, Granger DN, Kubes P. Inducible nitric oxide synthase (iNOS) and regulation of leucocyte/endothelial cell interactions: studies in iNOS-deficient mice. *Acta Physiol Scand.*2001;173:11 9-126.
4. Tapiero H, Mathe G, Couvreur P, Tew KD. I. Arginine. *Biomed Pharmacother.*2002; 56:439-445.
5. Moncada S. The L-arginine: nitric oxide pathway, cellular transduction and immunological roles. *Adv Second Messenger Phosphoprotein Res.* 1993;28:97-99.
6. Duda DG, Fukumura D, Jain RK. Role of eNOS in neovascularization: NO for endothelial progenitor cells. *Trends Mol Med.*2004; 10:143-145.
7. Szabo C. Multiple pathways of peroxynitrite cytotoxicity. *Toxicol Lett.*2003; 140–141:105-112.
8. Kurose I, Wolf R, Grisham MB, Granger DN. Modulation of ischemia/reperfusion-induced microvascular dysfunction by nitric oxide. *Circ Res.*1994; 74:376-382.
9. Kaminski A, Pohl CB, Sponholz C, et al. Up-regulation of endothelial nitric oxide synthase inhibits pulmonary leukocyte migration following lung ischemia-reperfusion in mice. *Am J Pathol.*2004; 164:2241-2249.
10. Wagner JG, Roth RA. Neutrophil migration mechanisms, with an emphasis on the pulmonary vasculature. *Pharmacol Rev.*2000; 52:349-374.
11. Fagan KA et al. Upregulation of nitric oxide synthase in mice with severe hypoxia-induced pulmonary hypertension. *Respir Res.*2001; 2:306-313.
12. Tedgui A, Mallat Z. Anti-inflammatory mechanisms in the vascular wall. *Circ Res.*2001; 88:877-887.
13. Bell TE, Kongable GL, Steinberg GK. Mild hypothermia: an alternative to deep hypothermia for achieving neuroprotection. *J Cardiovasc Nurs.*1998; 13:34-44.
14. Zhang L et al. Importance of endothelial nitric oxide synthase for the hypothermic protection of lungs against ischemia-reperfusion injury. *J Thorac Cardiovasc Surg.* 2006; 131:969-974.
15. Liu J, Narasimhan P, Yu F, Chan PH. Neuroprotection by hypoxic preconditioning involves oxidative stress-mediated expression of hypoxia-inducible factor and erythropoietin. *Stroke.*2005; 36:1264-1269.
16. Tritto I et al. Oxygen radicals can induce preconditioning in rabbit hearts. *Circ Res.*1997; 80:743-748.
17. Koti RS et al. Nitric oxide synthase distribution and expression with ischemic preconditioning of the rat liver. *FASEB J.* 2005;19:1155-1157.
18. Kaminski A et al. Endothelial nitric oxide synthase mediates protective effects of hypoxic preconditioning in lungs. *Respir Physiol Neurobiol.* 2007;155:280-285.
19. Blais V, Rivest S. Inhibitory action of nitric oxide on circulating tumor necrosis factor-induced NF-kappaB activity and COX-2 transcription in the endothelium of the brain capillaries. *J Neuropathol Exp Neurol.* 2001;60:893-905.
20. Guery B., Neviere R., Viget N. et al. Inhaled NO preadministration modulates local and remote ischemia-reperfusion organ injury in a rat model. *J Appl Physiol.*1 999;87:47-53
21. Hataishi R., Rodrigues A.C., Neilan T.G. et al. Inhaled nitric oxide decreases infarction size and improves left ventricular function in a murine model of myocardial ischemia-reperfusion injury. *Am J Physiol Heart Circ Physiol.* 2006; 291:H379-H384.
22. Fullerton DA, et al. Effective control of pulmonary vascular resistance with inhaled nitric oxide after cardiac operation. *J Thorac Cardiovasc Surg* 1996;111:753–762; discussion 762–763
23. Bloch KD, Ichinose F, Roberts JD Jr, Zapol WM. Inhaled NO as a therapeutic agent. *Cardiovasc Res.* 2007;75: 339-348.
24. Date H et al. Inhaled nitric oxide reduces human lung allograft dysfunction. *J Thorac Cardiovasc Surg.* 1996;111: 913-919.

25. Ardehali A et al. A prospective trial of inhaled nitric oxide in clinical lung transplantation. *Transplantation*. 2001;72:112-115.

26. Meade MO et al. A randomized trial of inhaled nitric oxide to prevent ischemia-reperfusion injury after lung transplantation. *Am J Respir Crit Care Med*. 2003;167:1483-1489.

27. Tornberg DC et al. Exhaled nitric oxide before and after cardiac surgery with cardiopulmonary bypass – response to acetylcholine and nitroglycerin. *Br J Anaesth*. 2005;94:174-180.

28. Humpl T et al. Levels of exhaled nitric oxide before and after surgical and transcatheter device closure of atrial septal defects in children. *J Thorac Cardiovasc Surg*. 2002;124:806-810.

Activity of Glutathione-Related Enzymes in Ischemia and Reperfusion Injury

13

Emmanuele Tafuri, Andrea Mezzetti, Antonio Maria Calafiore, and Francesco Cipollone

13.1 Introduction

Myocardial ischemic injury is caused by severe impairment of the coronary blood supply usually produced by thrombosis or other acute alterations of coronary atherosclerotic plaques. Intense investigation has led to considerable insight into the pathobiology of myocardial ischemic injury.[1,2]

Ischemia–reperfusion is a clinical problem associated with procedures such as thrombolysis, angioplasty, and coronary bypass surgery which are commonly used to establish the blood reflow and minimize damage to the heart due to severe myocardial ischemia.

The ischemia–reperfusion injury may include various events: (a) *reperfusion arrhythmias,* (b) *microvascular damage,* (c) *myocardial stunning "reversible mechanical dysfunction,"* (d) *cell death* occurring either together or separately.[3,4]

In humans, the formation and release of oxidized glutathione (GSSG) in the coronary sinus has been reported following myocardial IR. A positive correlation has been found between the release of GSSG and the duration of the ischemic period suggesting that glutathione (GSH) is employed during cardiac ischemia. Massive reduction of glutathione in myocardium has been observed during bypass surgery and such glutathione loss might be related to left ventricle dysfunction in ischemic human heart.[1]

In this section, we will review the mechanisms of the myocardial ischemia reperfusion injury and the role of the antioxidant enzyme systems, and in particular of the glutathione related enzymes.

13.2 Reperfusion and Reperfusion Injury: Role of Oxidative Stress

When research had established the impact of infarct size on prognosis, intensive investigation was focused on finding means of reducing the extent of infarct.

Pharmacological approaches have not generally been shown to have major clinically applicable effects on reducing infarct size with prolonged coronary occlusion.[1] In contrast, profound effects and have been found for reperfusion and preconditioning on the limitation of infarct size. Reperfusion can obviously limit the extent of myocardial necrosis, the magnitude of the damage being directly related to the timing of the intervention.[5] However, the effects of reperfusion are complex and include some deleterious effects collectively referred to as reperfusion injury. This reperfusion injury involves the activation of an inflammatory pathway which manifests as functional impairment, arrhythmia, and accelerated progression of cell death in certain critically injured myocytes. The major mediators of reperfusion injury are oxygen radicals, calcium loading, and neutrophils.

Oxygen radicals are generated by injured myocytes and endothelial cells in the ischemic zone, as well as neutrophils which enter the ischemic zone, and become activated on reperfusion. These oxygen radicals exacerbate membrane damage, which leads to calcium loading. The neutrophils collect in the microcirculation, release inflammatory mediators, and contribute to

E. Tafuri (✉)
Abruzzo section, Italian Society for the Study of Atherosclerosis,
Chieti, Italy
e-mail: e.tafuri@unich.it

E.A. Gabriel and T. Salerno (eds.), *Principles of Pulmonary Protection in Heart Surgery,*
DOI: 10.1007/978-1-84996-308-4_13, © Springer-Verlag London Limited 2010

microvascular obstruction and the no-reflow phenomenon in the reperfused myocardium.[6]

Myocardial stunning refers to the prolonged decrease in the contractile function of the spared myocardium that develops on reperfusion, even after relatively brief periods of coronary occlusion, amounting to about of 15 min, which are insufficient to cause myocardial necrosis. After longer intervals of coronary occlusion, i.e., 2–4 h, an even more severe and persistent decrease in contractile function occurs, although reperfusion allows significant sparing of the subepicardial myocardium.

Myocardial stunning is mediated by the effects of reperfusion, including free radicals and calcium loading, on myocytes which retain viability and ultimately recover contractile function. Hibernation consist of chronic depression of myocardial function due to chronic moderate reduction of perfusion.[5]

An essential role of ROS has been suggested in the pathogenesis of myocardial ischemia–reperfusion injury. A number of studies have shown that ROS, including hydrogen peroxide (H_2O_2), superoxide radical, hydroxyl radical and peroxynitrite, increase with reperfusion of the heart following ischemia. In ischemic-reperfused hearts, many alterations, such as decreased contractile function, arrhythmias, changes in gene expression, and loss of adrenergic pathways have been observed. Similar changes have been reported in hearts perfused with various ROS generating systems.[4]

Pretreatment of cardiac subcellular organelles with ROS as also produced similar changes. Alterations in the myocardium during ischemia–reperfusion were therefore suggested to be partially due to oxidative stress. It should be noted out that global ischemia (30 min) followed by reperfusion (60 min) in isolated rat hearts has been associated with depressed contractile function, as indicated by decreased left ventricular developed pressure (LVDP), 1dP/dt (rate of pressure development), 2dP/dt (rate of pressure decline) and increased left ventricular end-diastolic pressure (LVEDP).

Ischemia–reperfusion increases H_2O_2, [Ca^{2+}] and malondialdehyde (MDA) content in the heart. Treatment of the heart with antioxidant enzymes, superoxide dismutase (SOD) plus catalase, protected against these changes. The formation of ROS during ischemia–reperfusion has also been shown increased by means of the electron paramagnetic resonance technique.

ROS seem to increase significantly after a few minutes of reperfusion but their increase during ischemia alone is still controversial. In the light of these changes it has been suggested that the increase in H_2O_2 production

and other ROS during ischemia–reperfusion leads to lipid peroxidation and sulfhydryl group oxidation.

Damaging effects have recently been shown on the heart following by peroxynitrite ischemia–reperfusion. It is formed by a fast biradical reaction of nitric oxide and superoxide anion mainly in the endothelium, myocytes, and neutrophils. Although peroxynitrite is not a free radical, its intermediate can nitrate and hydroxylate phenolic compounds especially in tyrosine residues, which in turn alter the activities of essential proteins and enzymes. Peroxynitrite has been reported to produce cellular damage by lipid peroxidation and DNA fragmentation in the heart in addition to inducing depletion of antioxidants[4,7](Fig. 13.1).

13.3 The Protective Role of Antioxidants During Myocardial Ischemia–Reperfusion Injury

The beneficial effects of antioxidants, have been widely reported, as these agents provide the heart with resistance against the ischemic–reperfusion injury. However, other studies have failed to produce such findings. Several factors can contribute to this discrepancy such as differences, in species experimental, methods and techniques applied, and different time periods of ischemia–reperfusion insults, as well as different types of anti-oxidants with different properties. There is thus a clear need for a systematic study to exactly establish the protective role of antioxidants against ischemic–reperfusion injury.[8]

A recent investigation reported a depletion of endogenous antioxidants in the ischemic heart upon reperfusion; this change was dependent upon the severity of ischemia–reperfusion. Hydrophilic antioxidants such as ascorbate and glutathione, were decreased during 40 min of reperfusion, but not after ischemia; their oxidized forms (dehydroascorbate and glutathione disulfide) were markedly increased during reperfusion in the isolated rat hearts. At the same time, however, lipophilic antioxidants, such as ubiquinol 9 and vitamin E, did not change during Ischemia–reperfusion; but increasing the severity of ischemia–reperfusion by adding H_2O_2 resulted in tissue lipophilic antioxidant depletion. The addition of H_2O_2 (500 mM) during ischemia–reperfusion led to a decrease in tissue vitamin E and ubiquinol 9 by 65 and 95%, respectively.

These results suggest that ascorbate and a reduced form of glutathione may act as a first line of defense

Fig. 13.1 Pathophysiologic and therapeutic implications of oxidative stress in the myocardialinjury

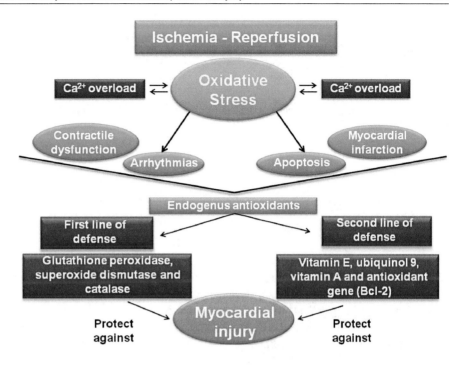

against oxidative stress during ischemia–reperfusion, while vitamin E may act later on during severe oxidative stress.[9]

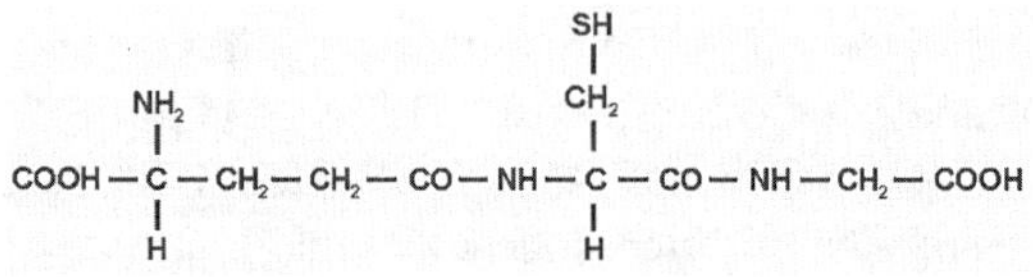

13.4 TheA ntioxidantSys tem: The Glutathione Superfamily

Glutathione plays a highly important role in the damage from reperfusion and ischemic injury. Low molecular weight sulfur containing compounds (thiols), such as thioredoxin and reduced glutathione (GSH), are easily oxidized and can be regenerated very rapidly.

These characteristics make them essential in many biochemical and pharmacological reactions. Although GSH has various functions, its main activities can be divided into three groups: (a) together with superoxide dismutase, it is the major intracellular antioxidant; (b) it modulates cell proliferation and immune responses; and (c) it helps to regulate signal transduction within cells through molecules such as nuclear factor-kappa B and protein tyrosine phosphatases 1-B.[10]

Glutathione is a tripeptide synthesized from the precursor amino acids cysteine, as illustrated in Fig. 13.2.

GSH is mainly synthesized within the liver, although scavenger pathways do exist, before being released

Fig. 13.2 Structureof gl utathione

into the blood and also the bile, which enables the upper jejunum to obtain GSH directly from the lumen of the gut.

The balance between the levels of oxidation and reduction is reflected by the redox state of cells. The GSH buffer system modulates cell response to redox changes. The GSH redox status is important in the regulation of most cellular metabolic processes including transcriptional activation. The GSH redox status is crucial in maintaining cellular viability because cells constantly generate reactive oxygen species during aerobic metabolism.

The reactive oxygen species includes hydroxyl radicals, superoxide anion, hydrogen peroxide and nitric oxide. They are a very transient species because of their high reactivity resulting in lipid peroxidation and the oxidation of DNA and proteins.

Oxidative stress is now known to be involved in the control of cell signaling and gene regulation systems.

Table 13.1 Harmful molecules and the protective effect of glutathione and glutathione-related reactions

Class of molecule	Toxic effect	Protective action of glutathione
Reactive oxygen species (ROS)	Oxidative damage to membrane lipids, DNA and proteins; peroxidation of lipoproteins	ROS are reduced or inactive through the generations of a disulfur bond between two glutathione molecules to form oxidized glutathione
ROS	Inactivation of respiratory chain complexes; inhibition of protein and DNA synthesis	ROS are reduced or inactivated through the generation of a disulfur bond between two glutathione molecules to form oxidized glutathione
Dietary oxidants	Generation of ROS	ROS are reduced or inactivated through the generation of a disulfur bond between two glutathione molecules to form oxidized glutathione
Xenobiotics	Induce cancer	Glutathione is involved in the conjugation of epoxides to less toxic compounds that will be eventually excreted

Glutathione peroxidases (GP), a major family of functionally important selenoproteins, catalyze the inactivation of reactive oxygen and nitrogen species. These enzymes create a disulfur bond between two GSH molecules and form oxidized glutathione (GSSG). GSH reductase then catalyzes the formation of two molecules of GSH from one molecule of GSSG. Glutathione peroxidises (GP) enzymes are: (1) classical GPX-1; (2) gastrointestinal GPX-GI; (3) plasma GPX-P; and (4) phospholipid hydroperoxide PHGPX; (5) GPX-5.

These isoenzymes are immunologically distinct and are encoded by different genes. (Table 13.1)

Members of the glutathione-S-transferase (GST) super family catalyze the conjugation of GSH with target compounds to form GSH conjugates (Table 13.2). These GSH conjugates are converted to mercapturic acids for excretion. The loci hat encode the GST enzymes are located on at least seven chromosomes (Tables 13.3). These structurally related molecules are involved in diverse functions that relate to the heat-shock response, the detoxification of electrophiles, drug resistance, carcinogenesis, and immunomodulatory functions. GST polymorphism is important in determining disease phenotypes and susceptibility to cancer.[11]

Serum gamma-glutamyl transferase (GGT) is used as an index of cholestatic liver disease, high alcohol consumption, and the use of enzyme-inducing drugs. Increases in serum GGT lead to a rise in the production of free radicals, particularly in the presence of iron. People with high serum GGT levels have an increased risk of death due to an association of GGT with other risk factors, and GGT is itself an independent predictor of ris k.

Various studies have reported the importance of glutathione peroxidase in preventing the damage from reperfusion of the ischemic myocardium.

Table 13.2 The gluta thionet ransferases uperfamily

Class	Chromosome	Protein(s)
Alpha	6p12	GSTA1
		GSTA2
		GSTA3
		GSTA4
Kappa	Unknown	GSTK1
Mu	1p13.3	GSTM1
		GSTM2
		GSTM3
		GSTM4
		GSTM5
Pi	11q13	GSTP1

Table 13.3 The gl utathionepe roxidases

Isoenzyme	Gene	Chromosome
Glutathione peroxidase-1 (GPX-1)	*Gpx1*	3, 21, and X
Gastrointestinal epithelium-specific glutathione peroxidase (GPX-GI)	*Gpx2*	14
Secreted plasma glutathione peroxidase (GPX-P)	*Gpx3*	5
Phospholipidh ydroperoxide glutathione peroxidase (PHGPX)	*Gpx4*	19

GPX are selenocysteine containing enzymes that are expressed in most tissues. As already mentioned, five GPX isoenzymes have been identified; cytosolic and mitochondrial GPX (GPX-1) was the first mammalian selenoprotein to be identified in 1957; it is expressed ubiquitously suggesting it plays a central role in cellular defense against hydroperoxides.

Phospholipid hydroperoxide GPX (GPX-4 or PHGPX) which was first described in 1982,is also present in most tissues; in contrast gastrointestinal GPX (GPX-2) and extracellular/plasma GPX (GPX-3) are localized only in the gastrointestinal tract and plasma, respectively. GPX-5 is a selenium-independent GPX specifically expressed in mouse epididymis.[12]

Although GPX isoenzymes reduce hydrogen peroxide and alkyl hydroperoxides, their specificities for hydroperoxide substrates differ markedly. GPX-1 and GPX-2 reduce only soluble hydroperoxides, such as H_2O_2, and some organic hydroperoxides, such as hydroperoxy fatty acids, cumene hydroperoxide or t-butyl hydroperoxide whereas GPX-4and to a small extent GPX-3 also reduce hydroperoxides of more complex lipids such as phosphatidylcholine hydroperoxide.

GPX-4 is also capable of reducing hydroperoxide groups of thymine, lipoproteins and cholesterol esters, and is the only enzyme acting on hydroperoxides integrated in membranes. Under adequate selenium supply, all cells express a certain amount of GPX-1. Tissues with a high rate of peroxide production, such as erythrocytes, liver, kidney and Lung, contain particularly high levels. Developmental changes in GPX-1 expression have also been observed in rat lungs, where it increases after birth, especially when exposed to high oxygen tensions. GPX-1 expression thus seems to parallel metabolic activity, which complies with an antioxidant function of the enzyme. Increased GPX-1 activity has also been shown to inhibit apoptosis, even under conditions of ROS production, showing that GPX is able to modulate apoptotic responses to a variety of stimuli.

The expression of GPX-2 is apparently limited to the epithelium of the gastrointestinal tract; in humans it is also found in the liver. GPX-3 is expressed in various tissues, including kidney, ciliary body and the maternal/fetal interface. GPX-3 is secreted from its origin into the extracellular environment. The activity of GPX-4 is generally lower than that of GPX-1 in all organs except the testis, which has the highest GPX-4 expression of all tissues studied. GPX-4 was previously thought to be a universal antioxidant protecting

membrane lipids; however, it appears to have roles also in redox regulation, silencing lipoxygenases, sexual maturation and differentiation. In addition, it can reduce hydroperoxides in high density lipoproteins (HDL) and low density lipoproteins (LDL) which infers may play a role in atherogenesis. GPX-1 exists as a homotetramer with each of its subunits containing a selenium atom incorporated within a catalytically active selenocysteine residue. This amino acid is sterically exposed on a flat lipophilic surface on the protein, allowing it to become oxidized by any hydroperoxide that may approach it. Although GPX-1, GPX-2 and GPX-3 are all homotetramers, GPX-4 is a monomer of lower molecular size than the subunits of the other isoenzymes. Because of its small size and hydrophobic surface has been implicated in its ability to react with complex hydroperoxides and lipids in membranes.

The catalytic mechanism proposed for reduction of hydroperoxide substrates by GPX involves the oxidation of the active site selenolate to selenoic acid. This results in GPX being oxidized to an inactive state, which then requires glutathione (GSH) for regeneration of its active state.[7]

Glutathione binds to two arginine residues adjacent to the catalytic center, which causes its SH group to be directed towards the oxidized selenium (selenoic acid), consequently forming a selenosulfide bridge. This bridge is split by a second GSH molecule which regenerates selenolate and reduces (active) GPX, by which process two molecules of GSH are oxidized to glutathione disulfide (GSSG).

These two molecules of oxidized glutathione (GSSG) are reconverted to their reduced state, GSH, by glutathione reductase (GSR) which uses electrons from NADPH. The hexose monophosphate shunt produces the NADPH reducing equivalents through glucose-6-phoshateoxida tion(Fig. 13.3).

Glutathione is not only a cofactor for GPX, but can also directly reduce reactive oxygen species such as the hydroxyl radical, N_2O_3 and peroxynitrite. It also reduces disulfide linkages between proteins and molecules, and acts in the synthesis of deoxyribonucleotide precursors of DNA.

Although glutathione, is used as a thiol substrate by all GPX isoenzymes, it is not the only possible reductant, GPX-3 has been shown to also use thioredoxin. Important information on cellular oxidative events is provided by changes in glutathione status, tissue accumulation or effluent release of GSSG being an accurate

Fig.13.3 Theme chanismof
glutathionea ction

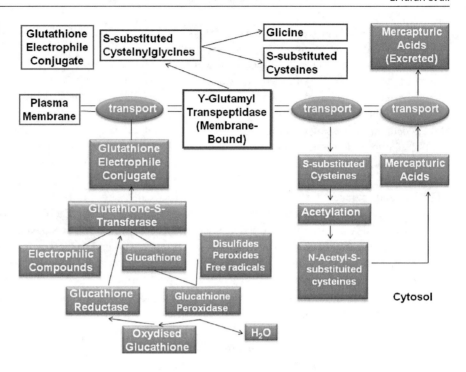

index of oxidative stress. When cells or tissues undergo oxidative stress, they are reported to export GSSG. The shift in ratio of [GSH]/[GSSG] changes the redox state to a more positive potential; if the potential rises too much it damages the cell. The export of GSSG prevents this shift, and helps maintain the redox balance of cells. This seems appears to contribute to the protection of cells and tissues against oxidative stress, and has been observed in hearts perfused with *t*-butyl hydroperoxide. The efflux of GSSG maintains the redox status during oxidative stress; it also results in the loss of GSH from the cell thus decreasing the reducing capacity of the cell, which can only be replaced by synthesis of new GSH[13] (Fig. 13.4).

Thus glutathione is an important antioxidant in the heart and a decrease in myocardial GSH content has been observed during ischemia and reperfusion of the ischemic myocardium.

Several studies have used inhibitors for glutathione peroxidase such as maleic acid diethyl ester, which reduce the recovery of contractile function in rat and cat's heart following ischemia or perfusion with peroxidase-derived free radicals. The deficiency of a coenzyme such as selenium, which is required in

maintaining the glutathione redox cycle, also renders the isolated rat heart more susceptible to oxidative injury.

These hypotheses have been supported by using knockout mice. These transgenic mice exhibited markedly depressed contractile function following 30 min of ischemia and 120 min of reperfusion. In addition, a significantly higher damage to cardiomyocytes was reported in transgenic mice compared to nontransgenic mice, demonstrated by creatine kinase release and size of infarction.

Moreover some studies suggest that endogenous glutathione has a role in providing protection against myocardial injury after a short period of ischemia and in protecting the coronary vasculature. It has been reported that lowering endogenous levels (without altering levels of glutathione peroxidase) impaired recovery of systolic function and increased coronary resistance and chamber stiffness. After ischemia, coronary perfusion increased the most in glutathione-depleted hearts suggesting a substantial rise in coronary resistance. The most likely explanation for the increase in coronary resistance in the glutathione-depleted hearts after ischemia–reperfusion is endothelial injury.[14,15]

Fig. 13.4 The antioxidant system

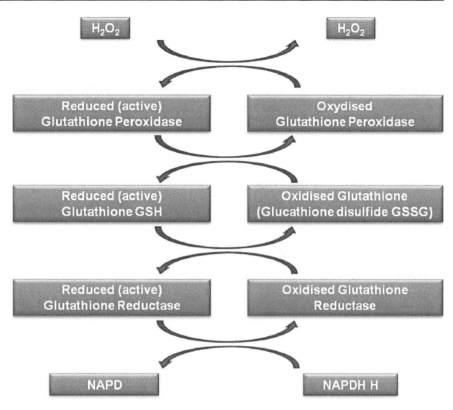

13.5 Conclusion

Oxidative stress plays an important role in the genesis of myocardial ischemia–reperfusion damage, and the potential beneficial effect of antioxidants, particularly glutathione, has been widely suggested. In this light, enhancing the activity of endogenous myocardial glutathione peroxide may be a promising avenue for protecting the heart against ischemia–reperfusion injury.

Nevertheless, many other aspects of the glutathione system still remain to be investigated, as studies involving antioxidants in the setting of ischemia–reperfusion have provided conflicting results. Future studies have to be designed to define the precise molecular targets as well as the ideal antioxidant in terms of molecule, dose,a bsorption,bioa vailabilitya ndpha rmacokinetic.

References

1. Buja LM. Myocardial ischemia and reperfusion injury. *Cardiovasc Pathol*.2005; 14:170-175.

2. Reimer KA, Ideker RE. Myocardial ischemia and infarction: anatomic and biochemical substrates for ischemic cell death and ventricular arrhythmias. *Hum Pathol*.1987; 18:462-475.

3. Marczin N, El-Habashi N, Hoare GS, Bundy RE, Yacoub M. Antioxidants in myocardial ischemia-reperfusion injury: therapeutic potential and basic mechanism. *Arch Biochem Biophys*.2003; 420:222-236.

4. Dhalla NS, Elmoselhi AB, Hata T, Makino N. Status of myocardial antioxidants in ischemia-reperfusion injury. *Cardiovasc Res*.2000; 47:446-456.

5. Maxwell SRJ, Lip GYH. Reperfusion Injury: a review of the pathophysiology, clinical manifestations and therapeutic options. *Int J Cardiol*.1997; 58:95-117.

6. Park JL, Lucchesi BR. Mechanism of myocardial reperfusion injury. *Ann Thorac Surg*.1998; 68:1905-1912.

7. Venardos KM, Perkins A, Headrick J, Kaye DM. Myocardial ischemia-reperfusion injury, antioxidant enzyme systems, and selenium: a review. *Cur Med Chem*. 2007;14:1539-1549.

8. Thomas J.P., Maiorino M., Ursini, F., and Girotti A.W. Protective action of Phospholipid Hydroperoxide Glutathione Peroxidase against membrane-damaging lipid peroxidation: in situ reduction of phospholipid and cholesterol hydroperoxides. J. Biol. Chem. 1990; 265: 454-461.

9. Marchioli R. Antioxidant vitamins and prevention of cardiovascular disease: laboratory, epidemiological and clinical trial data. *Pharm Res*.1999; 40:227-238.

10. Cheung PY, Wang W, Schulz R. Glutathione Protects again myocardial ischemia-reperfusion injury by detoxifyng peroxynitrite. *J Mol Cell Cardiol*.2000; 32:1669-1678.

11. Jefferies H, Coster J, Khalil A, Bot J, McCauley RD, Hall JC. Glutathione. ANZ J Surg 2003;73:517-522.
12. Brigelius-Flohe R. Tissue-specific functions of individual glutathione peroxidases. *Free Radic Biol Med*. 1999;27:951.
13. Schafer F. Q., Buettner G. R. Redox environment of the cell as viewed through the redox state of the glutathione disulfide/glutathione couple. Free Radical Biol. Med. 2001;30:1191–1212.
14. Konz KH, Haap M, Hill KE, Nurk RF, Walsh RA. Diastolic dysfunction of perfused rat hearts induced by hydrogen peroxide. Protective effect of selenium. *J Mol Cell Cardiol*. 1989;21:789-795.
15. Yoshida T, Watanabe M, Engelman DT. Transgenic mice overexpressing glutathione peroxidise are resistant to myocardial ischemia reperfusion injury. *J Mol Cell Cardiol*. 1996;28:1759-1767.

HeartHi stopathology
inl schemia-Reperfusionl njury

Paulo Sampaio Gutierrez and Márcia Marcelino de Souza Ishigai

Ischemic necrosis of a group of cells – infarct – develops if the blood flow is discontinued. The type of circulation of an organ influences the way such cell death occurs. Organs with double circulation, like lungs and bowel, usually resist the closure of one arterial channel, provided the other one is open. Thus, infarcts of these organs occur only when both territories are affected, most frequently due to a global circulatory collapse secondary to heart failure or shock. Anyway, these infarctions are commonly hemorrhagic. The heart has a single circulation with poor collateral branching. Thus, the closure at one point of the arterial tree is enough to cause myocardial infarct, which is usually anemic ("white" infarct).

There are two main morphological patterns of recent myocardial infarction (Fig. 14.1). In the first, the cells usually become thin, are strongly eosinophilic at hematoxylin-and-eosin staining, and finally lose their nuclei. This is the typical pattern found in acute myocardial infarction and is described as *myocellular irreversible relaxation injury*, an example of classical coagulative necrosis. Alternatively, there is an appearance of an exacerbation of the transversal striation-forming bands – an aspect called *contraction band necrosis*.

After the interruption of the flow, cell death is not instantaneous. The cells can survive without blood for some time, depending mostly on their metabolism. For example, massive neuronal necrosis may follow a circulatory arrest after around 10 min.[1] In the heart,

experimental studies in dogs demonstrated[2] that ischemia lasting less than 15 min caused no irreversible injury; if the arterial occlusion lasted 40 min or more, irreversible damage occurred, mostly at the subendocardial zone. Experimentally, it was demonstrated that the necrosis did not commit all fibers at one time but rather progressively, as a "wave" from the endocardium to the epicardium. so that about 3–6 h after ischemic injury, the transmural wave-front cell death was already been complete. Thus, the size of the lesion could still be reduced if reperfusion were provided within this period. In fact, in human beings the clinical experience indicates that myocardial cells eventually resist even more hours. That is the rationale behind the main therapeutic objective in the acute coronary syndromes: try to restore the blood flow,[3,4] either by chemical (with aspirin or other thrombolytic agents) or mechanical (with balloon angioplasty) destruction of the clot that caused the disease or by a surgical bypass. Spontaneous lysis of the thrombus may also occur.

Nevertheless, the susceptibility to myocardial cell death varies from individual to individual according to its previous status. It also varies with the situation of the cells: those near the border of the ischemic area without blood may be partially protected by a residual flow from the neighbor vessels. When reperfusion is achieved, its consequences depend on such variations and on the interval between the closure and the reopening of the artery. If it is early, the goal of myocardial salvage is accomplished, and the infarct is avoided or at least its area is diminished. However, frequently the return of the myocardium to the previous physiological conditions is not immediate. The challenged segment of the myocardium remains with a deficit in function that may last up to weeks, a condition called *stunning myocardium*. There are no morphological alterations clearly related to it. Baroldi et al.[5] argued that there is no

P. S. Gutierrez (✉)
Laboratory of Pathology – Heart Institute,
Hospital das Clínicas da Faculdade de Medicina da
Universidade de São Paulo
Department of Pathology
Federal University of Sao Paulo, Sao Paulo, Brazil
e-mail:a nppaulo@incor.usp.br

E.A. Gabriel and T. Salerno (eds.), *Principles of Pulmonary Protection in Heart Surgery*,
DOI: 10.1007/978-1-84996-308-4_14, © Springer-Verlag London Limited 2010

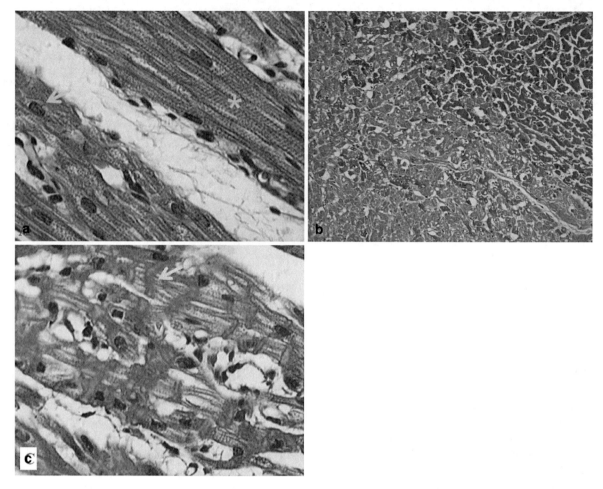

Fig. 14.1 Histological sections from pig heart (**a**, **c**), and dog heart (**b**). (**a**) Normal myocardiocytes (*arrow* and *asterisk*). (**b**) Border between preserved cells and myocardiocytes with coagulative necrosis, darker (more eosinophilic) and more homogeneous, at the right, upper zone of the picture. (**c**) Myocardiocytes showing contraction band necrosis (*arrow*). (**a**, **c**) From Gabriel et al.[25]

structural damage, and that the temporary blockage in myocardial function is likely at a molecular/ionic level, difficult to identify histologically. Probably, although the cells are alive, the broken contractile apparatus or energy resources demand some time to be rebuilt. Disturbances in calcium metabolism, lesions caused by oxide radicals, and apoptosis followed by hypertrophy of the adjacent myocardiocytes had been proposed to explain this situation.[6]

If the reperfusion occurs too late, the cells, or part of them, are already dead. The question thus is what happens in this situation. Does the presence of blood modify in any way the evolution of lesion? Is it beneficial, detrimental, or indifferent? One possibility is that lesions in the microcirculation, secondary to the ischemia, prevent the blood from reaching the cells – the *no-reflow phenomenon*. Another possibility is that the infarction is transformed into the hemorrhagic type (Fig. 14.2). Under certain circumstances, discussed further here, *reperfusion injury*, characterized by an evolution worse than would be expected if the blood flow had not been restored, can occur. Finally, if the flow is reintroduced very late – months or years after the ischemic necrosis – sometimes there is an improvement in that segmental area. The myocardium is considered to be *hibernating* during the period. Hibernation of the myocardium may correspond to a series of stunnings or a kind of atrophy of the myocardiocytes. It is noted when a surgical bypass or angioplasty is performed over an infarcted territory, and there is functional improvement. Histologically, it may be

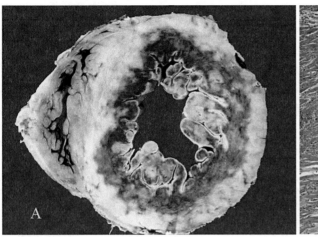
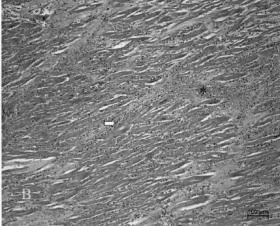

Fig. 14.2 (**a**) Transverse section of a human heart showing a circumferential hemorrhagic myocardial infarction. The patient died in the postoperative period after aortic valve replacement. (**b**) Histologic section of human heart presenting recent myocardium infarction, identified by the absence of nuclei and more related to myocellular vacuolization situated in areas preserved homogeneous, eosinophilic cytoplasms, surrounded by polymorphonuclear neutrophils (as exemplified by the *arrow*). The presence of many red blood cells (as exemplified by the *asterisk*) characterizest hei nfarctiona she morrhagic

Table14 .1 Consequencesof m yocardialr eperfusion

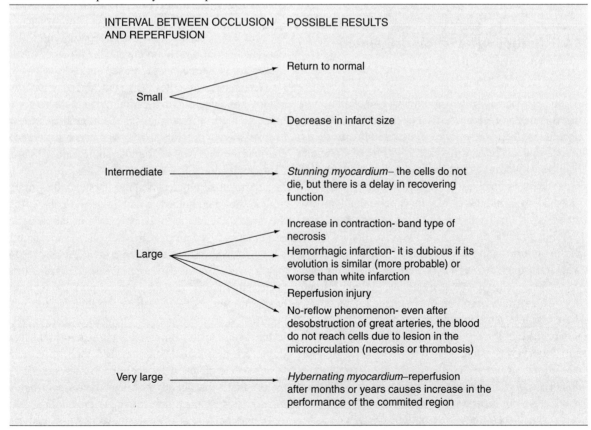

INTERVAL BETWEEN OCCLUSION AND REPERFUSION	POSSIBLE RESULTS
Small	Return to normal
	Decrease in infarct size
Intermediate	*Stunning myocardium*– the cells do not die, but there is a delay in recovering function
Large	Increase in contraction- band type of necrosis
	Hemorrhagic infarction- it is dubious if its evolution is similar (more probable) or worse than white infarction
	Reperfusion injury
	No-reflow phenomenon- even after desobstruction of great arteries, the blood do not reach cells due to lesion in the microcirculation (necrosis or thrombosis)
Very large	*Hybernating myocardium*–reperfusion after months or years causes increase in the performance of the commited region

related to myocellular vacuolization situated in areas preserved from previous ischemic damage, around vessels and in the subendocardial layer, without inflammation.[5]

The events related to myocardium reperfusion are summarized in Table 14.1 (adapted from Higuchi et al.[7]).

14.1 Causeso fR eperfusion

As stated, the most common cause of reperfusion is the dissolution of a clot by a drug or by a mechanical device. Coronary artery bypass surgery (CABG) during the acute phase of infarction also induces reperfusion. In addition, cardiac surgical procedures themselves, including CABG, if performed with circulatory arrest and extracorporeal circulation (ECC), are a cause of ischemia and, at their end and in return to regular circulation, reperfusion. A series of preventive actions is taken during surgery to avoid or minimize such effect: The duration of cardiac arrest and ischemia is as short as possible, the temperature of the heart is decreased, and a nutrient solution – cardioplegic solution – is applied at some intervals inside the coronary arteries. Cardiac surgery with ECC always represents a challenge to the myocardium, with a potential to lead to ischemia-reperfusion injury.

14.2 PathologicalFi ndingsR elated to Reperfusion

Although reperfusion has an unquestionable value in the treatment of myocardial infarct, in some conditions it could develop a series of detrimental effects on myocardial tissue, contributing to increase ischemic damage, myocardial dysfunction, and arrhythmia. This effect, known as *reperfusion injury*, was first detected by Jennings et al.[8] in experimental procedures. They realized that if the coronary flow was restored after the myocardial cells were already dead, the evolution of the lesion could be different from what occurred if no blood flow were reintroduced. One such consequence is that arrhythmias, including some severe forms, may become more frequent. Interestingly, there was less ventricular fibrillation after the restoration of the blood supply when the ligation of the coronary artery was released before 5–15 min or after 40–60 min than between these periods. Arrhythmias do not always represent an irreversible injury, and they may be present in an early phase of the ischemic process. The discussion of arrhythmias is beyond the scope of this chapter.

The morphological findings after reperfusion depend on a series of circumstances, the most important being the duration of the ischemia. The cause and situation of the interruption of the blood flow also affect its consequences; for example, when a thrombosis occurs outside the hospital, the conditions are much less controlled than during cardiac surgery. Even in this condition, as we discuss, there are different protocols that can potentially affect the evolution.[9]

The existence of transient episodes of ischemia before the definitive one improves the outcome by diminishing the infarct size. This effect, called *ischemic preconditioning*, was first noted by Murry et al.[10] in experimental animals; according to them, it results from rapid metabolic adaptation of the ischemic myocardium. The clinical correspondence of their finding is that patients with angina tend to have smaller infarcts than those without previous angina. An *ischemic postconditioning* has also been described: Brief periods of reocclusion after reperfusion are beneficial.[11] These endogenous mechanisms of myocardial protection are complex and can be influenced by conditions such as the period between the ischemic preconditioning stimulus and the subsequent infarct and the presence of risk factors for ischemic heart disease.[12]

The most remarkable change introduced in the morphology of a necrotic myocardium due to the return of blood is the transformation of the infarction into the hemorrhagic type (Fig. 14.2). The other differences concern the intensity of the alterations rather than in their quality.

The histopathological findings in myocardial infarction are not noted unless a certain period passes from the arterial occlusion to the obtention of the heart for examination. Accordingly, besides the hemorrhage, a period of evolution is required so that the discrepancies between lesions that are or are not reperfused can be noted. In the "classic" 1960 report by Jennings et al.,[8] the authors verified that, after 24 h in dogs with reperfusion, the myocardial fibers were disorganized in the whole lesion; in animals with permanent ligation, such disorganization – in fact, their description seems to characterize by the term *disorganization* a feature that subsequently has been named *contraction band necrosis* – is more restricted to the borders.

In another experimental study, Lopes[13] analyzed hearts from dogs submitted to three distinct protocols:

permanent occlusion of the anterior interventricular branch of the left coronary artery, reperfusion after 3 h, or reperfusion after 6 h. Specimens were examined by electron or light microscopy up to 30 days after infarction. At long-term evolution, more calcification was noted in the reperfused hearts.

In initial phases of myocardial infarction, the cells are swollen and present characteristic dense bodies in mitochondria (Fig. 14.3). If the necrotic area receives blood again, such alterations may be exacerbated into an "explosive swelling," and the quantity of dense bodies is increased. The sarcolemma is also severely damaged, becoming full of fluid or disrupted.[2] These findings seem to be related to the excess in oxygen and calcium in an already irreversibly damaged tissue, without energy supply to perform ion exchanges,[14,15] processes that have been called *oxygen paradox* and *calcium paradox*, respectively.[15,16] In addition, the reperfusion provokes a fall in lactate by "washing" the ischemic area, recovering the pH to a physiologic level, the *pH paradox*. It is the overload of calcium that leads to contraction band necrosis when it appears in myocardium reperfusion injury.[16]

Besides this mechanism of necrosis, apoptosis may also play a role in cell death caused by either the lack or the restoration of blood flow. As pointed out by Buja and Weerasinghe,[16] the rate and magnitude of ATP (adenosine triphosphate) burning up possibly determine

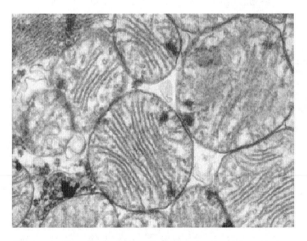

Fig. 14.3 Ultramicrography showing mitochondria with irreversible damage characterized by amorphous densities (gray structures inside the mitochondria) and loss of cristae in some of them. Original magnification ×1,000. From Dias et al.[9]

which pathway(s) of irreversible lesion will take place. This is important because therapeutic actions to reduce damage should target all of them. An increase in glucose uptake has also been investigated as a potential therapeutic goal.[17]

14.3 Ischemia-Reperfusion Injury and Cardiac Surgery with Extracorporeal Circulation

As mentioned, the cardiac surgery with ECC represents a challenge to the heart, which is submitted to ischemia followed by reperfusion. Therefore, myocardial infarcts may occur during such procedures, mainly in the less-protected subendocardial region,[18] even if protective measures are taken. It has been showed that ECC promotes a deleterious effect on myocardium by stimulating a repertory of inflammatory molecules that recruit neutrophils, generating reactive oxygen species and the action of proteolytic enzymes that amplify the heart tissue damage as well as injury to other organs, complicating the postoperative outcome.[19]

The ECC effects on myocardial cells have been reported for years. Balibrea et al.[20] found ultrastructural changes after 30 min of ECC with cardiac arrest in the absence of myocardial protection, which presented features of irreversibility when the ischemia was maintained for a longer period (60 min). The mitochondria showed edema and disruption of their membranes, developing a lamellar and granular degeneration, and the integrity of intercalated disks was lost.

Many techniques of cardioplegia have been proposed to minimize these negative effects and protect the heart from the ischemic-reperfusion injury.[19,21] An example is represented by a study in which one of us (PSG) was involved.[9] In this experiment, dogs were submitted to 120 min of ECC, with or without cardioplegic protection, including lidocaine. Animals that received cardioplegia had less contraction band necrosis. They also presented less coagulative necrosis and fewer ultrastructural lesions, but these differences were not statistically significant. However, none of the cardioplegic techniques conferred complete security, especially considering all the factors that can influence the inflammatory response, like surgical stress itself, temperature, anesthetics, and the conditions of the heart undergoing surgery.[21] For example, ischemic heart disease may alter the tolerance of myocardium to anoxia.[12,20] In accordance with these authors, Wheatley[22] pointed out that the heart condition is a limiting factor to be considered when planning the protective strategies of the surgery.

During ECC, oxygen may have a deleterious effect on microcirculation. In an animal model,[23] there was a reduction in functional capillary density and increase in adherent leukocytes in postcapillary venules and arterioles when surgery with ECC was performed under hyperoxia. Also, in patients with congenital cardiac defects, the use of hyperoxic cardiopulmonary bypass might be harmful for the hypoxic immature heart, although again there is controversy about its clinical significance in spite of the experimental findings.[24]

As stated, ECC conditions influence its detrimental effects. As an example, we present the evaluation made by one of us (MMI) of heart samples taken as part of a study conducted by Prof. Gabriel in a pig model.[25]

Myocardial samples were obtained before and after 30 min of ECC. The animals had been divided into two groups, one with and the other without cardioplegic arrest and moderate hypothermia; each group was separated into three subgroups, corresponding to animals receiving arterial blood, venous blood, or nothing within the pulmonary trunk. Different alterations were found on histological examination. The myocardium showed interstitial edema and hemorrhage with endothelial tumefaction of the capillaries and venules. They frequently showed leukocyte margination with occasional plugs (Fig. 14.4). Contracted myocells were present in almost all samples. In many of them, a pattern of contracted band necrosis with multifocal or diffuse distribution, sometimes associated with myocyte vacuolization, was also noted (Fig. 14.1c). As shown in Table 14.2, the differences between samples obtained before and after the procedure tissue varied according to the type of protocol.

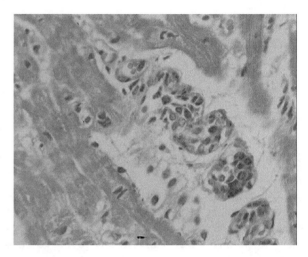

Fig. 14.4 Histologic section of pig heart submitted to extracorporeal circulation showing margination of polymorphonuclear neutrophils in a vessel of the myocardial microcirculation

Table14.2 Significant histopathological differences before and after 30 min of extracorporeal circulation

	No blood on pulmonary trunk	Arterial blood on pulmonary trunk	Venous blood on pulmonary trunk
Cardioplegic arrest and moderate hypothermia	Interstitial hemorrhage	Interstitial hemorrhage Contraction band necrosis Coagulativene crosis	Contractionba ndne crosis
Noc ardioplegica rrest	Coagulativene crosis	None	Myocardiali nflammatory infiltrate

14.4 ConcludingR emarks

The efficacy of the restoration of blood flow over an area of the myocardium challenged by ischemia has been proved; however, undesirable detrimental effects may prevent even better results, a point corroborated by experimental findings but not established yet in clinical investigation. The interruption of blood flow followed by reperfusion can be exemplified by cardiac surgery with ECC, in which different protocols influencethe pos toperativee volution.

References

1. Torp-Pedersen C, Birk-Madsen E, Pedersen A. The time factor in resuscitation initiated by ambulance drivers. *Eur Heart J*.1989;10:555-557 .
2. Jennings RB, Reimer KA. Factors involved in salvaging ischemic myocardium: effect of reperfusion of arterial blood. *Circulation*.1983;6 8:I25-I36.
3. Antman EM, Hand M, Armstrong PW, et al. 2007 focused update of the ACC/AHA 2004 guidelines for the management of patients with ST-elevation myocardial infarction: a report of the American College of Cardiology/American Heart Association Task Force on Practice Guidelines (Writing Group to Review New Evidence and Update the ACC/AHA 2004 Guidelines for the Management of Patients With ST-Elevation Myocardial Infarction). *J Am Coll Cardiol*.2008;51:210- 247.
4. Anderson JL, Adams CD, Antman EM, et al. 2007 guidelines for the management of patients with unstable angina/non-ST-elevation myocardial infarction: a report of the American College of Cardiology/American Heart Association Task Force on Practice Guidelines (Writing Committee to Revise the 2002 Guidelines for the Management of Patients with Unstable Angina/Non-ST-Elevation Myocardial Infarction) developed in collaboration with the American College of Emergency Physicians, the Society for Cardiovascular Angiography and Interventions, and the Society of Thoracic Surgeons endorsed by the American Association of Cardiovascular and Pulmonary Rehabilitation and the Society for Academic Emergency Medicine. *J Am Coll Cardiol* 2007;50:e1–e157. Erratum in: *J Am Coll Cardiol* 2008;51:974.
5. Baroldi G, Bigi R, Cortigiani L. Ultrasound imaging versus morphopathology in cardiovascular diseases. Myocardial cell damage. *Cardiovasc Ultrasound*.2005; 3:32-39.
6. Anselmi A, Abbate A, Girola F, et al. Myocardial ischemia, stunning, inflammation, and apoptosis during cardiac surgery: a review of evidence. *Eur J Cardiothorac Surg*. 2004; 25:304-311.
7. Higuchi ML, Aiello VD, Gutierrez PS. Coração. In: Brasileiro Filho G, ed. *Bogliolo – patologia (7ª Edição)*. Rio de Janeiro: Guanabara Koogan; 2006:408-456.
8. Jennings RB, Sommers HM, Smyth GA, Flack HA, Linn H. Myocardial necrosis induced by temporary occlusion of a coronary artery in the dog. *Arch Pathol*.1960; 70:68-78.
9. Dias AR, Gutierrez PS, Lourenção R, et al. Estudo experimental em cães da ação protetora de solução cardioplégica de lidocaína e potássio. *Rev Bras Cir Cardiovasc*. 2002;17: 79-89.
10. Murry CE, Jennings RB, Reimer KA. Preconditioning with ischemia: a delay of lethal cell injury in ischemic myocardium. *Circulation*.1986; 74:1124-1136.
11. Valen G, Vaage J. Pre- and postconditioning during cardiac surgery. *Basic Res Cardiol*.2005; 100(3):179-186.
12. Ferdinandy P, Schulz R, Baxter G. Interaction of cardiovascular risk factors with myocardial ischemia/reperfusion injury, preconditioning and postconditioning. *Pharmacol Rev*.2007; 59:418-458.
13. Lopes EA. Aspectos microscópicos e submicroscópicos do infarto do miocárdio experimental em cão submetido a revascularização precoce [thesis]. São Paulo: faculdade de Medicina da Universidade de São Paulo; 1972.
14. Khabbaz KR, Levitsky S. The impact of surgical and percutaneous coronary revascularization on the cardiac myocyte. *World J Surg*.2008; 32(3):361-365.
15. Yellon DM, Hausenloy DJ. Myocardial reperfusion injury. *N Engl J Med*.2007; 357:1121-1135.
16. Buja LM, Weerasinghe P. Unresolved issues in myocardial reperfusion injury. *Cardiovasc Pathol*.2010; 19:29-35
17. Webb IG, Williams R, Marber MS. Lizard spit and reperfusion injury. *J Am Coll Cardiol*.2009; 53:511-513.
18. Laurindo FR, Grinberg M. Campos de Assis RV, Jatene AD, Pileggi F. Perioperative acute myocardial infarction after valve replacement. *Am J Cardiol*.1987; 59:639-642.
19. Verma S, Fedak PW, Weisel RD, et al. Off-pump coronary artery bypass surgery: fundamentals for the clinical cardiologist. *Circulation*.2004; 109:1206-1211.
20. Balibrea L, Bullon A, DeLa Fuente A, et al. Myocardial ultrastructural changes during extracorporeal circulation with anoxic cardiac arrest and its prevention by coronary perfusion: experimental study. *Thorax*.1975; 30:371-381.
21. Suleiman MS, Zacharowski K, Angelini GD. Inflammatory response and cardioprotection during open-heart surgery: the importance of anaesthetics. *Br J Pharmacol*. 2008;153: 21-33.
22. Wheatley DJ. Protecting the damaged heart during coronary surgery. *Heart*.2003; 89:367-368.
23. Kamler M, Wendt D, Pizanis N, Milekhin V, Schade U, Jakob H. Deleterious effects of oxygen during extracorporeal circulation for the microcirculation in vivo. *Eur J Cardiothorac Surg*.2004; 26:564-570.
24. Allen BS. The reoxygenation injury: is it clinically important? *J Thorac Cardiovasc Surg*.2002; 124:16-19.
25. Gabriel EA, Locali RF, Matsuoka PK, et al. Lung perfusion during cardiac surgery with cardiopulmonary bypass: is it necessary? *Interact Cardiovasc Thorac Surg*. 2008;7:1089-1095.

Beating Heart Surgery and Pulmonary Ischemia and Reperfusion Injury

15

Tomas A. Salerno, Francisco Igor B. Macedo,
Maria R. Suarez, Marco Ricci, and Edward Gologorsky

15.1 Introduction

Much progress has occurred over the past two decades in cardiac surgery. Innovations abound in the clinical arena, with trends toward less-invasive approaches to ischemic and valvular heart disease and further evolution in techniques of heart transplantation. Despite improvements in techniques, early morbidity and mortality remain high in several procedures, mostly related to cardiopulmonary bypass and cardioplegic arrest.

Cardiac surgery was initially performed with cardiopulmonary bypass (CPB) in 1953.[1] This procedure has been associated with a postpump systemic inflammatory response syndrome (SIRS), which contributed to development of postoperative complications (i.e., cardiovascular instability, myocardial and renal dysfunction, severe respiratory insufficiency, bleeding disorders,

and multiple organ failure). Among many possible causes of SIRS, contact of blood components with the artificial surface of the bypass circuit, ischemia-reperfusion injury, endotoxemia, operative trauma, and blood loss were identified as underlying major factors.[2,3] Many strategies have been implemented to minimize these variables, including surface modifications of circuits, new pharmacological agents, and noncardioplegic techniques. However, several pathways are involved in the complex pathogenesis of the inflammatory response to CPB. The inhibition of a single mediator or of a single pathway may not achieve inhibition of the entire proinflammatory cascade to significantly improve clinical outcomes.

15.2 Pathogenesis: Stimuli and Mediators

The activation of acute-phase reaction induced by CPB is an extremely complex process, and it has various triggers: cytokines and the complement system, endotoxin, nuclear factor kappa B (NF-κB), oxygen free radicals, and adhesion molecules.

15.2.1 Cytokines

Exposure of blood to the nonphysiologic circuit activates the complement system through an alternative pathway. The extracorporeal circuit lacks endothelial cell (EC) surface inhibitors that regulate cofactor C3, resulting in stimulation of C3a and C5a with anaphylactic and chemotactic activity.[3] This activation is mediated by complement receptor type 1 (CR1), an important

T.A. Salerno (✉)
Division of Cardiothoracic Surgery, University of Miami Miller School of Medicine and Jackson Memorial Hospital, Miami, FL, USA

F.I.B. Macedo
University of Pernambuco, School of Medicine and Oswaldo Cruz University Hospital, Brazil

M.R. Suarez
Division of Cardiothoracic Surgery, University of Miami Miller School of Medicine and Jackson Memorial Hospital, Miami, FL, USA

M. Ricci
Division of Cardiothoracic Surgery, University of Miami Miller School of Medicine, Holtz Children's Hospital/Jackson Memorial Hospital, Miami, FL, USA

E.G. ologorsky
Department of Anesthesiology, University of Miami Miller School of Medicine and Jackson Memorial Hospital, Miami, FL, USA

E.A. Gabriel and T. Salerno (eds.), *Principles of Pulmonary Protection in Heart Surgery*,
DOI: 10.1007/978-1-84996-308-4_15, © Springer-Verlag London Limited 2010

factor in regulation of complement proinflammatory activity.[4] These complement factors and their degradation metabolites are responsible for inducing synthesis of proinflammatory cytokines.[5] These molecules are intercellular messengers of mature leukocytes, which may also be regulated by different cell lines, such as platelets.[3] Among various cytokines, tumor necrosis factor alpha (TNF-α), interleukin (IL) 6, IL-8, and IL-10 were extensively correlated to CPB-induced injury and to negative outcomes after cardiac surgery.[3]

15.2.2 Endotoxin

Bacterial lipopolysaccharide (LPS) is released by Gram-negative bacteria during their replication and growth. In plasma, endotoxin binds to LPS-binding protein, originating an endotoxin-LPS-binding protein complex. This complex binds to macrophage receptor CD14, thereby enhancing macrophage TNF-α synthesis and IL-6 by ECs.[6]

15.2.3 Nuclear Factor kappa B

Nuclear factor kappa B is a transcription factor involved in the regulation of several proinflammatory genes, and it is activated by stimuli of IL-1, TNF-α, LPS, and oxygen free radicals.[7] When stimulated, NF-κB is dissociated from an inhibitory IkB protein and translocates to the nucleus, where, binding to DNA, it is able to induce expression of several inflammatory mediators, including cytokines and adhesion molecules.[3]

15.2.4 Adhesion Molecules

Evidence have shown that the neutrophil is the main effector of the inflammatory response secondary to CPB,[8] and its activation is regulated by several proinflammatory mediators, including platelet-activating factor and IL-8, thereby increasing integrin on the leukocyte surface.[9] Cytokines stimulate the expression of intercellular (ICAM), vascular cell (VCAM), and platelet-endothelial cell (PECAM) adhesion molecules. The binding of integrins with adhesion molecules (i.e.,

ICAM and VCAM) results in strong adhesion of leukocytes on ECs, leading to their transendothelial migration into the interstitial fluid phase. Then, leukocytes release their lysosomal contents, which stimulates lipid peroxidation of ECs and myocyte membranes, leading to cellular dysfunction, edema, and cell death.[10] CPB is associated with increased levels of soluble adhesion molecules, which have been related to be responsible for the dysfunction of multiple organ systems.[3]

15.3 Ischemia-ReperfusionInjury

CPB and cardioplegia arrest with aorta cross clamping have been considered major factors associated with myocardial hypoxia and ischemia-reperfusion injury, both of which are proinflammatory stimuli. Ischemia contributes to the activation of ECs and leukocytes, the effectors of inflammatory cytotoxicity,[3] while reperfusion injury may be regulated by several factors, including platelets. The process initiates with formation of selectins – E- (EC), L- (leukocyte), and P- (platelet) selectins – which allows low-affinity binding among leukocytes, platelets, and ECs, thereby recruiting neutrophils. The binding between P-selectin and integrins on the platelet surface results in leukocyte-platelet microaggregates.[11] The vasoconstriction induced by oxygen free radicals and these microaggregates causes microvascular obstruction and the no-reflow phenomenon during reperfusion. Apoptosis induced by TNF-α also plays an important role in tissue damage related to ischemia-reperfusion injury.

In summary, while cardioplegia arrest and subsequent isquemia-reperfsion injury are associated with significant cytokine release and neutrophil activation,[12] the SIRS response to CPB alone results in myocardial inflammation, leukocyte activation, and cardiac enzyme release.[2]

Ischemia-reperfusion injury and CPB have also been correlated with reduction of the bronchial arterial blood flow, leading to low-flow ischemia in the lung. Since the beginning of open heart surgery, an association between these two phenomena has been recognized. The lungs have a bimodal blood supply from the pulmonary and bronchial arteries with extensive anastomotic connections. However, during CPB, these organs are purely dependent on bronchial arteries to provide the 5% of whole-body oxygen uptake that is necessary even under hypothermic conditions.[13] This results in a regional inflammatory response, leading to a significant accumulation of albumin, lactate dehydrogenase, neutrophils, and elastase in the bronchoalveolar lavage fluid.[14] CPB is also associated with significant pulmonary cytokine release (IL-8) and alveolar macrophage activation.[15] This inflammatory response in the lungs was demonstrated not to be caused by extracorporeal perfusion itself (i.e., artificial surfaces) but by changes in the regional perfusion patterns during CPB.[16]

15.4   Technical Strategies

Based on these facts, some strategies have been investigated to reduce the adverse effects of tissue injury related to CPB and cardioplegia arrest. Since most cardiac surgeries still require the use of CPB, many efforts have been made to diminish the effects of correlated variables, including pulsatile pulmonary perfusion. Pulsatile pulmonary perfusion such as occurs under physiological conditions was demonstrated to reduce inflammation more than a nonpulsatile model; therefore, it appears as a valuable tool to be implemented in cardiac surgeries in the near future.[16] Associated mechanical ventilation during CPB may also have protective effects if maintained together with pulmonary artery perfusion.[13] Cardiac surgeons have accepted the common practice of interrupting ventilation during CPB as blood oxygenation by the lungs is no longer required, and the movement from mechanical ventilation may interfere with the operation. However, hypoventilation during CPB is responsible for development of microatelectasis, hydrostatic pulmonary edema, poor compliance, and higher incidence of infection.[17] Therefore, combined lung ventilation and perfusion during CPB may have a beneficial role in preserving lung function by limiting platelet and neutrophil sequestration and attenuating the thromboxane 2 (TBX_2) response to CPB.[18]

The use of ultrafiltration during pediatric open heart surgery appeared to reduce excess body water accumulated during CPB and to improve hemodynamic parameters[19] and in adults to attenuate cytokine and adhesion molecules levels. Heparin-coated CPB circuits also aimed to reduce CPB-related complications by improving hemocompatibility. Hypothermia has been associated with reduced atrial fibrillation,[20] and it may delay but does not prevent expression of inflammatory mediators.[21] Despite efforts at identifying an optimal temperature for using CPB, studies have given conflicting results. Salerno et al.[22,23] demonstrated improvements in myocardial metabolism and function under warm cardioplegia, but hypothermia provided better neuroprotection in experimental studies.[24]

15.5   Beating Heart Technique

Conventional cardiac surgery and current myocardial protection are associated with varying degrees of myocardial injury, especially in patients with impaired ventricular function or right ventricular hypertrophy undergoing valve replacement. Both cold and warm cardioplegic strategies, used intermittently, have been shown to provide suboptimal myocardial protection. Conventional approaches lack sufficient oxygen delivery to the myocardium during cross clamping of the aorta between replenishments of the cardioplegic solution. Thus, cardioplegic arrest techniques will inevitably produce some degree of reperfusion injury, and they may result in significant risk of postoperative left ventricular dysfunction, requiring high-dose inotropic drug support, especially in those with prolonged CPB and cardioplegia arrest.[25]

Various surgical strategies have been developed in myocardial protection to prevent ischemia-reperfusion injury during cardiac surgery over the past decade. Several studies demonstrated the efficacy of using oxygenated blood supply to the heart throughout the operation to keep the heart in a more physiologic state. Good results were presented with perfusion in a retrograde fashion through the coronary venous system from the coronary sinus ostium.[26] Under this technique, there was less myocardial damage compared to cardioplegic arrest and a similar quality of visual field and technical accuracy. Other reports showed better results using antegrade myocardial perfusion since this procedure provides uniform distribution of the blood to every part of the myocardium, allowing longer operations.[27] Clinically, isolated antegrade perfusion through the aorta is used frequently; however, it does not ensure ideal blood delivery beyond eventual coronary stenoses or in the presence of aortic insufficiency. Retrograde techniques overcome these limitations, but they represent severe risk in patients with ventricular fibrillation.

In these cases, the technique should be abandoned because malperfusion is strongly suggested.[26]

Based on these limitations, Salerno and Buckberg[28,29] introduced a simultaneous antegrade/retrograde warm blood cardioplegia, which was subsequently proved to be safe and effective both experimentally and clinically. In this model, potassium was removed from the cardioplegic solution, allowing the surgery to be performed without cardioplegia by maintaining the heart in a perfused beating-empty state with normal electrocardiogram and sinus rhythm. This method of myocardial protection avoids ischemia-reperfusion injury, leaving the heart in a more physiologic condition during surgery. This technique has been investigated utilizing MRI (magnetic resonance imaging), which demonstrated a decrease of myocardial edema in hypertrophied beating hearts relative to conventional cardioplegic techniques.[30] The beneficial effects of the technique may be explained as a result of preservation of normal lymphatic flow[31] and prevention of inward movement of potassium chloride, leading to a reduction in accumulation of extracellular fluid and myocardial edema, thereby contributing to preserve myocardial function.

Several reports have appeared subsequently about surgical procedures utilizing beating heart techniques[25,26] in which cardioplegia is not used. Proinflammatory cytokines (i.e., IL-6, IL-8, and TNF-α) were significantly reduced in beating heart CABG (coronary artery bypass grafting).[32] In situ hybridization studies confirmed that myocardium is the main source of IL-6 synthesis after cold cardioplegic arrest and CPB.[33] IL-8 was shown to be released from the myocardium during ischemia-reperfusion,[34] and it has a positive correlation with troponin I after cardiac surgery. IL-10, an anti-inflammatory cytokine, was lower during beating heart surgery which can be explained by the decreased inflammatory response.[32]

Consequently, better early and midterm outcomes have been reported in patients receiving the beating heart technique; positive results included a reduced risk of stay in an intensive care unit, shorter total hospitalization time,[35] and use of inotropes.[25] Theoretically, by eliminating ischemia-reperfusion injury imposed by cardioplegia arrest, all cytokines and proinflammatory mediators should be attenuated. However, the use of CPB alone with both lungs ventilated results in a significant rise in all cytokines, which explains the great contribution of CPB in tissue injury. Although presently several cardiac operations cannot be performed without the use of CPB, beating heart surgeries appear as an intermediate option that continues to use CPB but eliminates the ischemic component.[26]

Almost all procedures already can be performed with beating heart technique under more physiologic states. There have been reported clinical trials with beating heart valve replacement of both mitral and aortic valves. Ricci and colleagues demonstrated the efficacy and safety of performing beating heart multiple valve surgery in a cohort of 59 patients with excellent outcomes.[37] Recently, Macedo et al. also demonstrated that beating heart surgery may be an attractive alternative to patients with impaired left ventricular function. In this series, it was reported an overall hospital mortality of 6% in patients with left ventricular ejection fraction (LVEF) < 30% undergoing beating heart valve replacements.[38] These results compare favorably with those utilizing conventional cardioplegia, with mortality between 6.4% and 12.5%. Beyond myocardial protective effects, in cases of mitral valve operations, beating heart surgery also provided a good opportunity to examine the mitral valve under more physiological conditions than the cardioplegic arrest state, when the valve becomes motionless and flaccid and may not accurately reflect its function.

Potential concerns related to warm beating-heart valve surgery include performance of surgery in a relatively blood-filled field, limited surgical precision due to difficult exposure, risk of air and debris embolization, a steep learning curve, and paradigm shift from arrested to beating heart valve surgery. The hypothetical increased risk of air embolism delayed this technique from implementation in routine cardiac practice. Brain ischemic injury during cardiac surgery may be induced by several perioperative events, such as global hypoperfusion or focal ischemia due to debris, especially air emboli. However, randomized studies[36] demonstrated no difference regarding neurological monitoring and major neurological outcomes between beating heart surgery and conventional arrested heart valve replacement.

15.6 ConcomitantL ungPer fusion/ventilation during Beating Heart Surgery

Although beating heart surgery with simultaneous antegrade/retrograde coronary perfusion has improved myocardial protection, there is still increased risk of pulmonary injury during CPB. Over the years, cardiac surgeons have accepted the common practice of stopping ventilation and perfusion during CPB as blood oxygenation by the lungs is no longer required and due to technical difficulties presented by the movement from mechanical ventilation. Consequently, it may result in atelectasis and parenchymal interstitial edema. Restoration of pulmonary artery blood flow at the end of cardiopulmonary bypass may further increase alveolar damage (ischemia-reperfusion injury).[14] This may translate into clinically significant increase in alveolar-arteriolar oxygen gradient, hypoxemia and pulmonary artery vasoconstriction.[39]

Cardiac and pulmonary dysfunction play a major role in limiting surgical outcomes, as the population of patients undergoing heart surgery changes and complexity of surgery increases. Lung perfusion and ventilation during cardiopulmonary bypass is a concept that has been gradually introduced as an 'ideal' modality of lung protection. Thus, beating heart valve surgery with concomitant continuous warm retrograde cardioplegia and continuous lung perfusion/ventilation, should be viewed conceptually at maintaining function and perfusion of organs that are susceptible to ischemia. Based on encouraging results of beating heart valve surgery with preserved ventricular function, and decreased need for inotropic support, continuous lung perfusion/ventilation, in our experience, allows for preservation of alveolar-arterial oxygen gradient, especially in patients considered at risk for post-cardiopulmonary bypass respiratory failure.

Our group has recently reported in a pilot study the role of lung perfusion/ventilation during warm beating heart valve surgery.[40] The technical aspects are summarized below:

Lungpe rfusion
A 14 gauge catheter, derived from the ascending aortic cannula, is inserted into the main pulmonary artery (PA). Pulmonary artery perfusion flows depend on the systemic perfusion pressure. At systemic flows of 5 L/min, and mean pressure of 60 mmHg, measured flows in the PA are maintained above 400 ml/min by Doppler flow measurement.

Alveolarv entilation
The lungs are ventilated with tidal volumes at 4-5 ml/kg of ideal body weight, frequency 5-6 breaths/min and PEEP (positive end-expiratory pressure) 5 cmH$_2$O. The heart is vented via the right superior pulmonary vein (Vent flow rates varied between 250-350 ml/min). Inspired and expired tidal flows are continuously analyzed with continuous side-stream capnography.

In near the future, cardiac surgeons have the challenge to attenuate the effects of CPB and pulmonary ischemia and therefore improve outcomes of patients undergoing beating heart surgery. An enormous experimental contribution has been provided with the assessment of maintained pulsatile pulmonary artery perfusion and lung ventilation throughout the operation, but further clinical studies have to confirm these potential beneficial effects.

References

1. Nolan SP, Zacour R, Dammann JF. Reflections on the evolution of cardiopulmonary bypass. *Ann Thorac Surg.* 1997;64: 1540-1543.
2. Murphy GJ, Angelini GD. Side effects of cardiopulmonary bypass: what's the reality? *J Card Surg.*2004; 19:481-488.
3. Paparella D, Yau TM, Young E. Cardiopulmonary bypass induced inflammation: pathophysiology and treatment. An update. *Eur J Cardiothorac Surg.*2002; 21:232-244.
4. Chenoweth DE, Cooper SW, Hugli TE, et al. Complement activation during cardiopulmonary bypass: evidence for generation of C3a and C5a anaphylotoxins. *N Engl J Med.* 1981;304:497-503.
5. Fischer WH, Jagels MA, Hugli TE. Regulation of IL-6 synthesis in human peripheral blood mononuclear cells by C3a and C3a (desArg). *J Immunol.*1999; 162:453-459.
6. Andersen LW, Landow L, Baek L, et al. Association between gastric intramucosal pH and splanchnic endotoxin, antibody to endotoxin, and TNF-α concentration in patients undergoing cardiopulmonary bypass. *Crit Care Med.* 1993;21:210-217.
7. Christman JW, Lancaster LH, Blackwell TS. Nuclear factor κ B: a pivotal role in the systemic inflammatory response syndrome and new target for therapy. *Intensive Care Med.* 1998;24:1131-1138.
8. Edmunds LH Jr. Inflammatory response to cardiopulmonary bypass. *Ann Thorac Surg.*1998; 66:S12-S16.
9. Ilton MK, Langton PE, Taylor ML, et al. Differential expression of neutrophil adhesion molecule during coronary artery surgery with cardiopulmonary bypass. *J Thorac Cardiovasc Surg.*1999; 118:930-937.
10. Jordan JE, Zhao ZQ, Vinten-Johansen J. The role of neutrophils in myocardial ischemia-reperfusion injury. *Cardiovasc Res.*1999; 43:860-878.
11. Zahler S, Massoudy P, Hartl H, et al. Acute cardiac inflammatory response to postischemic reperfusion during cardiopulmonary bypass. *Cardiovasc Res.*1999; 41:722-730.
12. Wan S, DeSmet JM, Barvais L, et al. Myocardium is a major source of proinflammatory cytokines in patients undergoing cardiopulmonary bypass. *J Thorac Cardiovasc Surg.* 1996; 112:806-811.

13. Ng CS, Wan S, Yim AP, Arifi AA. Pulmonary dysfunction after cardiac surgery. *Chest*.2002; 121:1269-1277.
14. Schlensak C, Doenst T, Preusser S, et al. Bronchial artery perfusion during cardiopulmonary bypass does not prevent ischemia of the lung in piglets: assessment of bronchial artery blood flow with fluorescent microspheres. *Eur J Cardiothorac Surg*. 2001;19:326-331.
15. Massoudy P, Zahler S, Becker BF, et al. Evidence for inflammatory responses of the lungs during coronary artery bypass grafting with cardiopulmonary bypass. *Chest*. 2001;119: 31-36.
16. Siepe M, Goebel U, Mecklenburg A, et al. Pulsatile pulmonary perfusion during cardiopulmonary bypass reduces the pulmonary inflammatory response. *Ann Thorac Surg*. 2008;86:115-122.
17. Magnusson L, Zemgulis V, Tehling A, et al. Use of a vital capacity maneuver to prevent atelectasis after cardiopulmonary bypass. *Anesthesiology*.1998; 88:134-142.
18. Friedman M, Sellke FW, Wang SY, et al. Parameters of pulmonary injury after total or partial cardiopulmonary bypass. *Circulation*.1994;90: 262-268.
19. Naik SK, Knight A, Elliot M. A prospective randomized study of a modified technique of ultrafiltration during pediatric open-heart surgery. *Circulation*. 1991;84:III422-III431.
20. Adams DC, Heyer EJ, Simon AE, et al. Incidence of atrial fibrillation after mild or moderate hypothermic cardiopulmonary bypass. *Crit Care Med*.2000; 28:309-311.
21. Le Deist F, Menaché P, Kucharsky C, et al. Hypothermia during cardiopulmonary bypass delays but does not prevent neutrophil-endothelial cell adhesion. A clinical study. *Circulation*. 1995;92:II354-III358.
22. Mezzetti A, Calafiore AM, Salerno TA, et al. Intermittent antegrade warm cardioplegia reduces oxidative stress and improves metabolism of the ischemic-reperfused human myocardium. *J Thorac Cardiovasc Surg*. 1995;109:787-795.
23. Wang J, Liu H, Salerno TA, et al. Does normothermic normokalemic simultaneous antegrade/retrograde perfusion improve myocardial oxygenation and energy metabolism for hypertrophied hearts? *Ann Thorac Surg*. 2007;83(5): 1751-1758.
24. Conroy BP, Lin CY, Jenkins LW, et al. Hypothermic modulation of cerebral ischemic injury during cardiopulmonary bypass in pigs. *Anesthesiology*.1998; 88:390-402.
25. Salerno TA, Panos AL, Tian G, et al. Surgery for cardiac valve and aortic root without cardioplegic arrest ("beating heart"): experience with a new method of myocardial perfusion. *J Card Surg*.2 007;22:459-464.
26. Matsumoto Y, Watanabe G, Endo M, et al. Efficacy and safety of on-pump beating heart surgery for valvular disease. *Ann Thorac Surg*.2002; 74:678-683.
27. Katircioglu SF, Cicekcioglu F, Tutun U, et al. On-pump beating heart mitral valve surgery without cross-clamping the aorta. *J Card Surg*.2008; 23:307-311.

28. Ihnken K, Morita K, Buckberg GD, Salerno TA, et al. The safety of simultaneous arterial and coronary sinus perfusion: experimental background and initial clinical results. *J Cardiac Surg*. 1994;9:15-25.
29. Ihnken K, Morita K, Buckberg GD, Salerno TA, et al. Simultaneous arterial and coronary sinus cardioplegic perfusion: an experimental and clinical study. *Thorac Cardiovasc Surg*.1994; 42(3):141-147.
30. Wang J, Liu H, Salerno TA, et al. Keeping heart empty and beating improves preservation of hypertrophied hearts for valve surgery. *J Thorac Cardiovasc Surg*. 2006;132:1314-1320.
31. Mehlhorn U, Allen SJ, Adams DL, et al. Normothermic continuous antegrade blood cardioplegia does not prevent myocardial edema and cardiac dysfunction. *Circulation*. 1995;92: 1940-1946.
32. Wan IY, Arifi AA, Wan S, et al. Beating heart revascularization with or without cardiopulmonary bypass: evaluation of inflammatory response in a prospective randomized study. *J Thorac Cardiovasc Surg*.2004; 127:1624-1631.
33. Dreyer WJ, Philips SC, Lindsey ML, et al. Interleukin-6 induction in the canine myocardium after cardiopulmonary bypass. *J Thorac Cardiovasc Surg*.2000; 120:256-263.
34. Ivey CL, Williams FM, Collins PD, et al. Neutrophil chemoattractants generated in two phases during reperfusion of ischemic myocardium in the rabbit: evidence for a role for C5a and interleukin-8. *J Clin Invest*. 1995;95:2720-2728.
35. Angelini GD, Taylor FC, Barnaby CR, et al. Early and midterm outcome after off-pump and on-pump surgery in Beating Heart against Cardioplegic Arrest Studies (BHACAS 1 and 2): a pooled analysis of two randomized controlled trials. *Lancet*.2002; 359:1194-1199.
36. Karadeniz U, Erdemli O, Yamak B, et al. On-pump beating heart versus hypothermic arrested heart valve replacement surgery. *J Card Surg*.2008; 23:107-113.
37. Ricci M, Macedo FI, Suarez MR, et al. Multiple valve surgery with beating heart technique. *Ann. Thorac. Surg* 2009; 87:527- 31.
38. Macedo FI, Carvalho EM, Hassan M, et al. Beating heart valve surgery in patients with low left ventricular ejection fraction. *J. Card. Surg*. 2010; 25(3):267–271.
39. Macedo FI, Carvalho EM, Gologorsky E, Salerno T. Lung ventilation/perfusion may reduce pulmonary injury during cardiopulmonary bypass. *J. Thorac Cardiovasc Surg*. 2010; 139(1):234- 6.
40. Macedo FI, Carvalho EM, Gologorsky E, et al. Gas Exchange during lung perfusion/ventilation during cardiopulmonary bypass: preliminary results of a pilot study. Open Journal of CardiovascularS urgery2010; 3: 1-7.

Si Pham and Eddie Manning

16.1 Introduction

Pulmonary edema is an abnormal collection of fluid in extravascular tissue or spaces of the lung.[1] The lungs have a dynamic water content; water and proteins continuously move into the interstitial lung spaces and return to the circulation via the lymphatic system. It is generally accepted that fluid movement between these spaces is governed by Starling's forces across semipermeable membranes. Pulmonary edema is the result of physiologic derangements that disrupt the normal circulation of fluids within the microstructure of the lung. This derangement can be an increase in pressures across the microvasculature (cardiogenic or high-pressure edema), a loss of integrity of the pulmonary capillary (increased permeability edema), or a combination of both. Pulmonary edema is associated with a variety of processes, including cardiac dysfunction, sepsis, traumatic injuries, occupational exposures, organ transplantation, blood transfusion, metabolic derangements, and fluid resuscitation. Although the clinical presentations of pulmonary edema, which manifests as signs and symptoms of hypoxia, may be similar, the treatments and prognosis of different types of pulmonary edema are quite different. This chapter reviews the different mechanisms that cause pulmonarye dema.

SiPha m(✉)
University of Miami, Jackson Memorial Hospital,
Miami, FL, USA
e-mail:s pham@med.miami.edu

16.2 Microstructureso ft heL ung that Participate in Normal Circulation of Fluids

The five microstructures that are important in the circulation of fluid within the lung are the pulmonary arterioles, capillaries, venules, lymphatics, alveolar wall interstitial spaces, and extra-alveolar interstitial spaces. Arterioles arise as terminations or lateral branches of the larger muscular pulmonary arteries.[2] Arterioles that participate in the formation of pulmonary edema have a near-identical microscopic appearance to their venous counterparts (the venules) and are only distinguishable by their position in the pulmonary lobule. The pulmonary arterioles and venules have external diameters of less than 100 μm, are devoid of a muscular layer, and consist of a single elastic lamina lined by endothelial cells. Pulmonary capillaries that arise from the arterioles form a web that covers the outer surface of the alveoli. They consist of a basement membrane lined by a single-cell layer of endothelium. The patency of any given capillary is dependent on its location on the surface of the alveolus. Those located on the alveolar wall of two adjacent alveoli are frequently collapsed when the intra-alveolar pressure exceeds the capillary hydrostatic pressure. In contrast, the capillaries present in regions where three or more alveoli meet are always patent.

The ultrastructure of the respiratory unit reveals that the alveolar wall is made up of a single layer of type I pneumocytes, a basement membrane, as well as a discontinuous layer of alveolar interstitium.[3] Along the periphery of the alveolar cells, the basal laminae of the endothelium and epithelium fuse together to constitute a thin layer of the alveolar wall without intestinal space. From this region toward the central portion of each alveolar cell, the basal epithelial and endothelial laminae separate, creating a space of extracellular matrix that is devoid of lymphatics.[2] These small pockets of matrix comprise the *alveolar interstitial space.* Fluid that accumulates in this space does not drain directly into the lymphatic system but must first travel to the extra-alveolar interstitial space. The *extra-alveolar interstitial space* is a continuous region that consists of the junctions where three or more alveoli meet and all of the connective tissue compartments that surround each pulmonary lobule. Within the extra-alveolar space reside the lymphatic microvessels, which have valves to allow unidirectional movement of fluid.[3] These lymphatic microvessels gradually increase in size as they join more centrally located ones. As the pulmonary lymphatics travel centrally toward the hilum, they increase in caliber and coalesce to form lymphatic trunks that drain into the central venous system at the convergence of the right subclavian and right internal jugular veins or on the left side via the thoracic duct or direct connection to the subclavian vein.

16.3 Physical Forces Governing Fluid Movement Within the Lung

The accumulation of fluid in the extra-alveolar interstitium is favored by both the physical forces acting on the pulmonary microvasculature and the active movement of fluid out of the alveolus by type I pneumocytes. There is convincing evidence that fluid developing within the alveolus is actively pumped into the alveolar interstitial space by sodium and potassium adenosine triphosphatase (ATPase) pumps located in the basolateral wall of type one pneumocytes.[3] The major barrier to fluid movement into the extra-alveolar space is the highly permeable capillary endothelium. Many small particles and water pass freely across this membrane, although the movement of protein is restricted. The movement of water out of the capillary lumen is governed by Starling's forces.[4] Generally, the hydrostatic forces within the capillary tend to favor fluid movement out, while the capillary oncotic pressure favors fluid movement into the lumen. On the contrary, the interstitial hydrostatic pressure favors fluid movement out of this space, while the oncotic

pressure draws fluid in. The net movement of fluid across the pulmonary microvascular endothelium is determined by Starling's equation, which states that fluid movement is equal to the product of the barrier conductance and driving pressure. The equation is expressed as follows[4]:

$$Q = K[(P_c - P_i) - \sigma(\pi_c - \pi_i)]$$

Q equals the net flow of fluid across the endothelium and out of the capillary lumen; K is the filtration coefficient; P_c and P_i are the hydrostatic pressures of the capillary and interstitium, respectively; σ is the reflection coefficient; and π_c and π_i are the oncotic forces of the capillary and interstitium, respectively.[4] K is the property of the system that describes how much water will flow across the membrane per unit change in pressure. This property is specific for the pulmonary capillary and is estimated to be 1 mL H_2O/mmHg min^{-1}.[1] σ is the reflection coefficient, which describes the effectiveness of the membrane in preventing the passage of protein compared with that of water across the membrane. The reflection coefficient of the pulmonary capillary is estimated to be 0.7–0.8, indicating that protein can cross the membrane, but the membrane is 70–80% effective as a barrier to this movement.

The pulmonary capillary hydrostatic pressure P_c is between the pulmonary artery and left atrial pressures. It can be calculated using the following formula[5]:

$$P_c = P_{CWP} + (P_{MPA} - P_{CWP})$$

P_{CWP} equals the pulmonary capillary wedge pressure or the pulmonary artery occlusion pressure, and P_{MPA} equals the mean pulmonary artery pressure. It should be noted, however, that the pulmonary capillary hydrostatic pressure is influenced by gravitational forces and remains higher in the lower portions of the upright lung when compared to the apex. The interstitial hydrostatic pressure is unknown, but it is generally accepted that it is well below atmospheric pressure. The colloid osmotic pressure of the interstitium has been derived from the protein concentration of lymph fluid from the lung. It is generally assumed that the protein composition of the interstitium is similar to that of the lymphatic fluid draining this space.[6,7] The colloid osmotic pressure of the pulmonary capillary is readily measured; its normal value is 25–28 mmHg.

Although the application of Starling's equation is purely theoretical, it gives us significant insight into the fluid dynamics of the pulmonary circulation and derangements that lead to the development of pulmonary edema. Substituting accepted normal values for each parameter in Starling's equation yields the following[8]:

$$Q = K[(P_c - P_i) - \sigma(\pi_c - \pi_i)]$$

$$Q = 1[(5-(-7)) - 0.8(25-12)] = 1.6$$

Therefore, in normal physiologic conditions there is a net positive flow of fluid from the microvascular lumen into the alveolar interstitium. In this compartment, pulmonary lymphatics remove fluid and return it to the venous circulation. The efficiency of the lymphatics is improved as the space expands, so that in many instances it appears that the fluid flows directly from the capillaries into the lymphatics.[2] When the rate of fluid accumulation in the extra-alveolar space exceeds the rate of lymphatic drainage, pulmonary edema will occur.

16.4 Pathophysiology

Pulmonary edema is the end result of fluid movement out of the microvasculature and into the extra-alveolar interstitial space at a rate beyond the drainage capacity of the pulmonary lymphatics. In addition to the lymphatics, there are two other mechanisms that protect against pulmonary edema within the interstitium. The first is the decreasing tissue oncotic pressure created by the dilutional effect of fluid moving into the interstitium. Because there is a relatively fixed complement of proteins within this space, the protein concentration decreases as water accumulates, thus decreasing the oncotic pressure. The second protective mechanism against the development of pulmonary edema is the increasing tissue hydrostatic pressure, which develops as water accumulates in the interstitium. Both of these protective mechanisms favor the movement of water out of the interstitium and into the pulmonary microvasculature.[2]

The development of pulmonary edema occurs in two stages. The first stage, as described, is the development of interstitial pulmonary edema, and the second stage is the progression to alveolar edema. Microscopically, the first stage is characterized by engorgement of the alveolar and extra-alveolar interstitiums with peribronchial and perivascular fluid accumulation and thickening of the alveolar wall (Fig. 16.1). Although pulmonary edema at this stage causes minimal impairment of pulmonary function, it does produce radiographic findings.[4] On the chest radiograph, short, linear, horizontal lines (Kerley's B lines) occur near the pleural surface of the lung in the lower zones as the result of fluid accumulation along the interlobar septum. Blotchy shadowing over most of the lung fields may occur in more severe interstitial edema (Fig. 16.2). Because this pattern usually originates from the hilar structures, it gives a butterfly appearance on chest X-rays.

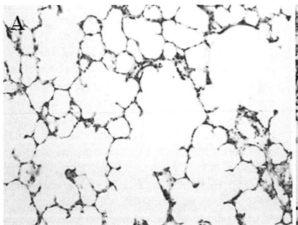
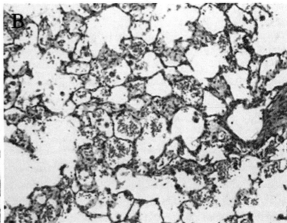

Fig. 16.1 Histology of pulmonary edema from increased capillary permeability. (**a**) Normal Lewis rat lung with preserved alveolar architecture; (**b**) increased capillary permeability after ischemia-reperfusion injury allows proteins and blood cells to leaki ntot hea lveolara irspace

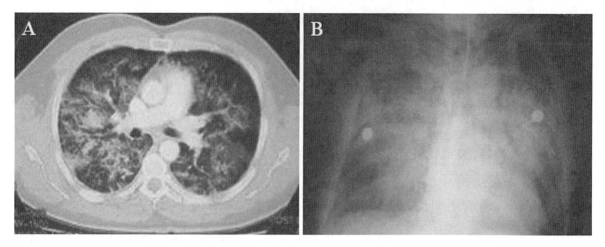

Fig. 16.2 Radiographic appearance of pulmonary edema. (**A**) Computed tomogram of the chest shows the bat's wing appearance of pulmonary edema; (**B**) chest radiograph shows the blotchy radiopaque densities in a butterfly wing configuration

As the interstitial fluid accumulates, the second stage of pulmonary edema, which is called *alveolar edema* (or alveolar flooding), occurs. In this stage, the alveolar airspaces are filled with fluid. The exact route of fluid movement into the alveolus is a topic of debate. As fluid moves into the alveolus, it covers the free surface and eventually fills the alveolar airspace. The force that keeps the alveolar space open is governed by Laplace's law:

$$P = 2T / R$$

where P equals pressure, T equals surface tension, and R equals radius. As the edema progresses, alveolar surfactant is replaced with edema fluid, causing an increase in the surface tension and a decrease in the alveolar radius. As the alveoli fill with fluid and shrink in size, ventilation becomes insufficient, and hypoxemia ensues. The continued accumulation of fluid in the alveolar edema leads to the movement of fluid into the small and large airways, eventually expelled as frothy sputum. It has been shown that protective mechanisms against alveolar flooding reside within the alveolar cells. There is ample evidence indicating that the alveolar epithelium actively reabsorbs fluid in the alveolar airspace.[8,9] This process involves vectorial transport of Na^+ out of alveolar airspaces, with water following the Na^+ osmotic gradient, and is regulated via apical Na^+ and chloride channels and the sodium pump (Na-K-ATPase) located on the basolateral surface of the alveolar epithelial cells. Emerging evidence suggests that augmenting the sodium

pump by pharmacologic approaches[10,11] or gene therapy[11,12] may improve pulmonary edema.

16.5 Pathogenesiso fPul monaryEdem a

Physiologically, pulmonary edema can be classified into two categories: cardiogenic pulmonary edema (also called hydrostatic pulmonary edema) and noncardiogenic pulmonary edema (also known as increased permeability pulmonary edema).[13] Pulmonary edema is the result of a disturbance of the Starling's forces that regulate the flux of fluid across the pulmonary microvasculature. In a normal homeostatic state, there is a balance among hydrostatic and oncotic forces within the pulmonary capillary bed and the interstitial spaces. There is a small positive flux of fluid across the capillary bed, which is removed by the lymphatic systems (Fig. 16.3a). Cardiogenic pulmonary edema occurs when there is an increase in capillary hydrostatic pressure that overcomes the intravascular oncotic pressures, resulting in an increase in the flux of fluid across the capillary bed of a magnitude that overcomes the ability of the lymphatics to drain the transudate fluid (Fig. 16.3b). On the other hand, noncardiogenic pulmonary edema occurs when there is an increase in the permeability of the pulmonary microvasculature (Fig. 16.3c). Table 16.1 summarizes common clinical conditions that cause pulmonary edema.[2,14]

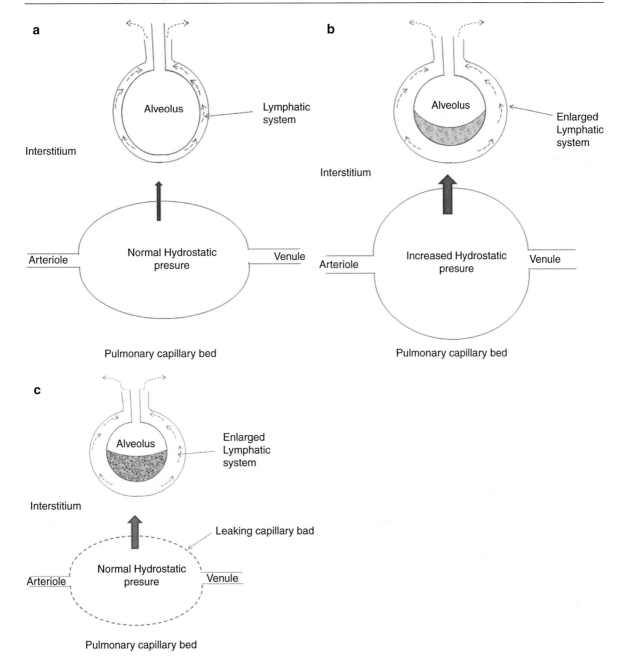

Fig. 16.3 Schematic representation of the mechanisms of pulmonary edema. (**a**) Normal physiological state; there is net positive outward flow of fluid from the pulmonary capillary, which is absorbed by the lymphatic system; (**b**) cardiogenic pulmonary edema with increased capillary hydrostatic pressure; (**c**) noncardiogenic pulmonary edema with increased capillary permeability

16.5.1 Cardiogenic Pulmonary Edema

Cardiogenic pulmonary edema is the most common form of pulmonary edema and is caused by cardiac dysfunction (such as acute myocardial infarction, aortic or mitral valve regurgitation, mitral valve stenosis, myocarditis, or primary cardiomyopathy) or other conditions that increase pulmonary capillary pressure (Fig. 16.3b). The common pathway of cardiogenic edema, regardless of the underlying causes, is the

Table 16.1 Clinical conditions associated with pulmonary edema

Cardiogenic pulmonary edema
Left heart failure
Mitrals tenosis
Fluido verload
Obstruction of pulmonary vein
Constrictivepe ricarditis
Noncardiogenic pulmonary edema
Pneumonia
Aspiration of gastric content
Sepsis
Inhalationi njury
Ischemia-reperfusioni njury
Cardiopulmonarybypa ss
Transfusion of blood products
Acutepa ncreatitis
Drugo verdose
High-altitude pulmonary edema

increase in left atrial pressure leading to an increase in pulmonary venous and capillary pressures. The absolute capillary pressure needed to produce alveolar edema is relative to the overall disease state. It is a rapid rate of rise of the capillary hydrostatic pressure, and not the absolute pressure, that produces the edema. For example, in a patient with chronic mitral valve stenosis, for which left atrial pressures (and pulmonary capillary pressures) increase gradually, the pulmonary lymphatics are allowed time to adapt to this increased interstitial edema by increasing in size and number. This adaptation prevents alveolar edema at relatively high capillary hydrostatic pressures. In contrast, when a young trauma patient, whose atrial pressure is normal, receives an excessive amount of intravenous fluids or blood products over a short period of time, the capillary hydrostatic pressure increases rapidly. This rapid rise in capillary pressure produces a large increase in the interstitial fluid that overwhelms the lymphatic drainage capacity, resulting in alveolar edema at a relatively low pulmonary capillary pressure. This mechanism also explains the development of acute pulmonary edema that occurs as a result of an acute myocardial infarction, which results in a rapid rise in pulmonary capillary

pressure.[15] If the rise in hydrostatic pressure in the capillary is of sufficient magnitude, it will also lead to capillary stress failure, causing disruption of the pulmonary microvasculature and the alveolar membrane and resulting in the presence of protein-rich fluid-containing blood cells in the airway.

16.5.2 Noncardiogenic Pulmonary Edema

Noncardiogenic pulmonary edema occurs in the absence of elevated capillary hydrostatic pressures. Some of the mechanisms responsible for this type of pulmonary edema are discussed next.

16.5.3 Increased Capillary Permeability

According to the Starling's equation, in addition to increased hydrostatic pressure, another way to increase fluid movement across the capillary bed is to alter the integrity of the endothelial barrier. The primary cause of noncardiogenic pulmonary edema is increased capillary permeability, which may occur as the result of disruption of the capillary membrane because of exposures to toxins, radiation, ischemia, free radicals, or cytokines released during active infections.[16] The ultrastructural disruption of the capillary membrane leads to the movement of fluids, solutes, and blood cells into the alveolus (Fig. 16.2). Compared to cardiogenic pulmonary edema, alveolar fluid of patients with noncardiogenic pulmonary edema has a high protein content because the damaged vascular membrane is permeable to plasma proteins.

16.5.4 Reduced Lymphatic Drainage

The lymphatic system is an important mechanism for maintaining the normal hydration state of the lung. Lymphatic flow can increase by a factor of 10 when there is an increase in the interstitial pressure.[17] Magno and associates demonstrated that animals with chronically interrupted lymphatic vessels developed more severe pulmonary edema for similar stress than those with intact lymphatic vessels.[18] In clinical settings, reduced lymphatic drainage may occur in conditions in which the central venous pressure is chronically elevated (such as congestive heart failure, restrictive cardiomyopathy, fibrosing mediastinitis), impeding the draining of lymphatic fluid into the central venous system. Obstruction of the lymphatic vessels can also be caused by metastatic cancer cells or radiation-induced mediastinitis. Lung transplantation is another clinical situation in which the lymphatic drainage of the lung graft is destroyed. The reduced lymphatic drainage in the transplanted lung may contribute appreciably to posttransplant pulmonary edema observed during the perioperativepe riod.

16.5.5 Decreased Interstitial Pressure

Decreased interstitial pressure has been shown experimentally to promote the formation of pulmonary edema in the rapidly expanding lung when a large, single-sided pleural collection or pneumothorax is evacuated.[19,20] Because this fluid is usually of the high-permeability type, it is believed to be the result of damage to the ultrastructure of the pulmonary capillary, resulting in plasma proteins and fluids leaking into the interstitial and alveolar spaces.[4]

16.5.6 Decreased Colloid Osmotic Pressure

There is both experimental and clinical evidence that link decreased colloid osmotic pressure with the development of pulmonary edema. In conditions when plasma oncotic pressure is reduced from 25 to 15 torr, measurable pulmonary edema occurs with small increases in left atrial pressure.[21] Clinical conditions such as liver failure, nephrotic syndrome, and excessive administration of crystalloid solution produce hypoalbuminemia, which results in pulmonary edema in patients with mildly elevated left atrial pressures.

16.5.7 Unclear Etiology

There are clinical conditions in which the pathogenesis of pulmonary edema is not clearly established. Some of these conditions are as follows:

(a) *High-altitude pulmonary edema*: High-altitude pulmonary edema occurs in susceptible individuals who ascend to altitudes greater than 2,500 m for an hour or longer.[22] There has been a significant amount of research on the pathophysiology of this type of noncardiogenic pulmonary edema. Bronchoalveolar lavage samples from patients with high-altitude pulmonary edema show the characteristics of increased capillary permeability with high protein concentrations as well as blood cells.[23,24] These findings indicate that capillary damage occurs in this disorder. West et al. have suggested that the capillary injury is the result of stress failure precipitated by the increase in pulmonary artery pressures.[25] When exposed to low oxygen tension, there is a rise in pulmonary artery pressure secondary to constriction of these vessels. This constriction usually serves to protect the capillaries by decreasing their exposure to elevated hydrostatic forces. Whayne et al.[26] suggested that edema develops as a result of ruptured arterial walls proximal to the areas of constriction. However, it is widely accepted that uneven constriction of the small pulmonary arterioles leaves portions of the capillary bed unprotected and thus exposed to high pressures, resulting in capillary rupture and leakage.[22] This type of stress failure, as it is termed, has been demonstrated to occur at transmural pressures that exceed 50 cm H_2O.[25]

(b) *Neurogenic pulmonary edema*: Another type of noncardiogenic pulmonary edema is neurogenic pulmonary edema. It has been demonstrated experimentally that neurogenic pulmonary edema is the result of increased hydrostatic pressure within the pulmonary vasculature leading to capillary damage.[27,28] This form of edema is seen most often in patients with increased sympathetic activity after suffering severe head trauma and intracranial hemorrhage.[29,30] The mechanism of neurogenic pulmonary edema is due to a sudden increase in intracranial pressure that induces an α-adrenergic catecholaminergic response, which in turn causes transient but intense increases in both pulmonary and systemic venous and arterial vasoconstrictions. The sudden massive increase in pulmonary hydrostatic pressure causes a shift of fluid into the pulmonary alveoli and the interstitial spaces. In addition, the increase in pulmonary vascular pressure also causes damage to the pulmonary capillary endothelium and alveolar epithelium, resulting in the leakage of red blood cells and proteins into the alveolar spaces.[28]

(c) *Transfusion-related acute lung injury (TRALI)*: TRALI is another cause of noncardiogenic pulmonary edema. TRALI is a clinical syndrome that consists of hypoxia and bilateral pulmonary edema that occurs during or within 6 h of a transfusion in the absence of cardiac failure or intravascular fluid overload.[31] Plasma-rich components of blood products such as fresh frozen plasma and apheresis platelets have been most frequently implicated as culprits. The pathogenesis of TRALI is not well understood. It is believed that antibodies against human leukocyte antigens (HLAs) class I and class II or neutrophil-specific antigens contained in the transfused blood products bind to the recipient's leukocytes, resulting in the activation and releases of biologic modifiers that cause damage to the pulmonary capillary bed.

Many other conditions associated with pulmonary edema have pathogenesis that is as yet unexplained or partially delineated. These conditions include drowning and secondary drowning, pulmonary embolism, cardioversion, eclampsia, cardiopulmonary bypass, overinflation of the lung, and heroin overdose. It is believed that the pulmonary edema associated with these conditions is primarily due to increased capillary permeability.

16.6 Summary

Pulmonary edema, which clinically manifests as hypoxemia, is an urgent clinical problem. The pathophysiological mechanisms that cause pulmonary edema are mainly due to an increased hydrostatic pressure in, or an increased permeability of, the pulmonary capillary bed. Understanding the underlying mechanisms that cause pulmonary edema will help guide clinicians to elicit the appropriate history and look for signs and symptoms that aid in the selection of proper confirmatory tests and plan for timely and appropriate treatments.

References

1. Noble WH. Pulmonary oedema: a review. *Canad Anaesth Soc J*.1980;27(3):2 86-302.
2. Hogg JC. Pulmonary edema. In: Churg AM, Myers JL, Tazelaar HD, Wright JL, eds. *Thurlbeck's pathology of the lung*. 3rd ed. New York: Thieme Medical; 2005:345-353.
3. Michel RP. Arteries and veins of the normal dog lung: qualitative and quantitative structural differences. *Am J Anat*. 1982;164:227-241.
4. West JB. *Pulmonary pathophysiology the essentials*. 6th ed. Baltimore: Lippincott; 2003:101-111.
5. Gaar KA Jr, Taylor AE, Owens LJ, et al. Pulmonary capillary pressure and filtration coefficient in the isolated perfused lung. *Am J Physiol*.1967; 213(4):910-914.
6. Permutt S, Caldini P. Tissue pressures and fluid dynamics of the lungs. *Fed Proc*.1976; 35:1876-1880.
7. Parker JC, Guyton AC, Taylor AE. Pulmonary interstitial and capillary pressures estimated from intra-alveolar fluid pressures. *J Appl Physiol*.1978; 44:267-276.
8. Dada LA, Sznajder JI, Dada LA, Sznajder JI. Mechanisms of pulmonary edema clearance during acute hypoxemic respiratory failure: role of the Na,K-ATPase. *Crit Care Med*. 2003;31(4s uppl):S248-S252.
9. Mutlu GM, Sznajder JI, Mutlu GM, Sznajder JI. Mechanisms of pulmonary edema clearance. *Am J Physiol Lung Cell Mol Physiol*.2005; 289(5):L685-L695.
10. Perkins GD, McAuley DF, Thickett DR, et al. The beta-agonist lung injury trial (BALTI): a randomized placebo-controlled clinical trial [see comment]. *Am J Resp Crit Care Med*.2006; 173(3):281-287.
11. Litvan J, Briva A, Wilson MS, et al. Beta-adrenergic receptor stimulation and adenoviral overexpression of superoxide dismutase prevent the hypoxia-mediated decrease in Na,K-ATPase and alveolar fluid reabsorption. *J Biol Chem*. 2006;281(29):19892-19898.
12. Mutlu GM, Machado-Aranda D, Norton JE, et al. Electroporation-mediated gene transfer of the Na⁺, K⁺-ATPase rescues endotoxin-induced lung injury. *Am J Resp Crit Care Med*.2007; 176(6):582-590.
13. Ware LB, Matthay MA, Ware LB, Matthay MA. Clinical practice. Acute pulmonary edema. *N Engl J Med*. 2005; 353(26):2788-2796.
14. Sibbald WJ, Anderson RR, Holliday RL, Sibbald WJ, Anderson RR, Holliday RL. Pathogenesis of pulmonary edema associated with the adult respiratory distress syndrome. *Can Med Assoc J*.1979; 120(4):445-450.
15. Graham SP, Vetrovec GW, Graham SP, Vetrovec GW. Comparison of angiographic findings and demographic variables in patients with coronary artery disease presenting with acute pulmonary edema versus those presenting with chest pain. *Am J Cardiol*.1991; 68(17):1614-1618.
16. Ware LB, Matthay MA, Ware LB, Matthay MA. The acute respiratory distress syndrome. *N Engl J Med*. 2000;342(18):1334-1349.
17. Parker JC, Falgout HJ, Grimbert FA, et al. The effect of increased vascular pressure on albumin-excluded volume and lymph flow in the dog lung. *Circ Res*. 1980;47(6):866-875.
18. Magno M, Szidon JP, Magno M, Szidon JP. Hemodynamic pulmonary edema in dogs with acute and chronic lymphatic ligation. *Am J Physiol*.1976; 231(6):1777-1782.
19. Ziskind MM, Wiel H, George RA. Acute pulmonary edema following the treatment of spontaneous pneumothorax with excessive negative intrapleural pressure. *Am Rev Respir Dis*. 1965;92:623-636.
20. Trapnell DH, Thurston JT. Unilateral pulmonary edema after pleural aspiration. *Lancet*.1970; 1:1367-1369.

21. Guyton AC, Lindsey AW. Effect of elevated left atrial pressure and decreased plasma protein concentration on the development pulmonary edema. *Circ Res*.1959; 7:649-657.
22. Stream JO, Grissom CK. Update on high-altitude pulmonary edema: pathogenesis, prevention, and treatment. *Wild Environ Med*.2008 ;293(4):293-303.
23. Schoene RB, Swenson ER, Pizzo CJ. The lung at high altitude, bronchoalveolar lavage in acute mountain sickness and pulmonary edema. *J Appl Physiol*.1988; 64:2605-2613.
24. Hackett PH, Bertman J, Rodriguez C. Pulmonary edema fluid protein in high-altitude pulmonary edema. *JAMA*. 1986;256:36.
25. West JB, Colice GL, Lee YJ. Pathogenesis of high altitude pulmonary oedema: direct evidence of stress failure of pulmonary capillaries. *Eur Respir J*.1995; 8:523-529.
26. Whayne TF, Severinghaus JW. Experimental hypoxia pulmonary edema in the rat. *J Appl Physiol*. 1968;25: 729-732.
27. Mickersie RC, Christensen JM, Lawrence H. Pulmonary extravascular fluid accumulation following intracranial injury. *J Trauma*.1993; 23:968-975.
28. Novitzky D, Wicomb WN, Rose AG, Cooper DK, Reichart B. Pathophysiology of pulmonary edema following experimental brain death in the chacma baboon. *Ann Thorac Surg*. 1987; 43:288-294.
29. Sedy J, Zicha J, Kunes J, et al. Mechanisms of neurogenic pulmonary edema development. *Physiol Res*. 2008;57(4): 499-506.
30. Baumann A, Audibert G, McDonnell J, et al. Neurogenic pulmonary edema. *Acta Anaesth Scand*. 2007;51(4):447-455.
31. Triulzi DJ, Triulzi DJ. Transfusion-related acute lung injury: current concepts for the clinician. *Anesth Analg*. 2009; 108(3):770-776.

Idiopathic Pulmonary Hypertension: NewC hallenges

17

Tomas Pulido and Julio Sandoval

17.1 Introduction

Idiopathic pulmonary hypertension (IPH), formerly known as primary pulmonary hypertension (PPH), is one of the most severe forms of pulmonary hypertension and is included as part of a group of disorders known as pulmonary arterial hypertension (PAH). The term IPAH refers to elevation of pulmonary pressure with no apparent cause; it is a chronic and progressive disease with a median survival, before the advent of specific targeted therapy, of 2.8 years, its incidence is about 1–2 cases per million people per year with a prevalence of 13.5 cases per million people per year in the United States and 6.5 cases per million per year in France. It is most commonly seen in women (male:female ratio of 1:2–2.9) of childbearing age but can occur in either gender and at any age.[1-3]

The clinical classification of pulmonary hypertension includes five main categories that share similar histological, physiopathological, and clinical characteristics, offering the possibility for similar treatment (Table 17.1).[4]

17.2 Geneticso fPA H

In the year 2000, the gene mutation responsible for familial pulmonary hypertension was identified by two separate groups (in North Carolina and New York).[5,6] This gene is located in the long arm of chromosome 2 and is called bone morphogenetic protein receptor 2

(BMPR2) which is part of the transforming growth factor beta (TGF-β) superfamily.[5,6] Familial PAH constituted approximately 6% of the cases of PAH in the National Institutes of Health (NIH) registry. The prevalence of the BMPR2 mutation in FPAH has been reported as between 50 and 75%. In patients with IPAH, the reported frequency of BMPR2 mutations ranges from 9 to 26%.[7-9] Evaluation of families of patients with hereditary hemorrhagic telangiectasia (HHT) syndrome has revealed mutations in a second gene, activin receptor-like kinase 1 (ALK-1). Approximately 10% of subjects with HTT develop IPAH. Also a member of the TGF-β superfamily, ALK-1 probably shares the same signals with the BMPR2 mutations.[10,11] Mutations in a third member of the TGF-β receptor superfamily, endoglin, have been implicated in the development of IPAH.[12]

17.3 Pathologyo fl PAH

The main abnormalities of the pulmonary vasculopathy of IPAH include medial hypertrophy, intimal and adventitial thickening, and plexiform lesions (Fig. 17.1). Medial hypertrophy is produced by hypertrophy and hyperplasia of smooth muscle fibers and an increase in connective tissue matrix and elastic fibers in the media of muscular arteries. Intimal thickening is characterized by infiltration of fibroblasts, myofibroblasts, and smooth muscle cells. The plexiform lesion is a focal proliferation of endothelial channels lined by fibroblasts, smooth muscle cells, and connective tissue matrix. Arteritis may be associated with plexiform lesions and is characterized by necrosis of the arterial wall with fibrinoid insudation and infiltration with inflammatory cells.[13]

T.Pulido (✉)
CardiopulmonaryD epartment, IgnacioC havez
NationalH eartI nstitute, MexicoC ity, Mexico
e-mail:t pulido@prodigy.net.mx

E.A. Gabriel and T. Salerno (eds.), *Principles of Pulmonary Protection in Heart Surgery*,
DOI: 10.1007/978-1-84996-308-4_17, © Springer-Verlag London Limited 2010

Table 17.1 Pulmonary hypertension clinical classification: Venice2004

Class 1: Pulmonary arterial hypertension (PAH)
Idiopathic(IPAH)
Familial(FP AH)
Associatedc onditions
Collagen vascular disease
Systemic-to-pulmonarys hunts
Portalh ypertension
HIVi nfection
Drugs or toxins
Other: thyroid diseases, glycogen storage disease, Gaucher's disease, hemorrhagic hereditary telangiectasia, hemoglobin diseases, myeloproliferative disorders Conditions associated with significant venous or capillary involvement:
Pulmonary veno-occlusive disease (PVOD)
Pulmonary capillary hemangiomatosis (PCH)
Persistent pulmonary hypertension of the newborn (PPHN)
Class 2: Pulmonary hypertension due to left-sided heart disease
Atrial or ventricular left-sided heart disease, including left ventricular diastolic dysfunction
Valvular heart disease
Class 3: Pulmonary hypertension due to lung disease or hypoxia
Chronic obstructive lung disease
Interstitial lung disease
Sleep-disorderedbr eathing
Alveolarh ypoventilation
Chronic exposure to high altitude
Developmenta bnormalities
Class 4: Pulmonary hypertension due to chronic embolic or thrombotic disease
Proximal obstruction of pulmonary arteries
Distal obstruction of pulmonary arteries
Nonthrombotic embolism (tumors, parasites, foreign body)
Class 5: Miscellaneous
Sarcoidosis, histiocytosis X, lymphangioleiomyomatosis, compression of pulmonary vessels (adenopathies, tumors, fibrosing mediastinitis)

17.4 Pathogenesiso fl PAH

It has been proposed that an initial insult to the endothelium may occur in susceptible individuals (genetic mutations) that results in the development of IPAH (Fig. 17.2). Pulmonary artery vasoconstriction is an early event, that in excess can be associated with an abnormal expression of potassium channels in the smooth muscle cell and

endothelial dysfunction.[13] In normal conditions, the vascular tone in the pulmonary circulation is kept by the close interaction of vasodilators and vasoconstrictors. In PAH, however, the endothelial cells fail to maintain this balance, with the consequent impaired production of vasodilators (i.e., nitric oxide (NO), prostacyclin) and overexpression of vasoconstrictors and proliferators (i.e., endothelin-1 (ET-1), thromboxane A_2).[13]

Three pathways have been thoroughly studied: prostacyclin, endothelin, and NO.

Prostacyclin: Identified by Moncada and Vane in 1976, prostacyclin is a member of the family of prostaglandins produced by the vascular endothelial cells. It is formed by the cyclo-oxygenase pathway and is a powerful vasodilator of the pulmonary and systemic vascular beds as well as an inhibitor of platelet aggregation. It also has antiproliferative properties and inotropic effects.[14] Circulating levels of prostacyclin are decreased in patients with IPAH, and prostacyclin synthase expression is reduced in pulmonary arteries of patients with IPAH. There is evidence derived from prostacyclin receptor knockout mice indicating that prostacyclin and its receptor play a role in regulation of the remodeling found in PAH. Patients with severe PAH also have reduced expression of prostacyclin receptors in remodeled areas. Also, there is a decrease in urinary metabolites of prostacyclin and increased urinary metabolites of thromboxane A_2 in patients with IPAH.[14]

Endothelin-1: ET-1 is one of the most potent endogenous vasoconstrictors. It is a 21-amino-acid peptide discovered in 1988.[15] It is produced in the vascular endothelium, pulmonary artery smooth muscle cells, and lung fibroblasts.[15,16] It can be produced by numerous stimuli, like hypoxia and sheer stress; its biosynthesis is inhibited by prostacyclin and NO.[15] There are three isoforms of endothelin that are encoded by different genes. The ET-1 isoform is considered the predominant and more important physiopathological form.[17] As mentioned, ET-1 is a potent vasoconstrictor whose effect is mediated by two receptors in the smooth muscle cell, ET_A and ET_B. In normal conditions, the ET_B receptor does not seem to contribute significantly to pulmonary vascular tone but has vasodilatory properties that are more apparent when the vascular tone is increased. ET-1 promotes a vascular and interstitial remodeling, stimulates the proliferation of smooth muscle cells, fibroblast activation, and proliferation, with extracellular matrix deposition and contraction.[17]

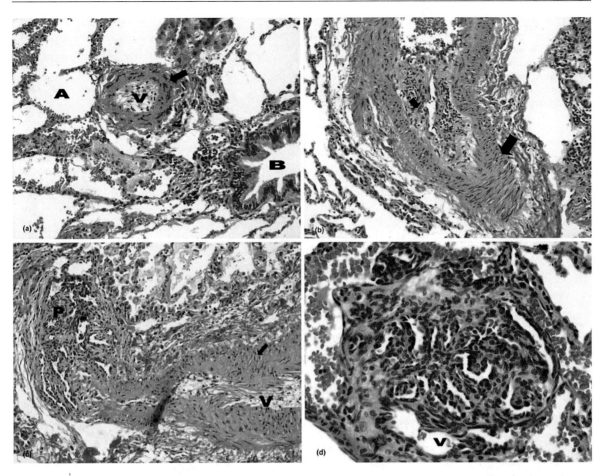

Fig. 17.1 Pathology of idiopathic pulmonary arterial hypertension. (**a**) Muscular pulmonary artery (*V*) showing marked medial thickening (*arrow*), *B* bronchiole, *A* alveolar space. (**b**) Small pulmonary artery showing medial thickening (*large arrow*) and intimal proliferation (*small arrow*). (**c**) Small pulmonary artery (*V*) showing intimal thickening (*arrow*) and a plexiform lesion (*P*). (**d**) Close-up of a plexiform lesion. (Hematoxylin and eosin, courtesy of Dr. Maria Virgilia Soto, National Heart Institute, Mexico City)

Nitric oxide: Formerly known as endothelium-derived relaxing factor, NO was identified in 1986.[18] NO is endogenously produced in the endothelial system, which plays an important role in the regulation of blood pressure and flow, inflammatory responses, and neurotransmission.[18] Its production depends on the cellular conversion of L-arginine to L-citruline, which is catalyzed by the nitric oxide synthases (NOSs). These enzymes can be divided in two major groups, constitutive and inducible forms. Once produced in the endothelial cell, NO travels to the smooth muscle cell to target the cytosolic enzyme guanylate cyclase. Stimulation of the latter increases the level of the second messenger cyclic guanosine monophosphate (cGMP) within vascular smooth muscle, promoting vasorelaxation. cGMP is rapidly hydrolyzed by cyclic

nucleotide phosphodiesterases (PDEs). In patients with IPAH, increased expression of NOS has been identified in plexiform lesions, suggesting that the pulmonary circulation responds to pulmonary hypertension by increasing synthesis of NO in an attempt to restore normal tone.[18]

IPAH requires an extensive workup to identify known causes of pulmonary hypertension (Fig. 17.3). Right heart catheterization is the standard test to identify patients with PAH. The presence of a mean pulmonary artery pressure (PAP) above 25 mmHg pulmonary capillary wedge pressure (PCWP) less than 15 mmHg and PVR 3 Wood units define PAH.[13] Increased mortality has been associated with a mean PAP above 85 mmHg, right atrial pressure greater than 20 mmHg and a cardiac index less than 2 L/m[2].[13] Catheterization

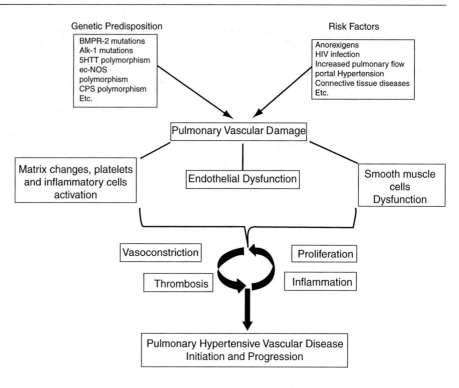

Fig. 17.2 Pulmonary arterial hypertension: potential pathogenetic and pathobiologic mechanisms. *BMPR-2* bone morphogenetic receptor protein 2 gene; *Alk-1* activin-receptor-like kinase 1 gene; *5-HTT* serotonin transporter gene; *ec-NOS* nitric oxide synthase gene; *CPS* carbamyl-phosphate synthetase gene. (Reprinted with permission from the Task Force on Diagnosis and Treatment of Pulmonary Arterial Hypertension of the European Society of Cardiology[13])

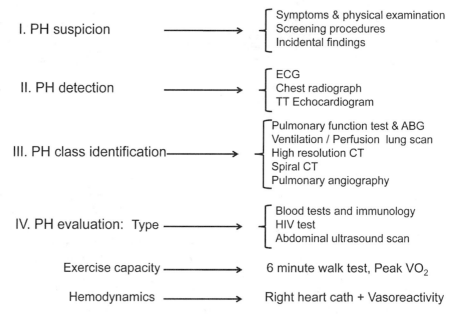

Fig. 17.3 Pulmonary hypertension diagnostic approach. *ABG* arterial blood gases; *CT* computerized tomography; *PH* pulmonary hypertension; *PAH* pulmonary arterial hypertension; *TT* transthoracic; *VO₂* oxygen consumption; *Cath* catheterization. (Reprinted with permission from the Task Force on Diagnosis and Treatment of Pulmonary Arterial Hypertension of the European Society of Cardiology[13])

is also useful for evaluating vasoreactivity in patients with IPAH to norm the initiation of therapy. The acute vasoreactivity test is performed with intravenous epoprostenol (prostacyclin analog), intravenous adenosine or inhaled NO. According to the guidelines of the American College of Chest Physicians and the European Society of Cardiology, a positive vasoreactive test is defined as a fall in 10 mmHg or more, to an mPAP of 40 mmHg or less with an unchanged or increased cardiac output.[13,19]

17.5 Managemento fl PAH

The management of IPAH can be divided into general measures, conventional therapy, and specific therapy.

General measures: General measures include fluid restriction, low salt intake, education, and support in managing complex drug therapies. Patients with IPAH should be counseled regarding the high risk of pregnancy (>30% mortality).[20] Patients should be given advice to vaccinate against influenza and pneumococcal pneumonia.[13]

Conventional therapy: Supplemental oxygen in patients with IPAH should be individualized to keep a saturation above 92% at all times.[13] Diuretics should be used in case of decompensation of right heart failure. The use of inotropes is somewhat controversial due to the lack of randomized controlled trials assessing this kind of drug and needs to be individualized.[13]

There is some retrospective evidence showing improved survival in patients with PPH who received long-term treatment with warfarin compared to patients who only received conventional therapy.[19] Unless contraindicated, oral anticoagulation is recommended to prevent in situ pulmonary artery thrombosis; the INR should be kept between 1.5 and 2.5.[13,20]

Calcium channel blockers: Uncontrolled studies suggested that the long-term administration of high doses of calcium channel blockers improved survival in those patients who are responders during an acute vasodilator challenge.[21] Unfortunately, the percentage of responders was less than 10%.[20]

Specific therapy: Specific therapy can be divided into three important groups: prostacyclin analogs, endothelin receptor antagonists (ERAs) and PDE-5 inhibitors[22](Fig. 17.4).

17.6 ProstacyclinA nalogs

The prostacyclin analog drugs have demonstrated improvement in hemodynamics, functional class, quality of life, and time to clinical worsening.[22] Class-related side effects (common to all prostanoids) are flushing, diarrhea, jaw pain, headache, and systemic hypotension.

Epoprostenol: Epoprostenol was the first drug approved for the treatment of PAH. It is administered intravenously through a permanent catheter. It is indicated for patients in functional class III or IV disease not responding to conventional therapy.[13] Epoprostenol improves survival, hemodynamics, and exercise capacity in patients with IPAH.[22,23] Two large observational studies showed that epoprostenol improved outcomes compared with historic controls, with survival rates of 85–88% at 1 year and 63% at 3 years.[24,25] Epoprostenol requires continuous intravenous infusion using a portable pump because of its instability and short half-life (3–5 min). Patients receiving epoprostenol can develop sepsis and central-line infection. Left heart failure secondary to a high-output state has also been reported.[26]

Iloprost: Iloprost It is available in both intravenous and aerosolized preparations. The aerosolized preparation causes preferential vasodilation in the more ventilated regions of the lung. In a 3-month, randomized, placebo-controlled trial, inhaled iloprost improved 6-min walk distances 36 m more than placebo.[27] In a separate open-label, uncontrolled study of patients with IPAH, inhaled iloprost improved both 6-min walk distance and pulmonary hemodynamics at 1 year.[28] Iloprost is associated with fewer systemic side effects when inhaled, but due to its short half-life it has to be administered seven to nine times a day.[13]

Treprostinil – Treprostinil is approved for patients in functional class II, III, and IV disease and can be administered intravenously or subcutaneously. In a placebo-controlled trial of subcutaneous treprostinil, patients in functional class II through IV disease experienced a dose-related improvement in 6-min walk distances.[29] In an open-label study by Tapson and colleagues,[30] improvements in mean PAP, cardiac index, and 6-min walk distance were observed after 12 weeks of intravenous treprostinil therapy. Common side effects include pain, erythema, induration, and rash at the infusion site. Local reactions can be treated with local anesthetics, nonsteroidal anti-inflammatories, and narcotics. Inhaled and oral formulations are currently under development.

17.7 EndothelinR eceptorA ntagonists

There are two FDA-approved agents in the ERA class approved by the Food and Drug Administration (FDA): bosentan and ambrisentan. A third agent, sitaxsentan, is approved in the European Union, Australia, and Canada.

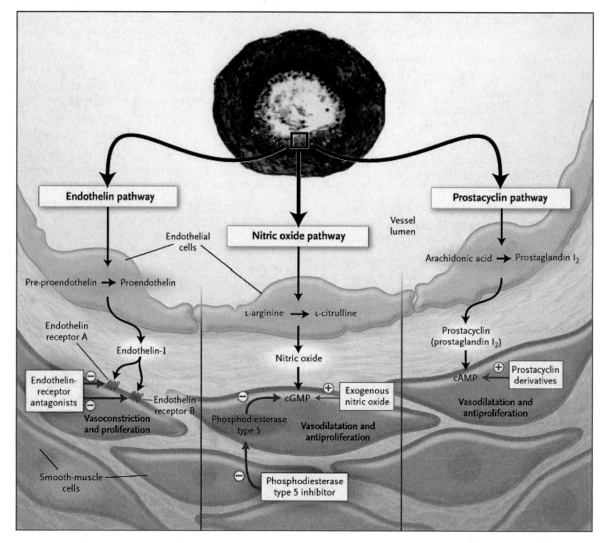

Fig. 17.4 Targets for current or emerging therapies in pulmonary arterial hypertension. Three major pathways involved in
abnormal proliferation and contraction of the smooth muscle
cells of the pulmonary artery in patients with pulmonary arterial
hypertension are shown. Dysfunctional pulmonary artery
endothelial cells (blue) have decreased production of prostacyclin and endogenous nitric oxide, with an increased production
of endothelin 1 – a condition promoting vasoconstriction and
proliferation of smooth muscle cells in the pulmonary arteries
(*red*). Current or emerging therapies interfere with specific targets in smooth-muscle cells in the pulmonary arteries. Plus signs
denote an increase in the intracellular concentration; *minus signs*
indicate blockage of a receptor, inhibition of an enzyme, or a
decrease in the intracellular concentration; cGMP cyclic
guanosine monophosphate. (Reprinted with permission from
Humbert et al[22])

Bosentan: *Bosentan* is a dual ERA approved for
functional class III and IV PAH. It has been shown to
improve exercise capacity, reduce symptoms, and
decrease the rate of clinical deterioration in patients
with PAH.[31] In a study conducted by McLaughlin and
colleagues,[32] patients treated with bosentan as first-line
therapy had a 95% survival at 1 year and 89% survival
at 2 years compared with predicted survival rates of 69
and 57%, respectively. Bosentan therapy requires

close monitoring of laboratory values, particularly
liver-associated enzymes.

Ambrisentan: Ambrisentan is a selective ETB receptor antagonist that has been approved by the FDA. It is
indicated for the treatment of patients in functional class
II and III disease. FDA approval was based on the results
of two 12-week, randomized, double-blinded, placebo-
controlled trials (ARIES-1 and ARIES-2) In these studies, average improvements in 6-min walk test were

between 23 ± 83 m and 49 ± 75 m for the 5-mg dose and 44 ± 63 m for the 10-mg dose (both formulations approved by the FDA). Time to clinical worsening was also improved in the ambrisentan group. Ambrisentan was also evaluated in an open-label, long-term follow-up trial of 383 patients previously treated in the ARIES-1 and ARIES-2 trials. In this cohort, subjects had a 95% 1-year survival, with 94% of patients still receiving ambrisentan monotherapy.[33,34]

Sitaxsentan: Sitaxsentan, also, a selective ETB antagonist, has shown improvement in exercise capacity and hemodynamics in patients with PAH. In the Sitaxsentan To Relieve Impaired Exercise (STRIDE)-1 trial, 178 New York Heart Association (NYHA) class II through IV patients with PAH had improvements in exercise capacity (35 m) and functional classification after 12 weeks of therapy with sitaxsentan. In a second double-blind, placebo-controlled trial (STRIDE-2), 247 patients were randomized to receive placebo, sitaxsentan, or bosentan. After 18 weeks, patients treated with sitaxsentan had increased 6-min walk distances when compared with patients who received placebo.[35,36]

17.8 Phosphodiesterase5I nhibitors

Sildenafil is the only oral agent approved for patients in functional class II disease. In the Sildenafil Use in Pulmonary Arterial Hypertension (SUPER-1) study,[37] 278 patients with symptomatic PAH were randomized to either sildenafil (20, 40, or 80 mg orally three times a day) or placebo for 12 weeks. Improvements in 6-min walk distance, functional class, and mean PAP were seen in all sildenafil groups compared with the placebo group. Patients who completed 1 year of sildenafil monotherapy improved their 6-min walk distance by 51 m from baseline. Common side effects were headache, flushing, epistaxis, dyspepsia, and diarrhea. There seems to be a dose-dependent effect of systemic blood pressure.

Tadalafil is currently approved for the treatment of erectile dysfunction and is being evaluated for its efficacy in PAH.

17.9 CombinationT herapy

To date, specific therapy for PAH acts through three different and potentially complementary mechanisms; combination therapy may provide additive benefit by simultaneously addressing multiple disease pathways. Combination of a PDE-5 inhibitor with a prostanoid has shown such potential via the sildenafil's inhibitory activity for of sildenafil PDE-1 as well as PDE-5, which mediates hydrolysis of both cyclic adenosine monophosphate (cAMP) and cGMP.[38] The other theoretically potential mechanism of synergy may be seen by combining a selective endothelin receptor antagonist (ERA) and a PDE-5 inhibitor. Stimulation of the endothelial ETB receptor leads to the release of NO as well as prostacyclin, and is important for clearance of ET-1. Addition of a PDE-5 inhibitor would augment the effects of increased NO production. So, theoretically, the use of a highly ETA-selective ETRA along with a PDE-5 inhibitor may be more effective.[39] Several studies have been developed to evaluate these theories, and the results look promising.[40-42]

17.9.1 Interventional Therapy for IPAH

Atrial septostomy (AS): Survival of patients with IPAH is determined by adequate right ventricular function and hypertrophy. Once right heart failure develops, survival is poor.[2] Through the creation of an orifice in the atrial septum, AS allows blood to shunt from the right to the left side of the heart. The rationale for the procedure is based in the survival of patients with Eisenmenger syndrome and IPAH with a patent foramen ovale. Both groups have improved survival and fewer symptoms of right heart failure than other patients with PAH.[43] Procedure-related mortality is about 5% and is related to the creation of a large shunt, decrease in oxygen saturation of 10% or more of the baseline value, or when the right atrial pressure 20 mmHg or more. Indications for AS are syncope or right heart failure despite optimal medical treatment; it could be the first line of treatment in countries that have limited access to new drugs and as a bridge to lung transplantation.[44]

Lung transplantation: The number of lung transplants for PAH has diminished due to the approval of new drugs; however, it remains as the last option for patients with IPAH. Either bilateral lung transplantation (BSLTx) or heart–lung transplantation (HLTx) is performed in most centers. An important improvement in the long-term outcome in patients with IPAH at 1, 5, and 10 years postprocedure has been reported in 86,

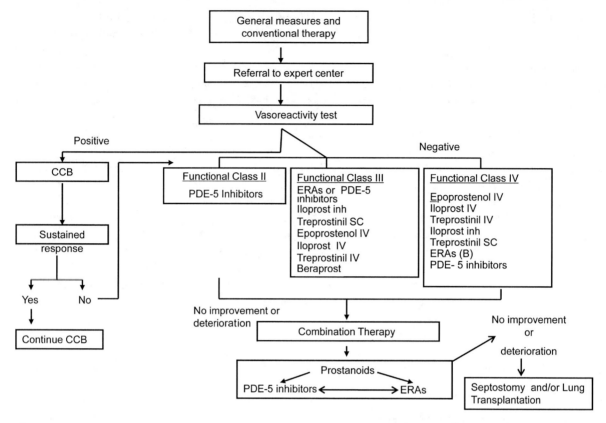

Fig. 17.5 Evidence-based treatment algorithm for pulmonary arterial hypertension. *CCB* calcium channel blockers; *inh* inhaled; *IV* continuous intravenous; *PDE* phosphodiesterase; *R* receptors. (Reprinted with permission from the Task Force on Diagnosis and Treatment of Pulmonary Arterial Hypertension of the European Society of Cardiology[13])

75, and 66% respectively. This improvement has been related to better immunosuppression, lung preservation, and postoperative management.[44]

Figure 17.5 shows the algorithm for treatment of IPAH.

17.10 FutureOp tionsf ort heT reatment of IPAH

Vasoactive intestinal polypeptide: Vasoactive intestinal polypeptide (VIP) is a substance that has vasodilating properties and antiproliferative effects and is produced by various cells.[45] VIP deficiency has been described in lung tissues from patients with IPAH. In a preliminary case series, eight patients with IPAH who were treated with inhaled VIP at daily doses of 200 mg in four single inhalations showed marked clinical and hemodynamic improvement.[46]

Serotonin receptor and transporter function: Serotonin (5-HT) is a potent vasoconstrictor and mitogen that may play a role in the pathogenesis of PAH.[47] In PAH, the serotonin receptor 5HT2 may be upregulated,[48] which can be a novel therapeutic target because antagonists to these receptors have been developed. The serotonin transporter, a molecule that facilitates transmembrane transport of serotonin into the cell, is also upregulated in PAH.[49] Drugs such as the selective serotonin reuptake inhibitors could potentially be useful, and their study is warranted.

Rho kinase inhibitors: Rho kinase is an enzyme that is involved in the processes of cellular growth and regulation of the smooth muscle tone. Fasudil has improved vascular injury and hemodynamics in an animal model of PAH, and a case report in patients with

IPAH showed that fasudil decreased pulmonary vascular resistance.[50,51]

Inhibitors of growth factor synthesis: Monoclonal expansion (a process reminiscent of malignant transformation) has been demonstrated in the plexiform lesion of IPAH.[52] Imatinib, a tyrosine kinase inhibitor that is approved for the treatment of hematopoietic malignancies, produced improvement in an animal model of pulmonary hypertension[53] and in three patients with PAH who had refractory symptoms despite optimal combination therapy suggest that this novel approach may be of benefit in PAH.[54]

Adrenomedullin is a peptide that causes vasodilation and inhibits proliferation of pulmonary vascular smooth muscle cells and has been used in patients with IPAH.[55]

Cellular therapy: Recent publications have demonstrated that infusions of endothelial progenitor cells in animal models of pulmonary hypertension attenuate the injury, particularly when these cells are transfected with NOS.[56] Safety and efficacy trials are under way with progenitor cell infusions in patients who have severe PAH refractory to medical therapy.[57]

Statins attenuate the pulmonary arteriopathy induced by the administration of monocrotaline to experimental animals.[58,59] Clinical studies that evaluate the efficacy of statins in patients with PAH are being developed.

References

1. D'Alonzo GE, Barst RJ, Ayres SM, et al. Survival in patients with primary pulmonary hypertension: results from a national prospective registry. *Ann Intern Med*. 1991;115:343-349.
2. Humbert M, Sitbon O, Chaouat A, et al. Pulmonary arterial hypertension in France. Results from a national registry. *Am J Respir Crit Care Med*.2006; 173:1023-1030.
3. Runo JR, Lloyd JE. Primary pulmonary hypertension. *Lancet*.2003;361:1533- 1544.
4. Simonneau G, Galiè N, Rubin LJ, et al. Clinical classification of pulmonary hypertension. *J Am Coll Cardiol*. 2004;43:5S-12S.
5. Lane KB, Machado RD, Pauciulo MW, et al. Heterozygous germline mutations in BMPR2, encoding a TGF-beta receptor, cause familial primary pulmonary hypertension. The International PPH Consortium. *Nat Genet*. 2000;26:81-84.
6. Deng Z, Morse JH, Cuervo N, et al. Familial pulmonary hypertension (gene PPH1) is caused by mutations in the bone morphogenetic protein receptor-II gene. *Am J Hum Genet*.2000; 67:737-744.
7. Hill NS, ed. *Pulmonary hypertension therapy*. New York: Summit Communications; 2006.
8. Newman JH, Trembath RC, Morse JC, et al. Genetic basis of pulmonary arterial hypertension: current understanding and future directions. *J Am Coll Cardiol*.2004; 43:33S-39S.
9. Thomson JR, Machado RD, Pauciulo MW, et al. Sporadic primary pulmonary hypertension is associated with germline mutations of the gene encoding BMPR-II, a receptor member of the TGF-beta family. *J Med Genet*. 2000;37:741-745.
10. Trembath RC, Thomson JR, Machado RD, et al. Clinical and molecular genetic features of pulmonary hypertension in patients with hereditary hemorrhagic telangiectasia. *N Engl J Med*.2001; 345:325-334.
11. Abdalla SA, Gallione CJ, Barst RJ, et al. Primary pulmonary hypertension in families with hereditary hemorrhagic telangiectasia. *Eur Respir J*.2004; 23:373-377.
12. Chaouat A, Coulet F, Favre C, et al. Endoglin germline mutation in a patient with hereditary hemorrhagic telangiectasia and dexfenfluramine associated pulmonary arterial hypertension. *Thorax*.2004; 59:446-448.
13. The Task Force on Diagnosis and Treatment of Pulmonary Arterial Hypertension of the European Society of Cardiology. Guidelines on diagnosis and treatment of pulmonary arterial hypertension. *Eur Heart J*.2004; 25:2243-2278.
14. Fortin TA, Tapson VF. Intravenous prostacyclin for pulmonary arterial hypertension. In: Peacock AJ, Rubin LJ, eds. *Pulmonary circulation. Diseases and treatment*. 2nd ed. London: Arnold; 2004:255-267.
15. Yanagisawa M, Kurihara K, Kimura S, et al. A novel potent vasoconstrictor peptide produced by vascular endothelial cells. *Nature*.1988; 332:411-415.
16. Markewitz BA, Farrukh IS, Chen Y, Li Y, Michael JR. Regulation of endothelin-1 synthesis in human pulmonary arterial smooth muscle cells. Effects of transforming growth factor- and hypoxia. *Cardiovasc Res*.2001; 49:200-206.
17. Shi-Wen X, Chen Y, Denton CP, et al. Endothelin-1 promotesmyofibroblast induction through the ETA receptor *via* a rac/phosphoinositide 3-kinase/Akt-dependent pathway and is essential for the enhanced contractile phenotype of fibrotic fibroblasts. *Mol Biol Cell*. 2004;15:2707-2719.
18. Dupuis J, Hoeper MM. Endothelin receptor antagonists in pulmonary arterial hypertension. *Eur Respir J*. 2008;31:407-415.
19. Badesch DB, Abman SH, Simonneau G, et al. Medical therapy for pulmonary arterial hypertension: updated ACCP evidence-based clinical practice guidelines. *Chest*. 2007;131:1917-1928.
20. National Pulmonary Hypertension Centres in the UK and Ireland. Consensus statement on the management of pulmonary arterial hypertension in clinical practice in the UK and Ireland. *Heart*.2008; 94:1-41.
21. Rich S, Kaufmann E, Levy PS. The effect of high doses of calcium-channel blockers on survival in primary pulmonary hypertension. *N Engl J Med*.1992; 327:76-81.
22. Humbert M, Sitbon O, Simonneau G. Treatment of pulmonary arterial hypertension. *N Engl J Med*. 2004;351:1425-1436.

23. Barst RJ, Rubin LJ, Long WA, et al. A comparison of continuous intravenous epoprostenol (prostacyclin) with conventional therapy for primary pulmonary hypertension. The Primary Pulmonary Hypertension Study Group. *N Engl J Med*.1996;334:296 -302.

24. McLaughlin VV, Genthner DE, Panella MM, Rich S. Reduction in pulmonary vascular resistance with long-term epoprostenol (prostacyclin) therapy in primary pulmonary hypertension. *N Engl J Med*.1998; 338:273-277.

25. McLaughlin VV, Shillington A, Rich S. Survival in primary pulmonary hypertension: The impact of epoprostenol therapy. *Circulation*.2002; 106:1477-1482.

26. Rich S, McLaughlin VV. The effects of chronic prostacyclin therapy on cardiac output in primary pulmonary hypertension. *J Am Coll Cardiol*.1999; 34:1184-1187.

27. Olschewski H, Simonneau G, Galie N, et al. Inhaled iloprost for severe pulmonary hypertension. *N Engl J Med*. 2002; 347:322-329.

28. Hoeper MM, Schwarze M, Ehlerding S, et al. Long-term treatment of primary pulmonary hypertension with aerosolized iloprost, a prostacyclin analogue. *N Engl J Med*. 2000;342:1866-1870.

29. Simonneau G, Barst RJ, Galie N, et al. Continuous subcutaneous infusion of treprostinil, a prostacyclin analogue, in patients with pulmonary arterial hypertension: a double-blind, randomized, placebo-controlled trial. *Am J Respir Crit Care Med*.2002; 165:800-804.

30. Tapson VF, Gomberg-Maitland M, McLaughlin VV, et al. Safety and efficacy of IV treprostinil for pulmonary arterial hypertension: a prospective, multicenter, open-label, 12-week trial. *Chest*. 2006;129:683-688.

31. Rubin LJ, Badesch DB, Barst RJ, et al. Bosentan therapy for pulmonary arterial hypertension. *N Engl J Med*. 2002;346: 896-903.

32. McLaughlin VV, Sitbon O, Badesch DB, et al. Survival with first-line bosentan in patients with primary pulmonary hypertension. *Eur Respir J*.2005; 25:244-249.

33. Galie N, Badesch D, Oudiz R, et al. Ambrisentan therapy for pulmonary arterial hypertension. *J Am Coll Cardiol*. 2005;46:529-535.

34. Galiè N, Olschewski H, Oudiz RJ, et al. Ambrisentan for the treatment of pulmonary arterial hypertension: Results of the ambrisentan in pulmonary arterial hypertension, randomized, double-blind, placebo-controlled, multicenter, efficacy (ARIES) study 1 and 2. *Circulation*.2008; 117:3010-3019.

35. Barst RJ, Langleben D, Frost A, et al. Sitaxsentan therapy for pulmonary arterial hypertension. *Am J Respir Crit Care Med*.2004;169:441- 447.

36. Barst RJ, Langleben D, Badesch D, et al. Treatment of pulmonary arterial hypertension with the selective endothelin-A receptor antagonist sitaxsentan. *J Am Coll Cardiol*. 2006;47:2049-2056.

37. Galie N, Ghofrani HA, Torbicki A, et al. Sildenafil citrate therapy for pulmonary arterial hypertension. *N Engl J Med*. 2005;353:2148-2157.

38. Rybalkin SD, Yan C, Bornfeldt KE, Beavo JA. Cyclic GMP phosphodiesterases and regulation of smooth muscle function. *Circ Res*.2003; 93:280-291.

39. Wedgwood S, Black SM. Endothelin-1 decreases endothelial NOS expression and activity through ETA receptor-

40. mediated generation of hydrogen peroxide. *Am J Physiol Lung Cell Mol Physiol*.2005; 288:L480-L487.

40. Humbert M, Barst RJ, Robbins IM, et al. Combination of bosentan with epoprostenol in pulmonary arterial hypertension: BREATHE-2. *Eur Respir J*.2004; 24:353-359.

41. McLaughlin VV, Oudiz RJ, Frost A, et al. Randomized study of adding inhaled iloprost to existing bosentan in pulmonary arterial hypertension. *Am J Respir Crit Care Med*. 2006; 174:1257-1263.

42. Simonneau G, Rubin LJ, Galiè N, et al. Addition of sildenafil to long-term intravenous epoprostenol therapy in patients with pulmonary arterial hypertension. A randomized trial. *Ann Intern Med*.2008; 149:521-530.

43. Sandoval J, Gaspar J, Pulido T, et al. Graded balloon dilation atrial septostomy in severe primary pulmonary hypertension: a therapeutic alternative for patients nonresponsive to vasodilator treatment. *J Am Coll Cardiol*. 1998;32:297-30424.

44. Klepetko W, Mayer E, Sandoval J, et al. Interventional and surgical modalities of treatment for pulmonary arterial hypertension. *J Am Coll Cardiol*.2004; 43:73S-80S.

45. Said SI. Mediators and modulators of pulmonary arterial hypertension. *Am J Physiol Lung Cell Mol Physiol*. 2006; 291:547-558.

46. Petkov V, Mosgeoller W, Ziesche R, et al. Vasoactive intestinal polypeptide as a new drug for treatment of primary pulmonary hypertension. *J Clin Invest*. 2003;111: 1339-1346.

47. Fanburg BL, Lee SL. A new role for an old molecule: serotonin as a mitogen. *Am J Physiol*.1997; 272:L795-L806.

48. Long L, MacLean MR, Jeffery TK, et al. Serotonin increases susceptibility to pulmonary hypertension in BMPR2-deficient mice. *Circ Res*.2006; 98:818-827.

49. Eddhaibi S, Humbert M, Fadel E, et al. Serotonin transporter overexpression is responsible for pulmonary artery smooth muscle hyperplasia in primary pulmonary hypertension. *J Clin Invest*.2001; 108:1141-1150.

50. Oka M, Homma N, Taraseviciene-Stewart L, et al. Rho kinase-mediated vasoconstriction is important in severe occlusive pulmonary arterial hypertension in rats. *Circ Res*. 2007;100:923-929.

51. Abe K, Shimokawa H, Morikawa K, et al. Long-term treatment with a Rho-kinase inhibitor improves monocrotaline-induced fatal pulmonary hypertension in rats. *Circ Res*. 2004;94:385-393.

52. Yeager ME, Halley GR, Golpon HA, et al. Microsatellite instability of endothelial cell growth and apoptosis genes within plexiform lesions in primary pulmonary hypertension. *Circ Res*.2001; 88:2-11.

53. Schermuly RT, Dony E, Ghofrani HA, et al. Reversal of experimental pulmonary hypertension by PDGF inhibition. *J Clin Invest*.2005; 115:2811-2821.

54. Ghofrani HA, Seeger W, Grimminger F. Imatinib for the treatment of pulmonary arterial hypertension. *N Engl J Med*. 2005;353:1412-1413.

55. Nagaya N, Kangawa K. Adrenomedullin in the treatment of pulmonary hypertension. *Peptides*.2004; 25:2013-2018.

56. Zhao YD, Courtman DW, Deng Y, et al. Rescue of monocrotaline-induced pulmonary arterial hypertension using bone marrow-derived endothelial-like progenitor cells: efficacy of

combined cell and eNOS gene therapy in established disease. *Circ Res*.2005; 96:442-450.

57. Wang XX, Zhang FR, Shang YP, et al. Transplantation of autologous endothelial progenitor cells may be beneficial in patients with idiopathic pulmonary arterial hypertension: a pilot randomized controlled trial. *J Am Coll Cardiol*. 2007;49:1566-1571.

58. Nishimura T, Faul JL, Berry GJ, et al. Simvastatin attenuates smooth muscle neointimal proliferation and pulmonary hypertension in rats. *Am J Respir Crit Care Med*. 2002; 166:1403-1408.

59. Nishimura T, Vaszar LT, Faul JL, et al. Simvastatin rescues rats from fatal pulmonary hypertension by inducing apoptosis in neointimal smooth muscle. *Circulation*. 2003;108:1640-1645.

18.1 Introduction

Pulmonary thromboendarterectomy (PTE) for the treatment of chronic thromboembolic pulmonary hypertension is an uncommon surgical procedure; however, it remains the only curative option that could provide immediate and permanent cure for this devastating disease. This condition is remarkably underdiagnosed, and as a result the procedure is uncommonly applied. Overall, patients with chronic pulmonary hypertension secondary to thromboembolic disease may present with a variety of debilitating cardiopulmonary symptoms. However, once the diagnosis is made, there is really no curative role for medical management, and medical management at best is only palliative. Surgical removal of the thromboembolic material by bilateral thromboendarterectomy is the only therapeutic option.

The exact incidence of pulmonary embolism remains unknown; however, there are some valid estimates. It is estimated that pulmonary embolism results in approximately 650,000 symptomatic episodes in the United States yearly. Acute pulmonary embolus is the third most common cause of death after heart failure and cancer. Interestingly, approximately 70% of autopsy-proven pulmonary embolisms were not detected clinically. Of course, the disease is particularly more common in hospitalized and elderly patients, and of all hospitalized patients who develop pulmonary

embolism, approximately 12–21% will die in the hospital, and another 24–39% will die within 12 months. Approximately 36–60% of patients who survive the initial episode live beyond 12 months and may present later in life with a variety of symptoms. Of those who survive the initial episode, approximately 3–5% will go on to develop chronic pulmonary hypertension.

It is well established that the mainstay of treatment for patients with acute pulmonary embolism and patients with deep venous thrombosis is medical management. In fact, in the majority of patients the treatment is anticoagulation with or without thrombolytics. In general, cardiac surgeons may rarely intervene in hospitalized patients who suffer a massive embolus that causes life-threatening acute right heart failure and severe hemodynamic compromise. In contrast, the only treatment for patients with chronic thromboembolic disease is surgical removal of the disease by pulmonary endarterectomy. Medical management in these patients is only palliative, and surgery by means of transplantation is an inappropriate use of resources, with less-than-satisfactory short- and long-term results for this population.

The prognosis for patients with pulmonary hypertension is poor, and it is worse for those who do not have intracardiac shunts. Thus, patients with primary pulmonary hypertension and those with pulmonary hypertension secondary to pulmonary emboli fall into a higher-risk category than patients with Eisenmenger syndrome and have a higher mortality rate. In fact, once the mean pulmonary artery pressure reaches greater than 50 mm mercury, the 3-year mortality approaches 90%. Surgical treatment by pulmonary endarterectomy can now be performed with very low risk of morbidity and mortality and excellent long-term outcome. What follows is the description of this procedure as it is performed at the University of California, San Diego (UCSD) as well as a

Michael M. Madani (✉)
Division of Cardiothoracic Surgery
University of California San Diego, Medical Center
200 West Arbor drive
San Diego, CA92101
e-mail:m madani@ucsd.edu

E.A. Gabriel and T. Salerno (eds.), *Principles of Pulmonary Protection in Heart Surgery*,
DOI: 10.1007/978-1-84996-308-4_18, © Springer-Verlag London Limited 2010

brief overview of the incidence, the clinical presentation, and the natural history of this disease.

18.2 Incidence

It is impossible to determine an accurate incidence of chronic thromboembolic pulmonary hypertension. Most patients with this condition do not have a clear history of deep venous thrombosis or pulmonary embolism. Furthermore, the majority, about 75%, of autopsy-proven pulmonary embolisms were not clinically diagnosed premortem. This makes the exact incidence of this disease even more difficult to determine. The incidence of chronic thromboembolic occlusion in the population depends on what proportion of patients failed to resolve acute embolic material. Recent studies have shown that, of these patients, up to 3.1% will have symptomatic chronic thromboembolic pulmonary hypertension at 1 year, and 3.8% will have it at 2 years. If these figures are correct and one only counts patients with symptomatic acute pulmonary emboli, approximately 15,000–19,000 individuals would progress to chronic thromboembolic pulmonary hypertension in the United States each year. However, because many, if not most, patients diagnosed with chronic thromboembolic disease have no antecedent history of acute embolism, the true incidence of this disorder is much higher.

Regardless of the exact incidence or the circumstances, it is clear that acute embolism and its chronic relation, fixed chronic thromboembolic occlusive disease, are both much more common than generally appreciated and are seriously underdiagnosed. Calculations extrapolated from mortality rates and the random incidence of major thromboembolic occlusions found at autopsy support a postulate that more than 100,000 patients in the United States currently have pulmonary hypertension that could be relieved by this operation.

18.3 NaturalHi story

For most episodes of pulmonary embolism, the natural history is generally total embolic resolution or resolution leaving minimal residua but with restoration of a normal hemodynamic status. However, for unknown reasons, embolic resolution is incomplete in a small subset of patients. If the acute emboli are not lysed in 1–2 weeks, the embolic material becomes attached to the pulmonary arterial wall at the main pulmonary artery, lobar, segmental, or subsegmental levels.[1] With time, the initial embolic material progressively becomes converted into connective and elastic tissue. Often, visualization of the pulmonary arteries by angioscopy a few weeks after unresolved pulmonary embolism reveals vessel narrowing at the site of embolic incorporation. In some patients, recanalization of some of the pulmonary arterial branches occurs, with the formation of fibrous tissue in the form of bands and webs.[2] By a mechanism that is poorly understood, this chronic obstructive disease may lead to a small-vessel arteriolar vasculopathy characterized by excessive smooth muscle cell proliferation around small arterioles in the pulmonary circulation.[3] This small-vessel vasculopathy is seen in the remaining open vessels, which are subjected to long exposure at high flow. Pulmonary hypertension results when the capacitance of the remaining open bed cannot absorb the cardiac output because of either the degree of primary obstruction by embolus or the combination of a fixed obstructive lesion and secondary small-vessel vasculopathy.

Once pulmonary hypertension has developed as the result of chronic thromboembolic material, patients will be in need of expeditious treatment. These patients do not generally respond to medical management as the underlying cause of the disease is vascular obstruction. The only curative option is to proceed with surgical removal of the scarred thromboembolic material by endarterectomy.

Unfortunately, in the last few years we have started to see a delay in referral of these patients for appropriate therapy. There seems to be a developing trend to start pulmonary vasodilator therapy before referring patients for surgical management, and in some cases this comes at a cost of significant delay in referral. We need to be clear that the appropriate treatment of chronic thromboembolic pulmonary hypertension is the surgical removal of the disease, and vasodilator therapy will not add any benefit for most patients. Of course, in a rare situation one may encounter a patient with long-standing disease and significant right heart failure secondary to significant pulmonary hypertension who only has a mild-to-moderate degree of obstructive disease. Such a patient may temporarily benefit from a trial of vasodilator therapy (e.g., epoprostenol) prior to surgery, but the benefit is generally temporary and should not delay referral for surgery.

Without surgical intervention, the survival of patients with chronic thromboembolic pulmonary hypertension is poor and is inversely related to the degree of pulmonary hypertension at the time of diagnosis. Riedel et al. [4] found a 5-year survival rate of 30% among patients with a mean pulmonary artery pressure greater than 40 mmHg at the time of diagnosis and 10% in those whose pressure exceeded 50 mmHg. In another study, a mean pulmonary artery pressure as low as 30 mmHg was identified as a threshold for poor prognosis.[5]

18.4 Pathophysiology

Although most individuals with chronic pulmonary thromboembolic disease are unaware of a past thromboembolic event and give no history of deep venous thrombosis, the origin of most cases of unresolved pulmonary emboli is acute embolic episodes. Why some patients have unresolved emboli is not certain, but a variety of factors must play a role, alone or in combination.

In certain patients, the volume of acute embolic material may simply overwhelm the lytic mechanisms. The total occlusion of a major arterial branch may prevent lytic material from reaching, and therefore dissolving, the embolus completely. In others, repetitive emboli may not be able to be resolved. Yet sometimes, the emboli may be made of substances that cannot be resolved by normal mechanisms (already well-organized fibrous thrombus, fat, or tumor). Furthermore, the lytic mechanisms themselves may be abnormal, or some patients may actually have a propensity for thrombus or a hypercoagulable state.

In general, after the clot becomes wedged in the pulmonary artery, if complete resolution does not take effect, one of two processes progresses:[6]

1. The organization of the clot proceeds to canalization, producing multiple small endothelialized channels separated by fibrous septa (i.e., bands and webs).
2. Complete fibrous organization of the fibrin clot without canalization may result, leading to a solid mass of dense fibrous connective tissue totally obstructingthe a rteriallume n.

In addition, there are other special circumstances. Chronic in-dwelling central venous catheters and pacemaker leads are sometimes associated with pulmonary emboli. More rare causes include tumor emboli; tumor fragments from stomach, breast, and kidney malignancies have also been demonstrated to cause chronic pulmonary arterial occlusion. Right atrial myxomas may also fragment and embolize.

As previously described and discussed, in addition to the embolic material, a propensity for thrombosis or a hypercoagulable state may be present in a few patients. This abnormality may result in spontaneous thrombosis within the pulmonary vascular bed, encourage embolization, or be responsible for proximal propagation of thrombus after an embolus. But, whatever the predisposing factors to residual thrombus within the vessels, the final genesis of the resultant pulmonary vascular hypertension may be complex. With the passage of time, the increased pressure and flow as a result of redirected pulmonary blood flow in the previously normal pulmonary vascular bed can create a vasculopathy in the small precapillary blood vessels similar to Eisenmenger syndrome.

Factors other than the simple hemodynamic consequences of redirected blood flow are probably also involved in this process. For example, after a pneumonectomy, 100% of the right ventricular output flows to one lung, yet little increase in pulmonary pressure occurs, even with follow-up to 11 years.[7] In patients with thromboembolic disease, however, we frequently detect pulmonary hypertension even when less than 50% of the vascular bed is occluded by thrombus. It thus appears that sympathetic neural connections, hormonal changes, or both might initiate pulmonary hypertension in the initially unaffected pulmonary vascular bed. This process can occur with the initial occlusion either in the same or in the contralateral lung.

Regardless of the cause, the evolution of pulmonary hypertension as a result of changes in the previously unobstructed bed is serious because this process may lead to an inoperable situation. Consequently, with our accumulating experience in patients with thrombotic pulmonary hypertension, we have increasingly been inclined toward early operation to avoid these changes.

18.5 ClinicalPr esentation

There are no signs or symptoms specific for chronic thromboembolism. The most common symptom associated with thromboembolic pulmonary hypertension, as with all other causes of pulmonary hypertension, is exertional dyspnea. This dyspnea is out of proportion to any abnormalities found on clinical examination. Like complaints of easy fatigability, dyspnea that initially occurs only with exertion is often attributed to anxiety or being "out of shape." Syncope or presyncope (light-headedness during exertion) is another common symptom in pulmonary hypertension. Generally, it occurs in patients with more advanced disease and higher pulmonary arterial pressures.

Nonspecific chest pains or tightness occur in approximately 50% of patients with more severe pulmonary hypertension. Hemoptysis can occur in all forms of pulmonary hypertension and probably results from abnormally dilated vessels distended by increased intravascular pressures. Peripheral edema, early satiety, and epigastric or right upper quadrant fullness or discomfort may develop as the right heart fails (cor pulmonale). Some patients with chronic pulmonary thromboembolic disease present after a small acute pulmonary embolus that may produce acute symptoms of right heart failure. A careful history brings out symptoms of dyspnea on minimal exertion, easy fatigability, diminishing activities, and episodes of angina-like pain or light-headedness. Further examination reveals the signs of pulmonary hypertension.

The physical signs of pulmonary hypertension are the same no matter what the underlying pathophysiology. Initially, the jugular venous pulse is characterized by a large A wave. As the right heart fails, the V wave becomes predominant. The right ventricle is usually palpable near the lower left sternal border, and pulmonary valve closure may be audible in the second intercostal space. Occasional patients with advanced disease are hypoxic and slightly cyanotic. Clubbing is an uncommon finding.

The second heart sound is often narrowly split and varies normally with respiration; P2 is accentuated. A sharp systolic ejection click may be heard over the pulmonary artery. As the right heart fails, a right atrial gallop usually is present, and tricuspid insufficiency develops. Because of the large pressure gradient across the tricuspid valve in pulmonary hypertension, the murmur is high pitched and may not exhibit respiratory variation. These findings are quite different from those usually observed in tricuspid valvular disease. A murmur of pulmonic regurgitation may also be detected.

18.6 DiagnosticSt udies

To ensure diagnosis in patients with chronic pulmonary thromboembolism, a standardized evaluation is recommended for all patients who present with unexplained pulmonary hypertension. Pulmonary vascular disease always must be considered in the differential diagnosis of unexplained dyspnea. The diagnostic evaluation serves three purposes: to establish the presence and severity of pulmonary hypertension; to determine its etiology; and, if thromboembolic disease is present, to determine whether it is surgically correctible.

Chest radiography is often unrevealing in the early stages of chronic thromboembolic pulmonary hypertension. As the disease progresses, several radiographic abnormalities may be found. These include peripheral lung opacities suggestive of scarring from previous infarction, cardiomegaly with dilation and hypertrophy of the right-sided chambers, and dilation of the central pulmonary arteries. *Pulmonary function tests* are often obtained in the evaluation of dyspnea and serve to exclude the presence of obstructive airways or parenchymal lung disease. There are no characteristic spirometric changes diagnostic of chronic thromboembolic pulmonary hypertension. Single-breath diffusing capacity for carbon monoxide (DLCO) may be moderately reduced, and it has been reported that 20% of patients have a mild-to-moderate restrictive defect caused by parenchymal scarring.[8] Arterial blood oxygen levels may be normal even in the setting of significant pulmonary hypertension. Most patients, however, experience a decline in Po_2 with exertion.

Transthoracic echocardiography is the first study to provide objective evidence of the presence of pulmonary hypertension. An estimate of pulmonary artery pressure can be provided by Doppler evaluation of the tricuspid regurgitant envelope. Additional echocardiographic findings vary depending on the stage of the disease and include right ventricular enlargement, leftward displacement of the interventricular septum, and encroachment of the enlarged right ventricle on the left ventricular cavity with abnormal systolic and diastolic function of the left ventricle.[9] Contrast echocardiography may demonstrate a persistent foramen ovale, the result of high right atrial pressures opening the previously closed intra-atrial communication.

Once the diagnosis of pulmonary hypertension has been established, distinguishing between major-vessel obstruction and small-vessel pulmonary vascular disease is the next critical step. *Radioisotope ventilation-perfusion (V/Q) lung scanning* is the essential test for establishing the diagnosis of unresolved pulmonary thromboembolism. The V/Q scan typically demonstrates one or more mismatched segmental defects caused by obstructive thromboembolism. This is in contrast to the normal or "mottled" perfusion scan seen in patients with primary pulmonary hypertension or other small-vessel forms of pulmonary hypertension.[10] It is important to note that V/Q scanning may underestimate the magnitude of perfusion defects with chronic thromboembolic pulmonary hypertension as partial recanalization of the vessel lumen can occur, resulting in some perfusion, although with significant obstruction to flow.[11]

Cardiac catheterization provides essential information in the evaluation of patients with suspected thromboembolic pulmonary hypertension. Right ventricular catheterization allows for the quantification of the severity of pulmonary hypertension and assessment of cardiac function. Measurement of oxygen saturations in the vena cava, right ventricular chambers, and the pulmonary artery may document previously undetected left-to-right shunting. Coronary angiography and left-sided heart catheterization provide additional information about patients at risk for coronary artery or valvular disease and establish baseline measurements for cardiac output and left ventricular function. This information is crucial in the preoperative risk assessment of patients deemed candidates for pulmonary endarterectomy.

Pulmonary angiography is the gold standard for defining pulmonary vascular anatomy and is performed to identify whether chronic thromboembolic obstruction is present, to determine its location and surgical accessibility, and to rule out other diagnostic possibilities. In angiographic imaging, thrombi appear as unusual filling defects, pouches, webs, bands, or completely thrombosed vessels that may resemble congenital absence of a vessel. Organized material along a vascular wall produces a scalloped or serrated luminal edge.[12] Despite concerns regarding the safety of performing pulmonary angiography in patients with pulmonary hypertension, with careful monitoring, pulmonary angiography can be performed safely even in patients with severe pulmonary hypertension. Biplane imaging is preferred, offering the advantage of lateral views that provide greater anatomical detail compared with the overlapped and obscured vessel images often seen with

the anterior–posterior view. Maturation, organization, and recanalization of clot produces angiographic patterns of the following: (1) pouch defects, (2) webs or bands, (3) intimal irregularities, (4) abrupt narrowing of major vessels, and (5) obstruction of main, lobar, or segmental pulmonary vessels.[13]

More recently, *helical computed tomography* scanning,[14] *SPECT-CT fusion imaging*,[15] and *magnetic resonance angiography*[16] have been used to screen patients with suspected thromboembolic disease. Features of chronic thromboembolic disease seen by these modalities include evidence of organized thrombus lining the pulmonary vessels in an eccentric fashion, enlargement of the right ventricle and central pulmonary arteries, variation in size of segmental arteries (relatively smaller in affected segments compared with uninvolved areas), and parenchymal changes compatible with pulmonary infarction.

18.7 PulmonaryEndar terectomy

Although there were previous attempts, Allison et al.[17] did the first successful pulmonary "thromboendarterectomy" through a sternotomy using surface hypothermia, but only fresh clots were removed. The operation was 12 days after a thigh injury that led to pulmonary emboli, and there was no endarterectomy. Since then, there have been many occasional reports of the surgical treatment of chronic pulmonary thromboembolism, but most of the surgical experience in pulmonary endarterectomy has been reported from the UCSD Medical Center. Braunwald commenced the UCSD experience with this operation in 1970, which now totals more than 2,500 cases. In the following discussion, the operation described, using deep hypothermia and circulatory arrest, is the standard procedure.

18.8 Indications

When the diagnosis of thromboembolic pulmonary hypertension has been firmly established, the decision for operation is made based on the severity of symptoms and the general condition of the patient. Early in the pulmonary endarterectomy experience, Moser et al.[18] pointed out that there were three major reasons for considering thromboendarterectomy: hemodynamic, alveolo-respiratory, and prophylactic.

The hemodynamic goal is to prevent or ameliorate right ventricular compromise caused by pulmonary hypertension. The respiratory objective is to improve respiratory function by the removal of a large ventilated but unperfused physiologic dead space, regardless of the severity of pulmonary hypertension. The prophylactic goal is to prevent progressive right ventricular dysfunction or retrograde extension of the obstruction, which might result in further cardiorespiratory deterioration or death. Our subsequent experience has added another prophylactic goal: the prevention of secondary arteriopathic changes in the remaining patent vessels.

Although most patients have a pulmonary vascular resistance (PVR) level in the range of 800 dyn/s/cm^{-5} and pulmonary artery pressures less than systemic, the hypertrophy of the right ventricle that occurs over time makes pulmonary hypertension to suprasystemic levels possible. Therefore, many patients (approximately 20% in our practice) have a PVR level in excess of 1,000 dyn/s/cm^{-5} and suprasystemic pulmonary artery pressures. There is no upper limit of PVR level, pulmonary artery pressure, or degree of right ventricular dysfunction that excludes patients from operation.

18.9 Operation

18.9.1 Principles

There are several guiding principles for the operation. Surgical treatment and endarterectomy must be bilateral because this is a bilateral disease in the vast majority of our patients. Furthermore, for pulmonary hypertension to be a major factor, both pulmonary vasculatures must be substantially involved. The only reasonable approach to both pulmonary arteries is through a median sternotomy incision. Cardiopulmonary bypass is essential to ensure cardiovascular stability when the operation is performed and to cool the patient to allow circulatory arrest. Excellent visibility is required, in a bloodless field, to define an adequate endarterectomy plane and then to follow the pulmonary endarterectomy specimen deep into the subsegmental vessels. Because of the copious bronchial blood flow usually present in these cases, periods of circulatory arrest are necessary to ensure perfect visibility. A true endarterectomy in the plane of the

media must be accomplished. It is essential to appreciate that the removal of visible thrombus is largely incidental to this operation. Indeed, in most patients, no free thrombus is present, and on initial direct examination, the pulmonary vascular bed may appear normal. The early literature on this procedure indicated that thrombectomy was often performed without endarterectomy, and in these cases the pulmonary artery pressures did not improve, often with the resultant death of the patient.

18.10 OperativeTechnique

After a median sternotomy incision is made, the pericardium is incised longitudinally and attached to the wound edges. Typically, the right heart is enlarged, with a tense right atrium and a variable degree of tricuspid regurgitation. There is usually severe right ventricular hypertrophy, and with critical degrees of obstruction, the patient's condition may become unstable with the manipulation of the heart.

Anticoagulation is achieved with the use of beeflung heparin sodium (400 units/kg IV) administered to prolong the activated clotting time beyond 400 s. Full cardiopulmonary bypass is instituted with high ascending aortic cannulation and two caval cannulae. The heart is emptied on bypass, and a temporary pulmonary artery vent is placed in the midline of the main pulmonary artery.

When cardiopulmonary bypass is initiated, surface cooling with both the head jacket and the cooling blanket is begun. The blood is cooled with the pump oxygenator. During cooling, a 10°C gradient between arterial blood and bladder or rectal temperature is maintained.[19] Cooling generally takes 45 min to an hour. When ventricular fibrillation occurs, an additional vent is placed in the left atrium through the right superior pulmonary vein. This prevents atrial and ventricular distension from the large amount of bronchial arterial blood flow that is common with these patients.

It is most convenient for the primary surgeon to stand initially on the patient's left side. During the cooling period, some preliminary dissection can be performed, with full mobilization of the right pulmonary artery from the ascending aorta. The superior vena cava is also fully mobilized. The approach to the right pulmonary artery is made medial, not lateral, to the superior vena cava. All dissection of the pulmonary arteries takes place intrapericardially, and neither pleural cavity should be entered.

There are four broad types of pulmonary occlusive disease related to thrombus that can be appreciated, and we use the following classification [13,20,21]: Type I disease (approximately 38% of cases of thromboembolic pulmonary hypertension; Fig. 18.1) refers to the situation in which a major-vessel clot is present and readily visible on the opening of the pulmonary arteries. As mentioned, all central thrombotic material has to be completely removed before the endarterectomy. In type II disease (approximately 42% of cases; Fig. 18.2), no major-vessel thrombus can be appreciated. In these cases, only thickened intima can be seen, occasionally with webs, and the endarterectomy plane is raised in the main, lobar, or segmental vessels. Type III disease (approximately 18% of cases; Fig. 18.3) presents the most challenging surgical situation. The disease is very distal and confined to the segmental and subsegmental branches. No occlusion of vessels can be seen initially. The endarterectomy plane must be carefully and painstakingly raised in each segmental and subsegmental branch. Type IV disease does not represent primary thromboembolic pulmonary hypertension and is inoperable. In this entity, there is intrinsic small-vessel disease, although secondary thrombus may occur as a result of stasis. Small-vessel disease may be unrelated to thromboembolic events ("primary" pulmonary

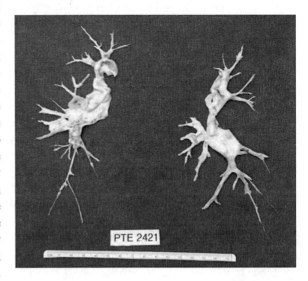

Fig. 18.2 Surgical specimen removed in a patient with type II disease. Both pulmonary arteries have evidence of chronic thromboembolic material, but there is no evidence of fresh thromboembolic material. Full resolution of pulmonary hypertension depends on complete removal of all the distal tails. The rulerm easures15c m

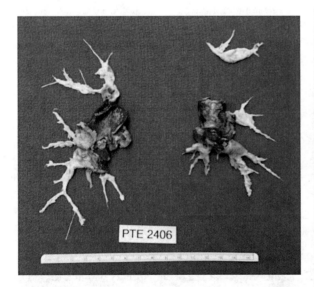

Fig. 18.1 Surgical specimen removed from a patient showing fresh and old thrombus in the main and both right and left pulmonary arteries. It is important to note removal of the proximal disease initially encountered on pulmonary arteriotomy will not be therapeutic and will certainly result in patient's demise unless a full endarterectomy is performed. The ruler measures 15 cm

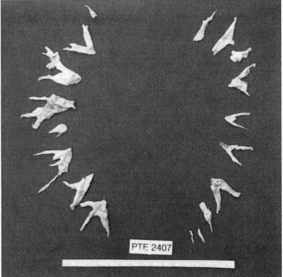

Fig. 18.3 Specimen removed from a patient with type III disease. Note that in this group of patients the disease is in the segmental and subsegmental branches, and the plane of dissection has to be raised individually at each segmental level. The ruler measures15c m

hypertension) or occur in relation to thromboembolic hypertension as a result of a high-flow or high-pressure state in previously unaffected vessels similar to the generation of Eisenmenger syndrome. We believe that there may also be sympathetic "cross talk" from an affected contralateral side or stenotic areas in the same lung.

When the patient's temperature reaches 20°C, the aorta is cross-clamped, and a single dose of cold cardioplegic solution (1 L) is administered. Additional myocardial protection is obtained using a cooling jacket. The entire procedure is now performed with a single aortic cross-clamp period with no further administration of cardioplegic solution.

A modified cerebellar retractor is placed between the aorta and superior vena cava. When blood obscures direct vision of the pulmonary vascular bed, thiopental is administered (500 mg to 1 g) until the electroencephalogram becomes isoelectric. Circulatory arrest is then initiated, and the patient undergoes exsanguination. All monitoring lines to the patient are turned off to prevent the aspiration of air. Snares are tightened around the cannulae in the superior and inferior vena cavae. It is rare that one 20-min period for each side is exceeded.

Any residual loose thrombotic debris encountered is removed. Then, a microtome knife is used to develop the endarterectomy plane posteriorly because any inadvertent egress in this site could be repaired readily or simply left alone. Dissection in the correct plane is critical because if the plane is too deep, the pulmonary artery may perforate, with fatal results, and if the dissection plane is not deep enough, inadequate amounts of the chronically thromboembolic material will be removed.

Once the plane is correctly developed, a full-thickness layer is left in the region of the incision to ease subsequent repair. The endarterectomy is then performed with an eversion technique. Because the vessel is everted and subsegmental branches are being worked on, a perforation here will become completely inaccessible and invisible later. This is why the absolute visualization in a completely bloodless field provided by circulatory arrest is essential. It is important that each subsegmental branch is followed and freed individually until it ends in a "tail," beyond which there is no further obstruction. Residual material should never be cut free; the entire specimen should "tail off" and come free spontaneously.

Once the right-sided endarterectomy is completed, circulation is restarted, and the arteriotomy is repaired with a continuous 6–0 polypropylene suture. The hemostatic nature of this closure is aided by the nature of the initial dissection, with the full thickness of the pulmonary artery preserved immediately adjacent to the incision.

After the completion of the repair of the right arteriotomy, the surgeon moves to the patient's right side. The pulmonary vent catheter is withdrawn, and an arteriotomy is made from the site of the pulmonary vent hole laterally to the pericardial reflection, avoiding entry into the left pleural space. Additional lateral dissection does not enhance intraluminal visibility, may endanger the left phrenic nerve, and makes subsequent repair of the left pulmonary artery more difficult.

The left-sided dissection is virtually analogous in all respects to that accomplished on the right. The duration of circulatory arrest intervals during the performance of the left-sided dissection is subject to the same restriction as the right.

After the completion of the endarterectomy, cardiopulmonary bypass is reinstituted, and warming is commenced. Methylprednisolone (500 mg IV) and mannitol (12.5 g IV) are administered, and during warming a 10°C temperature gradient is maintained between the perfusate and body temperature, with a maximum perfusate temperature of 37°C. If the systemic vascular resistance level is high, nitroprusside is administered to promote vasodilation and warming. The rewarming period generally takes approximately 90–120 min but varies according to the body mass of the patient.

When the left pulmonary arteriotomy has been repaired, the pulmonary artery vent is replaced at the top of the incision. The heart is retracted upward and to the left, and a posterior pericardial window is made between the aorta and the left phrenic nerve. Alternatively, prior to closure a posterior pericardial drain can be placed; it is removed once drainage has substantially decreased.

The right atrium is then opened and examined. Any intra-atrial communication is closed. Although tricuspid valve regurgitation is invariable in these patients and is often severe, tricuspid valve repair is not performed. Right ventricular remodeling occurs within a few days, with the return of tricuspid competence. If other cardiac procedures are required, such as coronary artery or mitral or aortic valve surgery, these are conveniently performed during the systemic rewarming period. Myocardial cooling is discontinued once all cardiac procedures have been concluded. The left atrial vent is removed, and the vent site is repaired. All air is removed from the heart, and the aortic cross-clamp is removed.

When the patient has rewarmed, cardiopulmonary bypass is discontinued. Dopamine hydrochloride is routinely administered at renal doses, and other inotropic agents and vasodilators are titrated as necessary to sustain acceptable hemodynamics. The cardiac output is generally high, with a low systemic vascular resistance. Temporary atrial and ventricular epicardial pacing wires are placed.

Despite the duration of extracorporeal circulation, hemostasis is readily achieved, and the administration of platelets or coagulation factors is generally unnecessary. Wound closure is routine. A vigorous diuresis is usual for the next few hours, also a result of the previous systemic hypothermia.

18.11   AdverseEf fects

Patients are subject to all complications associated with open heart and major lung surgery (arrhythmias, atelectasis, wound infection, pneumonia, mediastinal bleeding, etc.) but also may develop complications specific to this operation. These include persistent pulmonary hypertension, reperfusion pulmonary response, and very rarely disorders related to deep hypothermia and total circulatory arrest.

Severe reperfusion injury is the single most frequent complication after pulmonary endarterectomy, historically occurring in approximately 15% of patients, but now in a much smaller percentage of our patients (about 5–8%). Of patients with reperfusion injury, the majority resolve the problem with a short period of ventilatory support and aggressive diuresis. A minority of patients with severe lung reperfusion injury require prolonged periods of ventilatory support, while extreme cases require venovenous extracorporeal support for oxygenation and blood carbon dioxide removal.[22] Neurologic complications from circulatory arrest have mostly been eliminated by shorter circulatory arrest periods and the use of a direct cooling jacket placed around the head, which provides even cooling to the surface of the cranium. Perioperative confusion and stroke rates for pulmonary endarterectomy are similar to those seen with conventional open heart surgery. Since 2000, reexploration for bleeding has occurred at a rate of 3.3%,

and 29.1 of patients have required intraoperative or postoperative blood transfusion. Despite an average duration of surgery of 6.5 h, wound infection occurred only in 1.3% of patients.

The single greatest risk factor for operation remains the severity of pulmonary vascular resistance and the ability to lower it to a normal range at operation. Those patients with high pulmonary vascular resistance with minimal vascular obstruction on angiogram (type IV small-vessel vasculopathy indistinguishable from idiopathic pulmonary arterial hypertension) have the worst prognosis, and surgery does not correct pulmonary hypertension in this population. Arteriolar-capillary vasculopathy without larger-vessel thromboembolic disease was not influenced by blind endarterectomy of the proximal pulmonary arterial tree. The majority of early deaths after this operation are in this subgroup, and efforts are directed at better determining who these patients are in the preoperative setting to avoid unnecessaryope ration.

18.12   Results

Although pulmonary endarterectomy is now performed at several major cardiovascular centers throughout the world, the majority of experience with this operation has been at UCSD, where the technique of this operation was pioneered and refined. More than 2,500 pulmonary endarterectomy operations have been performed at UCSD since 1970, while the entire reported cases in the literature worldwide on this operation (exclusive of UCSD) are approximately 1,500 cases. Since 2000, the mean patient age has been 51.6 years with a range of 8.9–84.8 years. There is a slight male predominance, reflecting disease predilection, surgical bias, or both. In 40% of cases, at least one additional cardiac procedure was performed at the time of operation. Most commonly, the adjunct procedure was closure of a persistent foramen ovale or atrial septal defect (18.9%) or coronary artery bypass grafting (7.9%).[23]

With this operation, a reduction in pulmonary pressures and resistance to normal levels and corresponding improvement in pulmonary blood flow and cardiac output are generally immediate and sustained.[10,24] These changes are permanent.[25] Whereas before the operation, more than 78.7% of the patients were in the New York Heart Association (NYHA) functional class

III or IV in this series; at 1 year after operation 97% of patients were reclassified as NYHA functional class I or II. In addition, echocardiographic studies have demonstrated that, with the elimination of chronic pressure overload, right ventricular geometry rapidly reverts toward normal.[26] Right atrial and right ventricular hypertrophy and dilation regress. Tricuspid valve function returns to normal within a few days as a result of restoration of tricuspid annular geometry after the remodeling of the right ventricle; therefore, tricuspid valve repair is not performed with this operation.[27]

In the UCSD experience, overall perioperative mortality was 9% for the entire cohort of patients, encompassing a time span of more than 30 years. In the last 1,000 cases, surgical mortality for pulmonary endarterectomy was 4.7%. Since 2008, the operative mortality for isolated pulmonary endarterectomy cases at UCSD has been about 2.5%, despite a patient population with higher risk factors. This reflects the learning curve for safely performing this operation and the refinements in surgical technique that enhance patient outcome.

A survey of surviving patients who underwent pulmonary endarterectomy between 1970 and 1995 at UCSD has formally evaluated long-term outcome from this operation.[28] Questionnaires were mailed to 420 patients who were more than 1 year after operation, and responses were obtained from 308 patients. Survival, functional status, quality of life, and the subsequent use of medical assistance were assessed. Survival after pulmonary endarterectomy was 75% at 6 years or more. This survival exceeds single- or double-lung transplant survival for thromboembolic pulmonary hypertension. Ninety-three percent of the patients were found to be in NYHA class I or II, compared to about 95% of the patients being in NYHA class III or IV preoperatively. Of the working population, 62% of patients who were unemployed before operation returned to work. Patients who had undergone pulmonary endarterectomy scored several quality-of-life components slightly lower than normal individuals but significantly higher than the patients before operation. Only 10% of patients used oxygen after surgery. In response to the question, "How do you feel about the quality of your life since your surgery?" 77% replied much improved, and 20% replied improved. These data appear to confirm that pulmonary endarterectomy offers substantial improvement in survival, function, and quality of life.

18.13 Summary

Pulmonary hypertension due to chronic pulmonary emboli is a condition that is underrecognized and carries a poor prognosis. Medical therapy for this condition is ineffective and only transiently improves symptoms. The only therapeutic alternative to pulmonary endarterectomy is lung transplantation. The advantages of pulmonary endarterectomy include a lower operative mortality, better long-term results with respect to survival and quality of life, and the avoidance of chronic immunosuppressive treatment and allograft rejection. Currently, mortality rates for pulmonary endarterectomy are in the range of 2.5–4.7%, and the operation allows for sustained clinical benefit. These results make it the treatment of choice over transplantation for thromboembolic disease to the lung in both the short and the long term.

Although pulmonary endarterectomy is a technically demanding operation, excellent results can be achieved. Improvements in operative technique developed since the 1970's allow us to offer pulmonary endarterectomy to our patients with an acceptable mortality rate and anticipation of significant clinical improvement. With the increasing recognition of patients who have thromboembolic pulmonary hypertension and the realization that pulmonary endarterectomy is a safe and effective operation for this condition, it is anticipated that this will be an expanding area of surgical therapy in the future.

References

1. Bernard J, Yi JS. Pulmonary thromboendarterectomy: a clinicopathologic study of 200 consecutive pulmonary thromboendarterectomy cases in one institution. *Hum Pathol.*2007; 38:871-877.
2. Guillanta P, Peterson KL, Ben-Yehuda O. Cardiac catheterization techniques in pulmonary hypertension. *Cardiol Clin.* 2004;22:401-405.
3. Du L, Sullivan CC, Chu D, et al. Signaling molecules in nonfamilial pulmonary hypertension. *N Engl J Med.* 2003; 348:500-509.
4. Riedel M, Stanek V, Widimsky J, et al. Long-term follow-up of patients with pulmonary thromboembolism. Late prognosis and evolution of hemodynamic and respiratory data. *Chest.*1982; 81:151-158.
5. Lewczuk J, Piszko P, Jagas J, et al. Prognostic factors in medically treated patients with chronic pulmonary embolism. *Chest.*2001; 119:818-823.

6. Dibble JH. Organization and canalization in arterial thrombosis. *J Pathol Bacteriol*.1958; 75:1-4.

7. Cournad A, Rilev RL, Himmelstein A, Austrian R. Pulmonary circulation in the alveolar ventilation perfusion relationship after pneumonectomy. *J Thorac Surg*. 1950;19:80-116.

8. Morris TA, Auger WR, Ysrael MZ, et al. Parenchymal scarring is associated with restrictive spirometric defects in patients with chronic thromboembolic pulmonary hypertension. *Chest*.1996;1 10:399-403.

9. D'Armini AM, Zanotti G, Ghio S, et al. Reverse right ventricular remodeling after pulmonary endarterectomy. *J Thorac Cardiovasc Surg*. 2007;133:162-168.

10. Menzel T, Kramm T, Mohr-Kahaly S, et al. Assessment of cardiac performance using Tei indices in patients undergoing pulmonary thromboendarterectomy. *Ann Thorac Surg*. 2002;73:762-766.

11. Ryan KL, Fedullo PF, Davis GB, et al. Perfusion scan findings understate the severity of angiographic and hemodynamic compromise in chronic thromboembolic pulmonary hypertension. *Chest*.1988; 93:1130-1185.

12. Coulden R. State-of-the-art imaging techniques in chronic thromboembolic pulmonary hypertension. *Proc Am Thorac Soc*.2006;3:577-58 3.

13. Jamieson SW, Kapelanski DP. Pulmonary endarterectomy. *Curr Probl Surg*.2000; 37:165-252.

14. Reichelt A, Hoeper MM, Laganski M, et al. Chronic thromboembolic pulmonary hypertension: evaluation with 64-detector row CT versus digital subtraction angiography. *Eur J Radiol*.2008; 71(1):49-54.

15. Suga K, Kawakami Y, Hayashi N, et al. Comprehensive assessment of lung CT attenuation alteration at perfusion defects of acute pulmonary thromboembolism with breath-hold SPECT-CT fusion images. *J Comput Assist Tomogr*. 2006;30:83-91.

16. Nikolaou K, Schoenberg SO, Attenberger U, et al. Pulmonary arterial hypertension: diagnosis with fast perfusion MR imaging and high-spatial-resolution MR angiography – preliminary experience. *Radiology*.2005; 236:694-703.

17. Allison PR, Dunnill MS, Marshall R. Pulmonary embolism. *Thorax*.1960; 15:273.

18. Moser KM, Houk VN, Jones RC, Hufnagel CC. Chronic, massive thrombotic obstruction of the pulmonary arteries: analysis of four operated cases. *Circulation*. 1965;32:377-385.

19. Rohrer WMH, CH RSC, et al. Perfusion techniques of profound hypothermia and circulatory arrest for pulmonary thromboendarterectomy. *J Extra Corpor Technol*. 1990;22:57-60.

20. Madani MM, Jamieson SW. Pulmonary embolism and thromboendarterectomy. In: Cohn LH, ed. *Cardiac surgery in the adult*. 3rd ed. New York: McGraw Hill; 2007:1309-1331.

21. Jamieson SW. Pulmonary thromboendarterectomy. In: Franco KL, Putnam JB, eds. *Advanced therapy in thoracic surgery*. Hamilton, Ontario: Decker; 1998:310-318.

22. Thistlethwaite PA, Madani MM, Kemp AD, et al. Venovenous extracorporeal life support after pulmonary endarterectomy: indications, techniques, and outcomes. *Ann Thorac Surg*. 2006;82:2139-2145.

23. Thistlethwaite PA, Auger WR, Madani MM, et al. Pulmonary thromboendarterectomy combined with other cardiac operations: indications, surgical approach, and outcome. *Ann Thorac Surg*.2001; 72:13-17.

24. Thistlethwaite PA, Madani MM, Jamieson SW. Outcomes of pulmonary endarterectomy surgery. *Semin Thorac Cardiovasc Surg*.2006; 18:257-264.

25. Corsico AG, D'Armini AM, Cerveri I, et al. Long-term outcome after pulmonary endarterectomy. *Am J Respir Crit Care Med*2008; 178(4):419–424.

26. Ilino M, Dymarkowski S, Chaothawee L, et al. Time course of reversed remodeling after pulmonary endarterectomy in patients with chronic pulmonary thromboembolism. *Eur Radiol*.2008; 18:792-799.

27. Thistlethwaite PA, Jamieson SW. Tricuspid valvular disease in the patient with chronic pulmonary thromboembolic disease. *Curr Opin Cardiol*.2003; 18:111-116.

28. Archibald CJ, Auger WR, Fedullo PF, et al. Long-term outcome after pulmonary thromboendarterectomy. *Am J Respir Crit Care Med*.1999; 160:523-528.

Ruchi Gupta, Shirah Shore, Maria M. Rodriguez, and Marco Ricci

Eisenmenger syndrome results when there is a congenital heart defect that causes persistent shunting of blood from the left side to the right side of the heart, resulting in pulmonary vascular changes over time that eventually cause pulmonary artery hypertension and reversal of shunt flow from the right side to the left side of the heart.

In 1897, Dr. Viktor Eisenmenger published his paper on "congenital defects of the ventricular septum." He described a patient with breathing difficulty and cyanosis throughout life who eventually developed heart failure and then died suddenly of massive hemoptysis at 32 years of age. On autopsy, the patient was diagnosed with a ventricular septal defect and severe pulmonary vascular disease, which led to pulmonary infarction and fatal hemoptysis.[1] In 1958, Dr. Paul Wood defined the term *Eisenmenger complex* as "pulmonary hypertension at the systemic level, due to a high pulmonary vascular resistance (PVR), with reversed or bidirectional shunt through a large ventricular septal defect."[2] Wood also extended the definition to include different congenital heart defects that are responsible for left-to-right shunting and are associated with elevated pulmonary artery pressure and elevated PVR. Currently, the term *Eisenmenger syndrome* is used to describe the clinical features of patients who have such pulmonary vascular disease and oxygen-unresponsive cyanosis resulting from a ventricular septal defect or any other systemic-to-pulmonary shunt.[3]

The congenital heart defects that are responsible for shunting of blood from the left side of the heart to the right side are numerous. It is estimated that about 8% of patients with congenital heart defects and 11% of patients with left-to-right shunts develop Eisenmenger syndrome.[4] Unrepaired defects such as ventricular septal defects (VSDs), atrial septal defects (ASDs), atrioventricular septal defects (AVSDs), patent ductus arteriosus (PDA), and aortopulmonary windows (AP window) account for a large number of cases of Eisenmenger syndrome. However, other lesions, such as single-ventricle variants, transposition of the great arteries (TGA), truncus arteriosus, and surgically created aortopulmonary shunts, also can lead to pulmonary artery hypertension and Eisenmenger syndrome.[5] Studies done to associate the development of pulmonary artery hypertension with the type of congenital heart defect have concluded that the degree of pulmonary vascular disease and time of onset depends on the size of the anatomic defect, the type of the defect, and the magnitude of shunt flow. Three percent of patients with a small or moderate-size VSD (less than or equal to 1.5 cm in diameter by echocardiography) and about 50% of patients who have a large VSD (greater than 1.5 cm in diameter by echocardiography) develop Eisenmenger syndrome.[6] In patients with large-size defects, Eisenmenger syndrome develops in almost 100% of patients with truncus arteriosus, about 50% of patients with VSDs or PDAs, but only 10% of patients with ASDs.[7] The age at presentation is affected by the size of the lesion. The size of the defects in the ventricular septum and atrial septum correspond to the magnitude of shunting, and larger defects can present with shunt reversal earlier. The type of lesion also determines the time of onset.

M.R icci (✉)
DepartmentSur gery, Universityof M iami, Miami, FL, USA
e-mail:m ricci@med.miami.edu

Of patients who developed Eisenmenger syndrome, those with AVSD, truncus arteriosus, TGA, large PDA, and large VSD present the earliest – even as early as the first decade of life.[3] When patients with ASDs develop Eisenmenger syndrome, they usually present later on in adulthood – in the second or third decade.[4,5]

In patients with unrestricted left-to-right shunting and a high ratio of pulmonary blood flow to systemic blood flow (Qp:Qs), there will be more insult to the pulmonary vascular bed than in patients with a low Qp:Qs. It is still unknown if risk of development of Eisenmenger syndrome is completely proportional to degree of shunt flow or if there is an underlying genetic predisposition with so Eisenmenger syndrome is a disease me specific lesions. For example, individuals with some lesions, such as unrepaired truncus arteriosus, are at a very high risk of developing pulmonary artery hypertension compared to patients with VSDs and ASDs, who carry a relatively lower risk.[3,7] Although patients with unrepaired VSDs, ASDs, and PDAs have a relatively lower risk of developing Eisenmenger syndrome than patients with some more complex lesions, they account for a significant percentage of patients with Eisenmenger syndrome today.[8] One reason may be that VSDs, ASDs, and PDAs are much more prevalent in the population than the other more complex congenital heart defects.

Pulmonary vascular resistance can change throughout life. In utero, during fetal development, the lungs are filled with amniotic fluid, and the pulmonary arterioles are constricted; the PVR is high. Forty percent of the blood returning to the right atrium is shunted across the foramen ovale through the interatrial septum to the left atrium. Also, because of the high PVR, 90% of the blood leaving the heart through the pulmonary artery crosses the ductus arteriosus into the aorta and to the placenta, which is low resistance. As soon as the baby is born, the placenta is removed from the circulation, causing a rise in the systemic vascular resistance (SVR). Simultaneously, the PVR decreases due to lung expansion, causing physical expansion of pulmonary blood vessels as well as oxygen delivery to the pulmonary alveoli, which causes chemoreflex vasodilation. The sudden increase in SVR and drop in PVR cause reversal of flow through the ductus arteriosus and an increase in pulmonary blood flow. The left atrial pressure rises, and the right atrial pressure falls; the flap valve of the foramen ovale closes against the edge of the crista dividens, eliminating shunting at

the interatrial septum. The PVR continues to drop from birth until about 6–8 weeks of age.

When there is any persistent communication between the pulmonary and systemic circulations, the systolic blood pressures in the pulmonary artery and the aorta equalize. In infancy and early childhood, the PVR is lower than the SVR, blood flow follows the path of least resistance, and there is shunting of blood from the systemic circulation to the pulmonary circulation. As the pulmonary vascular bed is exposed to increased blood flow at high systemic-level pressures, there are changes in the pulmonary microvasculature. The appearance of the pulmonary vascular bed that results from unrestricted pulmonary blood flow from a congenital heart defect very closely resembles the changes seen in histological specimens of lungs with idiopathic pulmonary artery hypertension.[9]

Pulmonary biopsies should be stained with hematoxylin, eosin, and elastic van Gieson (EVG) to better demonstrate the internal and external *elastic laminae*. The changes in pulmonary hypertension include arteriolar medial hypertrophy, intimal proliferation and fibrosis, capillary and arteriolar occlusion, and eventually plexiform lesions and necrotizing arteritis. The result of these progressive changes is complete obliteration of pulmonary arterioles and capillaries.[9,10] Figure 19.1 depicts a normal bronchiolus and pulmonary artery stained with EVG. Figure 19.2a–f demonstrates the six grades of

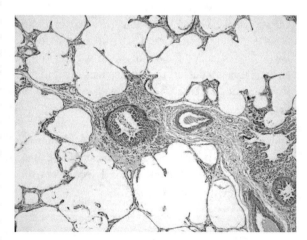

Fig. 19.1 Normal lung. Elastic Van Gieson stain (×10). Observe the bronchiolus lined by pseudostratified epithelium and next to it the pulmonary artery with an internal and an external elastic lamina. Both structures are approximately of the same diameter with an imperceptible intima (endothelial lining), and the muscularisi st hin

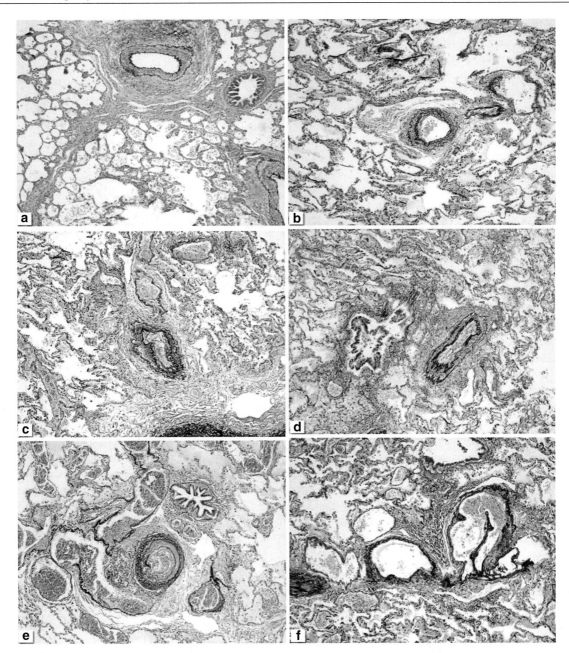

Fig. 19.2 Grades of severity of pulmonary hypertension. Elastic Van Gieson stain (×10). (**a**) *Grade 1*. Hypertrophy of muscularis with normal intima. There is a bronchiolus to the right and the artery to the left and slightly above. Observe the internal and external elastic laminae delimiting the thick muscularis. The vascular lumen is still widely patent. (**b**) *Grade 2*. Mild intimal proliferation. It narrows the arteriolar lumen clearly delimited by the internal elastic lamina. (**c**) *Grade 3*. Laminar intimal fibrosis. The intima has proliferated inside the vascular lumen to almost completely occlude it, leaving only two small vascular channels. These changes and higher grades of pulmonary hypertension are considered irreversible. (**d**) *Grade 4*. The arterial wall has been damaged. Notice the interruption of the internal elastic lamina. The intima is fibrotic and almost completely occluded. There is a bronchiolus to the left. (**e**) *Grade 5*. Plexiform lesions and vascular obstruction. Some vessels are dilated and congested, while the artery at the center is thrombosed with two smaller recanalized lumina. Observe that the elastic lamina is partly destroyed. It is believed that these changes are secondary to healed vascular fibrinoid necrosis that incompletely destroys the internal elastic lamina and occludes the lumen. (**f**) *Grade 6*. Angiomatoid changes. The arteries become dilated, thin walled, and tortuous. It may be difficult to appreciate the two elastic layers. These distended vessels may rupturea ndpr oducei ntra-alveolarhe morrhage

severity in pulmonary hypertension. Sometimes, there is overlap between two grades of pulmonary hypertension in the same biopsy. However, the grading should be given by the predominant lesion.

The mechanism of all of these changes in the microvasculature is not completely understood. Studies have been done in sheep to study the release of growth factors in response to microvascular injury. The production of elastase enzymes, insulin-like growth factor I, and transforming growth factor all may play a role in medial hypertrophy, intimal proliferation, and eventual arteriolar destruction.[11,12] In addition to changes in the histology, the microvasculature is altered in its ability to relax in response to mediators.[13]

With these changes in the microvasculature, pressure in the pulmonary vascular bed increases progressively and eventually irreversibly. The shunting of blood goes from being all left to right to bidirectional. Eventually, the pulmonary artery pressure is higher than the systemic arterial pressure. With the anatomic source still available, the shunt reverses, and the blood goes from the pulmonary circulation to the systemic circulation – permanently right-to-left shunting. The diastolic pressures in the pulmonary artery are also higher than the systemic arterial pressures in Eisenmenger syndrome.[5] With decreased pulmonary blood flow, there is decreased oxygenated hemoglobin and cyanosis. As in other cyanotic states, the physiologic response to hypoxemia is to produce more hemoglobin and more red blood cells, resulting in erythrocytosis. The last causes increased blood viscosity and sludging, which produces some of the complications seen in patients with Eisenmenger syndrome.

Since Eisenmenger syndrome is a disease that progresses as a result of congenital heart defects, the clinical presentation also changes with the progression of the disease. Initially in infancy and early childhood, when patients have a left-to-right shunt, they experience increased pulmonary blood flow and congestion with corresponding symptoms of tachypnea and poor feeding. Figure 19.3 shows the chest radiograph of an infant with a ventricular septal defect depicting pulmonary vascular congestion due to unrestricted left-to-right shunt. As the pulmonary vasculature changes and the PVR rises, the pulmonary blood flow decreases and even normalizes. The symptoms of pulmonary congestion resolve. This clinical presentation at the time of late infancy or early childhood is deceptive since the pulmonary blood flow is "normal," but correspondingly, the

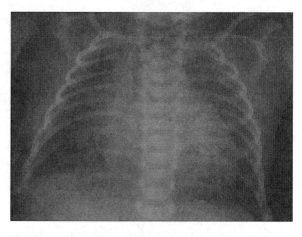

Fig. 19.3 Chest radiograph of a 2-month-old infant with a ventricular septal defect. There is cardiomegaly and increased pulmonary vascular markings consistent with pulmonary overcirculation from a left-to-right shunt

pulmonary vasculature is abnormal with high PVR and pressure. Finally, when the shunt reverses, the patient presents with Eisenmenger syndrome. Figure 19.4a, b shows the chest radiograph and left pulmonary artery angiogram of a 59-year-old man with an unrepaired atrial septal defect and Eisenmenger syndrome.

In addition to developing progressive cyanosis, patients may also present with signs of decreased systemic output and congestive heart failure due to abnormal ventricular function. In patients with Eisenmenger syndrome, as the right-sided or subpulmonary ventricle continues to be exposed to high pulmonary pressures, there is ventricular hypertrophy, dilation, and dysfunction. Symptoms include dyspnea on exertion, fatigue, edema, volume retention, palpitations, and syncopal episodes.[1,3–5] With volume overload, the systemic venous pressure can be abnormally high, and hepatic dysfunction can result. As the disease progresses, in the third decade of life morbidities become more apparent. Patients with more complex anatomical lesions, such as single-ventricle variants and double-outlet right ventricle, have earlier clinical deterioration than those with simple defects such as ASDs or VSDs.[14] As the right ventricle becomes more and more abnormal, it can become ischemic, and patients can experience angina. Also, chest pain can be a result of coronary artery compression from an enlarged, engorged pulmonary artery.[3]

Cyanosis and hypoxemia can cause the physiologic response of erythrocytosis with subsequent hyperviscosity

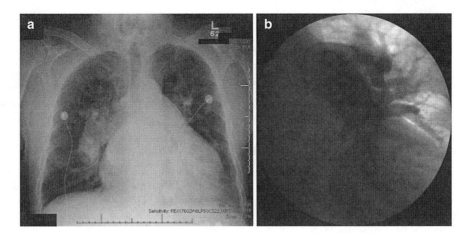

Fig. 19.4 (**a**) Chest radiograph of a 59-year-old man with Eisenmenger syndrome due to an unrepaired atrial septal defect. There is cardiomegaly, prominent central pulmonary arteries, and rapid tapering of distal pulmonary arteries. (**b**) Left pulmo- nary artery angiogram of the same patient with Eisenmenger syndrome. There is significant dilation of the central left pulmonary artery segments with "pruning" or tapering of the distal pulmonarya rteries

or intravascular sludging. Hyperviscosity can cause neurological symptoms such as headache or vision changes. In severe cases, organ damage such as cerebrovascular changes from strokes can occur. Cerebral vascular accidents result from hyperviscosity-related thrombosis or from peripheral embolism due to impaired ventricular function or arrhythmia.[14]

The disease progression of patients with Eisenmenger syndrome fluctuates.[15] There are periods of worsening and periods of improvement. The periods of deterioration are associated with any one of the complications discussed but also can occur in times of emotional disturbances, such as a parent's death or a divorce. Lifestyle changes can cause surges in pulmonary artery pressures, and patients can experience symptoms such as hemoptysis, increased dyspnea, or syncope.[14] In some cases, severe emotional distress can lead to sudden death. There are some states that can cause the SVR to fall and cause more right-to-left shunting. These include environmental heat, exercise, and fever.[4] With increased right-to-left shunting, patients will be more cyanotic and can suffer from any of the complications mentioned.

The prognosis of patients with Eisenmenger syndrome is improving with more specialized care and management by experts experienced in adult congenital heart disease. The prognosis for patients with Eisenmenger syndrome is better than for patients with primary pulmonary hypertension.[16] The long-term survival data are changing with new treatment modalities

and better understanding of the pulmonary disease process. When patients die, death is attributable to sudden cardiac deaths, congestive heart failure, and hemoptysis.[8,14] Patients with more advanced disease obviously have a poorer prognosis. Signs of advanced and irreversible pulmonary microvasculature changes and decreased ventricular function with poor cardiac output include syncopal episodes and severe hypoxemia with oxygen saturation less than 85%.[8]

Patients with Eisenmenger syndrome can have sudden death from a variety of etiologies, including arrhythmias, hemoptysis, and cerebrovascular accidents. Arrhythmias are prevalent in patients with Eisenmenger syndrome. Types of electrocardiographic disturbances include supraventricular and ventricular extrasystoles, atrial flutter, atrial fibrillation, and ventricular tachycardia. When arrhythmias present, usually clinical deterioration is imminent with heart failure, peripheral embolism, and sudden death.[14] Hemoptysis as described by Eisenmenger can be caused by pulmonary infarction, rupture of a pulmonary artery dilated by aneurysm, a thin-walled pulmonary arteriole, or bleeding diathesis.[1,4] As in the case described by Eisenmenger, hemoptysis can be acute in onset, severe, and fatal. The most common causes of death in patients with Eisenmenger syndrome include sudden cardiac death (from ventricular arrhythmias), right ventricular (or subpulmonary ventricular) failure, severe hemoptysis, cerebral vascular accidents, brain abscesses, or death during pregnancy or noncardiac surgery with general anesthesia.[4,8,14]

On physical examination, patients with Eisenmenger syndrome can have cyanosis and clubbing of the nail beds. They may also have signs of right heart failure, such as jugular venous distension, hepatic congestion, and hepatomegaly. Signs of pulmonary artery hypertension include palpable right ventricle with a prominent parasternal heave, palpable pulmonary artery, and a loud pulmonic component of the second heart sound. With volume overload in the pulmonary circulation and main pulmonary artery dilation, patients may develop a pulmonary ejection click and soft systolic ejection murmur. High-pitched, diastolic, decrescendo pulmonary regurgitant murmurs (Graham Steell murmurs) or holosystolic tricuspid regurgitant murmurs may also result. Lung auscultation is usually unremarkable, and patients may or may not have edema depending on the state of the right ventricle and the central venous pressures.[4]

In December 2008, the American College of Cardiology and the American Heart Association released guidelines for the management of adults with congenital heart disease. According to these guidelines, the evaluation (including noninvasive and invasive testing) of a patient with Eisenmenger syndrome should be conducted at a center with expertise in both adult congenital heart disease and pulmonary artery hypertension. It is necessary to document and follow the size and direction of the shunt. It is also necessary to document the degree of pulmonary artery hypertension, ventricular function, and presence of any secondary complications. The evaluation should include a noninvasive assessment of cardiovascular anatomy and lesions of potential shunting with the following: finger and toe pulse oximetry with and without supplemental oxygen; chest X-ray; electrocardiogram; diagnostic cardiovascular imaging (echocardiography, magnetic resonance imaging, or computed tomography [CT]); pulmonary function tests; pulmonary embolism-protocol CT with "chest windows"; complete blood count with indices; ferritin and iron studies; and renal and hepatic function tests. It is also reasonable to conduct a 6-min walk test with or without oximetry and cardiopulmonary testing. A complete cardiac catheterization is also recommended with potential for vasodilator testing at an appropriate center.

On follow-up, patients should have yearly comprehensive evaluations of functional capacity and assessment for any potential complications. Patients with Eisenmenger syndrome should have hemoglobin, platelet count, iron store, creatinine, and uric acid tests yearly.

Oximetry tests with and without supplemental oxygen should be at least yearly. All medication changes or planned interventions should be carefully discussed. Procedures such as noncardiac surgery and cardiac catheterization should only take place in centers with expertise in adult congenital heart disease and pulmonary artery hypertension physiology. Intravenous tubing should be rigorously checked for air bubbles in patients with Eisenmenger syndrome because of the potential for systemic peripheral embolization from right-to-left shunting. Patients should be instructed to seek prompt therapy for complications such as arrhythmias and infections. The following should be avoided in patients with Eisenmenger syndrome because they can cause destabilizing volume shifts: pregnancy, dehydration, moderate and severe strenuous exercise, acute exposure to excessive heat, and chronic high-altitude exposure. Pregnancy should be avoided in patients with Eisenmenger syndrome because it poses a significant risk of maternal death.[14] Contraception with agents that can aggravate the potential for thrombosis should also be avoided. Special considerations must be made to select an appropriate contraceptive method in women of reproductive age who have Eisenmenger syndrome. Consultation with a maternal fetal medicine expert may be required.[3]

When considering corrective cardiac surgery in a patient with a history of left-to-right shunt and potentially elevated pulmonary artery pressures, it is important to consider the degree of pulmonary vascular disease. If surgery is performed before the pulmonary vasculature has undergone irreversible changes, the pulmonary vascular bed may be able to reverse some of the changes that occurred with shunt-mediated pulmonary artery hypertension. If the changes in the pulmonary vasculature are irreversible, then pulmonary artery pressures will also be irreversibly elevated, and surgical outcomes will be poor. Hemodynamic measurements made by cardiac catheterization are useful for assessing the degree of disease. Calculations of pulmonary blood flow and PVR are used to assess whether the pulmonary vasculature has reversible changes. Inhaled nitric oxide or intravenous prostacyclin is used to determine the reactivity of the pulmonary vascular bed. The pulmonary vascular bed is considered acutely reactive if the vasculature relaxes with these agents and pulmonary artery pressures as well as calculation of PVR decrease after administration. Lower PVR and reactivity correspond to increased surgical success. If, however, the pulmonary vascular changes are "fixed" and irreversible, surgical intervention could cause the patient to suffer from diminished cardiac output with severe heart failure and death.[3]

The treatment of erythrocytosis with therapeutic phlebotomy should only be performed if the hemoglobin is more than 20 g/dL and the hematocrit is greater than 65%. It is important to screen for and treat iron deficiency anemia.[17,18] Medical therapies for patients with Eisenmenger syndrome include supplemental oxygen, anticoagulation with warfarin, intravenous epoprostenol, oral prostacyclin analogs, oral endothelin antagonists, oral phosphodiesterase antagonists, and transplantation. The use of any of these treatments is still under debate. The role of lung or heart-lung transplantation requires special consideration on a case-by-case basis. For medical management, randomized controlled trials need to be conducted in patients specifically with Eisenmenger physiology. One such trial published in 2006 was the BREATHE-5 (Bosentan Randomized Trial of Endothelin Antagonist Therapy 5) trial. Oral bosentan was compared with placebo in 54 adults with Eisenmenger syndrome due to ASD or VSD. After 16 weeks use of bosentan, patients with Eisenmenger syndrome had significant reduction in PVR and significant improvement in exercise capacity (assessed by the 6-min walk distance test). The trial showed therapeutic safety with no reduction in oxygen saturation in the bosentan treatment group.[19] Since there is lack of consensus on therapeutic mainstays for Eisenmenger syndrome, treatment should only be conducted at a specialized center.[3]

There is much that remains to be understood about Eisenmenger physiology and management. It is hoped that basic science research to further elucidate the pathophysiology of pulmonary microvasculature and genetic predispositions as well as clinical trials on new treatment modalities will help patients with Eisenmenger syndrome.

References

1. Eisenmenger V. Die angeborenen Defects des Kammerscheidewand des Herzen. *Z Klin Med*1897; 32(suppl):1–28.
2. Wood P. The Eisenmenger syndrome or pulmonary hypertension with reversed central shunt. *Br Med J*. 1958;46: 701-709.
3. Warnes CA et al. ACC/AHA 2008 guidelines for the management of adults with congenital heart disease. *Circulation*. 2008;118(23):e714-e833.
4. Vongpatanasin W, Brickner ME, Hillis LD, Lange RA. The Eisenmenger syndrome in adults. *Ann Intern Med*. 1998;128: 745-755.
5. Somerville J. How to manage the Eisenmenger syndrome. *Int J Cardiol*.1998; 63:1-8.
6. Kidd L, Driscoll DJ, Gersony WM, Hayes CJ, Keane JF, O'Fallon M, et al. Second natural history study of congenital heart defects. Results of treatment of patients with ventricular septal defects. *Circulation*1993; 87(2s uppl):138–151.
7. Gault JH, Morrow AG, Gay WA Jr, Ross J Jr. Atrial septal defect in patients over the age of forty years clinical and hemodynamic studies and the effects of operation. *Circulation*.1968; 37:261-272.
8. Saha A, Balakrishnan KG, Jaiswal PK, et al. Prognosis for patients with Eisenmenger syndrome of various aetiology. *Int J Cardiol*.1994; 45:199-207.
9. Tuder RM, Cool CD, Yaeger M, Taraseviciene-Stewart L, Bull TM, Voelkel NF. The pathobiology of pulmonary hypertension. Endothelium. *Clin Chest Med*. 2001;22:405-418.
10. Heath D, Edwards JE. The pathology of hypertensive pulmonary vascular disease. A description of six grades of structural changes in the pulmonary arteries with special reference to congenital cardiac septal defects. *Circulation*. 1958;18:533-547.
11. Perkett EA, Badesch DB, Roessler MK, Stenmark KR, Meyrick B. Insulinlike growth factor I and pulmonary hypertension induced by continuous air embolization in sheep. *Am J Respir Cell Mol Biol*.1992; 6:82-87.
12. Perkett EA, Lyons RM, Moses HL, Brigham KL, Meyrick B. Transforming growth factor-β activity in sheep lung lymph during the development of pulmonary hypertension. *J Clin Invest*. 1990;86:1459-1464.
13. Celermajer DS, Cullen S, Deanfield JE. Impairment of endothelium-dependent pulmonary artery relaxation in children with congenital heart disease and abnormal pulmonary hemodynamics. *Circulation*.1993; 87:440-446.
14. Daliento L, Somerville J, Presbitero P, et al. Eisenmenger syndrome. Factors relating to deterioration and death. *Eur Heart J*.1998; 19:1845-1855.
15. Galie N. Classification of patients with congenital systemic-to-pulmonary shunts associated with pulmonary arterial hypertension: current status and future directions. In: Beghetti M, Barst RJ, Naeije R, et al., eds. *Pulmonary arterial hypertension related to congenital heart disease*. Munich: Elsevier; 2006:11-17.
16. Hopkins WE, Ochoa LL, Richardson GW, Trulock EP. Comparison of the hemodynamics and survival of adults with severe pulmonary hypertension or Eisenmenger syndrome. *J Heart Lung Transplant*.1996; 15(pt1) :100-105.
17. Sondel PM, Tripp ME, Ganick DJ, Levy JM, Shahidi NT. Phlebotomy with iron therapy to correct the microcytic polycythemia of chronic hypoxia. *Pediatrics*.1981; 67:667-670.
18. Perloff JK, Marelli AJ, Miner PD. Risk of stroke in adults with cyanotic congenital heart disease. *Circulation*. 1993; 87:1954-1959.
19. Galie N, Beghetti M, Gatzoulis MA, et al. Bosentan therapy in patients with Eisenmenger syndrome: a multicenter, double-blind, randomized, placebo-controlled study. *Circulation*.2006; 114:48-54.

Disseminated Intravascular Coagulation inCardiacSurgery

20

Leticia Sandre Vendrame, Helio Penna Guimaraes, and Renato Delascio Lopes

20.1 Introduction

Disseminated intravascular coagulation (DIC) is a complex thrombohemorrhagic disease, secondary to an underlying clinical disease,[1] producing both thrombosis and hemorrhage. It is initiated by a number of defined disorders and consists of the following components[2]: exposure of blood to procoagulants; formation of fibrin in the circulation; fibrinolysis; depletion of clotting factors; and end-organ damage. Systemic activation of coagulation in its most extreme form is known as DIC,[3] which occurs in approximately 1% of hospital admissions.[4]

The majority of bleeding events in cardiovascular surgery are not due to surgical causes but are biological in origin, essentially the result of DIC in its later phases. To anticipate its occurrence and to prevent further deterioration of the hemostatic system, follow-up and treatment of DIC are extremely important.

After cardiac surgery, the administration of protamine potentially promotes the recovery of the coagulation pathways. In this situation, the patient is hypercoagulated as a result of surgery, the existence of thromboplastic material released during surgery, circulatory arrest and stasis, anoxia, acidosis, and other factors. Despite the presence of presumed adequate heparinization, large amounts of thrombin are generated, and subsequently fibrinogen is activated. Therefore, surgeons should be alerted to the potential risk for and likely occurrence of DIC, especially in the presence of severe hemodynamic instability, metabolic changes, or hepatic perturbation, as well as in cases of probable sepsis when a systemic inflammatory response syndrome (SIRS) is present, or during surgical reinterventions. It may often be necessary to administer heparin to neutralize the thromboplastic material released to break the vicious circle of a self-sustained activation of the coagulation system.[5]

20.2 Definition

The International Society on Thrombosis and Haemostasis (ISTH) defined DIC as an acquired syndrome characterized by the intravascular activation of coagulation with loss of localization arising from different causes. It can originate from and cause damage to the microvasculature, which if sufficiently severe can produce organ dysfunction.[6]

The DIC syndrome is characterized by a systemic activation of the coagulation system with laboratory evidence of the following[1]: procoagulant activation, fibrinolytic activation, inhibitor consumption, and biochemical evidence of endogen damage or failure.

DIC is classically characterized as the occurrence of widespread (micro)vascular thrombosis that compromises adequate blood supply to various organs and may contribute to organ failure.[3] At the same time, the use and subsequent depletion of platelets and coagulation proteins resulting from the ongoing coagulation may induce severe bleeding[7] (Fig. 20.1). Bleeding may be the presenting symptom in a patient with DIC, a factor that can complicate decisions about treatment.[7]

R.D.Lopes (✉)
Division of Cardiovascular Medicine,
Duke University Medical Center,
Duke Clinical Research Institute, Box 3850,
2400 Pratt Street, Room 0311 Durham, NC 27705, USA
e-mail:renato.lopes@duke.edu

E.A. Gabriel and T. Salerno (eds.), *Principles of Pulmonary Protection in Heart Surgery*,
DOI: 10.1007/978-1-84996-308-4_20, © Springer-Verlag London Limited 2010

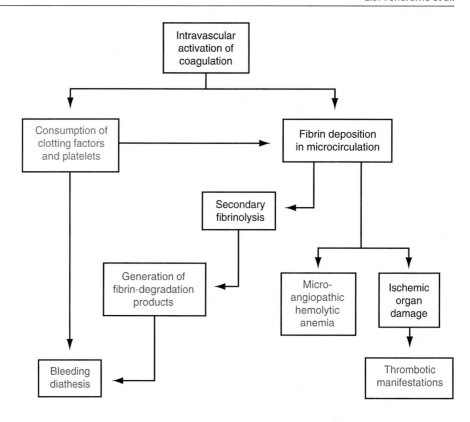

Fig.20.1 DICc ausing bleeding and thrombotic manifestations[2]

20.3 Etiologyandl ncidence

It is important to stress that DIC is not a disease by itself; it is always secondary to an underlying disorder that causes the activation of coagulation.[3] In general, there are two major pathways that may cause DIC: (1) a systemic inflammatory response that activates the cytokine network and coagulation cascade (such as in severe sepsis and major trauma); or (2) the release or exposure of procoagulant material into the bloodstream (such as in cancer or obstetric patients).[8]

Previous studies[9,10] demonstrated that 19–24% of patients who presented in-hospital with DIC were surgical or trauma patients. It was shown that the incidence of DIC is 50–70% among patients with major trauma who have resulting SIRS,[11] and the occurrence of DIC and SIRS are strong predictors for posttrauma multiple-organ dysfunction syndrome.[12] As a result, it was hypothesized that the release of tissue enzymes or phospholipids from damaged tissue into systemic circulation triggers activation of cytokine networks and the hemostatic system, leading to the occurrence of DIC secondary to large surgeries or trauma.[13] However, the precise prevalence of DIC in patients with severe

trauma is not known. It may be difficult to differentiate DIC from the coagulopathy due to massive blood loss and the dilutional coagulopathy that may occur in the first hours after major trauma.[3]

Specifically, it is known that large aortic aneurysms may result in local activation of coagulation. In patients with this condition, local activation of coagulation most commonly results in the systemic depletion of locally consumed coagulation factors and platelets. Heightened expression of coagulation factors is implicated in the development and propagation of DIC.[14] The incidence of clinically overt DIC is approximately 0.5–1% among patients with large aortic aneurysms.[15]

Approximately 30% of patients require a blood transfusion after coronary artery bypass graft (CABG) surgery.[16] In addition, bleeding is associated with a significant increase in transfusion rates, intensive care unit admissions, and prolonged hospital stays. To preoperatively identify patients at high risk for bleeding, one study of 1,007 patients undergoing a first CABG surgery developed a prediction rule based on data from two thirds of the sample and prospectively applied it to the remaining one third.[16-19] Independent factors predicting the need for transfusion were lower preoperative hemoglobin, lower weight, older age, and female sex. Additional risk factors for perioperative bleeding included preoperative use of antiplatelet or antithrombotic drugs, reoperation, coagulation abnormalities, and emergency operations.[20] Bleeding risk is also increased in patients who undergo off-pump CABG surgery.[20] Extensive bleeding is usually due to one or more of the following factors: incomplete surgical hemostasis; residual heparin effect after cardiopulmonary bypass; platelet dysfunction occurring as a result of cardiopulmonary bypass or preoperative aspirin use clotting factor depletion; hypothermia; postoperative hypotension; or hemodilution with both dilutional thrombocytopenia and coagulopathy.[21]

20.4 Pathogenesis

The pathogenesis of DIC involves several simultaneous mechanisms in the promotion of a procoagulant state. It is due to an uncontrolled and excessive production of thrombin, leading to widespread and systemic intravascular fibrin deposition. The systemic deposition of fibrin results from tissue factor (TF)-mediated thrombin generation with simultaneous suppression of physiological anticoagulation mechanisms and impaired fibrinolysis[7] (Fig. 20.2). Although they occur at the same time, these steps are described separately for didactic reasons.

20.4.1 Thrombin Generation

The initiation of coagulation activation leading to thrombin generation in DIC is exclusively initiated by TF-activated factor VII complex.[22] TF-mediated thrombin generation plays a central role in the pathogenesis of DIC.[23] Monocytes,[24] polymorphonuclear cells,[25] endothelial cells,[26] and cancer cells[3] express TF in response to proinflammatory cytokines (mainly interleukin 6). It is important to stress that interleukin 6 is the principal mediator of the activation of coagulation,

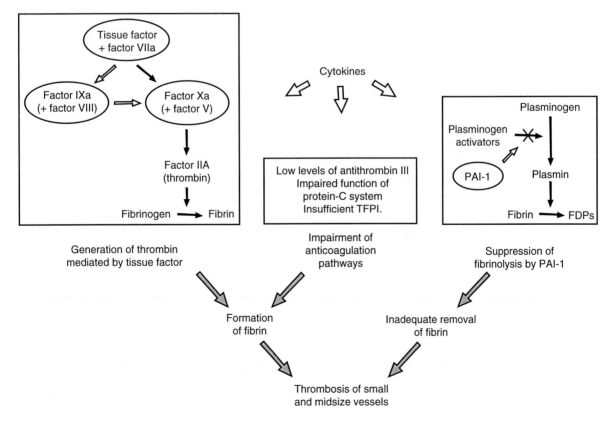

Fig. 20.2 Pathogenesis of DIC. *FDP* fibrin degradation product, *PAI-1* plasminogen activator inhibitor 1, *TFPI* tissue factor pathway inhibitor[7]

and tumor necrosis factor inhibits the physiological anticoagulation pathways and fibrinolysis.[1]

The TF-factor VIIa complex can activate factor X directly or indirectly by means of activated factor IX and factor VIII. In combination with factor V, activated factor X can convert prothrombin (factor II) to thrombin (factor IIa).[7] Thrombin converts fibrinogen to fibrin and is a potent platelet activator. Activated platelets form a phospholipid surface on which activated coagulation factor complexes assemble and accelerate coagulation activation.[27]

20.4.2 Inhibition of Physiological Anticoagulant Pathways

Despite the potent initiation of coagulation by TF, the activation of coagulation cannot be propagated if physiologic anticoagulant pathways function properly. In

DIC, however, all major natural anticoagulant pathways (antithrombin III, the protein C system, and TF pathway inhibitor) seem to be impaired.[28] These regulatory systems are defective as a result of endothelial dysfunction. Widespread thrombin generation occurs, and this leads to fibrin formation.[27]

Plasma levels of antithrombin III, the most important inhibitor of thrombin and factor Xa, are markedly reduced during DIC due to a combination of consumption, degradation by elastase from activated neutrophils, and impaired synthesis.[3,29]

A significant depression of the protein C system may further compromise an adequate regulation of activated coagulation. This impaired function of the protein C system is caused by a combination of impaired protein synthesis, cytokine-mediated downregulation of endothelial thrombomodulin (by proinflammatory cytokines, particularly tumor necrosis factor-α and interleukin 1β), and a decrease in the concentration of the free fraction of

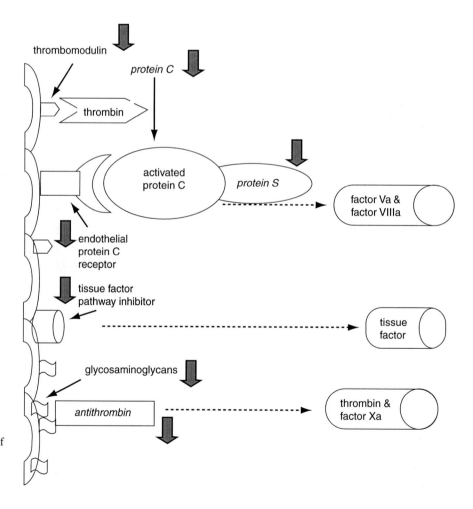

Fig.20.3 Representation of the endothelium and the three anticoagulant pathways[3]

protein S (the essential cofactor of protein C), resulting in reduced activation of protein C.[30]

In addition, there seems to be an imbalance of TF pathway inhibitor function in relation to the increased TF-dependent activation of coagulation.[31] The literature is controversial about the levels of this inhibitor. Some evidence[32] suggests that the endogenous concentration of TF pathway inhibitor is decreased in DIC. Others[33] found that the TF pathway inhibitor levels are only modestly reduced or even increased in some patients with DIC.

Interestingly, all of these anticoagulant pathways are linked to the endothelium (Fig. 20.3), and it is likely that endothelial cell perturbation and dysfunction are important for the impaired function of these anticoagulant systems.[3]

20.4.3 Defective Fibrinolysis

Experimental and clinical studies[8,34] indicate that during DIC, the fibrinolytic system is largely suppressed at the time of maximal activation of coagulation. This inhibition of fibrinolysis is caused by a sustained rise in the plasma level of plasminogen activator inhibitor 1 (PAI-1), the principal inhibitor of the fibrinolytic system. Low levels of plasmin-α2-antiplasmin complex, and high levels of PAI-1 are markers of escalating disease. Both endothelial cells and activated platelets release PAI-1 in DIC. In clinical studies, high levels of PAI-1 precede the onset of DIC and predict an adverse outcome.[35]

The combination of the increased formation of and inadequate removal of fibrin results in disseminated intravascular thrombosis. In some patients, the widespread deposition of fibrin results in tissue ischemia and consumption of platelets, fibrinogen, prothrombin, and factors V and VIII, which in turn may lead to bleeding. Moreover, the release of fibrin degradation products (FDPs) may enhance bleeding by interfering with normal fibrin polymerization and by binding to the platelet surface glycoprotein IIb/IIIa fibrinogen receptor, interfering with platelet aggregation. In addition, since plasmin can cleave proteins other than fibrin, excessive plasmin will lead to proteolytic degradation of fibrinogen and other clotting factors, thereby causing consumption coagulopathy and exacerbating the bleeding diathesis.[2]

20.5 InteractionB etween Coagulation and Inflammation

Coagulation activation produces proteases that interact with both the coagulation protein zymogens and cell receptors that induce inflammation-signaling pathways. Proinflammatory mediators induce the expression of TF on circulating monocytes, tissue macrophages, and neutrophils.[36,37] Coagulation proteins (such as factor Xa, thrombin, and fibrin) activate endothelial cells to release proinflammatory cytokines and growth factors.[38] The most important receptor involved is the protease-activated receptor (PAR).

In summary, coagulation proteases induce proinflammatory mediators that have procoagulant effects and amplify the cascade that leads to DIC.

20.6 Classification

In 2001, the ISTH Subcommittee of the Scientific and Standardisation Committee on DIC proposed that the working definition of DIC be delineated into two phases: acute or decompensated (overt) and chronic or compensated (nonovert).[6] As a result, a scoring system to aid in the diagnosis of DIC was proposed. The scoring system and its applicability are discussed elsewhere in this chapter.

20.6.1 Acute or Decompensated DIC

If the reaction is brisk and explosive, the clinical picture is dominated by intravascular coagulation, which can cause the depletion of platelets, fibrinogen, prothrombin, and factors V and VIII. In addition, the production of FDPs via the plasmin action will further interfere with hemostasis. The clinical consequence is a profound systemic bleeding diathesis with blood oozing from wound sites, intravenous lines, and catheters, as well as bleeding into deep tissues.[39]

20.6.2 Chronic or Compensated DIC

If the activation occurs slowly, an excess of procoagulants is produced, predisposing to thrombosis. At the same time, as long as the liver can compensate for the consumption of clotting factors and the bone marrow maintains an adequate platelet count, the bleeding diathesis will not be clinically apparent. Its clinical presentation consists of primarily thrombotic manifestations, which can be both venous and arterial.[39]

20.7 ClinicalMani festation

The coagulation disturbances associated with DIC can manifest as a wide spectrum of clinical signs and symptoms that vary from bleeding to thrombosis.

Associated with excessive plasmin formation, bleeding is the most dramatic physical manifestation of acute DIC. Patients may have ecchymoses at venipuncture and wound sites and petechiae on the soft palate and skin.[40] However, major bleeding occurs in only a minority of patients with DIC.[7] In recent studies, the prevalence of major bleeding in patients with DIC was 5–12%.[41] Critically ill patients with a platelet count of less than 50×10^9/L have a four- to fivefold higher risk of bleeding compared with patients with a higher platelet count.[42]

Less clinically obvious and more common is the microvascular thrombosis caused by fibrin deposition in various organs that leads to organ failure.[43] According to Bick et al., pyrexia occurs in 58% of patients, hypotension in 50%, and microangiopathic hemolytic anemia in 15%.[44]

Using the classification system described, two clinical forms of DIC, acute and chronic, have been delineated. Acute DIC is characterized by a profound systemic bleeding diathesis and is due to widespread intravascular fibrin deposition, tissue ischemic injury, and microangiopathic hemolytic anemia.[39] In one series of 118 patients with acute DIC,[10] the main clinical manifestations included the following:

- Bleeding (64%): Petechiae and ecchymoses in conjunction with blood oozing from wound sites, intravenous lines, catheters, and mucosal surfaces.
- Renal dysfunction (25–40%): Acute renal failure caused by microthrombosis of afferent arterioles that may produce cortical ischemia or necrosis (renal thrombotic microangiopathy) and hypotension that may lead to acute tubular necrosis.
- Hepatic dysfunction (19%): Jaundice is common in patients with DIC and may be due to both liver disease and increased bilirubin production secondary tohe molysis.

- Respiratory dysfunction (16%): Pulmonary hemorrhage and hemoptysis (damage to the pulmonary vascular endothelium), acute respiratory distress syndrome, or acute lung injury (due to diffuse pulmonarymic rothrombosis).
- Shock(14%).
- Thromboembolism(7%).
- Centralne rvouss ystemin volvement(2%).

Autopsy findings in patients with acute DIC include diffuse bleeding, hemorrhagic necrosis, microthrombi in small blood vessels, and thrombi in midsize and larger arteries and veins.[45,46] In these studies, fibrin deposition in small and midsize vessels in patients with DIC was invariably associated with ischemia and necrosis and with clinical dysfunction of organs.

Compensated or chronic DIC develops when blood is continuously or intermittently exposed to small amounts of TF and compensatory mechanisms in the liver and bone marrow are largely able to replenish the depleted coagulation proteins and platelets. Under these conditions, the patient is either asymptomatic with increased levels of FDPs or has manifestations of venous or arterial thrombosis. Patients with chronic DIC may also have minor skin and mucosal bleeding.[39] Autopsy findings in patients who have chronic DIC show diffuse bleeding at various sites, hemorrhagic tissue necrosis, and thrombosis in small and large blood vessels.[47]

20.8 Diagnosis

There is no single laboratory test that can establish or rule out the diagnosis of DIC.[7] However, a combination of test results in a patient with a clinical condition known to be associated with DIC can be used to diagnose the disorder. Various approaches have been recommended to evaluate the degree of dysfunction in DIC. These include laboratory tests of coagulation,[48] molecular markers in DIC, and scoring systems.[6,49-51]

In clinical practice, a diagnosis of DIC can often be made by a combination of platelet count, measurement of global clotting times (activated partial thromboplastin time [aPTT] and prothrombin time [PT]), measurement of one or two clotting factors and inhibitors (such as antithrombin [AT]), and a test for FDPs[3,7] (Table 20.1).

Coagulation tests can be classified as tests for intravascular fibrin formation and FDPs, markers of

Table 20.1 Laboratory tests used to confirm disseminated intravascular coagulation (DIC)[1]

Prothrombin time (PT)	↑
Activated partial thromboplastin time (aPTT)	↑
Plateletc ount	↓
Fibrinogenc oncentration	↑
D-dimer	↑
Fibrin(ogen) degradation products (FDPs)	↑
Fibrinm onomer	↑
Peripheralbl oodpi cture	Schistocytes

From Ho et al.[1] ↑ increased, ↓de creased

thrombin generation, platelet count, coagulation factors and inhibitors, and fibrinolytic parameters.[52]

20.8.1 Tests for Intravascular Fibrin Formation and Fibrin Degradation Products

Since the primary trigger in the pathogenesis of DIC is defective fibrin formation, the demonstration of soluble fibrin in plasma is essential for the diagnosis of DIC.[53,54] Clinical studies have shown that a raised soluble fibrin level yields a high sensitivity of 90–100% for the diagnosis of DIC[55]; however, it has a low specificity.

FDPs are formed when plasmin breaks down fibrin or fibrinogen. FDPs can be detected by enzyme-linked immunosorbent assay (ELISA) or latex agglutination. FDP levels were elevated in 80–100% of DIC patients.[56] However, several other conditions, such as trauma, recent surgery, inflammation, or venous thromboembolism may cause raised FDP levels. Moreover, FDPs are metabolized by the liver and secreted by the kidneys; therefore, plasma levels are dependent on hepatic and renal function.

Tests to specifically detect FDPs are more useful because these tests indicate that both clotting and fibrinolysis have occurred. The D-dimers of FDPs are derived from plasmin-degraded fibrin.[57] Although D-dimers are elevated in 95% of DIC patients, the test lacks specificity.[58]

Measurement of fibrinogen is often advocated as a useful tool for the diagnosis of DIC, but it is not helpful because it acts as an acute-phase reactant, and despite ongoing consumption, plasma levels can remain well within the normal range for a long time. In a consecutive series of patients, the sensitivity of a low fibrinogen level for the diagnosis of DIC was only 28%, and hypofibrinogenemia was detected in a small number of severe cases of DIC only. Sequential measurements of fibrinogen might be more useful.[3]

20.8.2 Markers of Thrombin Generation

Elevated plasma levels of thrombin may be reflected by increased levels of prothrombin activation fragment F1+2 (F1+2), thrombin–antithrombin (TAT) complex, and fibrinopeptide A. Elevated F1+2, TAT, and fibrinopeptide A levels are sensitive indicators of chronic DIC.[58] However, their usefulness is limited by the need for stringent sample handling and the lack of specificity. These assays are not widely available in routine diagnostic laboratories.[52]

20.8.3 Platelet Count

Thrombin-induced platelet aggregation accounts significantly for platelet consumption in DIC. However, impaired platelet production may occur simultaneously in the seriously ill patient.[59] Platelet levels repeated at 1- to 4-h intervals reflect the amount of ongoing thrombin formation. Thrombocytopenia (platelet count <100,000 or >50% drop from baseline values in the first 24 h) together with other laboratory tests (described further in this chapter) are key elements in diagnosing DIC.

20.8.4 Coagulation Factors and Inhibitors

The depletion of coagulation factors results in the prolongation of global clotting parameters such as PT and aPTT in only 50–70% of patients with DIC.[43] Therefore, normal values do not exclude the diagnosis of DIC. It is important to remember that the prolongation of the PT reflects reduced activity of the components of the extrinsic and common pathways. These include factors VII, X, V, and prothrombin, which are the most frequently decreased clotting proteins in DIC.[9] The aPTT measures the intrinsic and common pathways of coagulation. It is sensitive to deficiencies of factors XII, XI, IX, and VIII and less sensitive than the PT to deficiencies of components of the common pathway.[39]

The plasma concentrations of individual coagulation factors, such as factors V and VII, are usually low. However, factor VIII levels may be paradoxically elevated in most patients with DIC.[52]

Plasma levels of physiological inhibitors of coagulation, such as antithrombin III and protein C, are indirect indicators of coagulation activation. In acute DIC, the levels of AT, protein C, and protein S are reduced.[60] A low plasma protein C concentration is correlated with a poor outcome.[61]

20.8.5 Markers of Increased Fibrinolysis

Several tests can indicate the increase in fibrinolysis observed in DIC. The plasma levels of plasminogen and α2-antiplasmin are low in patients with DIC.[52] High concentrations of PAI-1 are found in patients with DIC; this is correlated with a poor outcome.[62]

A promising new development is the use of transmittance waveform analysis of routine coagulation tests. The transmittance waveform is the optical profile generated on standard coagulation assays such as the PT and aPTT, charting changes in light transmittance over the process and duration of clot formation. The normal aPTT transmittance waveform is a sigmoid-shaped curve. In patients with DIC, a biphasic waveform is observed.[63] The sensitivity and specificity of the association of the aPTT biphasic waveform with DIC are 97.6% and 98%, respectively.[64] Transmittance waveform analysis can be used to detect chronic DIC.[65] Although the clinical potential of this new diagnostic technique is great, the specialized equipment required is not widely available.

The laboratory findings used to confirm the diagnosis of DIC are different in acute and chronic disease (Table 20.2).[39] The chronic or compensated form of DIC frequently precedes the acute decompensated form. From a therapeutic point of view, it would be better to intercept the process before decompensation occurs. Unfortunately, chronic DIC is not evident clinically, and the usual laboratory tests can be normal.[1]

Table 20.2 Coagulation parameters in acute and chronic disseminated intravascular coagulation (DIC)[39]

Parameter	Acute (decompensated) DIC	Chronic (compensated) DIC
Platelet count	Reduced	Variable
Prothrombint ime	Prolonged	Normal
Activated partial thromboplastin time	Prolonged	Normal
Thrombint ime	Prolonged	Normal
Plasmafi brinogen	Reduced	Normal,e levated
Plasmaf actorV	Reduced	Normal
Plasmaf actorV III	Reduced	Normal
Fibrinde gradation products	Elevated	Elevated
D-dimer	Elevated	Elevated

FromL eung[39]

Table 20.3 International Society on Thrombosis and Haemostasis (ISTH) Scientific and Standardisation Committee (SSC) scoring system for overt DIC[50]

Risk assessment
Does the patient have an underlying disorder known to be associated with overt DIC
If yes, proceed; if no, do not use algorithm
Order global tests
Platelet count, prothrombin time, fibrinogen, soluble fibrin monomers, fibrin degradation products
Score global coagulation test results
Platelet c ount (>100=0; <100=1; <50=2)
Elevateds olublefi brin monomer or FDP (no increase=0; moderate i ncrease=2; s trong i ncrease=3)
Prolonged prothrombin time (<3 s=0; >3–6 s=1; >6 s=2)
Fibrinogen level (>1 g/L=0; <1 g/L=1)
Calculates core
>5=compatible with overt DIC
Repeat scoring daily
<5=suggestive for nonovert DIC Repeat next 1–2 days

From Toh et al.[50] *DIC* disseminated intravascular coagulation; *FDP*fi brin degradation products

20.8.6 Scoring System

In 2001, the ISTH Subcommittee on DIC proposed a five-step diagnostic algorithm to calculate a DIC score[6] (Table 20.3). This scoring system is based partly on a modification of the criteria for DIC proposed by the Japanese Ministry of Health and Welfare (JMWH).[66]

This system uses simple laboratory tests that are available in most hospital laboratories. A score of 5 or more is compatible with DIC. This scoring system has a sensitivity of 91% and a specificity of 97%.[49] It is a strong independent predictor of mortality in intensive care unit patients.[29]

For acute DIC, a cumulative score of 5 or more from prolonged PT, reduced platelets and fibrinogen,

and elevated fibrin-related markers was proposed. This required prospective confirmation. For chronic DIC, scoring would incorporate abnormal trends and results in both simple global tests and molecular markers of coagulation(T able 20.4).[50]

Both the acute and chronic scoring systems have been prospectively validated, and the acute DIC scoring system was demonstrated to be sufficiently accurate to diagnose DIC in intensive care unit patients. However, the chronic DIC algorithm could not clearly distinguish chronic DIC patients from the patients with acute DIC.[67] Based on this, the Japanese Association for Acute Medicine (JAAM) DIC Study Group announced new DIC diagnostic criteria for critically ill patients

Table 20.4 International Society on Thrombosis and Haemostasis (ISTH) Scientific and Standardisation Committee scoring system forn onovertD IC[50]

1. Risk assessment: does the patient have an underlying disorder known to be associated with DIC?
   yes = 2, no = 0

2.M ajorc riteria

Platelet Count	>100x10^9 l⁻¹ = 0	<100x10^9 l⁻¹ = 1	Rising = −1	Stable = 0	Falling = 1
PT Prolongation	<3 s = 0	<3 s = 1	Falling = −1	Stable = 0	Rising = 1
Fibrin related-markers	Normal = 0	Raised = 1	Falling = −1	Stable = 0	Rising = 1

3.S pecificc riteria

Antithrombin	Normal = −1	Low = 1
Protein C	Normal = −1	Low = 1
----------------	Normal = −1	Abnormal = 1

4. Calculate score:

From Toh et al.[50] *DIC* disseminated intravascular coagulation; *PT* prothrombin time

Table 20.5 Japanese Association for Acute Medicine (JAAM) scoring system for disseminated intravascular coagulation (DIC)[51]

I. Clinical conditions that may be associated with DIC
  A. Sepsis/severe infection (any microorganism)
  B. Trauma/burn/surgery
  C. Vascular abnormalities
     Large vascular aneurysms
     Giant hemangioma
     Vasculitis
  D. Severe toxic or immunological reactions
     Snakebite
     Recreational drugs
     Transfusion reactions
     Transplant rejection
  E. Malignancy (except bone marrow suppression)
  F. Obstetric calamities
  G. Conditions that may be associated with systemic
     inflammatory response syndrome
     Organ destruction (e.g., severe pancreatitis)
     Severe hepatic failure
     Ischemia/hypoxia/shock
     Heat stroke/malignant syndrome
     Fat embolism
     Rhabdomyolysis
     Other
  H. Other

II. Clinical conditions that should be carefully ruled out
  A. Thrombocytopenia
     1. Dilution and abnormal distribution
        Massive blood loss and transfusion, massive infusion
     2. Increased platelet destruction
        ITP, TTP/HUS, HIT, drugs, viral infection, alloim-
        mune destruction, APS, HELLP, extracorporeal
        circulation
     3. Decreased platelet production
        Viral infection, drugs, radiation, nutritional deficiency
        (vitamin B_{12}, folic acid), disorders of hematopoiesis,
        liver disease, HPS
     4. Spurious decrease
        EDTA-dependent gglutinins, nisufficient anticoagu-
        lation of blood samples
     5. Other
        Hypothermia, artificial devices in the vessel
  B. Prolonged prothrombin time
     Anticoagulation therapy, anticoagulant in blood
     samples, vitamin K deficiency, liver cirrhosis, massive
     blood loss and transfusion
  C. Elevated FDP
     Thrombosis, hemostasis and wound healing, hema-
     toma, pleural effusion, ascites, anticoagulant in blood
     samples, antifibrinolytic therapy
  D. Other

III. Diagnostic algorithm for systemic inflammatory response
   syndrome
  A. Temperature >38 or <36°C
  B. Heart rate >90 beats/min

(continued)

Table 20.5 (continued)

  C. Respiratory rate >20 breaths/min or $Paco_2$ <32 torr
     (<4.3 kPa)
  D. White blood cell >12,000 cells/mm³, <4,000 cells/mm³,
     or 10% immature (band) forms

IV. Diagnostica lgorithm
   Systemici nflammatory response syndrome criteria
     ≥3 = 1
     0–2 = 0
   Platelet counts (10⁹/L)
     <80 or >50% decrease within 24 h = 3
     ≥80 and <120 or >30% decrease within 24 h = 1
     ≥120 = 0
   Prothrombin time (value of patient/normal value)
     ≥1.2 = 1
     <1.2 = 0
   Fibrin/fibrinogen degradation products (mg/L)
     ≥25 = 3
     ≥10 and <25 = 1
     <10 = 0
   Diagnosis
     ≥4 points = DIC

From Gando et al.[51] *ITP* idiopathic thrombocytopenic purpura; *TTP* thrombotic thrombocytopenic purpura; *HUS* hemolytic uremic syndrome; *HIT* heparin-induced thrombocytopenia; *APS* antiphospholipid syndrome; *HELLP* hemolysis, elevated liver enzymes, and low platelet; *HPS* hemophagocytic syndrome; *EDTA* ethylenediaminetetraacetic acid; *FDP* fibrin/fibrinogen degradation product

(Table 20.5).[51] Both the JAAM and the ISTH scoring systems for DIC have been prospectively validated for their feasibility and DIC diagnostic property.[68] In 1,284 patients, Wada et al. found the rate of agreement between both ISTH and JAAM scores at 67.4%.[69]

20.9 Management

The fundamental principle in the treatment of DIC is prompt and aggressive treatment of the underlying disease process.[3] However, additional supportive treatment aimed specifically at the coagulation abnormalities may be required.[7]

20.9.1 Platelet and Plasma Replacement Therapy

Thrombocytopenia and low levels of coagulation factors place patients with DIC at risk of bleeding. Platelet and plasma replacement therapy is not indicated on the basis of laboratory results alone and is only indicated in patients who are actively bleeding and in those requiring an invasive procedure or surgery.[29] The threshold for transfusing platelets depends on the clinical situation of the patient. Based on expert opinion, platelet concentrate is generally transfused to patients who bleed and have a platelet count below $50 \times 10^9/L$.[70] In nonbleeding patients, a much lower threshold for platelet transfusion is used (usually $<10–20 \times 10^9/L$). The recommendation for platelet transfusion is 1–2 units/10 kg. After platelet transfusion, the platelet count should rise by at least $5 \times 10^9/L$/unit. Due to ongoing platelet consumption, patients with DIC typically show a less-than-expected rise in platelet count.[39]

With respect to replacement therapy, actively bleeding patients with a significantly elevated PT (international normalized ratio [INR]) or a fibrinogen concentration <50 mg/dL should receive fresh frozen plasma or cryoprecipitate, with the latter used for fibrinogen replacement. It is preferable to keep the fibrinogen level above 100 mg/dL.[70] The recommendation for fresh frozen plasma replacement is 15 mL/kg and for cryoprecipitate is 1 unit/5–10 kg.[39]

It may be necessary to use large volumes of plasma to correct the coagulation defect. Coagulation factor concentrates, such as prothrombin complex concentrate, will correct this defect, but these compounds lack essential factors such as factor V. Moreover, in older literature, caution was advised in the use of prothrombin complex concentrates in DIC because it may worsen the coagulopathy due to small traces of activated factors in the concentrate. However, it is not clear whether this is still relevant for the concentrates that are currently in use.[3] It is important to remember that these concentrates contain only selected coagulation factors, whereas patients with DIC usually have a deficiency of all coagulation factors.[7]

20.9.2 Anticoagulants

Based on the fact that DIC is characterized by extensive activation of coagulation, anticoagulant treatment may be a rational approach. Experimental studies have shown that heparin can at least partially inhibit the activation of coagulation in DIC.[71,72] A large trial in patients with severe sepsis supported a slight (not significant) benefit of low-dose heparin on 28-day mortality and underscored the importance of not stopping heparin in patients with DIC and abnormal coagulation variables.[3] The arguments against the routine use of heparin include potential aggravation of bleeding and the likelihood that heparin will have reduced effect due to the low levels of AT since it is known that the action of heparin requires an adequate plasma concentration of antithrombin III. As a result, once the clinical decision has been made to use heparin in a patient with DIC, it is important to be sure that the patient's AT level is near normal (80–100%) so that the biologically important heparin-AT complex can form and inactivate the serine protease procoagulants, particularly thrombin and factor Xa.[39] The usual intravenous bolus heparin injection of 5,000–10,000 units should be avoided. One may start with an intravenous dose of 300–500 units/h, aiming for an aPTT of about 45 s. Low molecular weight heparin may also be used as an alternative to unfractionated heparin.[73] Adequate prophylaxis is also needed to eliminate the risk of venous thromboembolism. In summary, treatment with heparin is probably useful in patients with DIC, particularly those with clinically overt thromboembolism or extensive deposition of fibrin.[7]

Theoretically, the most logical anticoagulant agent to use in DIC is directed against TF activity. Phase II trials of recombinant TF pathway inhibitor in patients with sepsis showed promising results, but a phase III trial did not show an overall survival benefit in patients who were treated with TF pathway inhibitor.[74,75]

20.9.3 Coagulation Inhibitors

Restoration of physiologic pathways of anticoagulation might be an appropriate aim of therapy. AT not only is an important physiological inhibitor of coagulation but also possesses anti-inflammatory properties.[57] AT concentrate has been available since the 1980s, and most trials with this compound showed some beneficial effect in terms of improvement of laboratory variables; however, none of the trials demonstrated a significant reduction in mortality. A large-scale, multicenter, randomized, controlled trial to directly address this issue also showed no significant reduction in mortality of septic patients who were treated with AT concentrate.[76] Interestingly, the subgroup of patients who had DIC and who did not receive heparin showed a survival benefit, but this finding needs to be prospectively validated.[77]

Protein C, a vitamin K-dependent serine protease, inhibits activated factors V and VIII, thereby preventing thrombin generation. Based on the finding of decreased plasma protein C levels in DIC, supplementation of activated protein C might potentially be of benefit. Indeed, in experimental sepsis studies, activated protein C was shown to be effective in reducing mortality and organ failure. The Recombinant Human Protein C Worldwide Evaluation in Severe Sepsis (PROWESS) trial, a large, multicenter, randomized, controlled study, demonstrated that recombinant human activated protein C (rhAPC) significantly reduced mortality from 30.8% to 24.7% at 28 days (relative risk [RR] reduction 19.4%; $p=0.005$) and improved the coagulation profile of the patients.[78] A post hoc analysis showed that patients with DIC had the highest benefit from activated protein C treatment.[79] Later studies confirmed the ability of activated protein C to normalize coagulation activation during severe sepsis.[80] Activated protein C seems to be relatively more effective in groups with higher disease severity, and a prospective trial in septic patients with relatively low disease severity did not show any benefit from activated protein C.[81] However, care should be undertaken when rhAPC is used in patients with thrombocytopenia (platelet count $<50 \times 10^9$/L) because there was an increasing trend toward intracranial hemorrhage with rhAPC treatment.

20.9.4 Antifibrinolytic Agents

The administration of antifibrinolytic agents, such as lysine analogs (aminocaproic acid or tranexamic acid) or aprotinin, is generally contraindicated in DIC since blockade of the fibrinolytic system may increase the risk of thrombotic complications.[82] Antifibrinolytic agents have been effective in the prevention of blood loss and transfusion in patients undergoing major surgical procedures and are relatively safe; however, there are no data in the context of DIC. The treatment of bleeding in cardiac surgery is frequently based on the antifibrinolytic agents aminocaproic acid, tranexamic acid, and aprotinin.[83-85] These three antifibrinolytic drugs were studied in a meta-analysis of 128 mostly small randomized controlled trials that compared the efficacy and safety of the three agents with placebo and with each other in patients

undergoing CABG surgery.[83] Compared with placebo, all agents were effective at reducing blood loss and at lowering the proportion of patients transfused with packed red blood cells. The meta-analysis found no statistically important worsening in the outcomes of mortality, stroke, myocardial infarction, or dialysis-dependent renal failure. However, high-dose aprotinin significantly increased the risk of *temporary renal dysfunction*, defined as an increase in serum creatinine (RR 1.47; 95% confidence interval [CI] 1.12–1.94). An increased likelihood of acute renal dysfunction with aprotinin was also seen in observational studies.[84-86] A randomized trial and two large observational studies published after the meta-analysis provided evidence for an increase in both short- and long-term mortality in patients who received aprotinin compared with aminocaproic acid, tranexamic acid, or placebo.[85,86] The Blood Conservation Using Antifibrinolytics in a Randomized Trial (BART) was designed to further evaluate the safety of aprotinin.[87] After enrollment of 2,331 of 3,000 patients scheduled to be randomly assigned to receive aprotinin, aminocaproic acid, or tranexamic acid, the trial was terminated early because of a significantly higher mortality rate in patients receiving aprotinin.

Similar results were found in a retrospective analysis of data from over 33,000 aprotinin recipients and over 44,000 aminocaproic acid recipients in which the unadjusted risk of death within the first 7 days after CABG surgery was 4.5% and 2.5%, respectively.[84] After adjustment for patient and hospital characteristics, the RR of death was significantly increased in the aprotinin group (RR 1.64; 95% CI 1.50–1.78). Another retrospective analysis found that the mortality risk with aprotinin remained significantly increased at 1 year.[85] The inability of the meta-analysis cited[86] to detect the mortality risk seen in BART illustrates the pitfalls of aggregating data from multiple small randomized trials.[87-89] The manufacturer has suspended marketing of aprotinin.

In general, the use of prohemostatic agents in patients with DIC is not recommended because, theoretically, they may worsen the coagulopathy.[3] Desmopressin (1-deamino-8-D-arginine vasopressin) is a vasopressin analog that induces release of the contents of endothelial cells, resulting in a marked increase in the plasma concentration of von Willebrand factor and, by as yet unexplained additional mechanisms, a potentiation of primary hemostasis. Relatively rare but important adverse effects of desmopressin include the occurrence of acute myocardial infarction (notably in patients with unstable coronary artery disease) and water intoxication with hyponatremia from its antidiuretic effect.[90] There are no data to support the use of desmopressin for patients with DIC. However, there are some reports of the successful use of prohemostatic agents, in particular recombinant factor VIIa, in patients with DIC and life-threatening bleeding.[91] Still, the efficacy and safety of this treatment in DIC is unknown. Interestingly, the administration of factor VIIa seemed not to result in an aggravation of DIC in these patients.[92] In addition, a trend toward a reduced incidence of multiple organ failure and acute respiratory distress syndrome was also observed in patients receiving recombinant factor VIIa. Surprisingly, a low incidence of thrombotic complications was observed in these patients. Based on this experience, some authors recommend off-label use of recombinant factor VIIa in the case of life-threatening bleeding.[90] Recombinant factor VIIa has a possible role in the treatment of otherwise-intractable, life-threatening bleeding after cardiac surgery, but randomized controlled trials are needed to prove its safety and efficacy.[93]

In summary, the recommendations concerning the management of coagulopathy associated with DIC are limited by the sparse number of controlled trials. Some authors suggested the use of one or more of the following supportive modalities for the symptomatic patient[39]:

- Treatment with platelets and coagulation factors is justified in patients who have serious bleeding, are at high risk for bleeding (after surgery), or require invasive procedures. Patients with marked or moderate thrombocytopenia (<50,000/μL) and serious bleeding should be given platelet transfusions.
- Actively bleeding patients with a significantly elevated PT (INR) or a fibrinogen concentration below 50 mg/dL should receive fresh frozen plasma or cryoprecipitate to keep the fibrinogen level above 100 mg/dL.
- The administration of heparin is generally limited to the subset of DIC patients who have predominantly thrombotic manifestations. It is important to be sure that the patient's AT level is near normal for heparintobe effective.

The ideal drug for prophylaxis and treatment of thrombotic disease remains an agent that will inhibit thrombosis but not hemostasis. Although not yet tested clinically, this observation suggests the possibility that pharmacologic inhibitors that disrupt the (P-selectin glycoprotein ligand) PSGL-1 interaction may have the potential to act as antithrombotic agents, particularly in disorders that are associated with activation of endothelial cells but in which the integrity of the endothelium is preserved.[94]

20.10 Prognosis

The contribution of DIC to morbidity and the risk of mortality varies depending on the underlying clinical condition and the intensity of the coagulation disorder.[7] In a large number of clinical studies, the occurrence of DIC appeared to be associated with an unfavorable outcome and was an independent predictor of mortality.[62] Prospective clinical studies have shown that the development of DIC in patients with severe trauma roughly doubles the risk of death.[95] The reported mortality rate from acute DIC ranges from 40% to 80% in patients with severe sepsis, trauma, or burns.[12]

20.11 Conclusions

DIC is a complex thrombohemorrhagic disease secondary to an underlying clinical disease, such as cardiac surgery, producing both thrombosis and hemorrhage. It occurs in approximately 1% of hospital admissions. The majority of the bleeding events in cardiovascular surgery are not due to surgical causes but are biological in origin, essentially the result of DIC in its later phases. After cardiac surgery, surgeons should be alerted to the potential risk for and likely occurrence of DIC, especially in the presence of severe hemodynamic instability, metabolic changes, or hepatic perturbation, as well as in cases of probable sepsis when SIRS is present or during surgical reinterventions. To anticipate its occurrence and to prevent further deterioration of the hemostatic system, the prompt diagnosis and treatment of DIC is extremely important to improve clinical outcomes.

References

1. Ho LW, Kam PC, Thong CL. Disseminated intravascular coagulation. *Curr Anaesth Crit Care*.2005; 16:151-161.
2. Leung LL. Pathogenesis and etiology of disseminated intravascular coagulation. UpToDate Web site. http://www.uptodate.

com/patients/content/topic.do?topicKey=~ourrinG/1tGmgs&s electedTitle=26~90&source=search_result. Accessed 9 Apr 2009

3. Levi M. Disseminated intravascular coagulation. *Crit Care Med.*2007;35:2191 -2195.

4. Matsuda T. Clinical aspects of DIC–disseminated intravascular coagulation. *Pol J Pharmacol.*1996; 48:73-75.

5. Raivio P, Suojaranta-Ylinen R, Kuitunen R. Recombinant factor VIIa in the treatment of postoperative hemorrhage after cardiac surgery. *Ann Thorac Surg.*2005; 80:66-71.

6. Taylor FB Jr, Toh CH, Hoots WK, Wada H, Levi M, Scientific Subcommittee on Disseminated Intravascular Coagulation (DIC) of the International Society on Thrombosis and Haemostasis (ISTH). Towards definition, clinical and laboratory criteria, and a scoring system for disseminated intravascular coagulation. *Thromb Haemost.* 2001;86:1327-1330.

7. Levi M, ten Cate H. Disseminated intravascular coagulation. *N Engl J Med.*1999; 341:586-592.

8. Levi M, van der Poll T, ten Cate H, van Deventer SJ. The cytokine-mediated imbalance between coagulant and anticoagulant mechanisms in sepsis and endotoxaemia. *Eur J Clin Invest.*1997;27:3-9.

9. Spero JA, Lewis JH, Hasiba U. Disseminated intravascular coagulation. Findings in 346 patients. *Thromb Haemost.* 1980;43:28-33.

10. Siegal T, Seligsohn U, Aghai E, Modan M. Clinical and laboratory aspects of disseminated intravascular coagulation (DIC): a study of 118 cases. *Thromb Haemost.* 1978;39:122-134.

11. Gando S. Disseminated intravascular coagulation in trauma patients. *Semin Thromb Hemost.*2001; 27:585-592.

12. Gando S, Nanzaki D, Kemmotsu O. Disseminated intravascular coagulation and sustained systemic inflammatory response syndrome predict organ dysfunctions after trauma: application of clinical decision analysis. *Ann Surg.* 1999;229:121-127.

13. Stéphan F, Hollande J, Richard O, Cheffi A, Maier-Redelsperger M, Flahault A. Thrombocytopenia in a surgical ICU. *Chest.*1999; 115:1363-1370.

14. Aboulafia DM, Aboulafia ED. Aortic aneurysm-induced disseminated intravascular coagulation. *Ann Vasc Surg.* 1996; 10:396-405.

15. Kazmers A, Jacobs L, Perkins A, Lindenauer SM, Bates E. Abdominal aortic aneurysm repair in Veterans Affairs medical centers. *J Vasc Surg.*1996; 23:191-200.

16. Karkouti K, Cohen MM, McCluskey SA, Sher GD. A multivariable model for predicting the need for blood transfusion in patients undergoing first-time elective coronary bypass graft surgery. *Transfusion.*2001; 41:1193-2003.

17. Sellman M, Intonti MA, Ivert T. Reoperations for bleeding after coronary artery bypass procedures during 25 years. *Eur J Cardiothorac Surg.*1997; 11:521-527.

18. Munoz JJ, Birkmeyer NJ, Dacey LJ, et al. Trends in rates of reexploration for hemorrhage after coronary artery bypass surgery. Northern New England Cardiovascular Disease Study Group. *Ann Thorac Surg.*1999; 68:1321-1325.

19. Fiser SM, Tribble CG, Kern JA, Long SM, Kaza AK, Kron IL. Cardiac reoperation in the intensive care unit. *Ann Thorac Surg.*2001;71:1888- 1892.

20. Ferraris VA, Ferraris SP, Saha SP, et al. Perioperative blood transfusion and blood conservation in cardiac surgery: the Society of Thoracic Surgeons and the Society of Cardiovascular Anesthesiologists clinical practice guideline. *Ann Thorac Surg.*2007; 83:S27-S86.

21. Woodman RC, Harker LA. Bleeding complications associated with cardiopulmonary bypass. *Blood.* 1990;76:1680-1697.

22. Hambleton J, Leung LL, Levi M. Coagulation: consultative hemostasis. Hematology Am Soc Hematol Educ Program 2002;335–352.

23. Gando S, Nanzaki S, Sasaki S, Kemmotsu O. Significant correlations between tissue factor and thrombin markers in trauma and septic patients with disseminated intravascular coagulation. *Thromb Haemost.*1998; 79:1111-1115.

24. Osterud B, Flaegstad T. Increased tissue thromboplastin activity in monocytes of patients with meningococcal infection: related to an unfavourable prognosis. *Thromb Haemost.* 1983;49:5-7.

25. Giesen PL, Rauch U, Bohrmann B, et al. Blood-borne tissue factor: another view of thrombosis. *Proc Natl Acad Sci U S A.*1999; 96:2311-2315.

26. Levi M, ten Cate H, van der Poll T. Endothelium: interface between coagulation and inflammation. *Crit Care Med.* 2002;30:S220-S224.

27. Esmon CT. The regulation of natural anticoagulant pathways. *Science.*1987; 235:1348-1352.

28. Levi M, de Jonge E, van der Poll T. Rationale for restoration of physiological anticoagulant pathways in patients with sepsis and disseminated intravascular coagulation. *Crit Care Med.*2001; 29:S90-S94.

29. Levi M. Current understanding of disseminated intravascular coagulation. *Br J Haematol.*2004; 124:567-576.

30. Esmon CT. Role of coagulation inhibitors in inflammation. *Thromb Haemost.*2001; 86:51-56.

31. Levi M. The imbalance between tissue factor and tissue factor pathway inhibitor in sepsis. *Crit Care Med.* 2002;30:1914-1915.

32. Creasey AA, Chang AC, Feigen L, Wün TC, Taylor FB Jr, Hinshaw LB. Tissue factor pathway inhibitor reduces mortality from Escherichia coli septic shock. *J Clin Invest.* 1993;91:2850-2860.

33. Shimura M, Wada H, Wakita Y, et al. Plasma tissue factor and tissue factor pathway inhibitor levels in patients with disseminated intravascular coagulation. *Am J Hematol.* 1997;55:169-174.

34. van Hinsbergh VW, Bauer KA, Kooistra T, et al. Progress of fibrinolysis during tumor necrosis factor infusions in humans. Concomitant increase in tissue-type plasminogen activator, plasminogen activator inhibitor type-1, and fibrin(ogen) degradation products. *Blood.* 1990;76:2284-2289.

35. Levi M, de Jonge E, van der Poll T, ten Cate H. Disseminated intravascular coagulation. *Thromb Haemost.* 1999;82: 695-705.

36. Collins PW, Noble KE, Reittie JR, Hoffbrand AV, Pasi KJ, Yong KL. Induction of tissue factor expression in human monocyte/endothelium cocultures. *Br J Haematol.* 1995;91: 963-970.

37. Todoroki H, Nakamura S, Higure A, et al. Neutrophils express tissue factor in a monkey model of sepsis. *Surgery.* 2000;127:209-216.

38. van der Poll T, de Jonge E, Levi M. Regulatory role of cytokines in disseminated intravascular coagulation. *Semin Thromb Hemost.*2001; 27:639-651.

39. Leung LL. Clinical features, diagnosis and treatment of disseminated intravascular coagulation in adults. UpToDate Web site. http://www.uptodate.com/patients/content/topic. do?topicKey=~eLIUMBy0Hvb0ZFS.A ccessed9A pr2009

40. Bick RL. Disseminated intravascular coagulation and related syndromes: a clinical review. *Semin Thromb Hemost.* 1988;14:299-338.

41. Bernard GR, Margolis BD, Shanies HM, et al. Extended Evaluation of Recombinant Human Activated Protein C United States Trial (ENHANCE US): a single-arm, phase 3B, multicenter study of drotrecogin alfa (activated) in severe sepsis. *Chest.*2004; 125:2206-2216.

42. Strauss R, Wehler M, Mehler K, Kreutzer D, Koebnick C, Hahn EG. Thrombocytopenia in patients in the medical intensive care unit: bleeding prevalence, transfusion requirements, and outcome. *Crit Care Med.* 2002;30: 1765-1771.

43. Bick RL. Disseminated intravascular coagulation current concepts of etiology, pathophysiology, diagnosis, and treatment. *Hematol Oncol Clin North Am.*2003; 17:149-176.

44. Bick RL. Disseminated intravascular coagulation. Objective criteria for diagnosis and management. *Med Clin North Am.* 1994;78:511-543.

45. Robboy SJ, Major MC, Colman RW, Minna JD. Pathology of disseminated intravascular coagulation (DIC). Analysis of 26 cases. *Hum Pathol.*1972; 3:327-343.

46. Shimamura K, Oka K, Nakazawa M, Kojima M. Distribution patterns of microthrombi in disseminated intravascular coagulation. *Arch Pathol Lab Med.*1983; 107:543-547.

47. Regoeczi E, Brain MC. Organ distribution of fibrin in disseminated intravascular coagulation. *Br J Haematol.* 1969;17:73-81.

48. Toh CH. Laboratory testing in disseminated intravascular coagulation. *Semin Thromb Hemost.*2001; 27:653-656.

49. Bakhtiari K, Meijers JC, de Jonge E, Levi M. Prospective validation of the International Society of Thrombosis and Haemostasis scoring system for disseminated intravascular coagulation. *Crit Care Med.*2004; 32:2416-2421.

50. Toh CH, Hoots WK. The scoring system of the Scientific and Standardisation Committee on Disseminated Intravascular Coagulation of the International Society on Thrombosis and Haemostasis: a 5-year overview. *J Thromb Haemost.* 2007;5:604-606.

51. Gando S, Saitoh D, Ogura H, et al. Natural history of disseminated intravascular coagulation diagnosed based on the newly established diagnostic criteria for critically ill patients: results of a multicenter, prospective survey. *Crit Care Med.* 2008;36:145-150.

52. Levi M, de Jonge E, Meijers J. The diagnosis of disseminated intravascular coagulation. *Blood Rev.*2002; 16:217-223.

53. Bredbacka S, Blombäck M, Wiman B. Soluble fibrin: a predictor for the development and outcome of multiple organ failure. *Am J Hematol.*1994; 46:289-294.

54. Okajima K, Uchiba M, Murakami K, Okabe H, Takatsuki K. Determination of plasma soluble fibrin using a new ELISA method in patients with disseminated intravascular coagulation. *Am J Hematol.*1996; 51:186-191.

55. Horan JT, Francis CW. Fibrin degradation products, fibrin monomer and soluble fibrin in disseminated intravascular coagulation. *Semin Thromb Hemost.*2001; 27:657-666.

56. Bick RL. Disseminated intravascular coagulation: pathophysiological mechanisms and manifestations. *Semin Thromb Hemost.*1998;24:3 -18.

57. Mammen EF. Disseminated intravascular coagulation (DIC). *Clin Lab Sci.*2000;13: 239-245.

58. Wada H, Minamikawa K, Wakita Y, et al. Hemostatic study before onset of disseminated intravascular coagulation. *Am J Hematol.*1993; 43:190-194.

59. Akca S, Haji-Michael P, de Mendonça A, Suter P, Levi M, Vincent JL. Time course of platelet counts in critically ill patients. *Crit Care Med.*2002; 30:753-756.

60. Fourrier F, Chopin C, Goudemand J, et al. Septic shock, multiple organ failure, and disseminated intravascular coagulation. Compared patterns of antithrombin III, protein C, and protein S deficiencies. *Chest.*1992; 101:816-823.

61. Mesters RM, Helterbrand J, Utterback BG, et al. Prognostic value of protein C concentrations in neutropenic patients at high risk of severe septic complications. *Crit Care Med.* 2000;28:2209-2216.

62. Gando S, Nakanishi Y, Tedo I. Cytokines and plasminogen activator inhibitor-1 in posttrauma disseminated intravascular coagulation: relationship to multiple organ dysfunction syndrome. *Crit Care Med.*1995; 23:1835-1842.

63. Toh CH, Downey C, Dwyre L. Thromboplastin sensitivity in waveform analysis. *Thromb Haemost.* 2000;84:517-518.

64. Downey C, Kazmi R, Toh CH. Early identification and prognostic implications in disseminated intravascular coagulation through transmittance waveform analysis. *Thromb Haemost.*1998; 80:65-69.

65. Toh CH. Transmittance waveform of routine coagulation tests is a sensitive and specific method for diagnosing nonovert disseminated intravascular coagulation. *Blood Rev.* 2002;16:S11-S14.

66. Wada H, Wakita Y, Nakase T, et al. Outcome of disseminated intravascular coagulation in relation to the score when treatment was begun. Mie DIC Study Group. *Thromb Haemost.*1995; 74:848-852.

67. Toh CH, Downey C. Performance and prognostic importance of a new clinical and laboratory scoring system for identifying non-overt disseminated intravascular coagulation. *Blood Coagul Fibrinolysis.*2005; 16:69-74.

68. Gando S, Iba T, Eguchi Y, et al. A multicenter, prospective validation of disseminated intravascular coagulation diagnostic criteria for critically ill patients: comparing current criteria. *Crit Care Med.* 2006;34:625-631.

69. Wada H, Gabazza EC, Asakura H, et al. Comparison of diagnostic criteria for disseminated intravascular coagulation (DIC): diagnostic criteria of the International Society of Thrombosis and Haemostasis and of the Japanese Ministry of Health and Welfare for Overt DIC. *Am J Hematol.* 2003;74:17-22.

70. Carey MJ, Rodgers GM. Disseminated intravascular coagulation: clinical and laboratory aspects. *Am J Hematol.* 1998;59:65-73.

71. Pernerstorfer T, Hollenstein U, Hansen J, et al. Heparin blunts endotoxin-induced coagulation activation. *Circulation.* 1999;100:2485-2490.

72. Feinstein DI. Diagnosis and management of disseminated intravascular coagulation: the role of heparin therapy. *Blood.* 1982;60:284-287.

73. Sakuragawa N, Hasegawa H, Maki M, Nakagawa M, Nakashima M. Clinical evaluation of low-molecular-weight heparin (FR-860) on disseminated intravascular coagulation (DIC)–a multicenter co-operative double-blind trial in comparison with heparin. *Thromb Res.*1993; 72:475-500.

74. Abraham E, Reinhart K, Svoboda P, et al. Assessment of the safety of recombinant tissue factor pathway inhibitor in

patients with severe sepsis: a multicenter, randomized, placebo-controlled, single-blind, dose escalation study. *Crit Care Med*.2001;29: 2081-2089.

75. Abraham E, Reinhart K, Opal S, et al. Efficacy and safety of tifacogin (recombinant tissue factor pathway inhibitor) in severe sepsis: a randomized controlled trial. *JAMA*. 2003; 290:238-247.

76. Warren BL, Eid A, Singer P, et al. Caring for the critically ill patient. High-dose antithrombin III in severe sepsis: a randomized controlled trial. *JAMA*.2001; 286:1869-1878.

77. Kienast J, Juers M, Wiedermann CJ, et al. Treatment effects of high-dose antithrombin without concomitant heparin in patients with severe sepsis with or without disseminated intravascular coagulation. *J Thromb Haemost*. 2006;4: 90-97.

78. Bernard GR, Vincent JL, Laterre PF, et al. Efficacy and safety of recombinant human activated protein C for severe sepsis. *N Engl J Med*.2001; 344:699-709.

79. Dhainaut JF, Yan SB, Joyce DE, et al. Treatment effects of drotrecogin alfa (activated) in patients with severe sepsis with or without overt disseminated intravascular coagulation. *J Thromb Haemost*.2004; 2:1924-1933.

80. de Pont AC, Bakhtiari K, Hutten BA, et al. Recombinant human activated protein C resets thrombin generation in patients with severe sepsis-a case control study. *Crit Care*. 2005;9:R490-R497.

81. Abraham E, Laterre PF, Garg R, et al. Drotrecogin alfa (activated) for adults with severe sepsis and a low risk of death. *N Engl J Med*.2005; 353:1332-1341.

82. Ratnoff OD. Epsilon aminocaproic acid – a dangerous weapon. *N Engl J Med*.1969; 280:1124-1125.

83. Brown JR, Birkmeyer NJ, O'Connor GT. Meta-analysis comparing the effectiveness and adverse outcomes of antifibrinolytic agents in cardiac surgery. *Circulation*. 2007;115: 2801-2813.

84. Sedrakyan A, Treasure T, Elefteriades JA. Effect of aprotinin on clinical outcomes in coronary artery bypass graft surgery:

a systematic review and meta-analysis of randomized clinical trials. *J Thorac Cardiovasc Surg*.2004; 128:442-448.

85. Ray MJ, O'Brien MF. Comparison of epsilon aminocaproic acid and low-dose aprotinin in cardiopulmonary bypass: efficiency, safety and cost. *Ann Thorac Surg*. 2001;71: 838-843.

86. Karkouti K, Beattie WS, Dattilo KM, et al. A propensity score case-control comparison of aprotinin and tranexamic acid in high-transfusion-risk cardiac surgery. *Transfusion*. 2006;46:327-338.

87. Fergusson DA, Hébert PC, Mazer CD, et al. A comparison of aprotinin and lysine analogues in high-risk cardiac surgery. *N Engl J Med*.2008; 358:2319-2331.

88. Ray WA. Learning from aprotinin–mandatory trials of comparative efficacy and safety needed. *N Engl J Med*. 2008;358:840-842.

89. Aranki S, Cutlip D, Aroesty JM. Early noncardiac complications of coronary artery bypass graft surgery. UpToDate Web site. http://www.uptodate.com/patients/content/topic.do?topicKey=~f55Cyv91Fhhx.I. Accessed 9 Apr 2009

90. Levi M, Opal SM. Coagulation abnormalities in critically ill patients. *Crit Care*.2006; 10:222.

91. Mannucci PM, Levi M. Prevention and treatment of major blood loss. *N Engl J Med*.2007; 356:2301-2311.

92. Levi M, Peters M, Büller HR. Efficacy and safety of recombinant factor VIIa for treatment of severe bleeding: a systematic review. *Crit Care Med*.2005; 33:883-890.

93. Pavie A, Szefner J, Leger P, Gandjbakhch I. Preventing, minimizing, and managing postoperative bleeding. *Ann Thorac Surg*.1999; 68:705-710.

94. Furie B, Furie BC. Mechanisms of thrombus formation. *N Engl J Med*.2008; 359:938-949.

95. Gando S, Kameue T, Nanzaki S, Nakanishi Y. Disseminated intravascular coagulation is a frequent complication of systemic inflammatory response syndrome. *Thromb Haemost*. 1996;75:224-228.

Julie John and Harold Palevsky

Pulmonary hypertension is a significant determinant of morbidity and mortality in patients undergoing cardiac surgery. The successful management of these patients requires an individualized and systematic approach. The analysis of preoperative risk factors, perioperative management of hemodynamics, and the prevention and early recognition of postoperative complications is imperative to successfully oversee the care of pulmonary hypertension patients undergoing cardiac surgery.

In this chapter, we first provide an overview of the current evaluation and available outpatient treatment options for pulmonary hypertension, using pulmonary arterial hypertension (PAH) as a paradigm. The risks of postoperative morbidity and mortality are greater in patients with PAH than in patients with other etiologies for their pulmonary hypertension. Optimization of the status of patients with pulmonary hypertension, using currently available medical therapies, should be undertaken prior to any elective cardiac surgery. The data regarding the management of pulmonary hypertension patients during the immediate preoperative, perioperative, and postoperative periods are limited but are discussed.

21.1 Classification of Pulmonary Hypertension

PAH is defined by a mean pulmonary artery pressure (mPAP) greater than 25 at rest or greater than 30 during activity; in these patients, the presence of a normal pulmonary capillary wedge pressure and an elevated pulmonary vascular resistance (PVR) (>3 Wood units) defines PAH.[1] Patients with pulmonary hypertension should be thoroughly evaluated to establish the etiology of their pulmonary hypertension. The most recent revision of the classification of the World Health Organization (WHO) of pulmonary hypertension divides pulmonary hypertension into five major groups: group 1, PAH; group 2, pulmonary hypertension secondary to left heart disease; group 3, pulmonary hypertension associated with intrinsic lung disease or hypoxia; group 4, pulmonary hypertension due to chronic thromboembolic disease; and group 5, miscellaneous causes such as sarcoidosis, histiocytosis, extrinsic compression of pulmonary vasculature, and lyphangiomatosis.[2] Once the etiology of the disease is determined, the patients are stratified using a functional classification that measures the physical limits the disease imposes on the patient. The WHO modification of the New York Heart Association functional classification (NYHA-FC) for pulmonary hypertension divides pulmonary hypertension patients into four functional classes; class I, patients without limitation of physical activity; class II, patients with slight limitation of physical activity; class III, patients with marked limitation of physical activity; and class IV, patients with inability to perform any physical activity. The assignment of patients within this schema is limited by the classification biases of physicians, which limits its utility as an endpoint.[3] Many studies have found that higher WHO/NYHA-FC class (III or IV), failing to improve by a WHO/NYHA-FC (functional class) with therapies, or deterioration (worsening WHO/NYHA-FC classification) are associated with increased mortality.[4] Clinical trials have established that the 6-min walk test (6MWT), in which the patient walks as far as possible for 6 min, may be considered a more

J.J ohn(✉)
Department of Medicine, Penn Presbyterian Medical Center, Philadelphia, PA, USA
e-mail:J ulie.John@uphs.upenn.edu

E.A. Gabriel and T. Salerno (eds.), *Principles of Pulmonary Protection in Heart Surgery*,
DOI: 10.1007/978-1-84996-308-4_21, © Springer-Verlag London Limited 2010

reliable and consistent assessment of the patients' functional status.[5,6]

Clinical evaluation, the history and physical examination, is the most important element of preoperative pulmonary risk assessment.[2] The symptoms associated with pulmonary hypertension are usually nonspecific. The National Institutes of Health (NIH) assessed 187 patients with primary pulmonary hypertension (PPH; now classified as idiopathic pulmonary arterial hypertension [IPAH]) in a prospective cohort study in which the mean interval from symptom onset to diagnosis was 2 years. In this study, the most common initial complaint was dyspnea (60%), followed by fatigue (19%). Fewer than 10% of patients initially experienced fatigue, syncope, chest pain, palpitations, or leg edema.[7] With progression of the disease, the patient may complain of progression of the initial symptom, the development of the symptoms noted here, and the development of signs of right heart failure with abdominal bloating, anorexia, right upper quadrant discomfort, and ascites. The presence of arthralgias and Raynaud's phenomenon may indicate a coexisting connective tissue disease. Orthopnea, dyspnea on exertion, and paroxysmal nocturnal dyspnea may indicate coexistent left ventricular dysfunction.[8] Family history should be queried because there are patients who have a genetic predisposition to develop PAH.[9] Physical examination of patients may reveal an elevated jugular venous pulse with a large V wave. Cardiac auscultation may demonstrate a prominent second heart sound, which is seen in more than 90% of patients with idiopathic (primary) PAH.[7] This may be associated with a holosystolic murmur (tricuspid regurgitation). Palpation over the parasternal area may demonstrate a right ventricular (RV) heave.[10] With progression of the disease and the development of RV failure, prominent jugular venous distension, tender hepatomegaly, and ascites will develop. A finding of pulmonary edema or crackles on auscultation of the lungs may indicate coexistent left heart disease or pulmonary venous hypertension.

Laboratory evaluation is not diagnostic of PAH but may aid in identifying associated conditions contributing to the pulmonary hypertension and in assessing disease severity. Laboratory tests include those for HIV, serologic markers for connective tissue disease, liver function and hepatitis panel, arterial blood gas, B-type natriuretic peptide (BNP), complete blood counts and coagulation profile, and cardiac enzymes. Plasma BNP (or N-terminal pro-BNP) levels may be used as a prognostic indicator for patients with worsening pulmonary hypertension.[4,11,12]

An *electrocardiogram* (EKG) is recommended by the American College of Physicians as a screening tool for cardiac anatomic and arrhythmic disorders.[8] Although the sensitivity for specific findings is restricted, there are certain EKG findings that are indicative of a poor prognosis, such as right axis deviation, P pulmonale or increased P-wave amplitude in lead 2, R/S wave more than 1 in V1, and WHO criteria for RV hypertrophy.[4,13,14]

Echocardiograms are usually obtained in patients as a screening tool to assess for pulmonary hypertension.[8] Echocardiogram is the most widely available noninvasive technology to estimate pulmonary artery pressure (PAP) and to evaluate cardiac structure and function.[8] Preoperatively, the echocardiogram can be used to estimate right atrial and pulmonary arterial pressures. It can evaluate the extent of right atrial and RV enlargement, estimate the degree of RV dysfunction (by global assessment of RV function and by use of recently described measures such as the TAPSE [tricuspid anular plane systolic excursion]), and reveal possible etiologies of pulmonary hypertension caused by valvular pathology or left-side heart disease.[15] Forfia and colleagues established that the degree of TAPSE (value less than 1.8 cm) can be used as a useful measure of RV systolic dysfunction and poor prognosis in PAH.[16] Patients who are going to surgery should be adequately volume resuscitated prior to echocardiography as severe hypovolemia can influence RV size and apparent function.[1,15]

The importance of RV function in patients undergoing cardiac surgery has been assessed by numerous studies. Preoperative RV systolic dysfunction is associated with poor outcome after cardiac surgery in patients with decreased left ventricular ejection fraction.[17,18] RV systolic overload prolongs the duration of RV systole, which reverses the left-to-right pressure gradient and results in septal dyskinesia.[1] Diastolic overload on the RV results in right atrial dilation, inferior vena caval dilation, and tricuspid regurgitation.[1] Echocardiac findings that predict poor prognosis in patients with severe PPH include right atrial enlargement, the development of pericardial effusion, septal dyskinesia, and elevated Doppler RV index.[4,19,20] Transesophageal echocardiogram may provide additional information regarding cardiac function in patients in intensive care and diagnose specific conditions that may contribute as etiologies to pulmonary hypertension.[21] Although right heart catheterization is the procedure of choice to diagnose pulmonary hypertension, echocardiography may serve as a noninvasive alternative to estimate PAPs (by allowing measurement of the peak systolic pressure gradient associated with tricuspid regurgitation and using that value in the modified Bernoulli equation).[22,23]

Pulmonary function testing is not recommended as a screening tool in assessing patients for high-risk surgery. Patients with unexplained dyspnea or exercise intolerance, underlying chronic obstructive pulmonary disease (COPD), or asthma may benefit from preoperative spirometry if there is evidence of clinical deterioration that can be treated when compared with baseline.[24] The American College of Chest Physicians (ACCP) evidence-based guidelines regarding PAH concluded that there are conflicting data about the prognostic implications of pulmonary function tests. Reduced diffusing capacity for carbon monoxide (DLCO) (<45% of predicted) in patients with scleroderma-associated PAH may be used to predict poor prognosis.[4]

Exercise tolerance testing in patients with PAH is often measured with the 6MWT. distance less than 332 m indicates a poor prognosis in patients with PAH.[4,5] Numerous clinical trials have established that the 6MWT may be a more convenient tool for the assessment of patients' functional status than cardiopulmonary exercise testing.[5,6] Wensel et al. demonstrated that peak VO^2 (peak oxygen consumption) and peak systolic blood pressure in cardiopulmonary exercise testing are strong predictors of survival in patients with PPH.[4,25]

Right heart catheterization is required for confirming the diagnosis of PAH (by measuring the mPAP, the pulmonary capillary wedge pressure, and the cardiac output and by calculating the PVR).[26] Quantitative hemodynamic data can be assessed immediately by a right heart catheterization. PAPs (systolic/diastolic and mean), systemic blood pressures, cardiac output, and pulmonary capillary wedge pressure are measured during catheterization; cardiac index, PVR, PVR index, and systemic vascular resistance can be calculated. Cardiac output can be determined by either thermodilution or by the Fick method (which is considered to be more accurate in critically ill patients when a direct measurement of oxygen

consumption is utilized).[1] It is also possible to diagnose intracardiac shunts during right heart catheterization (particularly left-to-right shunt lesions) using serial oxygen saturation measurements in the vena cava (superior and inferior) at different sites in the right atrium and RV and pulmonary artery. Pulmonary capillary wedge pressure values greater than 15 mmHg suggest contributions from left ventricular or pulmonary venous disease. The NIH PPH Registry found that right atrial pressure greater than 12 mmHg, reduced cardiac index below 2.2 L/min/m², and mPAP greater than 55 mmHg were poor prognostic indices.[27]

The response to vasodilators can be assessed with right heart catheterization. Vasodilator studies are considered the standard of care prior to elective surgery for patients with PAH.[28-30] A short-acting agent such as intravenous adenosine, intravenous or inhaled prostacyclin (PGI_2), inhaled iloprost, or inhaled nitric oxide (NO) is recommended to assess for pulmonary vasoreactivity as these will assess pulmonary vasoreactivity at doses that will have little systemic hemodynamic effects. Inhaled NO appears to have a greater effect on decreasing peripheral vascular resistance than the other pulmonary selective vasodilators,[31] and PGI_2 may have the greatest effect on augmenting cardiac output. The current guidelines define a positive pulmonary vasodilator response as a fall in mPAP greater than or equal to 10 mmHg, to a mPAP less than or equal to 40 mmHg with a stable or improved cardiac output.[32] There is a subset of PAH patients who are responsive and may have long-term survival benefit when treated with calcium channel blockers such as nifedepine, diltiazem, or amlodipine; these can only be identified by assessing for pulmonary vasoreactivity during right heart catheterization.[4,26,32] A study evaluated the effect of inhaled NO and 100% oxygen in decreasing PVR in cardiomyopathy patients who were being evaluated for heart transplantation. The patients were previously on maximal intravenous vasodilator therapy but continued to suffer from persistent moderate-to-severe pulmonary hypertension. Inhaled NO was observed to improve their RV hemodynamics.[33] Preoperative vasodilator trials in patients undergoing cardiac surgery (i.e., mitral valve repair or replacement) can screen for the reversibility of pulmonary hypertension present. The studies provide prognostic information to guide therapy to reduce elevated PAPs[4,34] and to decrease perioperative risk.

Assessment of patient-related risks, comorbid conditions, and procedure-related risks is crucial to decreasing the risks of morbidity and mortality from any surgery.[35] Active cardiac conditions contributing to pulmonary hypertension or RV dysfunction such as unstable coronary syndromes, decompensated heart failure, significant arrhythmias, and valvular disease are associated with an increased risk of morbidity and mortality.[36]

The following patient-related risk factors should be assessed:

1. Age: It is uncertain whether age is an independent predictor of major cardiac complications. However, increased age does correlate with length of hospital stay, mortality, and postoperative cardiac and noncardiac complications.[28]
2. Smoking: The risk of postoperative complications associated with smoking is highest in patients who have smoked within 2 months of surgery.[29,30] Indices for assessing risks of postoperative pulmonary complication after surgery consider smoking within the last 8 weeks a risk factor.[31,32]
3. Obstructive sleep apnea: Obstructive sleep apnea (OSA) correlates with increased postoperative morbidity and mortality; however, preoperative treatment with continuous positive airway pressure can reduce the risk.[37] Awareness of this condition and perioperative use of continuous positive airway pressure (CPAP) or bilevel positive airway pressure (BiPAP) are essential to minimizing the perioperative morbidity from OSA.
4. Metabolic risk factors: Increased uric acid levels and decreased serum albumin level (<3.5 mg/dL) are predictors of 30-day mortality.
5. General health status: If there is evidence of RV failure, consideration should be given to delaying surgery until the patient's health is optimized.[35]

21.2 Outpatient Treatment of Pulmonary Arterial Hypertension

In 2004, the American College of Physicians published a set of evidence-based guidelines for the treatment of PAH.[38] These recommendations for treatment were based on the quality of the evidence and the net benefit of therapy for the patient. They were subsequently updated to reflect the availability of new therapeutic agents.[32] Before the development of present therapeutic options, it was estimated that, following diagnosis, the median survival of patients with IPAH (then PPH) was 2.8 years.[27]

Warfarin, supplemental oxygen, diuretics, and digoxin are considered the standard therapies for pulmonary hypertension. It is recommended that patients with IPAH should receive anticoagulation with warfarin.[32,39,40] The risk-benefit ratio should be carefully considered before administering warfarin in patients with other etiologies of pulmonary hypertension. For example, patients with significant right-to-left shunting have an increased risk for paradoxical embolism and may benefit from anticoagulation, whereas warfarin is relatively contraindicated in patients with portopulmonary hypertension (underlying liver disease), who may be at an increased risk for gastrointestinal (GI) bleeding. Warfarin therapy in patients with IPAH appears to have a beneficial effect on long-term survival.[41,42] Patients receiving intravenous PAH medications should be on warfarin because of their additional risk of catheter-associated thrombosis. The target international normalized ratio (INR) generally recommended is 1.5–2.5.[38]

Hypoxemia is a vasoconstrictor that can worsen pulmonary hypertension. It is recommended that patients use supplemental oxygen to keep oxygen saturation greater than 90% at rest, with activity (exertion), and during sleep.[39] Diuretics are important in the long-term therapeutic management of patients with IPAH. Evidence of RV failure or significant peripheral edema is an indication for using diuretics. Spironolactone is frequently added to the diuretic regimen for both potassium-sparing effects and neurohormonal effects similar to those beneficial in patients with depressed left ventricular function. Digoxin may be considered for patients with PAH with a dilated RV with depressed function. Digoxin is an RV inotrope, resulting in an increase in cardiac output in patients with pulmonary hypertension and symptomatic heart failure.[43]

Calcium channel blockers: A subset of patients with PAH demonstrates a favorable response to acute vasodilator testing during cardiac catheterization. These patients (predominately patients with IPAH) are the only individuals likely to respond favorably to long-term calcium channel blocker therapy. The recommended agents for vasodilator testing in pulmonary hypertension are intravenous (IV) PGI_2, inhaled PGI_2 or iloprost, inhaled NO, or intravenous adenosine.[38,42] Patients are considered to have demonstrated acute vasoreactivity if the decrease in mPAP is 10 or more to 40 mmHg or less with an increased or unchanged cardiac output.[44] Only a small percentage of patients with IPAH will be true responders. The calcium channel blockers used chronically (in acute responders) include nifedipine, diltiazem, or amlodipine; verapamil should be avoided because of its negative inotropic effects. Patients are reassessed every 3 months and are monitored closely for deterioration. Calcium channel blockers should not be used as therapy for pulmonary hypertension in patients with PAH unless there is evidence of significant vasoreactivity demonstrated during right heart catheterization.

Endothelin (ET) receptor antagonists act as antagonists of ET receptor subtypes (ET_A or ET_B). Activation of ET_A receptors results in vasoconstriction and proliferation of vascular smooth muscle, while stimulation of ET_B receptors results in vasodilation and NO release. Increased levels of ET-1 contribute to the vascular abnormalities associated with pulmonary hypertension, and ET-1 levels correlate with PAH disease progression and severity.[45] Currently available endothelin receptor antagonists are bosentan (Tracleer), ambrisentan (Letairis), and sitaxentan (Thelin).[128] At present, only bosentan and ambrisentan have been approved by the Food and Drug Administration (FDA) for use in the United States; sitaxentan has been approved for use in Europe and Canada. Bosentan acts on both ET receptor subtypes, while sitaxentan sodium is said to be approximately 6,000-fold more selective as an antagonist for ET_A compared with ET_B. Ambrisentan appears to be in between these in terms of ET receptor selectivity.[46]

Bosentan: Bosentan was administered to 32 patients with PAH in a double-blind, placebo-controlled study. The patients were randomly assigned to bosentan (62.5 mg twice daily for 4 weeks followed by 125 mg twice daily) or placebo for a minimum of 12 weeks. The study found that bosentan increased exercise capacity and improved hemodynamic parameters in patients with pulmonary hypertension.[47] A second study evaluated the effect of different bosentan dosages (62.5 mg twice daily for 4 weeks followed by 125 or 250 mg twice daily) on exercise capacity in 213 patients with PAH for 12 weeks. The study concluded that bosentan was

beneficial in patients with PAH at a dose of 125 mg twice daily.[48] The results of the endothelin antagonist trial in patients with mildly symptomatic PAH (EARLY) study in patients with functional class II PAH found that, compared to placebo, treatment with bosentan (62.5 mg twice daily for 4 weeks, followed by 125 mg twice daily) improved patients' functional capacity and delayed clinical worsening.[49] Adverse effects with bosentan included abnormal liver function tests (increased transaminases), syncope, and flushing. The abnormal serum transaminases were found to be dose dependent, and the hepatic function abnormalities were generally transient. The FDA requires that liver function tests be performed monthly along with hemoglobin/hematocrit testing every 3 months because patients can develop dilutional anemia. Bosentan is contraindicated in women of childbearing age secondary to its potential teratogenic effects.[38]

Ambrisentan: Ambrisentan is an oral, once-daily, endothelin receptor antagonist that is more selective for ET_A receptors. In the initial clinical trial, patients with IPAH in functional class II and III or PAH associated with connective tissue disease, anorexigen use, or HIV infection were randomized to receive 1, 2.5, 5, or 10 mg of ambrisentan for a total of 12 weeks followed by 12 weeks of open-label ambrisentan in a double-blind study. After 12 weeks, the 1-mg dose was judged inadequate; 6MWT increased in all other groups, as did Borg dyspnea index, functional class, mPAP, and cardiac index. Adverse events were related to elevated transaminases and peripheral edema.[50] The ARIES (Ambrisentan in Pulmonary Arterial Hypertension, Randomized, Double-Blind, Placebo-Controlled, Multicenter, Efficacy Study 1 and 2) administered ambrisentan (ARIES-1, 5 or 10 mg; ARIES-2, 2.5 or 5 mg) orally once daily for 12 weeks. The authors concluded that patients who received ambrisentan (although the dose response is unclear due to different results observed in ARIES-1 and ARIES-2) demonstrated improved exercise capacity with low risk of aminotransferase abnormalities.[51] The FDA has approved both 5- and 10-mg once-daily dosing for PAH.

Sitaxsentan: Sitaxsentan is the most selective ET_A receptor antagonist in clinical development. The initial sitaxsentan study included 178 patients with IPAH or PAH related to connective tissues disease or PAH related to congenital systemic-to-pulmonary shunts that were NYHA class II, III, and IV. Sitaxsentan improved exercise capacity and functional class after 12 weeks of treatment. The most reported adverse clinical events were peripheral edema, headache, nausea, and dizziness. Increased international normalized ratio seen in patients on warfarin was the most reported adverse laboratory event.[52] In a second double-blind, placebo-controlled 18-week study, 247 patients with PAH were randomized to receiving placebo, sitaxsentan 50 or 100 mg, or oral bosentan. At 18 weeks, patients treated with 100 mg of sitaxsentan had improved exercise capacity and WHO functional class with a very low hepatic toxicity incidence rate.[50] FDA approval is pending for this drug.

Phosphodiesterase inhibitors: Phosphodiesterase (PDE) 5 inhibitors increase cyclic guanosine monophosphate (cGMP) levels by inhibiting PDE5 from degrading cGMP. Drugs that inhibit cAMP (cyclic adenosine monophosphate)-specific PDEs or nonspecific or other cGMP-specific phosphodiasterases have weak effects on the pulmonary circulation, whereas drugs that inhibit the cGMP-specific PDE5 (PDE5 inhibitors) increase the pulmonary vascular response to endogenous or inhaled NO.

Sildenafil: Sildenafil is a highly specific PDE5inhibitor. Sildenafil and inhaled NO were studied to determine if sildenafil was an effective acute pulmonary vasodilator. Sildenafil proved to be effective not only as a pulmonary vasodilator by decreasing mPAP but also as a drug that increased cardiac output.[53] When sildenafil was administered with NO, it prolonged the pulmonary vasodilator effects of NO and prevented rebound pulmonary vasoconstriction on termination of the NO inhalation.[54] In another study, 278 patients with PAH were treated with sildenafil 20, 40, or 80 mg or placebo orally three times daily in a double-blind manner for 12 weeks. This placebo-controlled study demonstrated that sildenafil improved functional capacity (as measured by the 6MWT), WHO functional class, and clinical worsening in a dose-dependent manner.[55] The side effects were flushing, dyspepsia, and diarrhea. The dosage subsequently approved by the FDA is 20 mg three times daily.

Tadalafil: Tadalafil, an analog of sildenafil, is a long-acting oral PDE5 inhibitor currently being studied for the treatment of PAH. It is metabolized by cytochrome P450 (CYP) 3A4.[56] A phase 3, double-blind,

placebo-controlled study compared patients with PAH who were randomized to placebo or tadalafil 2.5, 10, 20, or 40 mg orally once daily over 16 weeks. Tadalafil appeared to increase cardiac output and reduce PAP and PVR. The study has been presented in abstract form and appeared to demonstrate that tadalafil may be used as an alternative drug in the treatment of PAH.[57] The FDA has approved Tadalafil in the treatment of PAH. Tadalafil's longer half life compared to sildenafil allows the medication to be administered once daily.

Prostanoids: PGI2 is a metabolite of arachidonic acid. It is produced in the vascular endothelium and acts as a vasodilator, antiplatelet agent, and antiproliferative agent in both the pulmonary and systemic circulations. Currently, there are several different prostanoids available for use in the treatment of pulmonary hypertension.[58] These may be administered by continuous intravenous or continuous subcutaneous infusion, by inhalation, or by oral ingestion. Epoprostenol (Flolan and generic epoprostenol), treprostinil (Remodulin), and inhaled iloprost (Ventavis) are currently available in the United States; intravenous iloprost and beraprost are available in several other countries.

Epoprostenol: Barst et al. conducted a 12-week, prospective, open-label, randomized study comparing the effect of epoprostenol plus conventional therapy versus conventional therapy in patients with NYHA/WHO class III and IV PPH. The study concluded that continuous intravenous infusion of epoprostenol improved survival, hemodynamics, and symptoms in patients with severe PPH.[59] Since that initial study, additional studies have demonstrated that epoprostenol improves the long-term survival of patients with PAH.[60,61] Epoprostenol is administered through continuous intravenous infusion with a tunneled central venous catheter. Adverse effects of epoprostenol therapy included anorexia, nausea and vomiting, jaw pain, diarrhea, musculoskeletal aches and pains, and a blotchy erythematous rash.

Treprostinil: Treprostinil is another PGI_2 analog, less potent than intravenous epoprostenol and with a longer half-life.[62] Treprostinil can be used by either continuous intravenous infusion and a continuous subcutaneous infusion delivery. A study of 25 patients comparing intravenous and subcutaneous treprostinil demonstrated that either route of administration favorably affected cardiopulmonary hemodynamics.[38,62] In a large, randomized, multi-center trial, 470 patients with PAH received either continuous subcutaneous infusion of treprostinil or continuous infusion of placebo plus conventional therapy. Patients receiving treprostinil demonstrated improvements in hemodynamics, but 85% of patients complained of pain at the infusion site.[62] Subcutaneous treprostinil was approved by the FDA in 2002 for NYHA class II; intravenous treprostinil was approved in 2004 for patients in NYHA class II, III, and IV in whom subcutaneous infusion was not tolerated.[32]

Iloprost: Iloprost is a PGI_2 analog that is available in intravenous, inhalational, and oral dosing forms. Intravenous and inhalational iloprost were compared with intravenous PGI_2 in a study that found that inhaled iloprost exerted selective pulmonary vasodilation, which reduced PVR and PAP without the systemic vasodilation seen with the two intravenous agents.[63] Inhaled iloprost and intravenous nitroglycerin were compared in patients undergoing mitral valve surgery; during weaning from cardiopulmonary bypass, inhaled iloprost proved to be superior due to the selective pulmonary vasodilator effects of the drug.[64] The Aerosolized Randomized Iloprost Study (AIR) trial studied inhaled iloprost (2.5 or 5.0 μg of iloprost inhaled six to nine times a day) compared to placebo in the long-term treatment of primary or secondary pulmonary hypertension. The study demonstrated that inhaled iloprost improved NYHA functional class, dyspnea, and quality of life in patients with pulmonary hypertension.[65] The side effects of inhaled iloprost are cough, flushing, and headache. The FDA approved inhaled iloprost in 2004 for PAH functional class III and IV. Intravenous iloprost is used in Europe for the treatment of severe PAH. Inhaled iloprost has also been studied as an alternative agent for the assessment of acute vasoreactivity in patients with IPAH and those with chronic thromboembolic pulmonary hypertension.[66,67]

Beraprost: Beraprost is an orally active analog of PGI_2.[38] Beraprost has been evaluated not only in PAH, but also in peripheral vascular disorders such as Raynaud's phenomenon, intermittent claudication, and systemic sclerosis, with variable results.[68,69] Beraprost appears to have a beneficial effect on survival in pulmonary hypertension.[70] In a double-blind, randomized, placebo-controlled trial, the safety and efficacy of beraprost sodium were evaluated as a treatment for PAH. The study determined that beraprost was effective in WHO class II and III PAH; however, the effects seemed to attenuate over time.[71] Beraprost is currently approved for use in the treatment of PAH in Japan and Korea; it is being restudied in the United States and Europe for the treatment of PAH as part of a multidrug (combination) re gimen.

Treatment Based on Functional Class: The recommendations for treatment based on functional class are based on the published ACCP guidelines.[32] Clinical judgment, knowledge of the patient's condition, and their preferences should be considered before starting any of the chronic treatments. If patients fail to respond to initial therapies, agents can be used in combination, with inhaled and parenteral prostanoids generally reserved for patients with late class III or class IV disease.[72]

21.3 PreoperativeManag ement

The preoperative management of pulmonary hypertension is a challenge. High-risk patients need to be identified and treated to reduce postoperative complications and morbidity and mortality related to cardiothoracic surgery.[37,73] Although preoperative pulmonary risk assessment is well defined for noncardiac surgery, risk stratification in cardiac surgery is not as well defined. Ramakrishna et al. addressed the impact of pulmonary hypertension on the outcome of noncardiac surgery. This study evaluated 145 patients with pulmonary hypertension undergoing noncardiac surgery; the short-term perioperative mortality was 7%. Variables associated with increased morbidity, including NYHA functional class II or higher, history of pulmonary embolism, duration of anesthesia longer than 3 h, the presence of OSA, and the need for intermediate- to high-risk surgery. The use of intraoperative dopamine or epinephrine, lack of use of NO, and preoperative RV systolic pressure/systolic BP ratio greater than 0.66 were also associated with increased morbidity and mortality.[34,37]

Preoperative risk assessment is an individualized process taking into account the etiology of the patients' pulmonary vascular disease and their functional status, assessment of patient- and procedure-related risk factors, electrocardiography, echocardiography, pulmonary function testing, laboratory testing, exercise tolerance testing, and if available, preoperative right heart catheterization with or without vasodilator testing.[74]

Patients with preoperative pulmonary hypertension can be divided into three groups:

1. Patients with an incidental finding of pulmonary hypertension who are asymptomatic or who are compensated while currently on medications to treat pulmonary hypertension
2. Patients undergoing surgery to manage their pulmonaryh ypertension
3. Patients with decompensated right heart failure who are being evaluated for surgery not directed at managingt heirp ulmonaryh ypertension

Surgery to treat pulmonary hypertension includes atrial septostomy, pulmonary thromboendarterectomy (for chronic thromboembolic disease), closure of congenital systemic–pulmonary shunts, valve replacements in patients with PH secondary to left-sided valvular disease, and lung transplantation.[75,76] Atrial septostomy is a palliative option in patients with refractory and severe pulmonary hypertension with RV failure or recurrent syncope or as a bridge to transplantation.[77] A retrospective analysis of hemodynamic changes in patients with pulmonary hypertension who underwent atrial septostomy found that atrial septostomy provides improvement in cardiac index and right atrial pressure. However, there was increased mortality in patients undergoing surgery with elevated right atrial pressures (>18 mmHg) or a PVR index greater than 55 U/m[2.78,79] Pulmonary thromboendarterectomy is a high-risk procedure to treat proximal chronic (unresolved) pulmonary emboli.[80] It can result in dramatic hemodynamic and functional improvement if appropriate patients with chronic thromboembolic pulmonary hypertension are referred for the surgery. Mortality rates have been reduced to less than 10% in centers that are experienced with performing this procedure.[81,82] Lung transplantation and heart-lung transplantation are the primary palliative surgical options for patients with refractory PAH.[43,82]

In the absence of specific evidence-based literature, predictors of preoperative risk of surgery are those factors that correlate with survival in PAH.[74] Preoperatively, the goal should be to improve RV function and cardiac output by decreasing PVR and PAPs. The adequacy of the compensation of the RV to the increased PVR is assessed by evaluating right atrial pressure and cardiac output/cardiac index. These and functional status are the major predictors of perioperative risk in the surgical patient.[34] The goals of the preoperative evaluation of patients with PAH undergoing surgery are as follows:

1. To identify and appropriately classify patients with incidental pulmonary hypertension. Treatment should be started preoperatively and continued throughout the perioperative period.[27] The predictors of high risk and poor outcome should be improved or the need for surgery be reevaluated until the patient has improved significantly.[4,74]

   (a) NYHA/WHOf unctionalc lass
   (b) Hemodynamics: Right atrial pressure (RAP more than 12 mmHg, mPAP above 55 mmHg, reduced cardiac output (CI less than 2.2 L/min/m^2), abnormal RV stroke index
   (c) Echocardiography: severe right atrial enlargement, interventricular septal diastolic flattening, pericardial effusion, RV myocardial performance index greater than −0.75, RV hypertrophy, Right ventricular systolic pressure: systolic blood pressure (RVSP:SBP) ratio greater than 0.66, TAPSE score <0.8 cm
   (d) Electrocardiography: right axis deviation, P pulmonale or increased P-wave amplitude in lead 2, qR pattern in V1
   (e) LaboratoryB NPgr eatert han330ng/ mL

2. In patients undergoing surgery to correct pulmonary hypertension, it is high risk to perform corrective surgeries when there are predictors such as those mentioned and if there is a PVR index above 4,400 dyn/s/m^2 or a resting oxygen saturation less than 80%.[34,75] Consideration should be given to delaying surgery if predictors of poor prognosis are present and are not improved as the risk of morbidity and mortality from right heart failure may outweigh the potential benefits of the surgery.

3. Decompensated right heart failure is a contraindication to all but the most emergent surgery. Management of decompensated heart failure involves treating any causative conditions that can be corrected. Invasive hemodynamic monitoring may be required to guide the management of volume status. In patients with decompensated heart failure, useful agents may include diuretics, anticoagulants, inhaled NO, intravenous or inhaled epoprostenol, inhaled or intravenous iloprost, and inotropic support with dobutamine or milrinone.[83] Dobutamine, which is preferred over dopamine unless there is severe hypotension, can

restore adequate tissue perfusion in the setting of systemic hypotension/hypoperfusion.[74,84] Digoxin is an inotropic agent that may be effective in the setting of RV dilation and dysfunction due to pulmonary hypertension.[43] Levosimendan may be beneficial secondary to positive inotropic effects and interaction between the RV and pulmonary vascular system.[85] Nesiritide is generally not recommended in pulmonary venous hypertension and has proven to be of no appreciable benefit in pulmonary artery hypertension.[86] Patients who have RV failure from pulmonary causes other than PAH do not generally benefit from treatment with pulmonary vasodilators.[83] There is increased incidence of atrial tachyarrhythmias with RV failure.[83] Atrial flutter or atrial fibrillation is associated with an increased risk of death in patients with pulmonary hypertension in RV failure.[87]

21.4 Perioperative Management

Pulmonary hypertension is a major predictor of perioperative morbidity and mortality in cardiac surgery. The perioperative management of these patients requires frequent assessment of hemodynamics, administration of adequate oxygen, avoidance of volume depletion or volume overload, administration of pulmonary vasodilators, and the recognition and management of acute diastolic right ventricular failure (ADRVF).[74] Preoperative risk assessment is extremely important because risk stratification allows the surgeon and anesthesiologist to balance the hemodynamic demands of the surgery against the functional demands of the patient.

Perioperative management of PAH will be focused on the following:

1. Anesthetic management of pulmonary hypertension in patients undergoing surgery
2. Initial management of acute increases in PAP (with consequent RV failure)

21.4.1 Perioperative Assessment

Nearly all etiologies of pulmonary hypertension ultimately result in increased PVR, which is considered to be an independent risk factor for morbidity and mortality in patients undergoing heart surgery.[88] Therapy should be directed at reversing any acute increase in

PVR and in optimizing control of chronically elevated PVR perioperatively. Acute increases in PVR can be a result of hypercarbia (goal P_{CO_2}: 30–35), acidosis (goal pH: higher than 7.4), hypoxia (goal arterial oxygen saturation >90%), hypothermia, increased sympathetic tone, and endogenous or exogenous pulmonary vasoconstrictors such as catecholamines, serotonin, thromboxane, and endothelin.[34,89,90] These factors can also be acute precipitants of diastolic left ventricular or RV failure that must be avoided. In the asymptomatic patient with pulmonary hypertension, control of the precipitating factors with continuous monitoring of ventilation, pulse oximetry, or arterial blood gas are required for perioperative management.

21.4.2 Anesthetic Management

PAH during the perioperative period is a challenge for anesthesiologists. To detect complications of increased PVR, monitoring is needed using continuous pulse oximetry, arterial blood gas sampling, continuous electrocardiogram monitoring, and vital signs. Accurately assessing the preload status of the patient involves closely monitoring central venous pressure and pulmonary artery occlusive pressure and observing the response to controlled challenges of fluid administration.[87] Transesophageal echocardiogram is often used intraoperatively to observe both the RV and left ventricular response to fluid expansion. Patients who are on pulmonary hypertension medications should not discontinue the medications prior to surgery.

General anesthesia has risks in patients with pulmonary hypertension; as a result, regional anesthesia is used when possible. In centers with experience, thoracic epidural anesthesia may be preferred for cardiac surgery.[88] Spinal anesthesia is avoided in patients with pulmonary hypertension due to sympatholytic effects, which may cause decreased systemic (and pulmonary) vascular resistance and provoke hypotension. Epidural anesthesia has been used successfully in patients with pulmonary hypertension. The onset of drug effect action is relatively slow, and the extent of the epidural block can be titrated. The effect of anesthetic drugs on the pulmonary circulation needs to be monitored closely as the effect of these agents on the pulmonary circulation may be different from their effects on the systemic circulation.[91]

During anesthetic induction, patients with pulmonary hypertension patients may develop systemic hypotension and cardiovascular collapse. Etomidate appears to be an appropriate agent to use because it maintains systemic hemodynamics without directly affecting PVR.[34] Rich et al. demonstrated that midazolam, smaller doses of etomidate (0.3 mg/kg), and propofol (2 mg/kg) do not affect PVR, whereas propofol significantly increased PVR after endothelial injury in isolated rat lungs.[92] Ketamine is also considered one of the appropriate drugs for the anesthetic management of patients with pulmonary hypertension. It has been shown that ketamine can produce pulmonary vasodilation in humans.[93] Fentanyl does not appear to affect pulmonary vascular tone. With respect to inhalational anesthesia, halothane is frequently poorly tolerated, and isoflurane, sevoflurane, and desflurane can cause pulmonary vasodilation. Sevoflurane can be used for anesthesia in patients with compensated heart failure because it is more titratable than isoflurane and does not produce tachycardia with rapid increases in concentration.[91,94,95] Riabova et al. demonstrated that isoflurane is favored over sevoflurane to maintain anesthesia in patients with cardiopulmonary disease during operations under prolonged artificial one-lung ventilation.[96]

Ventilatory management is difficult in patients with pulmonary hypertension. High concentrations of oxygen, low levels of positive end-expiratory pressure (PEEP) to decrease FRC (functional residual capacity; PVR is dependent on FRC), and moderate tidal volumes must be sufficient to produce hyperventilation. After surgery, a narcotic-oxygen anesthetic technique followed by postoperative mechanical ventilation appears appropriate.[34]

Patients with pulmonary hypertension undergoing surgery may experience progressive hemodynamic deterioration with additional increases in PVR combined with decreased RV function secondary to perioperative hypotension.[34] Perioperative hypotension in pulmonary hypertension patients can be treated with several different types of agents:

1. Inotropic drugs: Dobutamine, isoproterenol, and milrinone are indicated when there is decreased cardiac output and increased PVR. These agents increase cardiac output and decrease PVR. Isoproterenol can cause tachycardia and tachyarrhythmias, which limits its use. Dobutamine produces vasodilation when used in a dose range of 5–20 µg/kg/min. Dobutamine and amrinone were compared in a randomized, double-blind trial, which determined that the use of amrinone was associated with a reduction in pulmonary arterial pressures and increased cardiac index after separation from bypass in patients with severe preoperative pulmonary hypertension.[97] Milrinone can cause severe systemic hypotension; its administration must be carefully monitored.

   Low-dose epinephrine, dopamine, and dobutamine can be used for inotropic effect in patients with pulmonary hypertension undergoing surgery. If the patient is still hypotensive and higher doses of epinephrine or dopamine are needed, then selective pulmonary vasodilators may be needed to counter pulmonary vasoconstriction.[91]

2. Vasopressors: Norepinephrine, phenylephrine, and vasopressin are all vasopressors that can be used in patients with pulmonary hypertension. Norepinephrine is preferred over phenylephrine in patients with chronic pulmonary hypertension who require hemodynamic support after induction of anesthesia.[91,98] Vasopressin has proved to be effective in patients with pulmonary hypertension undergoing spinal anesthesia.[99]

Dopamine is considered to be as effective as norepinephrine in patients with pulmonary hypertension with septic shock.[100] Epinephrine and dopamine produce dose-dependent effects on PVR; alpha effects increase PVR with dosages of epinephrine greater than 0.05 µg/kg/min and dopamine greater than 5 mg/kg/min.[91]

21.4.3 Management of Perioperative Pulmonary Hypertension

Pulmonary vasodilator therapy reduces PVR, which decreases PAP and may increase cardiac output. The ideal pulmonary vasodilator should decrease PVR without causing systemic effects. Agents that cause dilation of both pulmonary and systemic vascular beds may be useful if pulmonary hypertension is associated with systemic hypertension or with left heart disease. The pulmonary vasodilators used in the management of perioperative pulmonary hypertension include inhaled NO, intravenous NO donors such as nitroprusside and nitroglycerin (which may also affect the systemic arterial and venous beds), and prostanoids (prostaglandins) by inhalation or intravenous administration, including prostaglandin E1 (PGE1), epoprostenol, and iloprost.

Intravenous vasodilators available perioperatively to reduce decreased PAPs are nitroprusside, nitroglycerin, epoprostenol (PGI_2), iloprost, and PGE1. The nonselective NO donors nitroprusside and nitroglycerin have been available for the longest time period and can be used to decrease PVR in patients with pulmonary hypertension undergoing surgery. Unfortunately, these agents decrease both systemic and pulmonary vascular resistances and systemic blood pressure, which may predispose the RV to ischemia.

Inhaled NO does not produce the systemic vasodilation that is seen with intravenous nitroprusside and nitroglycerin. Inhaled NO is delivered to pulmonary vessels that are perfusing well-ventilated lung units, which helps augment blood flow to ventilated areas of the lung. Inhaled NO has more effect in patients with increased PVR than in those with more normal PVR.[62] Many studies demonstrated benefit from the use of inhaled NO in patients with pulmonary hypertension undergoing cardiac surgery to control pulmonary hypertension perioperatively.[35,101,102] Although intravenous PGI_2 is considered the most effective vasodilator in postoperative cardiac surgery patients, inhaled NO is recommended in patients with systemic hypotension complicating pulmonary hypertension and RV failure.[101] Different dosages of inhaled NO are associated with significant reductions in PVR. In one study, subjects were randomized to receive five doses of inhaled NO ranging from 10 to 40 ppm; the authors found that there was no further significant reduction in PVR with dosages greater than 10 ppm.[102] The toxicity related to NO is dose related; it has been recommended that patients should not be treated with doses higher than 20 ppm if undergoing cardiac surgery.[102] NO has also been used to prevent the inflammatory response from cardiopulmonary bypass. The recommended dose is 20 ppm of NO through the cardiopulmonary bypass machine throughout the procedure.[103] Although there are reports of NO inhibiting platelet function, there has been no evidence of clinical bleeding related to the inhalation of NO in patients who underwent cardiac surgery patients.[105]

Milrinone is a PDE3inhibitor that increases cAMP by inhibiting its breakdown and thereby promoting vasodilation. It is available as an inhaled medication and intravenous solution. Inhaled milrinone potentiates the vasodilation induced by inhaled PGI_2 and results in additional reduction in PAP and increased RV stroke volume. This study also showed that inhaled milrinone decreased PVR without systemic effects.[105] Milrinone is a useful additive to NO and prostaglandins in the management of pulmonary hypertension.[91] It can also be used to wean patients from the cardiopulmonary bypass circuit. The recommended dose is a bolus of 25–50 µg/kg followed by a continuous infusion of 0.375–0.750 µg/kg/min.[103]

Dipyridamole is a PDE5 inhibitor. It has been used primarily as an antiplatelet agent, but studies have demonstrated its vasodilating effects when used intravenously. Ziegler et al. demonstrated that diypridamole augmented the vasodilator response to inhaled NO.[106] Although clinical experience is limited, the combination of inhaled NO and dipyridamole decreased PAPs and resistance in refractory pulmonary hypertension in patients undergoing cardiac valvular surgery.[107] Dipyridamole is recommended at a dose of 0.2–0.6 mg/kg IV over 15 min to be repeated after 12 h when administered with NO.[103]

Prostacyclins are important therapeutic agents for the management of perioperative pulmonary hypertension.[88] Intravenous prostanoids are limited by the systemic effects they have, promoting systemic vasodilation and systemic hypotension and interfering with hypoxic vasoconstriction, thereby promoting intrapulmonary shunting and systemic hypoxemia. One study assessed the effects of intravenous sodium nitroprusside, intravenous PGI_2, intravenous PGE_1, and inhaled NO (5, 10, and 20 ppm) in patients after heart transplantation. The authors concluded that PGI_2 is the best choice for an intravenous pulmonary vasodilator after heart transplantation. Compared to the other agents, PGI_2 (dosages of 16 ± 2 ng/kg/min) decreased systemic vascular resistance and pulmonary vascular resistance and increased cardiac output, stroke volume, and central filling pressures.[101] However, systemic hypotension may limit the use of prostanoids in cardiac surgery.

Alternative modes of administering PGI_2 is by inhalation, by mask, or through a ventilator circuit. The advantages of inhaled PGI_2 are minimization of systemic effects, with no toxic metabolic by-products or known toxic effects. The disadvantages are that the aerosolized dose varies with alteration in minute ventilation, with variations in flow rates, and with nebulizer driving pressure. Inhaled PGI_2 may cause systemic hypotension if there is systemic absorption, although this may be controlled by reducing the dosage; the frequency of this effect is not established.[91] One study compared the hemodynamic effects of inhaled PGI_2 and inhaled NO and intravenous sodium nitroprusside in patients undergoing mitral valve replacement secondary to mitral valve stenosis. The study determined that inhaled NO and inhaled PGI_2 have similar effectiveness for treatment of pulmonary hypertension after mitral valve replacement.[88] The plasma half-life of PGI_2 is approximately 3–6 min, so it requires continuous administration to be effective. Iloprost is a stable analog of PGI_2 with a half-life of 20–30 min; it may be administered intermittently. Various studies comparing inhaled iloprost, inhaled NO, and inhaled PGI_2 have concluded that all three agents have similar pulmonary and hemodynamic effects in treating pulmonary hypertension.[108-110] PGE1, or alprostadil, is another prostaglandin that causes pulmonary vasodilation. It is used intravenously in neonatal intensive care units to maintain patency of patent ductus arteriosus until surgery is performed.[108] There are limited studies and published reports with inhaled PGE1. One study compared inhaled NO, intravenous PGE1, and aerosolized PGE1 in patients with acute respiratory distress syndrome (ARDS). Inhaled PGE1 is effective in improving PVR and decreasing mPAP and in improving RV ejection fraction.[104] Inhaled PGI_2 is our first choice agent for managing pulmonary hypertension in patients undergoing cardiac surgery and has similarly been recommended by others.[108]

Inhaled nitroprusside and nitroglycerin are agents that may be used in managing perioperative pulmonary hypertension. Yurtseven et al. demonstrated that inhaled nitroglycerin produced a reduction in mPAP and PVR in patients after mitral valve operations without reducing mean arterial pressure and systemic vascular resistance.[105] Inhaled nitroprusside has only been studied in newborns with persistent pulmonary hypertension or refractory hypoxia.[106]

Other drugs under investigation include adenosine; sildenafil; PDE6 inhibitors such as zaprinast, recombinant BNP, or Nesiritide; NO donors such as L-arginine or NONOates; and 3-hydroxy-3-methylglutaryl-coenzyme A (HMG-CoA) reductase inhibitors such as simvastatin and atorvastatin. Adenosine activates adenylate cyclase and stimulates the generation of cAMP, but it is rapidly inactivated, with a plasma half-life of less than 10 s.[91] Sildenafil was studied as an adjunct to inhaled NO in the management of pulmonary hypertension and was beneficial.[111] Aerosolized zaprinast proved to be effective as a selective pulmonary vasodilator but needs to be studied further in humans.[129] Nesiritide was studied in patients from the preoperative period to the postoperative period and proved to effective; it decreased PAPs and myocardial oxygen consumption. The authors recommended that further evaluation of its role in cardiac surgery is warranted.[130] The use of HMG-CoA reductase inhibitors in patients with pulmonary hypertension is under investigation, and their use in patients with pulmonary hypertension undergoing surgery also requires further study.

The goal of managing perioperative pulmonary hypertension is to reduce PVR PAPs and increase cardiac output without causing systemic side effects, which can complicate the surgical and postoperative course of the patient. Different drugs can be combined to act synergistically to increase efficacy and decrease the dose of individual drugs to reduce side effects.[91,105,114] Various management options exist for the intraoperative and perioperative management of pulmonary hypertension. We favor the use of inhalational agents (inhaled NO at 10–40 ppm or inhaled PGI_2 starting at 50 mg/kg/min and then decreasing to the minimum effective dose), supplementing them with PDE5 inhibitor if synergy is required.

21.5 PostoperativeManag ement of Pulmonary Hypertension

The period following cardiac surgery is particularly tenuous as many patients die in the postoperative period from progressive increases in PVR, decreased myocardial function, right heart failure, and sudden death. The goals in the treatment of postoperative pulmonary hypertension (with or without RV failure) should be the following[111]:

1. Optimize preload to the RV (central venous pressure [CVP] should be greater than 10 mmHg)
2. DecreasePV Rtode creaseR Va fterload
3. Use high inspired oxygen concentrations, increased tidal volumes, end-expiratory pressure ventilation, and generation of a mild respiratory alkalosis to

limit hypoxic pulmonary vasoconstriction

4. Maintain systemic blood pressure and tissue perfusion

The ultimate treatment goal is to dilate pulmonary vasculature and reduce PVR while maintaining systemic blood pressure.

The following agents have been studied in the management of postoperative pulmonary hypertension and right heart failure:

1. Isoproterenol is a nonselective beta agonist that can increase cardiac output at therapeutic doses while decreasing pulmonary and systemic vascular resistance.[112,113] Systemic hypotension and tachycardia may limit the usefulness of isoproterenol. Once initiated, isoproterenol infusions should be titrated down carefully since systemic vascular resistance may rebound after the drug has been discontinued.[111]

2. Dobutamine is useful in patients in whom the goal is to increase cardiac output and decrease systemic vascular resistance since this drug is primarily a beta agonist. Although it is useful in patients with pulmonary hypertension and heart failure, levosimendan has proven more effective in achieving pulmonary artery vasodilation and improving cardiac output in patients when compared to dobutamine.[115]

3. Adenosine is a pulmonary vasodilator used in the preoperative evaluation for vasoreactivity in patients with pulmonary hypertension. Adenosine acts through activation of adenyl cyclase and release of cAMP. It has a very short plasma half-life, being cleared from the circulation by adenosine deaminase after a single pass through the lungs. Adenosine may be used in patients with right heart failure to selectively lower RV afterload after cardiac surgery.[116] Since adenosine increases pulmonary capillary wedge pressure and the risk of inducing pulmonary edema, it is not recommended for long-term therapy.

4. Inhaled NO is a rapidly acting, potent, and selective pulmonary vasodilator that decreases PVR and PAPs without affecting systemic vascular resistance. Inhaled NO only dilates blood vessels in ventilated regions of the lung; this improves ventilation perfusion matching. Nonselective intravenous vasodilators can lead to ventilation perfusion mismatch (and intrapulmonary shunting) by increasing pulmonary blood flow to regions of poorly ventilated lung. In the immediate postoperative period, inhaled NO has demonstrated significant decreases in PVR with increased cardiac index.[117]

5. Milrinone is a PDE3inhibitor that acts through the cAMP pathway to produce vasodilation. Milrinone is effective in patients with heart failure because it does not increase myocardial oxygen demand by decreasing afterload. Bolus doses of 12.5–75 µg/kg continued over 48 h did not demonstrate tolerance to the effects of milrinone in patients with heart failure.[118] This agent can be used synergistically with dobutamine because it avoids stimulation of desensitized beta receptors, which may be seen in patients with heart failure managed on dobutamine.[119] Milrinone has been studied in cardiac surgical patients who develop RV failure after left ventricular assist device implantation as an inotropic agent that acts as a direct vasodilator.[120]

6. Prostanoids include PGI_2 (epoprostenol), iloprost, treprostinil, and PGE1. These agents are naturally occurring substances (PGI_2 and PGE1), with short half-lives, or with modifications of prostacylin to increase the half-life, that are all potent pulmonary vasodilators. These agents may be administered intravenously or by inhalation. Inhaled administration tends to minimize systemic side effects, such as hypotension or hypoxemia (due to intravenous prostanoids interfering with hypoxemic vasoconstriction and resulting in intrapulmonary shunting). Studies have shown that prostanoids are effective in patients with right heart failure with implanted RV assist devices.[121] PGE1 has been extensively used in cardiac surgery not only for the preoperative treatment of pulmonary hypertension but also for perioperative and postoperative treatment.[122] One study demonstrated successful weaning from cardiopulmonary bypass, with central venous PGE1 administered simultaneously with left atrial norepinephrine infusion in patients with acute pulmonary hypertension.[123] Inhaled prostanoids are increasingly used after cardiac surgery (i.e., mitral valve surgery, pulmonary thromboendarterectomy) and after thoracic transplantation (heart, lung, and heart-lung transplantation) to prevent pulmonary vasoconstriction or rebound pulmonary hypertension and to improve ventilation-perfusion matching and arterial oxygenation.

If specific drug therapies do not control postoperative pulmonary artery hypertension, right heart failure can develop. Available mechanical therapies include RV assist devices, extracorporeal membrane oxygenation, and pulmonary arterial counterpulsations.[111] Ozdogan et al. have found that decompressing the RV by creating a patent foramen ovale (PFO; atrial septostomy) and concurrent prostanoid inhalation (in this report, inhalation of iloprost) can control postoperative pulmonary hypertension during weaning from cardiopulmonary bypass. The PFO created may be closed using a transcatheter septal occlusion device when the patient's condition is more stable.[124]

21.5.1 Agents Under Development

Although considerable progress has been made in the pharmacologic management of pulmonary hypertension, there is still need for additional therapeutic options. Many agents are under clinical investigation, some in pharmacologic classes mentioned, others, such as statins, vasoactive intestinal peptide (VIP), adrenomedullin, cicletanine, and Rho kinase inhibitors, represent novel agents or potential therapeutic pathways.[125,126] Additional studies evaluating these agents as therapies for pulmonary hypertension, particularly in pre-, peri-, and postoperative cardiac surgerypa tients,w illbe re quired.

References

1. Zamanian R, Haddad F, Doyle RL, Weinacker A. Management strategies for patients with pulmonary hypertension in the intensive care unit. Crit Care Med. 2007;35(9): 9037–9050.
2. Smetana G. Preoperative pulmonary evaluation. N Engl J Med.1999;340:937- 944.
3. Humbert M, Sitbon O, Simonneau G. Treatment of pulmonary arterial hypertension. N Engl J Med. 2004;351: 1425-1436.
4. McLaughlin VV, Presberg KW, Doyle RL, et al. Prognosis of pulmonary arterial hypertension: ACCP evidence-based clinical practice guidelines. Chest.2004; 126:78-92.
5. Miyamoto S, Nagaya N, Satoh T, et al. Clinical correlates and prognostic significance of six-minute walk test in patients with primary pulmonary hypertension: comparison with cardiopulmonary exercise testing. Am J Respir Crit Care Med.2000;161: 487-492.
6. Villalba WO, Sampaio-Barros PD, Pereira MC, et al. Six-minute walk test for the evaluation of pulmonary disease severity in scleroderma patients. Chest. 2007;131(1):217-222.
7. Rich S, Dantzker DR, Ayres SM, et al. Primary pulmonary hypertension. A national prospective study. Ann Intern Med. 1987;107(2):216-223.
8. McGoon M, Gutterman D, Steen V, et al. Screening, early detection, and diagnosis of pulmonary arterial hypertension. Chest.2004; 126:145-305.
9. Davies RJ, Morrell NW. Molecular mechanisms of pulmonary arterial hypertension: role of mutations in the bone morphogenetic protein type II receptor. Chest. 2008;134(6):1271-1277.
10. Bates B, Bickley LS, Hoekelman RA. A guide to physical examination and history taking. 6th ed. Philadelphia: Lippincott;1995.
11. Leuchte HH, Holzapfel M, Baumgartner RA, et al. Clinical significance of brain natriuretic peptide in primary pulmonary hypertension. J Am Coll Cardiol. 2004;43(5): 764-770.
12. Nagaya N, Nishikimi T, Uematsu M, et al. Plasma brain natriuretic peptide as a prognostic indicator in patients with primary pulmonary hypertension. Circulation. 2000;102(8): 865-870.
13. Bossone E, Paciocco G, Iarussi D, et al. The prognostic role of the ECG in primary pulmonary hypertension. Chest. 2002;121:513-518.
14. Henkens IR, Mouchaers KT, Vliegen HW, et al. Early changes in rat hearts with developing pulmonary arterial hypertension can be detected with three-dimensional electrocardiography. Am J Physiol Heart Circ Physiol. 2007;293: H1300-H1307.
15. Viellard-Baron A, Prin S, Chergui K, et al. Echo-Doppler demonstration of acute cor pulmonale at the bedside in the medial intensive care unit. Am J Respir Crit Care Med. 2002;166:1310-1319.
16. Forfia P, Fisher MR, Mathai SC, et al. Tricuspid annula displacement predicts survival in pulmonary hypertension. Am J Respir Crit Care Med. 2006;174:1034-1041.
17. Maslow AD, Regan MM, Panzica P, et al. Precardiopulmonary bypass right ventricular function is associated with poor outcome after coronary artery bypass grafting in patients with severe left ventricular systolic dysfunction. Anesth Analg. 2002;95:1507-1518.
18. Reichert CL, Visser CA, van den Brink RB, et al. Prognostic value of biventricular function in hypertensive patients after cardiac surgery as assessed by transesophageal echocardiography. J Cardiothorac Vasc Anesth. 1992;6: 429-432.
19. Raymond RJ, Hinderliter AL, Willis PW, et al. Echocardiographic predictors of adverse outcomes in primary pulmonary hypertension. J Am Coll Cardiol. 2002;39(7): 1214-1219.
20. Yeo T, Dujardin KS, Tei C, et al. Value of a Doppler-derived index combining systolic and diastolic time intervals in predicting outcome in primary pulmonary hypertension. Am J Cardiol.1998; 81:1157-1161.
21. Hüttemann E. Transesophageal echocardiography in the intensive care unit. Minerva Anestesiol. 2006;72: 891-913.
22. Berger M, Haimowitz A, Van Tosh A. Quantitative assessment of pulmonary hypertension in patients with tricuspid regurgitation using continuous wave Doppler ultrasound. J Am Coll Cardiol.1985; 2:359-365.

23. Currie PJ, Seward JB, Chan K-L. Continuous wave Doppler determination of right ventricular pressure: a simultaneous Doppler-catheterization study in 127 patients. *J Am Coll Cardiol*.1985;6:750- 756.

24. Smetana GW. Preoperative pulmonary assessment of the older adult. *Clin Geriatr Med*.2003; 19:35-55.

25. Wensel R, Opitz CF, Anker SD, et al. Assessment of survival in patients with primary pulmonary hypertension: importance of cardiopulmonary exercise testing. *Circulation*. 2002;106:319-324.

26. Barst R, McGoon M, Torbicki A, et al. Diagnosis and differential assessment of pulmonary arterial hypertension. *J Am Coll Cardiol*.2004; 43:40-47.

27. D'Alonzo GE, Barst RJ, Ayres SM, et al. Survival in patients with primary pulmonary hypertension: results from a national prospective registry. *Ann Intern Med*. 1991;115:343-349.

28. Rodriguez R, Pearl R. Pulmonary hypertension and major surgery. *Anesth Analg*.1998; 87:812-815.

29. Haraldsson A, Kieler-Jensen N, Nathorst-Westfelt U. Comparison of inhaled nitric oxide and inhaled aerosolized prostacyclin in the evaluation of heart transplant candidates with elevated pulmonary vascular resistance. *Chest*. 1998; 114:780-786.

30. Adatia I, Perry S, Landzberg M, et al. Inhaled nitric oxide and hemodynamic evaluation of patients with pulmonary hypertension before transplantation. *J Am Coll Cardiol*. 1995;25:1656-1664.

31. Sitbon O, Brenot F, Denjean A, et al. Inhaled nitric oxide as a screening vasodilator agent in primary pulmonary hypertension. A dose-response study and comparison with prostacyclin. *Am J Respir Crit Care Med*. 1995;151: 384-389.

32. Badesch DB, Abman SH, Simonneau G. Medical therapy for pulmonary arterial hypertension: updated ACCP evidence-based clinical practice guidelines. *Chest*. 2007;131: 1917-1928.

33. Mahajan A, Shabanie A, Varshney SM, et al. Inhaled nitric oxide in the preoperative evaluation of pulmonary hypertension in heart transplant candidates. *J Cardiothorac Vasc Anesth*.2007;1:51-56.

34. Pearl R. Perioperative management of pulmonary hypertension: covering all aspects from risk assessment to postoperative considerations. *Adv Pulm Hypertens*W inter2005: 1–19

35. Solina AR, Ginserg SH, Papp D, et al. Response to nitric oxide during cardiac surgery. *J Invest Surg*.2002; 15:5-14.

36. Mauck KF, Manjarrez EC, Cohn SL. Perioperative cardiac evaluation: assessment, risk reduction, and complication management. *Clin Geriatr Med* 2008;24(4): 595–605, vii.

37. Bapoje SR, Whitaker JF, Schulz T, et al. Preoperative evaluation of the patient with pulmonary disease. *Chest*. 2007;132:1637-1645.

38. Badesch DB, Abman SH, Ahearn GS, et al. Medical therapy for pulmonary arterial hypertension. *Chest*. 2004;126:35-62.

39. Badesch DB, Abman SH, Simonneau G, et al. Medical therapy for pulmonary arterial hypertension: summary of recommendations from the chapter on medical therapies. *Chest*. 2002;131:1917-1928.

40. Johnson SR, Metha S, Granton JT. Anticoagulation in pulmonary arterial hypertension: a qualitative systematic review. *Eur Respir J*.2006; 28:999-1004.

41. Rich S, Kaufmann E, Levy PS. The effect of high doses of calcium-channel blockers on survival in primary pulmonary hypertension. *N Engl J Med*.1992; 327:76-81.

42. Frank H, Mlczoch J, Huber K, et al. The effect of anticoagulant therapy in primary and anorectic drug-induced pulmonary hypertension. *Chest*.1997; 112:714-721.

43. Rich S, Seidlitz M, Dodin E, et al. The short-term effects of digoxin in patients with right ventricular dysfunction from pulmonary hypertension. *Chest*.1998; 114:787-792.

44. Sitbon O, Humbert M, Jais X, et al. Long-term response to calcium channel blockers in idiopathic pulmonary arterial hypertension. *Circulation*.2005; 111:3105-3111.

45. Giaid A, Yanagisawa M, Langleben D, et al. Expression of endothelin-1 in the lungs of patients with pulmonary hypertension. *N Engl J Med*.1993; 328:1732-1739.

46. Galie N, Badesch D, Oudiz R, et al. Ambrisentan therapy for pulmonary arterial hypertension. *J Am Coll Cardiol*. 2005;46:529-535.

47. Channick RN, Simonneau G, Sitbon O, et al. Effects of the dual endothelin-receptor antagonist bosentan in patients with pulmonary hypertension: a randomized placebo-controlled study. *Lancet*.2001; 358:1119-1123.

48. Rubin LJ, Badesch DB, Barst RJ, et al. Bosentan therapy for pulmonary arterial hypertension. *N Engl J Med*. 2002;346:896-903.

49. Galie N, Rubin LJ, Hoeper MM, et al. Treatment of patients with mildly symptomatic pulmonary arterial hypertension with bosentan (EARLY study): a double-blind randomised controlled trial. *Lancet*.2008; 371:2093-2100.

50. Barst RJ, Langleben D, Badesch D, et al. Treatment of pulmonary arterial hypertension with the selective endothelin-A receptor antagonist sitaxsentan. *J Am Coll Cardiol*. 2006;47:2049-2056.

51. Galie N, Olshewski H, Oudiz RJ. Ambrisentan for the treatment of pulmonary arterial hypertension: results of the ambrisentan in pulmonary arterial hypertension, randomized, double-blind, placebo-controlled, multicenter, efficacy (ARIES) study 1 and 2. *Circulation*.2008; 117:3010- 3019.

52. Barst RJ, Langleben D, Frost A, et al. Sitaxsentan therapy for pulmonary arterial hypertension. *Am J Respir Crit Care Med*.2004; 169:441-447.

53. Michelakis E, Tymchak W, Lien D, et al. Oral sildenafil is an effective and specific pulmonary vasodilator in patients with pulmonary arterial hypertension: comparison with inhaled nitric oxide. *Circulation*.2002; 105:2398-2403.

54. Lepore JJ, Maroo A, Pereira NL, et al. Effect of sildenafil on the acute pulmonary vasodilator response to inhaled nitric oxide in adults with primary pulmonary hypertension. *Am J Cardiol*.2002; 90:677-680.

55. Galie N, Ghofrani HA, Torbicki A, et al. Sildenafil citrate therapy for pulmonary arterial hypertension. *N Engl J Med*. 2005;353:2148-2157.

56. Wrishko RE, Dingemanse J, Yu A, et al. Pharmacokinetic interaction between tadalfil and bosentan in healthy male subjects. *J Clin Pharmacol*.2008; 48:610-618.

57. Barst RJ, Brundage BH, Ghofrani A, et al. Tadalafil improves exercise capacity, health related quality of life and delays time to clinical worsening in patients with symptomatic pulmonary arterial hypertension (PAH). CHEST 2008: American College of Chest Physicians 74th Annual Scientific Assembly: Abstract AS2244. Presented 28 Oct 2008

58. Strauss WL, Edelman JD. Prostanoid therapy for pulmonary arterial hypertension. *Clin Chest Med.*2007; 28:127-142.
59. Barst RJ, Rubin LJ, Long WA, et al.; The Primary Pulmonary Hypertension Study Group. A comparison of continuous intravenous epoprostenol (prostacyclin) with conventional therapy for primary pulmonary hypertension. *N Engl J Med.* 1996;334:296-335.
60. McLaughlin VV, Genthner DE, Panella MM, et al. Reduction in pulmonary vascular resistance with long-term epoprostenol (prostacyclin) therapy in primary pulmonary hypertension. *Chest.*1998;338: 273-277.
61. McLaughlin VV, Shillington A, Rich S. Survival in primary pulmonary hypertension. The impact of epoprostenol therapy. *Circulation.*20 02;106:1477-1482.
62. McLaughlin VV, Gaine SP, Barst RJ, et al. Efficacy and safety of treprostinil: an epoprostenol analog for primary pulmonary hypertension. *J Cardiovasc Pharmacol.* 2003;41:293-299.
63. Opitz CF, Wensel R, Bettmann M, et al. Assessment of the vasodilator response in primary pulmonary hypertension: comparing prostacyclin and iloprost administered by either infusion or inhalation. *Eur Heart J.*2003; 24:356-365.
64. Rex S, Schaelte G, Metzelder S, et al. Inhaled iloprost to control pulmonary artery hypertension in patients undergoing mitral valve surgery: a prospective randomized-controlled trial. *Acta Anaesthesiol Scand.*2008; 52:65-72.
65. Olshewski H, Simonneau G, Galie N, et al. Inhaled iloprost for severe pulmonary hypertension. *N Engl J Med.* 2002;347:322-329.
66. Jing ZC, Jiang X, Han ZY, et al. Iloprost for pulmonary vasodilator testing in idiopathic pulmonary arterial hypertension. *Eur Respir J.*2009; 33(6):1354-1360.
67. Ulrich S, Fischler M, Speich R, et al. Chronic thromboembolic and pulmonary arterial hypertension share acute vasoreactivity properties. *Chest.*2006; 130:841-846.
68. Lievre M, Morand S, Besse B, et al.; Beraprost et Claudication Intermittente (BERCI) Research Group. Oral Beraprost sodium, a prostaglandin I(2) analogue, for intermittent claudication: a double-blind, randomized, multicenter controlled trial. *Circulation.* 2000;102:426-431.
69. Vayssairat M. Preventive effect of oral prostacyclin analog, beraprost sodium, on digital necrosis in systemic sclerosis. French Microcirculation Society Multicenter Group for the Study of Vascular Acrosyndromes. *J Rheumatol.* 1999;26: 2173-2178.
70. Nagaya N, Uematsu M, Okano Y, et al. Effect of orally active prostacyclin analogue on survival of outpatients with primary pulmonary hypertension. *J Am Coll Cardiol.* 1999;34: 1188-1192.
71. Barst RJ, McGoon M, McLaughlin V, et al. Beraprost therapy for pulmonary arterial hypertension. *J Am Coll Cardiol.* 2003;41:2119 2125.
72. O'Callaghan DS, Gaine SP. Combination therapy and new types of agents for pulmonary arterial hypertension. *Clin Chest Med.*2007;2 8:169-185.
73. Ferguson MK. Preoperative assessment of pulmonary risk. *Chest.*1999;115:58 S-63S.
74. McGlothlin D, De Marco T. Preoperative risk assessment of pulmonary arterial hypertension patients undergoing general surgery. *Adv Pulm Hypertens*Sum mer2007: 67–72
75. Olsson JK, Zamanian RT, Feinstein JA, Doyle RL. Surgical and interventional therapies for pulmonary arterial hypertension. *Semin Respir Crit Care Med.*2005; 26:417-428.

76. Sager JS, Ahya VN. Surgical therapies for pulmonary arterial hypertension. *Clin Chest Med.*2007; 28:187-202.
77. Rothman A, Sklansky MS, Lucas VW, Kashani IA. Atrial septostomy as a bridge to lung transplantation in patients with severe pulmonary hypertension. *Am J Cardiol.* 1999; 84:682-686.
78. Law MA, Grifka RG, Mullins CE, Nihill MR. Atrial septostomy improves survival in select patients with pulmonary hypertension. *Am Heart J.*2007; 153:779-784.
79. Sandova J, Rothman A, Pulido T. Atrial septostomy for pulmonary hypertension. *Clin Chest Med.* 2001;22(3):547-560.
80. Auger WR, Kim NH, Kerr KM. Chronic thromboembolic pulmonary hypertension. *Clin Chest Med.* 2007;28: 255-269.
81. Dartevelle P, Facel E, Mussot S, et al. Surgical treatment of pulmonary arterial hypertension. *Rev Prat.* 2008;58(18): 2031-2035.
82. Klepetko W, Mayer E, Sandoval J, et al. Interventional and surgical modalities of treatment of pulmonary arterial hypertension. *J Am Coll Cardiol.*2004; 43:73S-80S.
83. Haddad F, Doyle R, Murphy DJ, Hunt SA. Right ventricular function in cardiovascular disease, part 2: pathophysiology, clinical importance, and management of right ventricular failure. *Circulation.*2008; 117:1717-1731.
84. Greyson C. Pathophysiology of right ventricular failure. *Crit Care Med.*2008; 36:57-65.
85. Kerbaul F, Rondelet B, Demester JP, et al. Effects of levosimendan versus dobutamine on pressure load-induced right ventricular failure. *Crit Care Med.*2006; 34:2814-2819.
86. Michaels AD, Chatterjee K, De Marco T. Effects of intravenous nesiritide on pulmonary vascular hemodynamics in pulmonary hypertension. *J Card Fail.* 2005;11:425-431.
87. Tongers J, Schwerdtfeger B, Klein G, et al. Incidence and clinical relevance of supraventricular tachyarrhythmias in pulmonary hypertension. *Am Heart J.*2007; 153:127-132.
88. Fattouch K, Sbraga F, Bianco G, et al. Inhaled prostacyclin, nitric oxide, and nitroprusside in pulmonary hypertension after mitral valve replacement. *J Card Surg.* 2005;20: 171-176.
89. Hohn L, Schweizer A, Morel D, et al. Circulatory failure after anesthesia induction in a patient with severe primary pulmonary hypertension. *Anesthesiology.* 1999;91:1943-1945.
90. Via G, Braschi A. Pathophysiology of severe pulmonary hypertension in the critically ill patient. *Minerva Anestesiol.* 2004;70:233-237.
91. Subramniam K, Yared JP. Management of pulmonary hypertension in the operating room. *Semin Cardiothorac Vasc Anesth.*2007; 2:119-136.
92. Rich GF, Roos CM, Anderson SM, et al. Direct effects of intravenous anesthetics on pulmonary vascular resistance in the isolated rat lung. *Anesth Analg.*1994; 78:961-966.
93. Wiedemann K, Diestelhorst C. The effect of sedation on pulmonary function. *Anaesthesist.*1995; 44:588-593.
94. Malan TP, DiNardo JA, Isner RJ, et al. Cardiovascular effects of sevoflurane compared with those of isoflurane in volunteers. *Anesthesiology.*1995; 83:918-928.
95. Bennett SR, Griffin SC. Sevoflurane versus isoflurane in patients undergoing valvular cardiac surgery. *J Cardiothorac Vasc Anesth.*2001; 15:175-178.
96. Riabova OS, Vyzhigina MA, Zhukova SG, et al. Sevoflurane and isoflurane during thoracic operations under artificial one-lung ventilation in patients at a high surgical and anesthesiological risk. *Anesteziol Reanimatol.*2007; 2:15-21.

97. Jenkins IR, Dolman J, O'Connor JP, Ansley DM. Amrinone versus dobutamine in cardiac surgical patients with severe pulmonary hypertension after cardiopulmonary bypass: a prospective, randomized double-blinded trial. *Anaesth Intensive Care*. 1997;25:245-249.

98. Kwak YL, Lee CS, Park YH, Hong YW. The effect of phenylephrine and norepinephrine in patients with chronic pulmonary hypertension. *Anaesthesia*.2002; 57:9-14.

99. Braun EB, Palin CA, Hoque CW. Vasopressin during spinal anesthesia in a patient with primary pulmonary hypertension treated with intravenous epoprostenol. *Anesth Analg*. 2004;99:36-37.

100. Schreuder WO, Schneider AJ, Groeneveld AB, Thijs LG. Effect of dopamine vs. norepinephrine on hemodynamics in septic shock. Emphasis on right ventricular performance. *Chest*.1989;95:12 82-1288.

101. Kieler-Jensen N, Lundin S, Ricksten SE. Vasodilator therapy after heart transplantation: effects of inhaled nitric oxide and intravenous prostacyclin E1, and sodium nitroprusside. *J Heart Lung Transplant*.1995; 14:436-443.

102. Solina AR, Ginsberg SH, Papp D. Dose response to nitric oxide in adult cardiac surgery. *J Clin Anesth*. 2000;13: 281-286.

103. Blaise G, Langleben D, Hubert B. Pulmonary arterial hypertension: pathophysiology and anesthetic approach. *Anesthesiology*.2003; 99:1415-1432.

104. Samama CM, Diaby M, Fellahi JL, et al. Inhibition of platelet aggregation by inhaled nitric oxide in patients with acute respiratory distress syndrome. *Anesthesiology*. 1995;83:56-65.

105. Yurtseven N, Karaca P, Uysal G, et al. A comparison of the acute hemodynamic effects of inhaled nitroglycerin and iloprost in patients with pulmonary hypertension undergoing mitral valve surgery. *Ann Thorac Cardiovasc Surg*. 2006;12:319-323.

106. Ziegler JW, Ivy DD, Fox JJ. Dipyridamole, a cGMP phosphodiesterase inhibitor, causes pulmonary vasodilatation in the ovine fetus. *Am J Physiol*. 1995;269:473-479.

107. Fullerton DA, Jaggers J, Piedalue F, et al. Effective control of refractory pulmonary hypertension after cardiac operations. *J Thorac Cardiovasc Surg* 1997;113:363–368, 368–370

108. Siobal M. Aerosolized prostacyclins. *Respir Care*. 2004;6:640-652.

109. Olscheweski H, Walmrath D, Schermuly R, et al. Aerosolized prostacyclin and iloprost in severe pulmonary hypertension. *Ann Intern Med*. 1996;9:820-824.

110. Hoeper MM, Olschewski H, Ghofrani HA, et al.; German PPH Study Group. A comparison of the acute hemodynamic effects of inhaled nitric oxide and aerosolized iloprost in primary pulmonary hypertension. *J Am Coll Cardiol*. 2000;35:176-182.

111. Stoberska-Dzierzek B, Awad H, Michler RE. The evolving management of acute right-sided heart failure in cardiac transplant recipients. *J Am Coll Cardiol*. 2001;38: 923-931.

112. Mentzer RM, Alegre CA, Nolan SP. The effects of dopamine and isoproterenol on the pulmonary circulation. *J Thorac Cardiovasc Surg*.1976; 71:807-814.

113. Camara ML, Aris A, Alvarez J. Hemodynamic effects of prostaglandin E1 and isoproterenol early after cardiac operations for mitral stenosis. *J Thorac Cardiovasc Surg*. 1992;103:1177-1185.

114. Bigatello L, Hess D, Dennehy K, et al. Sildenafil can increase the response to inhaled nitric oxide. *Anesthesiology*. 2000;92:1827-1829.

115. Kerbaul F, Rondelet B, Demester JP. Effects of levosimendan versus dobutamine on pressure load-induced right ventricular failure. *Crit Care Med*.2006; 34:2814-2819.

116. Fullerton DA, Jones SD, Grover FL, et al. Adenosine effectively controls pulmonary hypertension after cardiac operations. *Ann Thorac Surg*.1996; 61:1118-1124.

117. Auler JO, Carmona MJ, Bocchi EA, et al. Low doses of inhaled nitric oxide in heart transplant recipients. *J Heart Lung Transplant*.1996; 15:443-450.

118. Rettig GF, Schieffer HJ. Acute effects of intravenous milrinone in heart failure. *Eur Heart J*.1989; 10:39-43.

119. Colucci WS. Cardiovascular effects of milrinone. *Am Heart J*.1991; 121:1945-1947.

120. Kihara S, Kawai A, Fukuda T, et al. Effects of milrinone for right ventricular failure after left ventricular assist device implantation. *Heart Vessels*.2002; 16:69-71.

121. Fonger JD, Borkon AM, Baumgartner WA, et al. Acute right ventricular failure following heart transplantation: Improvement with prostaglandin E1 and right ventricular assist. *J Heart Transplant*.1986; 5:317-321.

122. Weiss CI, Park JV, Bolman RM. Prostaglandin E1 for treatment of elevated pulmonary vascular resistance in patients undergoing cardiac transplantation. *Transplant Proc*. 1989; 21:2555-2556.

123. Tritapepe L, Voci P, Cogliati A, et al. Successful weaning from cardiopulmonary bypass with central venous prostaglandin E1 and left atrial norepinephrine infusion in patients with acute pulmonary hypertension. *Crit Care Med*. 1999;27:2180-2183.

124. Ozdogan ME, Erer D, Iriz E, et al. Right-to-left shunt through a patent foramen ovale left open in the management of acute right heart failure after heart transplantation. *J Heart Lung Transplant*.2008; 27:135.

125. Safdar Z. Phase 2 and 3 clinical trials in pulmonary arterial hypertension. *Adv Pulm Hypertens*.2008; 7(1):228-234.

126. NIH Clinical Trials. http://clinicaltrials.gov/ct2/results?term=pulmonary+hypertension. Accessed online 01 Apr 2009

127. Langleben D. Endothelin receptor antagonists in the treatment of pulmonary arterial hypertension. *Clin Chest Med*. 2007;28:117-125.

128. Ichinose F, Adrie C, Hurford WE, et al. Selective pulmonary vasodilatation induced by aerosolized zaprinast. *Anesthesiology*.1998; 88:410-416.

129. Salzberg SP, Filsoufi F, Anyanwu A, et al. High-risk mitral valve surgery: perioperative hemodynamic optimization with nesiritide (BNP). *Ann Thorac Surg*. 2005;80: 502-506.

130. Ramakrishna G, Sprung J, Ravi BS, et al. Impact of pulmonary hypertension on the outcomes of noncardiac surgery: predictors of perioperative morbidity and mortality. *J Am Coll Cardiol*.2005; 10: 1691-1699.

Cardiopulmonary Bypass and Pulmonary Injury

The Extracorporeal Circulation Circuit VersusB ioengineeringB iomaterials

22

José Francisco Biscegli, Fábio Nunes Dias, Cynara Viterbo Montoya, Sergio Luiz Nogaroto, and Edmo Atique Gabriel

During cardiopulmonary bypass (CPB), interaction of blood with nonbiological surfaces of the materials, like the tubing, oxygenator, and heart-lung machine cannula, results in the activation of several humoral cascades, such as the kallikrein-kinin system, coagulation and fibrinolytic system, and complement system.[1]

The extracorporeal circulation (ECC) procedure is associated with a range of operatory trauma-related side effects, blood contact with the surface of medical devices, heparin neutralization by protamine, and ischemia and reperfusion, which are caused by blood in bypassed tissues such as the heart and the lungs. The result of humoral and cell defense reactions is called the *systemic inflammatory response syndrome*. This syndrome comprises the hemostatic disturbances that are manifested as bleeding, platelet activation, and generation of macrothrombi and microthrombi, which may consequently result in thrombotic events, such as cerebral vascular accidents, which may cause such severe neurological symptoms as cognitive dysfunction. The activation of the complement system has often been deemed responsible for many of these occurrences associated with ECC.[2]

Complement is a multicomponent, complex, and highly evolved system that not only protects against invading pathogens but also contributes to regulate other internal defense systems.[3] The complement system is comprised of about 30 proteins (both receptor and regulating) present in the plasma and cell membrane and acting on the defense against foreign substances, including microorganisms, foreign bodies, and the remains of apoptotic cells.[4,5] The clinical consequences for complement system activation associated with incompatibility during ECC draws our attention to a better knowledge about how complement activation is caused by the contact with biomaterials, motivating the search and development of materials with little or no possibility of activating complement.[2] If there is also activation of cellular components of the defense systems, including neutrophils, platelets, and endothelial cells,[6] the inflammatory response is responsible for the "postperfusion syndrome," characterized by renal, pulmonary, cardiac, and cerebral dysfunction.[7]

Bioengineering always searches for a negative outcome that should be dealt with accordingly during complex procedures like an extracorporeal circuit in cardiopulmonary surgery. The following negative outcomes were considered: mortality; morbidity; prolonged stay in the intensive care unit (ICU) and hospital; neurological injuries (stroke, longer confusion); reduced quality of life (QOL) after surgery.

To minimize the negative outcomes of cardiopulmonary surgery, hemodialysis procedures, and liver transplantation systems, biomedical actions will reduce the contact surface with blood and develop new biomaterials for use in this blood-and-device circuit. In addition, the manufacture of the synthetic surfaces of the extracorporeal circuit used in cardiac surgery and hemodialysis must incorporate techniques that improve biocompatibility in an effort to minimize the rheological disturbances associated with blood extracorporealization. While considering design characteristics, focus must be given to minimize the dynamics forces of shear stress in a moving fluid column[8,9] and blood stasis, both of which enhance trauma to the blood cells and noncell elements. However, the ability of a blood gas exchange device to transfer gas is still the ultimate priority in determining its clinical utility.[10]

E.A.G abriel(✉)
Department of Surgery, Division of Cardiovascular Surgery
FederalU niversityof Sa oP aulo, SaoP aulo, Brazil
e-mail:e dag@uol.com.br

E.A. Gabriel and T. Salerno (eds.), *Principles of Pulmonary Protection in Heart Surgery*,
DOI: 10.1007/978-1-84996-308-4_22, © Springer-Verlag London Limited 2010

Material *biocompatibility*, defined as its capacity to minimize the reaction when in contact with biological tissues or fluids in a specific application, basically refers to inflammatory responses induced by such material. One example is the material incompatibility of cardiovascular devices that might cause several clinical manifestations during ECC, causing immediate and late sequelae that may be temporary or permanent, such as sudden and complete stent obstruction, acute and subacute thrombotic occlusion in grafts and angioplasty, and embolic and thrombotic complications.[11]

In recent years, the mortality rates have remained the same although patient risks are rising continuously. Stroke and neurologic injury are the "hot topics," especially as stroke is connected to mortality since almost one third of the same 7% of patients that have it after heart surgery will die in the first postoperative month.[8]

Neurologic injuries are obviously associated with atheromatous plaque, which is found in the aorta before surgery and is displaced during surgery. In this case, a new generation of special aorta cannula to catch the debris and microemboli (Embolex®, Edwards Lifesciences, Irvine, CA, USA) was developed by the aorta protection experts at Edwards.

CPB, liver transplantation procedure, and hemodialysis are subject to adverse effects (AEs) due to ECC of blood in stranger surface (non-endothelial).

Hemodialysis was once associated with severe anaphylactic reactions, in which complement activation was connected to so-called first-use syndrome whenever patients used a new dialyzer. With the practice of reusing dialyzers, this reaction was calmed; it still occurs, but less frequently. These inflammatory responses still contribute to the occurrence of arteriosclerosis in uremic patients.[2]

Due to improvements in CPB and hemodialysis, the focus of AEs has shifted from fatal complications, like death, toward more subtle effects, like neurological pulmonary dysfunction.

Cardiac surgery is associated with pulmonary and systemic inflammatory response. The pulmonary effects of this inflammatory reaction are often simple and include decreased lung compliance, pulmonary edema, increased intrapulmonary shunt fraction, and decreased functional residual capacity (FRC).[12]

Considering the ECC circuit used in cardiac surgery, the typical patient enters the system complaining of angina. Then, the patient usually is referred to a cardiologist, who guides this case through the system. The system pathway may be described as a decision-making tree starting with the least-invasive treatment and perhaps ending with the most invasive. The typical treatment path is shown in the flowchart of Fig. 22.1.[13] Table 22.1 compares some of these procedures and defines omeofthe te rmsus ed.

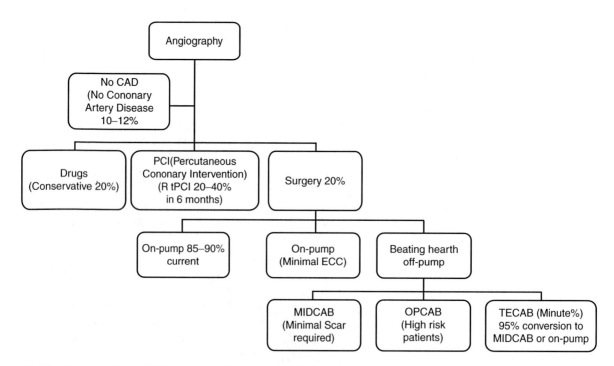

Fig.22.1 Patientpa thway. *ECC* extracorporeal circulation, *MIDCAB* minimally invasive coronary artery bypass, *OPCAB* off-pump coronary artery bypass, *TECAB*t otallye ndoscopicc oronarya rterybypa ss

Table 22.1 Comparison of prodedures and definition of terms used

MIDCAB: minimal invasive direct coronary artery bypass (CAB)	Originally on pump Today some cases off pump Commonly all coronary artery bypass grafting (CABG) with mini-incisions on or off pump are called MIDCAB
Port access	System by heart port with flexible endoscopes Commonly on pump
Endoscopic surgery	Suitable for both CABG and valve procedures Commonly on pump
TECAB:tota lly endoscopic CAB	Robot-assisted and computer-enhanced surgery through three or four ports; mostly on pump Recentlyfi rst off-pump procedures
Beating heart surgery: off-pump CAB	Originally off-pump coronary artery bypass (OPCAB; CTS, Cupertino, CA, USA) performed through ministernotomy Today commonly full sterno-tomy; more or less all off-pump CAB grouped under this term

Cardiac artery bypass graft (CABG) with ECC and cardioplegia often causes inflammatory responses that might affect the postoperative period. CABG without ECC has drawn attention since it results in significant reduction of ECC-related AEs.[14] The worst-case scenario in these procedures is the surgery on pump current and minimal ECC on pump due to biggest contact surface in the ECC circuit with the oxygenator, tubing, filters, cannulae, and blood aspirator during ECC.

With that in mind, and since one of the largest contact surfaces in ECC is the oxygenators, manufacturers have tried to reduce the contact surface in oxygenators in a systemic fashion. As an example, the Vital oxygenator (Nipro Medical, São Paulo, Brazil), by significantly reducing the contact surface with the oxygenator, eliminated siliconized sponge and filters with large surfaces from the venous drainage blood line and changed of the heat exchanger position to inside the prepump venous container, which means, the blood is not subjected to a pressure chamber, like in models having heat exchanger in the postpump are next to the oxygenation chamber. In the case of the Vital oxygenator, a significant reduction in shear stress, which causes critical cell damage in the ECC circuit, was possible.[15] This design conceived for the Vital oxygenator allowed a reduction of about 120 mL of the priming volume in the oxygenation chamber, with the advantages associated with this improvement.[16]

Most "beating hearts" do not use ECC (perfusion). The off-pump beating heart procedure seems to be growing in heart surgery, basically CAB without ECC, which means a great reduction of surface contact with blood, which means a decreased inflammatory response in the postoperative period.

22.1 Reductiono fExp osure to a Synthetic Surface

These is no doubt that the exposure of blood to synthetic surfaces is related to onset of a massive inflammatory response to CPB,[16] and it is interesting to relate the reduction in circuit volume to this decreased response. In practice, however, it is highly unlikely that such a simple maneuver will produce such a result. Most of the surface area involved is connected to the oxygenator, container, and any additional filters in the extracorporeal blood circuit, devices whose contact surface is basically made of plastic. A large surface area is currently mandatory as adequate stimulus for inflammation.

22.2 Advantageso fPl astics in Bioengineering

For thousands of years, in ancient cultures like Egypt, Babylon, and others, materials like gold, silver, copper, and lead were used as part of the skeletons of mummies. Certainly, this was done without any concerns regarding biocompatibility, a concept that was introduced only 50 years ago.[17] The use of biomaterials could only become a safe practice with the arrival of aseptic surgical techniques, developed in mid-1860s. Previous surgical procedures, either involving biomaterials or not, generally failed due to infection, which was aggravated by the presence of biomaterial.

The first biomaterials to succeed were those connected to the skeletal system, including several materials, such as vanadium and stainless steel. In World War II, the importance of polymers was noticed when it was verified that pilots wounded by plastic fragments from combat airplanes did not present chronic AEs from the presence of these fragments in their bodies.

So, methyl polymethacrylate (acrylic) became widely used as a biomaterial.[18]

Even though completely biocompatible materials have not yet been found, materials with low risk of complication in the cardiovascular area have been researched, developed, and utilized for years. Bioengineering or biomedical engineering has combined engineering knowledge with medical needs to develop new materials, devices, and machines to fulfill medical needs regarding health care improvement.

Medical products are responsible for about 60% of the entire volume of plastic material consumed every year, and according to a report from the Business Communications Company (*RP-121U – Plastics for Medical Devices*), the North American market of plastic for medical goods was estimated as approximately 1 billion kg annually until the end of 2002, with a growth of about 4.3% per year, with prospects of consumption of 1.3 billion kg annually until 2008.[19]

The attraction of plastic materials for biomedical applications lies in the diversity of types and properties available. In theory, it should be possible to tailor the material used to each particular application, but in general other important properties are sacrificed for economic reasons.

It is essential in medical use to guarantee that a product is not changed both in formulation and in properties. The same properties are attainable with different formulations, but this is often unacceptable for medical use. For example, polyacetal has a large number of additives permitted for food contact use, and a given product may show considerable batch-to-batch variations. When used inside the body, as this material is, the user must know that the same additives are always present, or tissue reaction studies become meaningless and possibly dangerously misleading.

Additives may be bad news, as in the case of polyvinyl chloride (PVC), which is the most widely applied blood-contacting material for the production of blood and blood component storage bags, catheters, and tubing for CPB devices.[20] PVC is widely used in the production of a number of medical devices, being responsible for about 25% of the whole plastic material utilized in medical applications, but it requires the use of plastificants in its composition. The main plastificants available are based on phthalate esters, including di-2-ethylhexyl phthalate (DEHP), also known as dioctylphthalate (DOP), one of the most commonly utilized plastificants in the production of medical devices.

Studies have shown that DEHP, besides being objectionable and controversial, might migrate from medical devices in different levels, exposing patients to toxicity risks. However, the development of plastificants alternatives to DEHP, such as trioctyl trimellitate, di(*n*-decyl) phthalate, polyadipates, and poly(ethylene oxide), in copolymers does not hinder the possibility of migration of plastificant from the PVC composition.[21]

In certain cases, the leaching of these with blood contact or body tissues may have a harmful effect, and for an already ill patient it may be just the final insult, as evidenced by inflammatory responses due to surface contact with blood for a long time.[22] In practice, certain materials have become prominent in use because they are completely satisfactory or because they offer the most acceptable compromise (e.g., polycarbonate, PVC, polyethylene, and polypropylene).

The judgment on how satisfactory a material is will include consideration of end-use properties and user acceptance; processability, including sterilization where necessary; and availability at an acceptable cost and sterilizable.

To sterilize medical devices, the most used sterilization technologies are vapor, ethylene oxide (EO), gamma irradiation, and electron beam. For medical devices, specially the thermosensitive ones, EO is the best choice as it is a sterilizing agent with great bactericide, sporicide, and virucide action, which significantly allowed and contributed to evolution of more complex and delicate medical devices. However, after the sterilization process, residual concentrations of EO and its derivatives ethylene chloridrine (ECH) and ethylene glycol (EG) may be left in medical devices. These are potentially toxic, mutagenic, and carcinogenic residues and must be removed from medical devices to avoid AEs in patients.[24,25]

ISO 10993-7 (*Biological Evaluation of Medical Devices – Ethylene Oxide Sterilization Residuals*) specifies maximum limits allowed for these substances based on a risk analysis to the patient, which mainly relates the concentration of these residues to the exposure time of the patient to the device.[26]

Other consideration about the combination of plastic, contact surface, and plastic processability for use in disposable medical devices is whether the product has a relatively low cost and high volume or a low product volume with a high markup to make sure disposable medical application is possible. The high-volume group is represented by disposable items like oxygenators, infusion sets, storage containers, and tubing.

In the other hand, the development of medical devices that contact physiological fluids is a rapidly increasing field of study.

However, different reactions of device surfaces in contact with blood components, like in an extracorporeal circuit during cardiac surgery, are still important factors that set limitations to the use of synthetic polymeric materials in contact with blood.

To ensure the possibility of using these plastic materials, those in the bioengineering field research various methods and device designs to achieve low surface contact with blood.

Other methods of surface modification have been proposed to improve hemocompatibility of plastic materials. Most of them are based on grafting from antithrombogenic biomolecules (mainly heparin).

Since 1980, heparinized ECC surfaces were largely researched, both experimentally and clinically, and the research showed them to be efficient in reducing the systemic inflammatory response, reducing morbidity and mortality, besides providing other complement activation-related benefits.[27]

The inflammatory response, mainly in the lungs and in the blood lost in heart surgery using the current ECC or mini-extracorporeal circuit of blood with an oxygenator, reservoir, and filter, is due to the large area of surface contact. Consequently, device design, such as the Nipro Vital oxygenator concept, is an improvement compared to other oxygenators.

Every medical article, before commercialization, must be approved by regulating bodies such as Food and Drug Administration (FDA) in the United States, European Medicines Agency (EMEA) in the European Community, and the National Sanitary Surveillance Agency (ANVISA) in Brazil. This approval is based on the presentation of data, from biological essays, ensuring the safety of the use of the medical device. These essays determine whether the contact with the material used in the medical device has any AE on patients. Thus, the essays include cytotoxicity tests, sensitization, irritation, systemic toxicity, and implants tests, required by ISO 10993-1, which besides confirming the safety of materials individually or in group, also confirm whether manufacturing processes hinder product safety for use.[28]

The selection of materials for developing medical devices must have criteria regarding use adjustment, physical and chemical properties, and their interaction with bodily fluids and tissues. So, ISO 10993-1:2003 indicated a selection of tests that involve biological evaluation and must be conducted by considering exposure of the device or material to the body, which must be classified as limited exposure (<24 h), prolonged exposure (24 h to 30 days), or permanent contact (>30 days).

Depending on the purpose and exposure time for the device, there may need to be tests for cytotoxicity, sensitization, irritation, intracutaneous reactivity, systemic acute toxicity, subacute and subchronic toxicity, genotoxicity, implantation reaction, and hemocompatibility. The tests may involve *in vitro, ex vivo, in vivo* assays and animal trial and clinical evaluation.

However, biologic evaluation is not limited to new developments. Any changes to a final product, such as in the formulation of materials used or in the manufacturing and sterilization processes, requires a new biologic evaluation.

ECC devices, such as oxygenators and hemodialyzers, may potentially activate complements and result in pulmonary injury. Therefore, platelet function tests and complement activation tests are extremely useful for the development of new materials and devices.

When tests involve blood interaction with devices or materials, the tests may fit in the following categories: thrombosis, coagulation, platelets, hematology, or complement. However, both in the development of new products and materials and in any changes having an impact on the final product, the analysis must be always performed under ISO 10993-1:2003.[29]

The flowchart in Fig. 22.2 summarizes the decision-making process for determining the need to perform testsin volvingbloodi nteractionw ithbi omaterials.

According to Block (1972), the characteristics of an ideal hemocompatible biomaterial are sterilizability; easy and low-cost manufacture; resistance to mechanical strengths; lack of allergenic or hypersensitivity properties; noncarcinogenic properties; lack of inciting an inflammatory response; and no physical modification in vivo.[30] According to Hastings (1983), the main concerns in biomaterial development are fatigue failure; surface wear; corrosion/degradation; deformation or creep; AEs to tissues; ion sensitization; wear debris.[22]

Considering these types of biomaterials and the design of devices, bioengineering development research to decrease the inflammatory response in the postoperative period of cardiac surgery considers the most aggressive device with blood contact. Some studies

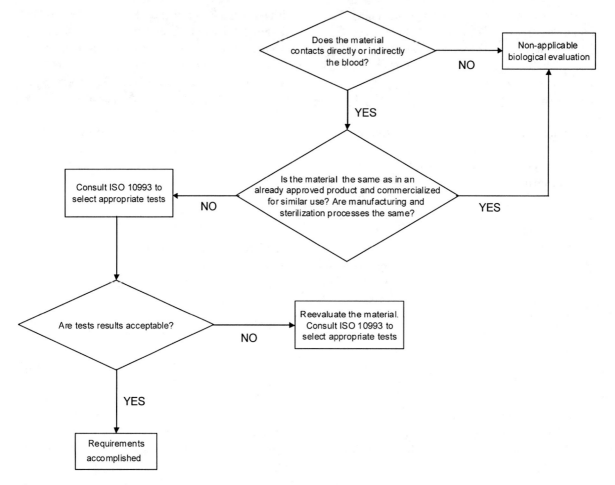

Fig.22.2 Flowchart of medical device biological evaluation. (Adapted from ISO 10993-1:2003(E)[29])

supported that variances in membrane oxygenator hemolysis are a function of design variables, such as membrane surface area, prime volume, and blood path length, rather than of pressure drop. The plasma hemoglobin freed from each membrane oxygenator was negligible when compared with typical plasma hemoglobin levels generated during routine CPB.[9]

22.3 TheFut ureo fB iomaterials

After about 60 years of innovation and development, biomaterials is a promising field, but regenerative medicine will considerably reduce the need for synthetic materials in the human body.[31]

In the future, use will be made of the so-called smart biomaterials, composed of structural elements capable of interpreting biological signals and responding appropriately (e.g., regenerative implants made of autologous cells cultured on a matrix scaffolding.[32]

According to JANdt (2007), the future of biomaterials is related to the recognition of biological and biochemical conditions of the human body, in processes involving proteins and cells, at a nanoscale biointerface. These biomaterials will be not able to induce inflammatory responses during and after implantation. The proposed biomaterials involve biological material, DNA, and stem cells, however, require rigorous criteria and should be carefully evaluated because there are still technical and ethical conflicts to be overcome.[33]

References

1. Hoel TN, Videm V, Baksaas SV, Mollnes TE, Brosstad F, Vennevig JLS. Comparison of Duraflot II – coated cardiopulmonary bypass circuit and atrillium-coated-oxygenator during open-heart surgery. *Perfusion*.2004; 1:177-184.

2. Nilsson B, Ekdahl KN, Mollnes TE, Lambris JD. The role of complement in biomaterial-induced inflammation. *Mol Immunol*.2007;44: 82-94.

3. Lambris JD, Reid KBM, Volanakis JE. The evolution, structure, biology and pathophysiology of complement. *Trends Immunol Today*199 9;20(5):207

4. Morikis D, Lambris JD. Structural aspects and design of low molecular-mass complement inhibitors. *Biochem Soc Trans* 2001;30:1026–1036

5. Sahu A, Lambris JD. Complement inhibitors: a resurgent concept in anti-inflammatory therapeutics. *Immunopharmacology*.2000;49:13 3-148.

6. van Oeveren W, Kazatchkine MD, Descamps-Latscha B, Maillet F, Fischer E, Carpentier A, Wildevuur CR. Deleterious effects of cardiopulmonary bypass. A prospective study of bubble versus membrane oxygenation. *J Thorac Cardiovasc Surg*19 85;89(6):888–899

7. Kirklin JK, Westaby S, Blackstone EH, Kirklin JW, Chenoweth DE, Pacifico AD. Complement and the damaging effects of cardiopulmonary bypass. *J Thorac Cardiovasc Surg*.1983;86(6):845- 857.

8. De Somer D, Foubert L, Vanackere M, Dujardin D, Delanghe J, Van Nooten G. Impact of oxygenator design on hemolysis, shear stress, and white blood cell and platelet counts. *J Cardiothorac Vasc Anesth*.1996; 10(7):884-889.

9. Bearss MG. The relationship between membrane oxygenator blood path pressure drop and hemolysis: an in-vitro evaluation. *J Extra Corpor Technol*.1993; 25(3):87-92.

10. Fried DW, Bell-Thomson J. Oxygen transfer efficiency of three microporous polypropylene membrane oxygenators. *Perfusion*.1991;6:105- 114.

11. Gorbet MB, Sefton MV. Biomaterial-associated thrombosis: roles of coagulation factors, complement, platelets and leukocytes. *Biomaterials*.2004; 25:5681-5703.

12. Miranda DR, Gommers D, Papadakos PJ, et al. Mechanical ventilation affects pulmonary inflammation in cardiac surgery patients: the role of the open-lung concept. *J Cardiothorac Vasc Anesth*.2007; 21:279-284.

13. Butler B, Kurusz M. Gaseous microemboli: a review. *Perfusion*.1990;5:81-99.

14. Czernya M, Baumera H, Kiloa J, et al. Inflammatory response and myocardial injury following coronary artery bypass grafting with or without cardiopulmonary bypass. *Eur J Cardiothorac Surg*.2000; 17:737-742.

15. Brian BF. *Comparative analysis of shear stress and pressure drop in membrane oxygenators*. White paper. ARVADA, CO: Cobe Laboratories Inc; 1995

16. Finn A, Rebuck N, Strobel S, Moat N, Elliott M. Systemic inflammation during paediatric cardiopulmonary bypass: changes in neutrophil adhesive properties. *Perfusion* 1993; 89(1):39–48

17. Hildebrand HF, Blanchemain N, Mayer G, Chai F, Lefebvre M, Boschin F. Surface coatings for biological activation and functionalization of medical devices. *Surf Coatings Technol*. 2006;200:6318-6324.

18. Park JB. The biomedical engineering handbook. 2nd ed. In: Bronzino JD, ed. *Biomaterials*. Boca Raton: CRC Press; 2000

19. North American medical device plastics market continues to rise. Plastics Additives & Compounding. September/October 2003

20. Granados DL, Jiménez A, Cuadrado TR. Assessment of parameters associated to the risk of PVC catheter reuse. *J Biomed Mater Res (Appl Biomater)*.2001; 58:505-510.

21. Messori M, Toselli M, Pilati F, et al. Prevention of plasticizer leaching from PVC medical devices by using organic–inorganic hybrid coatings. *Polymer*.2004; 45:805-813.

22. Hastings GW. *Medical application of plastics*. Hartshill: Bio-Medical Engineering Unit Medical Institute; 1983

23. Mendes GCC, Brandão TRS, Silva CLM. Ethylene oxide sterilization of medical devices: a review. *Am J Infect Control*.2007; 35:574-581.

24. Lucas AD, Merritt K, Hitchins VM, et al. Residual ethylene oxide in medical devices and device material. *Journal of Biomedical Materials Research, Part B Applyed Biomaterials*. 2003;66B(2):548-552.

25. ISO (International Standards Organization). Sterilization of health care products – requirements for validation and routine control – industrial moist heat sterilization. ISO 11134. Geneva;1994

26. ISO (International Standards Organization). Biological evaluation of medical devices – ethylene oxide sterilization residuals. ISO 10993-7. Geneva; 1995

27. Hsu C. Heparin-coated cardiopulmonary bypass circuits: current status. *Perfusion*2001; 16(5):417–428

28. Dunne P. Design and manufacture of a multiple material sample for implantation testing of thermoplastic materials used in a medical device. *Polym Test*.2005; 24:684-687.

29. ISO (International Standards Organization). 10993-1. Biological evaluation of medical devices – part 1: evaluation and testing. Geneva; 2003

30. Bloch B, Hastings GW. *Plastic materials in surgery*. 2nd ed. Springfield: Thomas; 1972

31. Ratner BD, Bryant SJ. Biomaterials: where we have been and where we are going. Annu Rev Biomed Eng 2004;6: 41–75

32. Friedman CD. Future directions in biomaterial implants and tissue engineering. *Arch Facial Plast Surg*2001,3: 136–137

33. Jandt KD. Evolutions, revolutions and trends in biomaterials science – a perspective. *Adv Eng Mater* 2007;9(12): 1035–1050

David J. Chambers, Hazem B. Fallouh and Nouhad A. Kassem

23.1 Introduction

Postoperative lung complications, arising from lung injury, occur during conventional cardiac surgery and during transplantation of the lung; both these procedures involve cardiopulmonary bypass (CPB). Lung injury is associated with various pathophysiological events that occur during CPB or the long-term storage of lungs during preservation. These events include ischemia-reperfusion (I/R)/hypoxia-reoxygenation, inflammation, and generation of reactive oxygen species (ROS). To counteract these adverse pathophysiological effects, there are a number of techniques currently in use to protect the lung during cardiac surgery and lung transplantation. These include the use of continuous inflation or ventilation, various protective or preservation solutions, together with the potential for exploiting the endogenous protective mechanism of preconditioning. This chapter briefly reviews the causes and mechanisms of lung injury and the techniques introduced to ameliorate this injury but focuses predominantly on the current evidence for preconditioning protection of the lung, including methods of initiating preconditioning in the lung (with emphasis on potentially clinically relevant triggers) to improve lung protection or preservation.

D. J. Chambers (✉)
CardiacSur gicalR esearch/CardiothoracicS urgery,
The Rayne Institute
(King's College London), Guy's and St Thomas' NHS
Foundation Trust, St Thomas' Hospital, London, UK
e-mail:da vid.chambers@kcl.ac.uk

23.2 Lungl njury

Lung injury resulting in pulmonary dysfunction occurs in many clinical conditions, including trauma, chronic obstructive pulmonary disease (COPD), cardiac surgery involving CPB, and lung transplantation.[1-4] This lung injury (Fig. 23.1) occurs predominantly as a result of ischemia-reperfusion, with the consequent effects of inflammation (particularly during CPB) and the generation and release of ROS.[1,5,6] This review concentrates on the surgically induced causes of lung injury that occur as a result of either CPB or transplantation.

23.2.1 Cardiac Surgery

During cardiac surgery, CPB is used for the majority of operations, and postoperative pulmonary dysfunction represents a significant problem. It manifests as abnormal gas exchange and poor lung mechanics arising from an increased pulmonary edema and vascular resistance, resulting in reduced lung compliance.[5] The severity of lung dysfunction varies within a wide spectrum, between an asymptomatic low-grade acute lung injury (ALI), which occurs in most surgical patients, to a less-common but severe condition of acute respiratory distress syndrome (ARDS).[4,5] Lung tissue is supplied with blood from two arterial networks; the predominant circulation (90–95%) from the pulmonary artery supplies deoxygenated blood from the right side of the heart (which becomes oxygenated via ventilation from the alveoli), and the bronchial circulation supplies oxygenated blood from the left side of the heart, with the two systems having

E.A. Gabriel and T. Salerno (eds.), *Principles of Pulmonary Protection in Heart Surgery*,
DOI: 10.1007/978-1-84996-308-4_23, © Springer-Verlag London Limited 2010

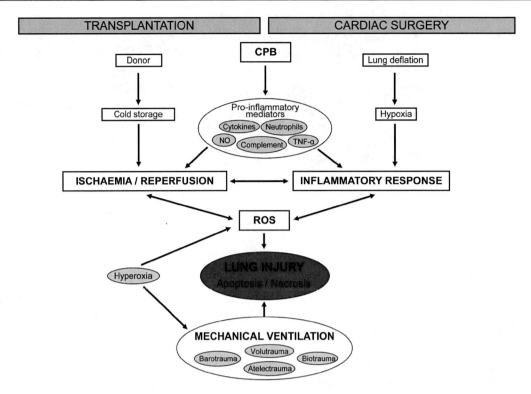

Fig. 23.1 Schematic diagram of the potential pathways inducing lung injury during either cardiac surgery or lung transplantation, highlighting the interrelationship between these two procedures. *CPB* cardiopulmonary bypass, *ROS* reactive oxygen species, *TNF-α* tumor necrosis factor alpha

anastomotic connections between them.[4,5]. The mechanism of oxygenation in lung tissue is therefore complicated and largely dependent on alveolar ventilation.[7]

During CPB, pulmonary circulation and alveolar ventilation are stopped, and the lungs are (generally) deflated. Studies from our laboratory[8] have demonstrated that lung deflation induces an injury per se that can be ameliorated by addition of phosphodiesterase (PDE) inhibitors to the perfusate. The maintained bronchial circulation represents only a small fraction (~5%) of the normal supply; thus, during CPB the deflated lungs will be subjected to a degree of ischemia or hypoxia. However, this is unlikely to be the only mechanism inducing lung injury during CPB, and others are well recognized, such as the effect of mechanical ventilation[9] during anesthesia and hyperoxic ventilation[10] inducing oxygen injury from high F_{IO_2} (with increasing ROS). Most important, however, CPB is known to induce a systemic inflammatory response that can have a severe impact on lung function.[4,5] CPB induces a cascade of proinflammatory mediators (such as cytokines, complement, neutrophil activation, together with increased elastase activity, arachidonic acid derivatives, platelet-activating factors, and excess nitric oxide [NO] and endothelin 1), which all promote lung injury and postoperative lung dysfunction.[1,4,5,7] Associated with all of these mediators is the initiation of ROS, which will have an impact on the lung during reoxygenation or reperfusion,[6,7] leading to increased lung apoptosis or necrosis. As a consequence of this multifactorial etiology of lung injury during cardiac surgery, attempting to dissect out a single mechanism is probably impractical. The widely used term *ischemia-reperfusion* injury would inevitably include effects of other mechanisms (such as mechanical ventilation, hyperoxia, deflation, and inflammation) (Fig. 23.1).

23.2.2 Transplantation

Lung transplantation, the therapy of choice for end-stage lung disease since the early 1980s, presents additional problems to those seen during cardiac surgery and CPB.[1,11] Donor lung selection is critical, and the success of a donor lung depends on many factors inherent in the characteristics of the donor,[12] which makes for donor lung shortages. The use of donor lungs from non-heart-beating donors (NHBDs) has increased with considerable success, but again with characteristic additional factors for lung injury.[13] Donor lungs usually require cold ischemic storage prior to implantation and will thus experience all the features associated with ischemia-reperfusion injury; these include sodium pump inactivation, cellular ionic overload, oxidative stress during both ischemia and reperfusion with the associated mitochondrial injury and the inflammatory response associated with I/R and CPB.[1,4,7,11] All of these events can lead to either apoptosis or necrosis, which will cause lung dysfunction (primary graft failure) or acute rejection.[6,14]

23.3 CurrentT echniques for Lung Protection

The protection of lungs during transplantation is associated with a number of problems in addition to that of the lung being subjected to CPB. Initially, the lung donor must be carefully assessed to ensure that the donor lung is in optimal condition and able to withstand prolonged ischemia-reperfusion. Thus, donor history is important, with factors such as smoking, race, gender, and lung disease primary considerations. Other important examinations for the assessment include arterial blood gases, chest X-ray, bronchoscopy, lung examination when removed from the donor, whether the donor was brain dead, whether mechanical ventilation has occurred and might have induced injury, and any trauma to the lung suffered by the donor.[1,12] Lungs deemed suitable for transplantation are generally subjected to relatively prolonged ischemic storage; the choice of storage or flush solution becomes critical to the recovery of the lung. Most centers select a single preservation or flush solution for technical simplicity; most of these solutions were originally designed for abdominal organ or heart preservation. Thus, the intracellular-type solutions (such as the Euro-Collins® solution [kidney preservation] or University of Wisconsin® [UW[solution [liver]) or extracellular-type solutions (such as the Celsior® solution) have been adapted for use in the lung. More recently, the low-potassium dextran (LPD) solution (Perfadex®) developed for lung preservation has been increasingly used in transplant centers.[11] In our

laboratory, we have utilized the extracellular-type low-potassium St. Thomas's Hospital cardioplegic solution as a combination heart-lung preservation solution and shown that, in rat lungs stored for 6 h, it can be used with considerable success compared to Euro-Collins solution.[15] In addition, use of protective additives (such as PDE inhibitors, which increase intracellular cyclic adenosine monophosphate [cAMP] levels) further enhances the efficacy of this solution.[16] Other important factors during the storage of lungs include the pressure, volume, and temperature of the flush solution; the temperature during storage; and whether the lungs are stored inflated and oxygenated.[1,11] Inflation of lungs during storage improves aerobic metabolism and preserves lung surfactant integrity and epithelial fluid transport. However, it is important to limit the inflation volume as well as the oxygen content to avoid exacerbating injury.[1,11]

Despite the evidence that lung inflation during storage is beneficial, during CPB lungs are generally maintained in a deflated state, and we[8] have demonstrated that deflation per se causes lung injury, with addition of PDE inhibitors to the perfusate reducing injury. It is possible, therefore, that mechanical ventilation during CPB could also improve lung protection, but this may cause technical problems for the surgeon during cardiac surgery[4] as well as the potential for additional injury.[9] Other potentially beneficial techniques include modifications to the CPB circuit by heparin coating so that neutrophil activation is minimized, as is the inflammatory response (cytokine release, etc.). In addition, hemofiltration during CPB may limit edema formation as well as remove cytokines and other detrimental inflammatory mediators.[4]

As well as limiting injury to the lung during storage (ischemia) or CPB when the lung is ischemic or hypoxic and deflated, there are a number of strategies that have been suggested for the reperfusion/reoxygenation phase. These include procedures such as reduced reperfusion pressure for a short period in an attempt to limit edema formation, leukocyte sequestration, and a protective ventilation strategy with lower ventilation volumes and positive end-expiratory pressure (PEEP).[11] In addition, pharmaceutical strategies such as the application of endogenous NO, either directly or by NO donors, to compensate for the reduced NO induced by ischemia-reperfusion of lungs, the use of prostaglandins to increase cAMP and to inhibit cytokine production, inhibition of the complement cascade, and surfactant therapy may all have beneficial effects.[1,11]

More recently, the endogenous protective technique of preconditioning has been advocated as a potential therapy against lung injury during both cardiac surgery (with CPB) and during lung transplantation.

23.4 Preconditioning

Ischemic preconditioning (IPC) was first described in the heart in 1986 [17]; it was shown to be an endogenous mechanism of protection by which myocardial infarction could paradoxically be limited by several brief periods of ischemia and reperfusion before an extended period of "lethal" ischemia.[18] Ischemic preconditioning was found to be effective in all species examined (including humans) and has also been shown to be effective in other organs, including the lung. Preconditioning protection can be induced both acutely and chronically. In acute (classic) preconditioning, protection is effective for only 2–3 h after the triggering signal. Multiple triggers can activate the preconditioning pathway, which can be additive to reach a threshold for preconditioning protection to occur[19]; however, it is often necessary to reach this threshold by multiple trigger cycles. Preconditioning also has a chronic response (termed the second window of protection, SWOP) that is manifest 24–72 h after the triggering signal.[18] A vast number of studies have been conducted to characterize the mechanism of action of ischemic preconditioning[19,20]; the signaling pathways proposed to be involved in activation of the mechanism include a number of sarcolemmal receptors linking to intracellular proteins such as protein kinase C (PKC); activation of specific mitochondrial channels, including the mitochondrial adenosine triphosphate (ATP)-sensitive potassium channel (mK_{ATP}-channel), that trigger mitochondrial ROS release, which ultimately influences the mitochondrial permeability transition pore (mPTP), shown to be significantly important in tissue development of either apoptosis or necrosis and hence tissue injury.

Elucidation of the increasingly complex signaling pathways involved in ischemic preconditioning[20] have initiated studies by which components of these pathways can be activated by pharmacological means (pharmacological preconditioning). This would potentially enhance the therapeutic impact of this protective mechanism without adding to the ischemia-reperfusion load

of the organ, which may already be compromised from ischemia-reperfusion injury.[18] In addition, studies have indicated that remote preconditioning may be possible by which initiating the triggering mechanism in one organ can stimulate the preconditioning signaling pathway of another, remote, organ. All these types of preconditioning have also been demonstrated in the lung.

23.4.1 Ischemic/Hypoxic Preconditioning of the Lung

Ischemic preconditioning of the lung has been demonstrated as an effective mechanism to improve lung protection during prolonged storage. Du et al.[21] subjected rat lungs to brief (5-min) bronchus and pulmonary artery occlusion followed by 10-min reperfusion and ventilation before perfusion and storage in UW solution for 6 or 12 h. Preconditioned lungs showed significantly improved gas exchange after 12 h of storage as well as reduced thiobarbituric acid (TBA) reactive substance, indicating lower ROS generation. Similarly, canine lungs subjected to preconditioning by 10-min occlusion of the left hilus and 15-min release before flush and storage in Euro-Collins solution for 2.5 h[22] demonstrated improved gas exchange and reduced lung injury after transplantation. Preconditioning reduced influx of neutrophils into lung interstitium, and this was associated with lower thromboxane B_2 (TXB_2) and malondialdehyde (MDA) levels (indicative of reduced ROS generation) and hence lower pulmonary artery pressure (PAP).

Similar to the multiple triggering requirements of ischemic preconditioning in the heart,[19] studies in the lung have investigated the effect of multiple episodes of ischemia and reperfusion (for various durations) required to induce preconditioning protection in the lung. Gasparri et al.[23] used an isolated rabbit lung preparation to examine the effects of either one or three cycles of 5-min ischemia and 10-min reperfusion or five cycles of 3-min ischemia and 6-min reperfusion before flush and storage for 2 h at 37°C in a buffer solution. Significant improvement in lung function during reperfusion was demonstrated for the multiple-cycle preconditioning groups; despite lung hemodynamic (PAP, pulmonary artery flow [PAF], and pulmonary vascular resistance [PVR]) being similar in all groups, static compliance and gas exchange were significantly improved and were probably associated with the reduced edema formation in these lungs. Similar results were seen in a study using isolated guinea pig lungs subjected to two cycles of 5-min ischemia and 5-min reperfusion before 3 h of 37°C ischemic storage[24]; reduced PAP and lower levels of MDA and glutathione (GSH) indicated reduced ROS generation during reperfusion in the preconditioned lungs.

We[25] have investigated the importance of ventilation or perfusion on the induction of preconditioning protection in isolated rat lungs subjected to 6 h of hypothermic (4°C) flush and storage in buffer solution. Cessation of both ventilation and perfusion induced significant preconditioning protection of both pulmonary compliance and vascular resistance; however, there were no differences between single cycles of 5 or 10 min of ventilation and perfusion cessation or two cycles of 5-min cessation and 5-min reperfusion (despite a trend for improvement in the latter). Additional studies demonstrated that, with a two-cycle preconditioning protocol, protection was maintained if ventilation was stopped but perfusion was maintained, whereas cessation of perfusion with continued ventilation abolished preconditioning protection.

Ucar and coworkers[26] confirmed these results in an isolated rat lung preparation subjected to two cycles of 5-min ischemia and 5-min reperfusion before 2 h of 4°C ischemic storage and 30-min reperfusion; the preconditioned lungs had significantly reduced ROS production (lipid peroxidation [MDA] and reduced/oxidized glutathione ratio [GSH/GSSG]) and reduced lung antioxidant enzyme depletion.

Additional studies by this group[27] have examined the role of excess ROS production and preconditioning protection of the lung. These studies focused on the enzyme semicarbazide-sensitive amine oxidase (SSAO), which converts amines to aldehydes with hydrogen peroxide (H_2O_2) as a by-product. Inhibition of SSAO, in combination with the preconditioning protocol described previously,[26] significantly reduced excess ROS generation to baseline levels and maintained lung antioxidant content. This is of interest in the context of studies in the heart, which have demonstrated an important role for mild ROS generation as part of the triggering mechanism in the preconditioning signal transduction cascade.[18-20] Ischemic preconditioning of the lung appears to involve a protective mechanism that results in significant reduction in ROS generation.

In contrast to the requirement for multiple trigger episodes in these studies, Friedrich et al.[28] were unable to observe a protective effect with a two-cycle preconditioning protocol (two episodes of 10-min ischemia and 10-min reperfusion of the pulmonary artery and lung hilus) before 3 h of "warm" ischemia and 8-h reperfusion in in vivo canine lungs. However, a preconditioning protocol of 5-min ischemia and 15-min reperfusion prevented decline in gas exchange and pulmonary compliance, and this was associated with reduced alveolar protein content and messenger RNA (mRNA) expression of tumor necrosis factor alpha (TNF-α) in bronchoalveolar lavage (BAL) cells from these lungs. These differences may be associated with the extended duration of reperfusion after the trigger ischemia.

Hypoxia occurs with relative frequency in animals; fetal life tends to be relatively hypoxic, and newborns exposed to normal room air can be thought of as hyperoxic. Provision of higher oxygen levels (for premature babies) can be extremely damaging, with induction of an inflammatory response that can lead to subsequent chronic lung problems. In addition, for those animals living at altitude, the chronic hypoxia leads to acclimatization and suggests that a protective mechanism may be invoked that may be similar to that observed with ischemic preconditioning. Hence, studies have examined the potential for hypoxia to induce a preconditioning protection in the lungs, either against hyperoxia or against hypoxia per se. Ahmad et al.[29] demonstrated that a prolonged (24-h) hypoxic preexposure of human lung microvascular endothelial cells (HLMECs) improved survival of these cells when exposed to a subsequent lethal hyperoxia. This protection was demonstrated to be mediated via the phosphatidylinositol 3-kinase (PI3-K) signaling pathway since specific PI3-K inhibitors blocked the protection. PI3-K has previously been demonstrated to be an integral component of the ischemic preconditioning signaling pathway elucidated for the myocardium.[20,30] In similar studies, [31] cultured human type II alveolar epithelial cells subjected to a preconditioning protocol before a hypoxia-reoxygenation-induced cell death protocol enhanced cell survival; this enhanced survival was prevented by a PKC inhibitor and a mK_{ATP}-channel blocker as well as a blocker of heat shock protein 70 (HSP70). Whole-body hypoxic preconditioning (six cycles of 10-min hypoxia and 10-min normoxia) has been shown to increase survival in mice subjected to a subsequent lethal hypoxic insult and to improve lung function (increased gas exchange, reduced pulmonary edema, and decreased pulmonary vascular permeability) after a sublethal hypoxic insult.[32] Subsequent studies[33] demonstrated that the protection induced by whole-body hypoxic preconditioning appeared to target alveolar type I cells and vascular endothelial cells, whereas alveolar type II cells appeared unaffected.

23.4.2 Pharmacological Preconditioning of the Lung

Although preconditioning with short periods of ischemia or hypoxia is an effective means of inducing additional protection to the lung, it would be preferable to avoid these potentially additional injurious triggers for preconditioning and utilize pharmacological means to activate trigger receptors. In the heart, this has been successfully demonstrated using a variety of compounds[18,19,34]; activation of the adenosine A_1 receptor was shown to have a major role in triggering preconditioning in the heart, with preconditioning protection induced by an A_1 receptor agonist. In contrast, Neely et al.[35] suggested that, in the lung, receptor desensitization using A_1 adenosine receptor antagonism could induce preconditioning of the lung. Cat lungs were treated with the selective A_1 receptor antagonists xanthine amine congener (XAC) or 1,3-dipropyl-8-cyclopentylxanthine (DPCPX) for 30 min before 2 h of ischemia and 2 h of reperfusion with significant reduction in alveoli injury (such as neutrophil, macrophage, red blood cell influx; alveoli edema) that was similar to lungs preconditioned by a cycle of 10-min ischemia and 10-min reperfusion. We[36] examined this further in rat lungs subjected either to preconditioning protection or to treatment with XAC or PDE inhibitors (such as theophylline, a nonspecific PDE inhibitor with additional adenosine receptor antagonism activity; Rolipram, a specific PDE-IV inhibitor; and enprofylline, a selective PDE inhibitor only) before ischemic storage (8 h) and reperfusion. However, we were unable to confirm the protective effect of XAC, whereas theophylline and enprofylline treatment enhanced protection.

NO appears to have a significant role in the induction of SWOP in the heart.[18] NO has also been shown to induce preconditioning protection of the lung, apparently via the classic preconditioning pathway. Thus, Waldow et al.[37,38] used an in situ porcine lung to demonstrate that inhalation of NO (15 ppm) for 10 min prior to a 90-min period of ischemia (left main bronchus occlusion and pulmonary artery and vein clamping) followed by 5 h of reperfusion increased pulmonary venous oxygenation (PVO_2) and decreased PVR to control (nonischemic) levels compared to ischemia alone. In addition, inflammatory response (measured by levels of interleukin [IL] 1β, IL-6, and transforming growth factor beta 1 [TGF-β1]) as well as release of ROS (measured by chemiluminescence) were reduced by NO treatment. The same group[39] examined the effect of NO inhalation (15 ppm for 10 min) on activity of matrix metalloproteinases (MMPs) in rat lungs subjected to 60 min of in situ ischemia (clamping of the left pulmonary hilum) and reperfusion for up to 4 h. There was an early (30 min of reperfusion) rise in MMP-2 and MMP-7 in BAL fluid that was attenuated (delayed) by NO treatment (at 4 h of reperfusion, MMP levels were similar to no treatment). This attenuation of the protein extravasation induced by I/R appeared to be via an effect on the lung permeability barrier. Increases in MMP-9 and neutrophil elastase (associated with increased neutrophil activity) continued with time and were not influenced by NO treatment, suggesting that infiltration of neutrophils into the lung was unaffected; in addition, tissue inhibitors of matrix proteases (TIMPs) were not influenced by NO treatment. Additional studies in this rat lung model of preconditioning[40] demonstrated that the protective effects of NO described were associated with changes in components of signaling pathways (such as extracellular-signal regulated kinase [ERK], c-Jun N-terminal kinase [JNK], p38 mitogen-activated protein kinase [MAPK], protein kinase B [AKT], and glycogen synthase kinase 3-beta [GSK-3β]) that were similar to those seen with ischemic preconditioning in the heart. Interestingly, peroxynitrite (ONOO$^-$), a powerful oxidant formed by a combination of NO and superoxide radical that can exert protective effects at physiological levels but be cytotoxic at high concentrations, has been shown to induce preconditioning protection in the heart with activation of stress response pathways. It has also been shown to be an effective trigger for preconditioning protection in isolated rat lungs[41] and mimics the beneficial effects of ischemic preconditioning in lungs.

Sildenafil, a PDE-5 inhibitor that prevents cyclic guanosine monophosphate (cGMP) breakdown, resulting in increased cGMP levels with consequent maintenance of NO levels, has also been used as a preconditioning agent in the lung, which could improve lung function after lung transplantation.[42] Donor pigs were either pretreated systemically with sildenafil (0.15 mg/kg IV) for 20 min prior to lung harvest (flush and 24 h storage at 5°C with LPD solution) or sildenafil was added to the LPD flush and storage solution. Transplanted lungs were observed for 6 h of reperfusion, and it was shown that improved lung function (PVR, PAP, gas exchange, and edema formation) occurred only when the donor animal was preconditioned.

One of the mechanisms by which ischemic preconditioning is proposed to initiate protection is by activation of the ATP-sensitive potassium channel (K_{ATP}-channel). Many studies in the heart have demonstrated the efficacy of K_{ATP}-channel openers, in particular the mK_{ATP}-channel.[18,19] In contrast, in the lung, pinacidil (a predominantly sarcolemmal K_{ATP}-channel opener) has been demonstrated to improve lung function after long-term preservation. Thus, Fukuse et al.[43] pretreated rat lungs with an intravenous infusion of pinacidil 5 min before flush with phosphate-buffered saline (PBS), storage for 9 h, and 2 h of reperfusion; compared to control or glibenclamide (a K_{ATP}-channel blocker) treatment, pinacidil improved lung function (peak inspiratory pressure [PIP] and PAP), reduced lung edema and lipid peroxidation, and maintained mitochondrial respiration (state III). Similar results were seen in rat lungs flushed with lactated Ringer's solution containing pinacidil (100 µM), storage at 37°C for 2.5 h, and 2 h of reperfusion.[44] Lung function (gas exchange) was significantly improved, lung injury (measured histologically) was reduced, and myeloperoxidase (MPO) was also reduced in the pinacidil-treated lungs.

Other pharmacological agents that may be involved in the amelioration of ROS-induced injury have been shown to induce preconditioning protection in the lung. Thus, the protective property of glycine (a nonessential amino acid and a component of glutathione and hence thought to have free radical scavenging properties) was examined in a pig model of lung transplantation.[45] Glycine was either used as an intravenous pretreatment to the donor pig for 1 h prior to flushing and storage (for 24 h) of the transplanted lung with LPD at 4°C or used as a supplement to the LPD flush solution before storage. During 7 h of reperfusion, lung function was evaluated; preconditioning of the donor with glycine prior to lung transplantation provided a significant improvement in lung function (gas exchange, PVR, PAP, and lung edema) compared to the control group and (for some parameters) to the glycine-supplemented LPD group. N-Acetyl cysteine (NAC; a precursor of GSH in its reduced form and a well-known antioxidant) has also been used to precondition lungs subjected to normothermic ischemia.[46] In a complex experimental protocol in which isolated perfused rat lungs were subjected to perfusion with effluent from rat livers subjected to ischemia-reperfusion injury, the pretreatment of lungs with NAC (at 3.7 mmol/L) before liver effluent perfusion protected against the damaging effects of the liver effluent, shown by a reduced ventilatory and perfusion pressure, reduced lung weight gain (edema), and reduced xanthine oxidase release in BAL fluid.

23.4.3 Heat Preconditioning of the Lung

The evidence for preconditioning protection by short periods of hyperthermia (heat shock) remains controversial, even in the heart.[18] It has been shown to initiate the induction of HSPs (primarily HSP70/72), which some studies have shown to be associated with SWOP. In the lung, evidence for this technique of preconditioning protection is also controversial and has recently been reviewed.[3] Javadpour and coworkers[47] investigated the effect of hyperthermia preconditioning using rats subjected to an increase in core body temperature (to ~41°C for 15 min) 18 h prior to induction of lower-body ischemia by 30-min aortic cross clamping and reperfusion for 2 h. Lungs from these animals had significantly reduced leakage of protein (as well as neutrophil count) in BAL fluid, reduced lung edema, lung MPO activity, and increased HSP72 expression compared to nonpreconditioned lungs. Studies from the same group,[48] examining a more clinically relevant preconditioning protocol (a once-daily increase of core body temperature by 1°C for 15 min for 5 days) in rats, showed similar results to those described.

Acute effects of hyperthermia have also been demonstrated in lungs. In a study designed to simulate clinical intestinal examination and the potential effects on remote organs (lung), rats were subjected to 15 min of whole-body hyperthermia (40°C), allowed to recover for 30 min, and then subjected to laparotomy and intestinal handling before sacrifice and measurements of injury to lung and intestines.[49] Preconditioning with heat reduced lung injury assessed histologically, as well as reducing neutrophil infiltration with associated lower MPO activity, reduced BAL protein leakage, and lower MDA activity. Pigs, subjected to two cycles of 15 min of hyperthermic (40°C) and normothermic (36°C) gas ventilation, were also shown to benefit from lungs subsequently subjected to 90 min of ischemia and 4 h of reperfusion.[50] Lung function (PAP, PVR, and gas exchange) was significantly improved, and oxidative stress and inflammatory cytokines were reduced. Hence, the data suggest that short durations of hyperthermia can induce both classic preconditioning and SWOP and may be an additional therapeutic means of protecting organs during surgical intervention.

23.4.4 Remote Preconditioning of the Lung

Preconditioning of one region of the heart was shown (by Przyklenk et al.[51]) to protect another, remote, region of the heart; this phenomenon was termed *remote preconditioning*. It remains little understood, with no consensus regarding a mechanism of action or how this might be achieved.[52] There have, however, been a number of studies demonstrating remote protection of the lung by preconditioning of other organs.

Lung injury is a common problem after intestinal ischemia and reperfusion, and this may be generated by increased ROS production. Ito and coworkers[53] conducted a study in rats to investigate the protective effect of pharmacological induction of heme oxygenase 1 (HO-1) by the anticancer drug doxorubicin following intestinal ischemia-reperfusion. HO-1 generates carbon monoxide (CO), biliverdin, and bilirubin, leading to lung protection via their antioxidant effects. Rats were treated with doxorubicin at 2 days before intestinal ischemia (120 min) and reperfusion (120 min); both intestine and lung injury were assessed. Results showed that lung injury was ameliorated (alveolar cells remained normal, MPO activity was reduced, and lung edema was prevented) by the drug treatment compared to no treatment. In a similar study in rats, Kalb et al.[54] showed the combined effect of remote and pharmacological preconditioning on lung protection; preconditioning by ventilation with the volatile anesthetic sevoflurane followed by 5 min washout prior to 2 h of hind limb ischemia and 3 h of reperfusion improved postischemic oxygen tension and reduced neutrophil infiltration.

In a model of off-pump coronary artery bypass (OPCAB) revascularization in sheep, Xia et al.[55] investigated the effect of three cycles of 5-min ischemia and 5-min reperfusion of the iliac artery followed by subsequent 10-min occlusion and reperfusion of coronary arteries (left anterior descending [LAD], diagonal, and circumflex arteries) on lung injury. It was shown that, in the remote preconditioned group, lung gas exchange was significantly improved, and associated PVR was reduced when compared to nonpreconditioned lungs. Similar studies in dogs[56] examined the effect of three cycles of 5-min occlusion and 10-min reperfusion of the femoral artery (i.e., hind-limb ischemia) applied 30–40 min before subjecting lungs to 90-min ischemia and 5-h reperfusion. Preconditioning of the hind limb significantly improved lung function, with reduced PAP and PVR, improved gas exchange, and reduced cytokine expression (IL-1β but not IL-6) and reduction in associated macrophage infiltration. However, preconditioning did not influence ROS production. This may be a novel and effective method for improving the protection of lungs during storage prior to transplantation.

Clinical studies have also demonstrated the potential for remote preconditioning protection of the lung. Patients undergoing valve replacement underwent CPB and were immediately subjected to two cycles of 3-min aortic cross-clamping and 2-min reperfusion before cardioplegic arrest, global ischemia (~68 min), and reperfusion.[57] Results showed that preconditioning limited oxidative injury of the lung, improved gas exchange and lung function, and decreased alveolar injury and neutrophil infiltration. In a study in children undergoing repair for congenital defects with CPB,[58] remote preconditioning was induced in the lower limb (four cycles of 5-min ischemia and 5-min reperfusion using a blood pressure cuff) before the initiation of CPB and global ischemia of about 80 min. Postoperative airway resistance was reduced at 6 h, but other lung parameters were not different from the control (nonpreconditioned) patients. There were also reductions in troponin I release and inotropic support, suggesting protection of the myocardium.

23.5 Conclusion

Ischemic preconditioning, first described in the heart in 1986, has become an established technique for inducing endogenous organ protection against ischemia and reperfusion injury and is recognized as one of the most efficacious methods of myocardial protection. A considerable body of work has been generated demonstrating that the protection is effective not only in the heart but also in other organs in which it has been investigated, including the lung (as described). In addition, details of the mode of action of preconditioning, and the triggers, mediators, and effectors involved, have been determined. These details allow speculation about alternative means of inducing the protection that avoids the potential for additional injury that may be

induced if the only trigger signal is ischemia-reperfusion. Pharmacological agents that act at various points of the signaling pathway have also been shown to induce the protection, and this opens the way for therapeutic treatment in the clinical arena.

The lung, as an organ that can benefit from preconditioning, has not been studied in anywhere near the detail of other organs; the mechanism of preconditioning protection in the lung remains unclear. For other organs that require aerobic perfusion, a powerful preconditioning trigger is ischemia; however, the lung is fundamentally different in that it is perfused mainly with hypoxic blood. The O_2 supply (to both blood and lung tissue) is via the O_2-rich alveolar space and the minimal arterial blood from the bronchial arteries. Hence, induction of "ischemia" is difficult

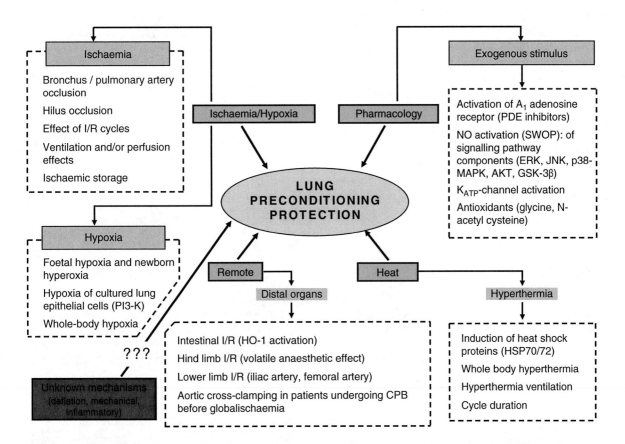

Fig. 23.2 Schematic diagram summarizing the potential mechanisms by which preconditioning protection may be induced in the lung and the various strategies that have been investigated. *CPB* cardiopulmonary bypass, *I/R* ischemia-reperfusion, K_{ATP}-*channel* adenosine triphosphate-sensitive potassium channel,

NO nitric oxide, *PDE* phosphodiesterase, *PI3-K* phosphatidylinositol 3-kinase, *SWOP* second window of protection, ERK extracellular-signal regulated kinase, JNK c-Jun N-terminal kinase, p38-MAPK p38-mitogen-activated protein kinase, AKT protein kinase B, GSK-3β glycogen synthase kinase-3β

and requires that both ventilation and perfusion of both circulatory networks be stopped. This is problematic to achieve as a trigger mechanism; even during lung transplantation involving storage of the isolated lung (with no perfusion or ventilation), the lungs are usually inflated, and this may provide sufficient O_2 to the thin-walled lung tissue to prevent the effect of ischemia. Thus, it is important to carefully establish the appropriate conditions when investigating preconditioning protection of the lung. Alternative means of inducing preconditioning protection in the lung may have more relevance than in other organs, and this has been demonstrated in studies described with protection induced by pharmacological agents, by heat, or by remote means (Fig. 23.2). However, the possibility also exists that other maneuvers, such as deflation, mechanical ventilation, or inflammatory stress, may act as preconditioning triggers. Many of these may be suitable as therapeutic mechanisms to improve lung protection during cardiac surgery or lung transplantation. Currently, there is a lack of mechanistic studies to determine the signaling pathways associated with lung preconditioning protection. Are these pathways similar to those established in the heart (and other aerobic organs), or do the fundamental differences in lung physiology result in alternative signaling pathway characteristics (triggers, mediators, and effectors)? This area remains a considerable challenge for the future.

References

1. de Perrot M, Liu M, Waddell TK, Keshavjee S. Ischemia-reperfusion-induced lung injury. *Am J Respir Crit Care Med.* 2003;167(4):490-511.

2. Troosters T, Gosselink R, Decramer M. Chronic obstructive pulmonary disease and chronic heart failure: two muscle diseases? *J Cardiopulm Rehabil.* 2004; 24(3):137-145.

3. Pespeni M, Hodnett M, Pittet JF. In vivo stress preconditioning. *Methods.* 2005;35(2):158-164.

4. Carvalho EM, Gabriel EA, Salerno TA. Pulmonary protection during cardiac surgery: systematic literature review. *Asian Cardiovasc Thorac Ann.* 2008; 16(6):503-507.

5. Ng CS, Wan S, Yim AP, Arifi AA. Pulmonary dysfunction after cardiac surgery. *Chest.* 2002; 121(4):1269-1277.

6. Ng CS, Wan S, Yim AP. Pulmonary ischaemia-reperfusion injury: role of apoptosis. *Eur Respir J.* 2005; 25(2):356-363.

7. Ng CS, Wan S, Arifi AA, Yim AP. Inflammatory response to pulmonary ischemia-reperfusion injury. *Surg Today.* 2006; 36(3):205-214.

8. Balogun E, Featherstone RL, Chambers DJ. Lung injury during cardiopulmonary bypass: characteristics of deflation-induced injury and attenuation with theophylline. *Interact Cardiovasc Thorac Surg.* 2006; 5(suppl2) :S198-S199.

9. Slutsky AS. Lung injury caused by mechanical ventilation. *Chest.* 1999; 116(1s uppl):9S-15S.

10. Li LF, Liao SK, Ko YS, Lee CH, Quinn DA. Hyperoxia increases ventilator-induced lung injury via mitogen-activated protein kinases: a prospective, controlled animal experiment. *Crit Care.* 2007; 11(1):R25.

11. de Perrot M, Keshavjee S. Lung preservation. *Semin Thorac Cardiovasc Surg.* 2004; 16(4):300-308.

12. de Perrot M, Bonser RS, Dark J, et al. Report of the ISHLT Working Group on Primary Lung Graft Dysfunction part III: donor-related risk factors and markers. *J Heart Lung Transplant.* 2005; 24(10):1460-1467.

13. de Antonio DG, de Ugarte AV. Present state of nonheart-beating lung donation. *Curr Opin Organ Transplant.* 2008; 13(6):659-663.

14. Tang PS, Mura M, Seth R, Liu M. Acute lung injury and cell death: how many ways can cells die? *Am J Physiol Lung Cell Mol Physiol.* 2008; 294(4):L632-L641.

15. Featherstone RL, Kelly FJ, Shattock MJ, Hearse DJ, Chambers DJ. Hypothermic preservation of isolated rat lungs in modified bicarbonate buffer, EuroCollins solution or St Thomas' Hospital cardioplegic solution. *Eur J Cardiothorac Surg.* 1998; 14(5):508-515.

16. Featherstone RL, Kelly FJ, Chambers DJ. Theophylline improves functional recovery of isolated rat lungs after hypothermic preservation. *Ann Thorac Surg.* 1999;67(3): 798-803.

17. Murry CE, Jennings RB, Reimer KA. Preconditioning with ischemia: a delay of lethal cell injury in ischemic myocardium. *Circulation.* 1986; 74(5):1124-1136.

18. Yellon DM, Downey JM. Preconditioning the myocardium: from cellular physiology to clinical cardiology. *Physiol Rev.* 2003;83(4):1113-1151.

19. Downey JM, Davis AM, Cohen MV. Signaling pathways in ischemic preconditioning. *Heart Fail Rev.* 2007;12(3–4): 181-188.

20. Downey JM, Krieg T, Cohen MV. Mapping preconditioning's signaling pathways: an engineering approach. *Ann N Y Acad Sci.* 2008; 1123:187-196.

21. Du ZY, Hicks M, Winlaw D, Spratt P, Macdonald P. Ischemic preconditioning enhances donor lung preservation in the rat. *J Heart Lung Transplant.* 1996; 15(12):1258-1267.

22. Li G, Chen S, Lu E, Hu T. Protective effects of ischemic preconditioning on lung ischemia reperfusion injury: an invivo rabbit study. *Thorac Cardiovasc Surg.* 1999;47(1): 38-41.

23. Gasparri RI, Jannis NC, Flameng WJ, Lerut TE, Van Raemdonck DE. Ischemic preconditioning enhances donor lung preservation in the rabbit. *Eur J Cardiothorac Surg.* 1999;16(6):639-646.

24. Soncul H, Oz E, Kalaycioglu S. Role of ischemic preconditioning on ischemia-reperfusion injury of the lung. *Chest.* 1999;115(6):1672-1677.

25. Featherstone RL, Chambers DJ, Kelly FJ. Ischemic preconditioning enhances recovery of isolated rat lungs after
hypothermic preservation. *Ann Thorac Surg.* 2000;69(1):
237-242.
26. Ucar G, Topaloglu E, Kandilci HB, Gumusel B. Effect of
ischemic preconditioning on reactive oxygen species-medi-
ated ischemia–reperfusion injury in the isolated perfused rat
lung. *Clin Biochem.*2005; 38(7):681-684.
27. Ucar G, Topaloglu E, Burak Kandilci H, Gumusel B.
Elevated semicarbazide-sensitive amine oxidase (SSAO)
activity in lung with ischemia-reperfusion injury: protective
effect of ischemic preconditioning plus SSAO inhibition.
*Life Sci*2005;78(4): 421–427
28. Friedrich I, Spillner J, Lu EX, et al. Ischemic pre-condition-
ing of 5 minutes but not of 10 improves lung function after
warm ischemia in a canine model. *J Heart Lung Transplant.*
2001;20(9):985-995.
29. Ahmad S, Ahmad A, Gerasimovskaya E, Stenmark KR,
Allen CB, White CW. Hypoxia protects human lung microvascular endothelial and epithelial-like cells against oxygen
toxicity: role of phosphatidylinositol 3-kinase. *Am J Respir
Cell Mol Biol.*2003 ;28(2):179-187.
30. Costa AD, Pierre SV, Cohen MV, Downey JM, Garlid KD.
cGMP signalling in pre- and post-conditioning: the role of
mitochondria. *Cardiovasc Res.*2008; 77(2):344-352.
31. Wang W, Jia L, Wang T, Sun W, Wu S, Wang X. Endogenous
calcitonin gene-related peptide protects human alveolar epithelial cells through protein kinase C epsilon and heat shock
protein. *J Biol Chem.*2005; 280(21):20325-20330.
32. Zhang SX, Miller JJ, Gozal D, Wang Y. Whole-body hypoxic
preconditioning protects mice against acute hypoxia by
improving lung function. *J Appl Physiol.* 2004;96(1):
392-397.
33. Zhang SX, Miller JJ, Stolz DB, et al. Type I epithelial cells
are the main target of whole-body hypoxic preconditioning
in the lung. *Am J Respir Cell Mol Biol.* 2009;40(3):
332-339.
34. Cohen MV, Baines CP, Downey JM. Ischemic preconditioning:
from adenosine receptor to KATP channel. *Annu Rev
Physiol.*2000;62:79- 109.
35. Neely CF, Keith IM. A1 adenosine receptor antagonists
block ischemia-reperfusion injury of the lung. *Am J Physiol.*
1995;268(6 pt 1):L1036-L1046.
36. Featherstone RL, Chambers DJ. Long-term hypothermic
lung preservation: does adenosine A1 receptor antagonism
have a role in ischemic preconditioning protection? *Interact
Cardiovasc Thorac Surg.*2004; 3(1):182-187.
37. Waldow T, Alexiou K, Witt W, et al. Attenuation of reperfusion-induced systemic inflammation by preconditioning
with nitric oxide in an in situ porcine model of normothermic lung ischemia. *Chest.*2004; 125(6):2253-2259.
38. Waldow T, Alexiou K, Witt W, et al. Protection of lung tissue against ischemia/reperfusion injury by preconditioning
with inhaled nitric oxide in an in situ pig model of normothermic pulmonary ischemia. *Nitric Oxide.* 2004;10(4):
195-201.
39. Waldow T, Witt W, Buzin A, Ulmer A, Matschke K.
Prevention of ischemia/reperfusion-induced accumulation
of matrix metalloproteinases in rat lung by preconditioning
with nitric oxide. *J Surg Res*2009; 152:198–208

40. Waldow T, Witt W, Ulmer A, Janke A, Alexiou K, Matschke
K. Preconditioning by inhaled nitric oxide prevents hyperoxic and ischemia/reperfusion injury in rat lungs. *Pulm
Pharmacol Ther.*2008; 21(2):418-429.
41. Turan NN, Demiryurek AT. Preconditioning effects of
peroxynitrite in the rat lung. *Pharmacol Res.* 2006;54(5):
380-388.
42. Pizanis N, Milekhin V, Tsagakis K, Aleksic I, Kamler M,
Jakob H. PDE-5 inhibitor donor intravenous preconditioning
is superior to supplementation in standard preservation solution in experimental lung transplantation. *Eur J Cardiothorac
Surg.*2007; 32(1):42-47.
43. Fukuse T, Hirata T, Omasa M, Wada H. Effect of adenosine
triphosphate-sensitive potassium channel openers on lung
preservation. *Am J Respir Crit Care Med.* 2002;165(11):
1511-1515.
44. Tang DG, Pavot DR, Mouria MM, Holwitt DM, Cohen NM.
Warm ischemia lung protection with pinacidil: an ATP regulated potassium channel opener. *Ann Thorac Surg*
2003;76(2):385–389; discussion 389–390
45. Gohrbandt B, Fischer S, Warnecke G, et al. Glycine intravenous donor preconditioning is superior to glycine supplementation to low-potassium dextran flush preservation and
improves graft function in a large animal lung transplantation model after 24 hours of cold ischemia. *J Thorac
Cardiovasc Surg.*2006; 131(3):724-729.
46. Weinbroum AA, Kluger Y, Ben Abraham R, Shapira I,
Karchevski E, Rudick V. Lung preconditioning with
N-acetyl-L-cysteine prevents reperfusion injury after liver
no flow-reflow: a dose-response study. *Transplantation*
2001;71(2):300–306
47. Javadpour M, Kelly CJ, Chen G, Stokes K, Leahy A,
Bouchier-Hayes DJ. Thermotolerance induces heat shock
protein 72 expression and protects against ischaemia-reper-
fusion-induced lung injury. *Br J Surg.*1998; 85(7):943-946.
48. McCormick PH, Chen G, Tlerney S, Kelly CJ, Bouchier-Hayes
DJ. Clinically relevant thermal preconditioning attenuates
ischemia-reperfusion injury. *J Surg Res.* 2003;109(1):24-30.
49. Thomas S, Pulimood A, Balasubramanian KA. Heat preconditioning prevents oxidative stress-induced damage in the
intestine and lung following surgical manipulation. *Br J
Surg.*2003; 90(4):473-481.
50. Luh SP, Kuo PH, Kuo TF, et al. Effects of thermal preconditioning on the ischemia-reperfusion-induced acute lung
injury in minipigs. *Shock.*2007; 28(5):615-622.
51. Przyklenk K, Bauer B, Ovize M, Kloner RA, Whittaker P.
Regional ischemic "preconditioning" protects remote virgin
myocardium from subsequent sustained coronary occlusion.
*Circulation.*1993; 87(3):893-899.
52. Ambros JT, Herrero-Fresneda I, Borau OG, Boira JM.
Ischemic preconditioning in solid organ transplantation: from
experimental to clinics. *Transpl Int.* 2007;20(3):219-229.
53. Ito K, Ozasa H, Kojima N, et al. Pharmacological preconditioning protects lung injury induced by intestinal ischemia/
reperfusion in rat. *Shock.*2003; 19(5):462-468.
54. Kalb R, Schober P, Schwarte LA, Weimann J, Loer SA.
Preconditioning, but not postconditioning, with Sevoflurane
reduces pulmonary neutrophil accumulation after lower
body ischaemia/reperfusion injury in rats. *Eur J Anaesthesiol.*
2008;25(6):454-459.

55. Xia Z, Herijgers P, Nishida T, Ozaki S, Wouters P, Flameng W. Remote preconditioning lessens the deterioration of pulmonary function after repeated coronary artery occlusion and reperfusion in sheep. *Can J Anaesth.* 2003;50(5):481-488.
56. Waldow T, Alexiou K, Witt W, et al. Protection against acute porcine lung ischemia/reperfusion injury by systemic preconditioning via hind limb ischemia. *Transpl Int.* 2005; 18(2):198-205.
57. Li G, Chen S, Lu E, Luo W. Cardiac ischemic preconditioning improves lung preservation in valve replacement operations. *Ann Thorac Surg.* 2001; 71(2):631-635.
58. Cheung MM, Kharbanda RK, Konstantinov IE, et al. Randomized controlled trial of the effects of remote ischemic preconditioning on children undergoing cardiac surgery: first clinical application in humans. *J Am Coll Cardiol.* 2006;47(11):2277-2282.

Impact of Cardiopulmonary Bypass onPul monaryHem odynamicV ariables

24

Edmo Atique Gabriel and Tomas Salerno

Ischemia reperfusion can be the triggering factor of lung injury; subsequently, high pulmonary vascular resistance (PVR) is a crucial risk factor of lung injury after cardiopulmonary bypass (CPB).[1]

In addition, endothelial dysfunction of the pulmonary arterial tree occurring after CPB contributes to pulmonary hypertension postoperatively. Total CPB shunts the majority of blood flow away from the pulmonary arterial tree, resulting in secondary vasoconstriction and increased vascular permeability.[2] Nyhan et al. pointed out that long exposure to CPB can determine a selective endothelial dysfunction to acetylcholine; therefore, the physiological impact of CPB on pulmonary vessels tends to occur in the acute phase following surgery.[3]

During partial CPB, regional blood flow to lungs becomes quite decreased to 40% of the prebypass values as, under such condition, lung perfusion is dependent on bronchial arterial flow.[4,5] Based on this finding, some authors have advocated that inducing the augmentation of bronchial flow could be optimizing the lung lymph flow, which would be essential for attenuating the inflammatory response and endothelial damage.[6]

Alternatively, Mendler et al.[7] proposed, in an experimental model, the use of biventricular CPB as a useful approach for ameliorating lung function. On one hand, it generates an uninterrupted flow through the lungs, which can be beneficial to avoid stasis and hence reperfusion injury (Fig. 24.1). Conversely, prolonged circulatory assist on either side of the heart is easily

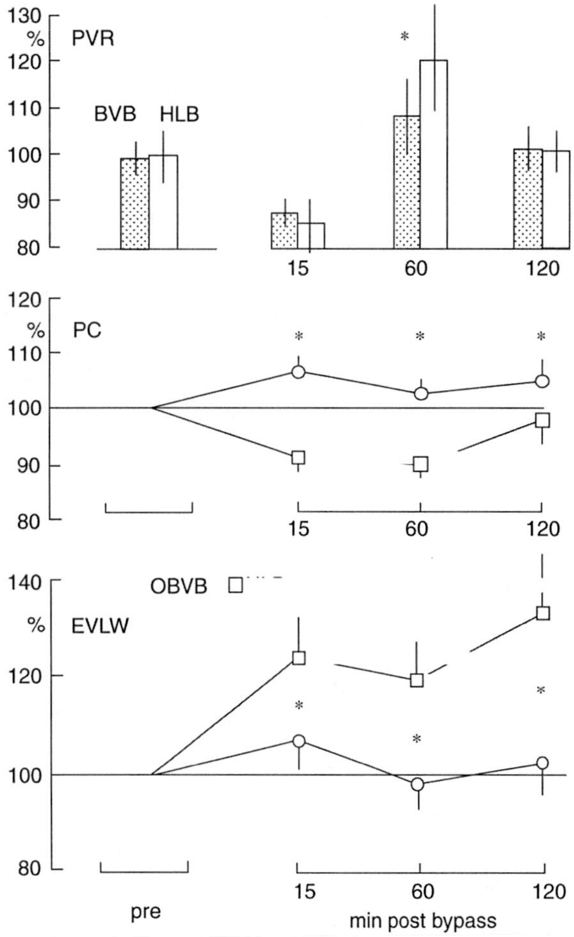

Fig. 24.1 Pulmonary vascular resistance (PVR) before and after 120 min of extracorporeal circulation (90 min cardioplegia, 30 min reperfusion) using a hollow-fiber membrane oxygenator (HLB) or biventricular cardiac bypass with autologous lung perfusion (BVB). All data given in percentage of prebypass values. (This figure was published in Mendler et al.[7] Copyright 2000, EuropeanA ssociationof C ardio-ThoracicS urgery)

E.A.G abriel(✉)
Federal University of Sao Paulo, Sao Paulo, Brazil
e-mail:e dag@uol.com.br

E.A. Gabriel and T. Salerno (eds.), *Principles of Pulmonary Protection in Heart Surgery,*
DOI: 10.1007/978-1-84996-308-4_24, © Springer-Verlag London Limted 2010

maintained when coming off bypass is difficult. On the other hand, there are a couple of surgical limitations of the technique. Indeed, placing four cannulae in the operating field is a strategy that may make difficult the management of flow rates and perfusion pressures as well as hamper manipulation of the heart without obstructing systemic or pulmonary venous drainage. Moreover, this technique may not be safe in terms of adequate control of air trapping in the heart.[7-10]

Sievers et al.[11] demonstrated that there is a relationship between lung perfusion during CPB and modifications of lung temperature. Moreover, these authors postulated that lung perfusion can be classified as a novel perfusion strategy during total CPB. Twenty-four patients were enrolled prospectively and alternately to three groups as follows: Seven patients were assigned to group I (controls: no lung perfusion, no ultrafiltration), nine patients to group II (those patients undergoing lung perfusion), and eight patients to group III (those patients undergoing lung perfusion plus ultrafiltration). As the aim of this chapter does not include the issue of ultrafiltration, our purpose is to highlight some aspects regarding perfused lungs and nonperfused lungs during CPB. After systemic heparinization, CPB with moderate systemic hypothermia (28–30°C nasopharyngeal temperature) was initiated by cannulating the ascending aorta and right atrial appendage. Lung perfusion was started once total pump flow was achieved by cannulating the main pulmonary artery. Pulmonary artery perfusion was maintained for 10 min with 1 L/min of arterial blood from the CPB circuit cooled to 15°C by a separate heat exchanger; the impact of lung perfusion on lung temperature was evaluated by sensors placed between the left lung lobes (Fig. 24.2). In nonperfused lungs, drop in lung temperature was less marked when compared to perfused lungs in which lung temperature decreased during lung perfusion to 18°C, remained stable for about 15 min, and increased to 33°C at the end of CPB. One of the most striking conclusions of this research was the absence of elevation of pulmonary artery pressure in patients whose lungs were perfused, implying that lung ischemia can be attenuated during on-pump cardiac surgery without posing additional hemodynamic damage to pulmonary vasculature.[11]

Techniques of controlled lung reperfusion can be employed to obtain better results at the time of aortic declamping. There are a lot of experimental models for illustrating this concept, but steady clinical tests are lacking in the literature.

When one mentions something about controlled lung reperfusion, the immediate image that comes to mind is the need for lung preservation for lung transplantation or maybe for heart-lung transplantation. However, lung preservation should be faced as a cornerstone issue in any cardiac surgery requiring use of conventional CPB in which uncontrolled lung perfusion may be considerably deleterious and substantially compromise short- and long-term postoperative outcomes.[12,13]

Because reperfusion injury is an extremely devastating condition for the pulmonary endothelium and subsequently for optimal hemodynamic performance following CPB, we can follow some pathways in pursuit of lung preservation during heart surgery with CPB. One option, and we believe that this is the best approach to achieve protective goals, is to perfuse the lungs using controlled lung perfusion pressure throughout CPB. There are different strategies to perfuse the lungs during CPB, such as intermittent or continuous perfusion; however, this matter is the subject for another chapters 30 and 36. Another approach is to bestow the concept of controlled reperfusion on lung preservation as proposed in several experimental models.[12,13]

Halldorsson et al.[14] created a model in which 20 pigs (25–35 kg) were studied using either uncontrolled lung reperfusion or controlled reperfusion. All hemodynamic measurements were taken with perfusion to the left lung only by clamping the right pulmonary artery. Ten animals were used as donors, and another ten pigs were

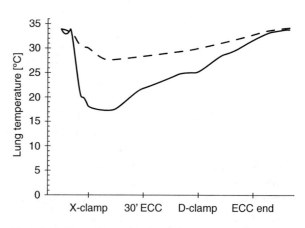

Fig. 24.2 Effect of lung perfusion on lung temperature as exemplified in two patients. *Solid line* lung perfusion; *broken line* no lung perfusion. *30′ ECC* after 30 min of ECC, *D-clamp* after release of the aortic clamp, *ECC* extracorporeal circulation, *ECC end* after end of ECC, *X-clamp* at the time of aortic cross clamping. (This figure was published in Sievers et al.[11] Copyright 2002, the Society of Thoracic Surgeons)

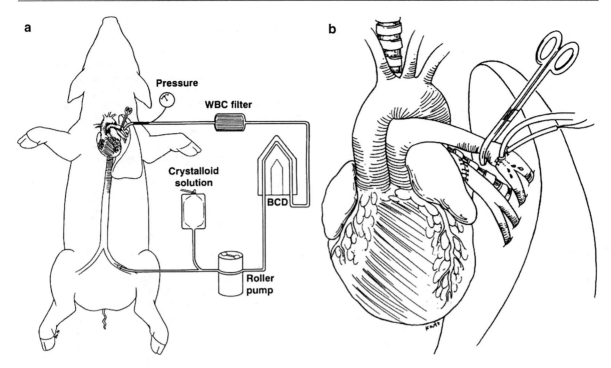

a

b

Fig. 24.3 (a) Experimental model of controlled pulmonary reperfusion. Blood is taken from the femoral artery, combined with a modified crystalloid solution using a BCD as a mixer, and then passed through a white blood cell (WBC) filter before it is returned to the pulmonary artery. The pressure in the distal pulmonary artery is constantly measured and kept between 20 and 30 mmHg. (b) The modified reperfusate is given into the left pulmonary artery distal to the clamp and is allowed to return to the pig through the pulmonary veins. (This figure was published in Halldorsson et al.[14] Copyright 2002, the Society of Thoracic Surgeons)

used as recipients for a left lung, which was harvested after cannulating the main pulmonary artery and giving cold modified Euro-Collins solution (4°C) to the lungs, using at least 50 mL/kg. In five pigs, the pulmonary artery clamp was removed, and the transplanted lung was reperfused using the native pulmonary circulation as is routinely done in clinical heart surgery (uncontrolled lung reperfusion). In five other pigs, the technique used for reperfusing the left lung in a controlled manner for 10 min is depicted in Fig. 24.3. The most important aspect of this technique was to strictly control left pulmonary artery pressure during reperfusion in such a way that pressure was kept between 20 and 30 mmHg, resulting in flows of 40–60 mL/min. Following a period of controlled reperfusion, the pulmonary artery clamp was removed, and native circulation was restored. A favorable impact on PVR was detected in the controlled perfused lungs, as demonstrated in Fig. 24.4.[14]

Gabriel et al.[12] advocated that uncontrolled lung perfusion pressure provided by conventional CPB does not prevent ischemia-reperfusion injury from jeopardizing lung function during and after heart surgery with CPB. Furthermore, these authors have pointed out that some pulmonary hemodynamic variables, such as mean pulmonary artery pressure, pulmonary capillary wedge pressure, and mainly PVR, can be considerably affected by inadequate flow to the lungs during CPB. It is noteworthy to emphasize that, experimentally, PVR was compromised by the absence of controlled lung perfusion in cardioplegic CPB as well as in beating heart CPB (Fig. 24.5).

In summary, conventional CPB itself can be deleterious to both hemodynamic performance during heart surgery with CPB and optimal hemodynamic recovery in the postoperative period, resulting in compromising damages to pulmonary vasculature. We believe that the best approach for solving this trouble or at least attenuating its consequences would be to adjust and particularly monitor lung perfusion pressure throughout heart surgery with CPB, aiming at preventing severe ischemia-reperfusion injury and its ultrastructural and clinicalc complications.

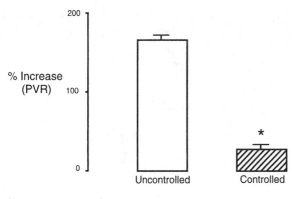

References

1. Suzuki T, Fukuda T, Inoue Y, Aki A, Cho Y. Effectiveness of continuous pulmonary perfusion during total cardiopulmonary bypass to prevent lung reperfusion injury. *Nippon Kyobu Geka Gakkai Zasshi*. 1997;45(1):31-36.
2. Lamarche Y, Gagnon J, Malo O, Blaise G, Carrier M, Perrault LP. Ventilation prevents pulmonary endothelial dysfunction and improves oxygenation after cardiopulmonary bypass without aortic cross-clamping. *Eur J Cardiothorac Surg*.2004; 26(3):554-563.
3. Nyhan D, Gaine S, Hales M, et al. Pulmonary vascular endothelial responses are differentially modulated after cardiopulmonary bypass. *J Cardiovasc Pharmacol*. 1999;34(4):518-525.
4. Onorati F, Cristodoro L, Bilotta M, et al. Intraaortic balloon pumping during cardioplegic arrest preserves lung function in patients with chronic obstructive pulmonary disease. *Ann Thorac Surg*.2006; 82(1):35-43.
5. Kuratani T, Matsuda H, Sawa Y, Kancko M, Nakano S, Kawashima Y. Experimental study in a rabbit model of ischemia-reperfusion lung injury during cardiopulmonary bypass. *J Thorac Cardiovasc Surg*.1992; 103(3):564-568.
6. Wagner EM, Blosser S, Mitzner W. Bronchial vascular contribution to lung lymph flow. *J Appl Physiol*. 1998;85(6):2190-2195.
7. Mendler N, Heimisch W, Schad H. Pulmonary function after biventricular bypass for autologous lung oxygenation. *Eur J Cardiothorac Surg*.2000; 17:325-330.
8. Schlensak C, Beyersdorf F. Lung injury during CPB: pathomechanisms and clinical relevance. *Interact Cardiovasc Thorac Surg*.2005; 4(5):381-382.
9. Shivaprakasha K, Rameshkumar I, Kumar RK, et al. New technique of right heart bypass in congenital heart surgery with autologous lung as oxygenator. *Ann Thorac Surg*. 2004;77(3):988-993.
10. Pepino P, Oliviero P, Petteruti F, Tommaso L, Monaco M, Stassano P. Left heart pump-assisted beating heart coronary surgery in high-risk patients. *Asian Cardiovasc Thorac Ann*. 2008;16(2):159-161.
11. Sievers HH, Freund-Kaas C, Eleftheriadis S, et al. Lung protection during total cardiopulmonary bypass by isolated lung perfusion: preliminary results of a novel perfusion strategy. *Ann Thorac Surg*.2002; 74:1167-1172.
12. Gabriel EA, Locali RF, Matsuoka PK, et al. Lung perfusion during cardiac surgery with cardiopulmonary bypass: is it necessary? *Interact Cardiovasc Thorac Surg*. 2008;7:1089-1095.
13. Carvalho EMF, Gabriel EA, Salerno TA. Pulmonary protection during cardiac surgery: systematic literature review. *Asian Cardiovasc Thorac Ann*.2008; 16:503-507.
14. Halldorsson AO, Kronon M, Allen BS, et al. Controlled reperfusion prevents pulmonary injury after 24 hours of lung preservation. *Ann Thorac Surg*.1998; 66:877-885.

Fig. 24.4 Postreperfusion pulmonary vascular resistance (PVR) expressed as percentage increase compared with baseline values. The PVR increased significantly when the lung was reperfused with unmodified blood in an uncontrolled fashion. Conversely, lungs undergoing controlled reperfusion by delivering a modified reperfusate at a low pressure for 10 min before restoring native circulation experienced minimal change in pulmonary vascular resistance (SE = standard error; *$p<0.001$) (This figure was published in Halldorsson et al.[14] Copyright 2002,t heSoc ietyof Thor acicSur geons)

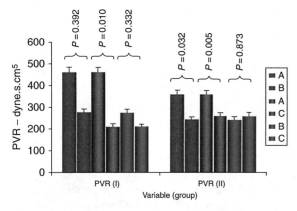

Fig. 24.5 Hemodynamic parameters in groups I and II postoperatively. *PVR* pulmonary vascular resistance. *Group I* cardioplegic group: *A* no lung perfusion, *B* lung perfusion with arterial blood, *C* lung perfusion with venous blood. *Group II* beating heart group: *A* no lung perfusion, *B* lung perfusion with arterial blood, *C* lung perfusion with venous blood. (Reproduced with permission from Gabriel et al.[12] Copyright 2008, European Association of Cardio-Thoracic Surgery. http://icvts.ctsnetjournals.org/)

Impact of Cardiopulmonary Bypass onG asExc hangeFeat ures

Edmo Atique Gabriel and Tomas Salerno

The lungs are effectively excluded from the circulation during cardiopulmonary bypass (CPB); therefore, inadequate pulmonary blood flow may result in postoperative impairment of pulmonary vascular endothelial function and inability for optimal gas exchange. Blood is shunted through the lungs, either perfusing inadequately ventilated alveoli or not sufficiently oxygenated because of alveolar-capillary block. The pathogenesis usually is multifactorial, involving intrinsic aspects of CPB and inflammatory mechanisms.[1] Although the vast majority of cases feature subclinical changes, the most complex manifestation of this endothelial injury is acute respiratory distress syndrome, which accounts for fewer than 2% of cases and usually has a mortality rate greater than 50%.[2,3]

Protective ventilatory strategies such as low tidal volume, positive end-expiratory pressure, and inhalation of pulmonary vasodilators are commonly used for management of CPB-related lung dysfunction postoperatively. Cessation of ventilation throughout CPB tends to be harmful to pulmonary parenchyma and induces structural damage and release of inflammatory mediators within the lung. However, this issue is still controversial, and some authors postulated that, in some instances, keeping ventilation active during heart surgery with CPB can produce proinflammatory effects.[4,5] As the relationship between ventilation and lung perfusion during heart surgery with CPB is the topic of another chapter, we call attention to the impact of ischemic lungs or perfused lungs during CPB on gas exchange postoperatively.

Although there are some pulmonary and bronchial connections for provision of adequate flow, optimal gas exchange, and prevention of hypoxia, bronchial circulation itself is not enough to support the respiratory functions of pulmonary tissue. Thereafter, some respiratory variables, such as pulmonary venous oxygen pressure (PvO_2), pulmonary venous oxygen saturation (SvO_2), arterial oxygen pressure (PaO_2), arterial oxygen saturation (SaO_2), oxygen index (OI), alveolar-arterial oxygen gradient, intrapulmonary shunt, and pulmonary compliance, can be deleteriously affected in the postoperative period.[6,7]

Ege et al.[8] investigated the importance of pulmonary artery perfusion in patients who underwent elective on-pump coronary artery bypass graft (CABG) regarding hemodynamic, inflammatory, and gasometric parameters. Twenty-two patients were assigned to two groups as follows: For group 1, only the aorta was cross clamped; for group 2, the aorta and pulmonary artery were cross clamped. CABG was done at moderate hypothermia and the cannulating aorta and right atrium. The ratio PaO_2/FiO_2 (fraction of inspired oxygen), which reflects the OI, was significantly higher in group 1 than group 2 at 2 h following aortic declamping, suggesting that aortic cross clamping can be less deleterious than aortic cross clamping associated to pulmonary artery cross clamping in terms of preservation of blood flow through connections between bronchial and pulmonary circulation and integrity of the blood-air barrier.[8]

Some respiratory abnormalities, such as elevation of alveolar-arterial oxygen pressure difference and pulmonary shunt fraction and reduction of carbon monoxide transfer factor and functional residual capacity, have been documented postoperatively in patients who underwent heart surgery requiring CPB.[9,10] CPB

E.A.G abriel (✉)
FederalU niversityof Sa oP aulo, SanP aulo, Brazil
e-mail:e dag@uol.com.br

E.A. Gabriel and T. Salerno (eds.), *Principles of Pulmonary Protection in Heart Surgery*,
DOI: 10.1007/978-1-84996-308-4_25, © Springer-Verlag London Limited 2010

and its intrinsic mechanisms compromise lung physiology, resulting in increased lung permeability and pulmonary vascular resistance, and particularly in neonates and children, dynamic lung compliance is considerably affected due to lung surfactant changes.[11,12] When pulmonary endothelial permeability is unbalanced as a result of the inflammatory response induced by CPB in neonates and children, pulmonary edema, alveolar protein accumulation, and inflammatory cell sequestration are exacerbated, altering lung surfactant composition and jeopardizing lung function, particularly in the initial stages after CPB. The immature lung is more vulnerable to ischemia-reperfusion injury; therefore, neonates tend to have a greater number of respiratory troubles postoperatively.[11,13,14]

Serraf et al.[14] performed meticulous studies to evaluate the possible mechanisms of lung dysfunction associated with alterations of neonatal pulmonary physiology in heart surgery with CPB. In one of these studies, 32 neonatal piglets were placed on CPB by cannulating the right atrium and ascending aorta. The animals were assigned to five groups as follows: group I, control group with no lung protective intervention during CPB; group II, lung perfusion with venous blood using a mean flow of 35 mL/min and mean perfusion pressure of 14 mmHg; group III, no lung perfusion and continuous ventilation throughout CPB; group IV, main pulmonary artery cross clamped and perfused with Cambridge solution; and group V, nitric oxide used for lung ventilation at the time of pulmonary reperfusion. Once CPB was instituted, mechanical ventilation was discontinued except in group III. The heart was kept beating at 28 °C without aortic cross clamping, and the main pulmonary artery was cross clamped during CPB of 90 min so that antegrade flow to the lungs was not allowed. Some pulmonary arterial segments were cut into rings and properly prepared to be evaluated regarding contractile response to phenylephrine and maximum relaxation to acetylcholine. Figure 25.1 demonstrates that in groups I and III, in which CPB was employed with no association to protective lung interventions, there were decreased oxygen tension values after weaning from CPB. Regarding endothelium-dependent relaxation in pulmonary and systemic vessels, following precontraction with phenylephrine and use of cumulative doses of acetylcholine, the pattern of response

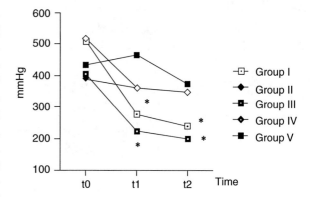

Fig. 25.1 Variations in the oxygen tension values. *t0*, before CPB; *t1*, 30 min after weaning from CPB; *t2*, 60 min after weaning from CPB. The groups are those described in the text. *$p = 0.001$ versus *t0*. (This figure was published in Serraf et al.[14] Copyright 1997, the American Association for Thoracic Surgery)

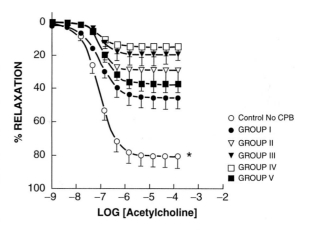

Fig. 25.2 Endothelium-dependent relaxation in pulmonary vessels. The vessels were precontracted with phenylephrine, and cumulative doses of acetylcholine were added to the bath. The groups are those described in the text. *$p = 0.01$ versus control no cardiopulmonary bypass (CPB). (This figure was published in Serraf et al.[14] Copyright 1997, the American Association for ThoracicS urgery)

was different between the two types of vessels (Figs. 25.2 and 25.3).[14]

It is mandatory to recognize that the advent of CPB made the lungs bypassed in terms of perfusion and oxygenation in such a way that gas exchange during heart surgery with CPB is essentially dependent on oxygenator performance. Over the last few decades,

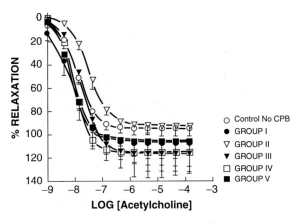

Fig. 25.3 Endothelium-dependent relaxation in systemic vessels. The vessels were precontracted with phenylephrine, and cumulative doses of acetylcholine were added to the bath. The groups are those described in the text. (This figure was published in Serraf et al.[14] Copyright 1997, the American Association for ThoracicSur gery)

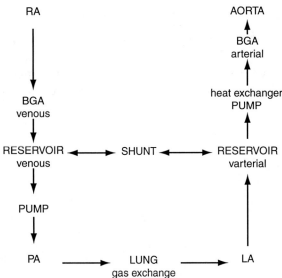

Fig. 25.4 Drew-Anderson technique. Principle of bilateral extracorporeal bypass without oxygenator. *BGA* blood-gas analysis, *LA* left atrium; *PA* pulmonary artery, *RA* right atrium. (This figure was published in Richter et al.[19] Copyright 2000, the Societyof T horacicS urgeons)

there has been development of oxygenators with better quality and biocompatibility; nonetheless, this did not prevent all degrees of inflammatory response produced by the interface between the extracorporeal circuit and the blood.[15]

On the assumption that oxygenators can play a substantial inflammatory role, we propose to revisit and reinvestigate the eventual benefits of the technique of biventricular heart bypass using a patient's own lungs for gas exchange. This technique was originally described by Charles Drew in the late 1950s especially for repair of congenital heart diseases using deep hypothermia.[16,17] Some authors have postulated that this technique can be helpful for heart surgery in which air embolism is not a life-threatening condition.[18]

Richter et al.[19] devised interesting clinical research in which 30 adult patients underwent elective CABG and were assigned to two equal groups as follows: The Drew group had bypass without an oxygenator, and the control group had regular CPB using a membrane oxygenator. The Drew-Anderson technique consisted of aortic cannulation, right atrium and inferior vena cava cannulation using a two-stage venous cannula, and main pulmonary artery cannulation distal to the pulmonary valve. Lung ventilation over the procedure was strictly controlled such that alveolar ventilation was adjusted to

temperature. Right-heart bypass flow was higher than left-side circulation, remaining fairly stable (0.2–0.3 L/min) throughout the operation. Opening and clamping the shunt were strategies used for, respectively, adjusting the level in reservoirs and stopping either bypass. The sequence for weaning from bilateral bypass was first right-side bypass and second left-side bypass. A schematic drawing of the Drew group technique is depicted in Fig. 25.4, and the resulting respiratory benefits can be viewed in Table 25.1.[19]

Further efforts and more functional maneuvers should be adopted during heart surgery requiring CPB so that there are better outcomes regarding lung function postoperatively. We believe that lung perfusion using controlled pressure is of paramount importance for optimizing gas exchange as it can attenuate the inflammatory response, ensure the integrity of the blood-air barrier, and reduce the accumulation of extravascular water. Furthermore, ongoing modifications of the extracorporeal circuit and revisiting old techniques can improve the quality of oxygen transport and be helpful as an increment to minimize inflammatory insult induced by conventional CPB.

Table 25.1 Perioperative gas exchange and pulmonary function[a]

Characteristic	Drew group ($n = 15$)	Control group ($n = 15$)	p Value[b] (t test)
Age (yr)	66.4 ± 2.2	61.7 ± 2.3	NS
Body weight (kg)	80.4 ± 2.9	80.9 ± 2.5	NS
Height (cm)	174 ± 2.1	173 ± 1.2	NS
Duration of operation (min)	263 ± 8	254 ± 14	NS
CPB time (min)	9.5 ± 7	101 ± 8	NS
Aortic cross-clamp time (min)	61.5 ± 5	63 ± 6	NS
Number of grafts			
Vein grafts	3.5 ± 0.3	3.6 ± 0.2	NS
LIMA used for CABG (yes/no)	14/15	15/15	NS
Blood loss			
6 h postop (mL)	319 ± 44	568 ± 72	0.006
ICU total (mL)	647 ± 69	965 ± 104	0.016
Allogenic blood requirement			
Intraop transfusion (U)	0.8 ± 0.3	1.4 ± 0.4	NS
ICU (U)	0.1 ± 0.1	1.4 ± 0.4	0.012
Time to extubation (h)	5.2 ± 0.4	9.5 ± 1.2	0.0025

[a]Data are shown as the mean ± standard error of mean

[b]Significance $p < 0.005$; Student t test was used

CABG coronary artery bypass grafting, *CPB* cardiopulmonary bypass, *ICU* intensive care unit, *intraop* intraoperative, *LIMA* left internal mammary artery, *NS* not significant, *postop* postoperative

PaO_2-PaO_2 alveolar-arterial oxygen tension difference, PaO_2 arterial oxygen tension, *respiratory index* alveolar-arterial oxygen pressure difference/PaO_2, $Q's/Q't$ intrapulmonary right-to-left shunt (%). This table was published in Richter et al.[19] Copyright 2000, the Society of Thoracic Surgeons

References

1. Richter JA, Meisner H, Tassani P, Barankay A, Dietrich W, Braun SL. Drew-Anderson technique attenuates systemic inflammatory response syndrome and improves respiratory function after coronary artery bypass grafting. *Ann Thorac Surg*.2000;69:77-83.
2. Jiang L, Wang Q, Liu Y, et al. Total liquid ventilation reduces lung injury in piglets after cardiopulmonary bypass. *Ann Thorac Surg*.2006;82: 124-130.
3. Asimakopoulos G, Smith PLC, Ratnatunga CP, Taylor KM. Lung injury and acute respiratory distress syndrome after cardiopulmonary bypass. *Ann Thorac Surg*. 1999;68:1107-1115.
4. Slutsky AS. Lung injury caused by mechanical ventilation. *Chest*.1999;116(1 suppl):9S-15S.
5. Chiumello D, Pristine G, Slutsky AS. Mechanical ventilation affects local and systemic cytokines in an animal model of acute respiratory distress syndrome. *Am J Respir Crit Care Med*.1999;16 0(1):109-116.
6. Schlensak C, Beyersdorf F. Lung injury during CPB: pathomechanisms and clinical relevance. *Interact Cardiovasc Thorac Surg*.2005; 4(5):381-382.
7. Gabriel EA, Locali RF, Matsuoka PK, et al. Lung perfusion during cardiac surgery with cardiopulmonary bypass: is it necessary? *Interact Cardiovasc Thorac Surg*. 2008;7: 1089-1095.
8. Ege T, Huseyin G, Yalcin O, Us MH, Arar C, Duran E. Importance of pulmonary artery perfusion in cardiac surgery. *J Cardiothorac Vasc Anesth*.2004; 18(2):166-174.
9. Macnaughton PD, Evans TW. The effect of exogenous surfactant therapy on lung function following cardiopulmonary bypass. *Chest*.1994; 105(2):421-425.
10. Taggart DP, el-Fiky M, Carter R, Bowman A, Wheatley DJ. Respiratory dysfunction after uncomplicated cardiopulmonary bypass. *Ann Thorac Surg*.1993; 56(5):1123-1128.
11. Ng CS, Wan S, Yim AP, Arifi AA. Pulmonary dysfunction after cardiac surgery. *Chest*. 2002;121(4):1269-1277. Review.
12. McGowan FX Jr, Ikegami M, del Nido PJ, et al. Cardiopulmonary bypass significantly reduces surfactant

activity in children. *J Thorac Cardiovasc Surg*. 1993;106(6): 968-977.

13. Haslam PL, Baker CS, Hughes DA, et al. Pulmonary surfactant composition early in development of acute lung injury after cardiopulmonary bypass: prophylactic use of surfactant therapy. *Int J Exp Pathol*.1997; 78(4):277-289.

14. Serraf A, Robotin M, Bonnet N, et al. Alteration of the neonatal pulmonary physiology after total cardiopulmonary bypass. *J Thorac Cardiovasc Surg*.1997; 114:1061-1069.

15. Dobell AR, Bailey JS. Charles Drew and the origins of deep hypothermic circulatory arrest. *Ann Thorac Surg*. 1997;63: 1193-1199.

16. Drew C, Keen G, Benazon D. Profound hypothermia. *Lancet*.1959; 1:745-747.

17. Drew C, Anderson I. Profound hypothermia in cardiac surgery. Report on three cases. *Lancet*.1959; 1:748-750.

18. Bodnar E, Ross D. Bilateral cardiac bypass without oxygenator for coronary surgery. *Prog Artif Org*. 1983;3: 379-382.

19. Richter JA, Meisner H, Tassani P, Barankay A, Dietrich W, Braun SL. Drew-Anderson technique attenuates systemic inflammatory response syndrome and improves respiratory function after coronary artery bypass grafting. *Ann Thorac Surg*.2000; 69:77-83.

Pulmonary Energy Metabolism and Multiple InflammatoryR epercussions

26

Edmo Atique Gabriel and Tomas Salerno

Deprivation of pulmonary flow is closely related to several limitations of bronchial flow to ensure effective lung perfusion during cardiopulmonary bypass (CPB). Likewise, ischemia-reperfusion injury is an augmenting factor for lung injury following CPB, and it can compromise pulmonary energy metabolism as well as cause multiple inflammatory repercussions.[1,2]

Optimizing pulmonary energy metabolism depends on characteristics of pulmonary circulation during CPB and the capacity of preserving tissue adenosine triphosphate (ATP) stores.[3] Kuratani et al.[4] have pointed out, in an experimental study using rabbits, that pulmonary blood flow and ATP reserves in the lungs dropped to 11% and 50% of values before bypass, respectively, during total CPB. On the other hand, pulmonary blood flow dropped only to 41% of the value before bypass, and there were no modifications in ATP reserves in the lungs during partial CPB.[1,4] Moreover, some authors have advocated that conventional CPB, even when hypothermia to 28°C is used, induces loss of intracellular high-energy phosphates, glycolysis, elevation of tissue lactate, and production of cytotoxic enzymes.[3]

The initial phase of CPB is characterized by a period of warm ischemia; that is, the organs tend to remain warmer while core temperature is being reached. As the lungs can be affected by this transient thermic process, aerobic metabolism can be converted into an anaerobic one; with this, ATP levels will decrease, and

dysfunction of enzymes dependent on ATP will certainly take place. Furthermore, the metabolism shifting can promote accumulation of intracellular calcium ions and activate some enzymes, such as xanthine dehydrogenase/oxidase, which in turn can damage pulmonary parenchymal and endothelial cells as well as activate different systems.[1,5-7]

Apoptosis and acute inflammation are two different types of tissue injury that can occur during ischemia and reperfusion of lung tissue. Apoptosis is usually mediated by activation of a transcriptional program controlled by nuclear factor kappa B (NFκB); acute inflammation is a complex process resulting from activation of alveolar macrophages, polymorphonuclear cells (pulmonary neutrophils), as well as expression of proinflammatory cytokines, chemokines, and cell surface adhesion molecules.[8,9]

Shimamoto et al.[8] demonstrated experimentally that lung ischemia-reperfusion injury is mediated by an upregulated receptor named toll-like receptor 4 (TLR4); in a similar manner, it has been demonstrated in hepatic and cardiac ischemia-reperfusion injury. TLR4 knockout mice were marked by less lung vascular permeability, myeloperoxidase activities, and inflammatory cytokine release following ischemic insult.[8,10,11] Likewise, Wei et al.[12] analyzed the impact of pulmonary artery perfusion on apoptosis of lung parenchymal cells during CPB. Forty children with tetralogy of Fallot were equally aligned into two groups: the control group without lung perfusion and the protective group with lung perfusion with a protective solution at 4°C). Pulmonary specimens were taken to evaluate apoptosis of lung parenchymal cells through tunnel techniques. The rate of apoptosis of lung parenchymal cells was significantly greater in the control group, implying that pulmonary artery perfusion with hypothermic solution can be an alternative strategy

26

26

E.A.G abriel(✉)
FederalU niversity ofSa oP aulo, SanP aulo, Brazil
e-mail:e dag@uol.com.br

E.A. Gabriel and T. Salerno (eds.), *Principles of Pulmonary Protection in Heart Surgery*,
DOI: 10.1007/978-1-84996-308-4_26, © Springer-Verlag London Limited 2010

for reducing the rate of apoptosis and attenuating CPB-induced lung ischemia-reperfusion injury.[12,13]

CPB activates neutrophils through mechanical shear stress and interface with the artificial extracorporeal circuit.[9,14,15] Thereafter, proteolytic enzymes and oxidative chemicals are released into the systemic and pulmonary circulation; these enzymes and chemicals include metalloproteinases (especially metalloproteinase 9), elastase, and oxygen free radicals (myeloperoxidase, hydrogen peroxide, and superoxides).[16,17] Several inflammatory markers have been believed to play a proinflammatory role, particularly in terms of neutrophilic activation, recruitment, and adhesion, such as interleukins (ILs) 1, 2, 6, and 8; tumor necrosis factor alpha (TNF-α); cell adhesion molecules (CD 18, CD 11b); platelet-activating factor; leukemia inhibitory factor; caspases; and the arachidonic acid derivative leukotriene.[9,18-20] It is noteworthy to emphasize that, from the functional point of view, there are different arachidonic acid metabolites; that is, prostacyclin and prostaglandin E2 can cause pulmonary vasodilation, whereas leukotrienes and thromboxane B_2 (TXB_2) can cause pulmonary vasoconstriction. Furthermore, TXB_2 is mostly found in the lungs, particularly after ischemic injury.[9,21]

In addition to proinflammatory cytokines, there are some regulatory cytokines that play an anti-inflammatory role in the face of ischemia-reperfusion injury and thereby contribute to attenuate endothelial and parenchymal damage.[22,23] We can include as modulating cytokines IL-4 and IL-10, which are T helper type 2 cells (Th-2) cytokines, although some researchers have demonstrated that the most anti-inflammatory effects have been exerted by IL-10.[24,25]

Farivar et al.[22] devised an experimental study to demonstrate protective effects of IL-10 and IL-4 in the face of lung ischemia-reperfusion injury.

Rats underwent left anterolateral thoracotomy through which the left lung was mobilized, after heparinization, the left pulmonary artery, vein, and main stem bronchus were clamped for 90 min. Following this ischemic period, the left lung was ventilated and reperfused for up to 4 h. These authors found that IL-10 and IL-4 can be detected 2 h after beginning reperfusion (Figs. 26.1 and 26.2), and they speculated that use of polyclonal antibodies to IL-10 and IL-4 did increase lung injury severity (Fig. 26.3).

Another essential concept should not be overlooked, although results of some reports about this topic can

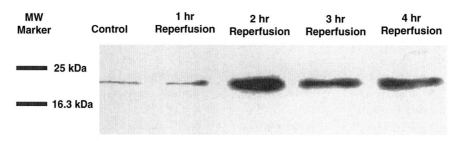

Fig. 26.1 Western blot analysis for interleukin 10. In the far *left lane,* the molecular weight (MW) markers are represented, as referenced from the kaleidoscope marker. There is minimal interleukin 10 protein in negative controls and 1-h reperfused lungs. At 2, 3, and 4 h of reperfusion, there is significantly increased expression of interleukin 10 protein in left lung homogenates. *hr* hour, *kDa* kilodaltons. (This figure was published in Farivar et al.[22] Copyright 2003, the Society of Thoracic Surgeons)

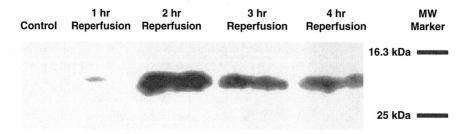

Fig. 26.2 Western blot analysis for interleukin 4. In the far *right lane,* the molecular weight (MW) markers are represented, as referenced from the kaleidoscope marker. There is no detectable interleukin 4 protein in negative controls or 1-h reperfused lungs. At 2, 3, and 4 h of reperfusion, there is significant expression of interleukin 4 protein in left lung homogenates. *hr* hour, *kDa* kilodaltons. (This figure was published in Farivar et al.[22] Copyright 2003, t heS ocietyof T horacicS urgeons)

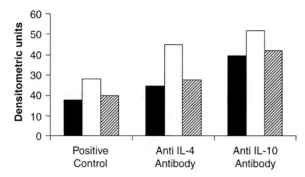

Fig. 26.3 Ribonuclease protection assay densitometry for cytokine messenger RNA (mRNA) using Image J software. Densitometric analysis reveals increased mRNA expression for tumor necrosis factor-α (*black*), interleukin 1β (*white*), and interferon-λ (*gray*) in animals treated with antibody to interleukin 4 and interleukin 10. *IL* interleukin. (This figure was published in Farivar et al.[22] Copyright 2003, the Society of Thoracic Surgeons)

still be conflicting, regards leukocyte depletion during CPB. Following aortic declamping, throughout lung reperfusion, activation of leukocytes and leukocyte-endothelium interaction are exacerbated. On the assumption that lung ischemia-reperfusion injury is closely associated with inflammatory mechanisms produced by leukocytes (particularly neutrophils), adopting techniques to attenuate this neutrophil-induced lung inflammatory insult during heart surgery requiring CPB can be promising and helpful.[26] Leukocyte-removal filters were first employed in blood banks to prevent transfusion complications caused by neutrophils; however, unintended effects can occur, such as simultaneous removal of platelets and ensuing hemostasis imbalance.[27,28] Taking into consideration different types of heart surgery requiring CPB, use of these devices as arterial line filters with leukocyte-depleting capacity can be an interesting strategy for attenuating the inflammatory response caused by neutrophilic activity. Moreover, as leukocyte-depleting filters are able to remove particles less than 5 μm in diameter, microaggregates generated during CPB, which are smaller than 30 μm in diameter and are barely caught by a cardiotomy filter, can be effectively removed, alleviating lung injury.[26-31]

Gu et al.[26] proposed a clinical study in which 30 patients were aligned into two groups – the leukocyte-depletion group or the control group – during elective heart surgery as such as coronary artery bypass grafting (CABG), valve replacement, or a combined procedure. All the procedures were performed using CPB and cardioplegic arrest. On weaning from CPB,

residual blood in the extracorporeal circuit was filtered to be reinfused before the end of the operation in the leukocyte-depletion group. By contrast, in the control group, residual blood was reinfused through the central venous line without leukocyte filtration. Following filtration, more than 97% of the leukocytes and nearly 60% of the platelets were taken from residual blood in the leukocyte-depletion group. Leukocyte and granulocyte counts decreased significantly in the depletion group, which is different from findings in the control group(Fig. 26.4).

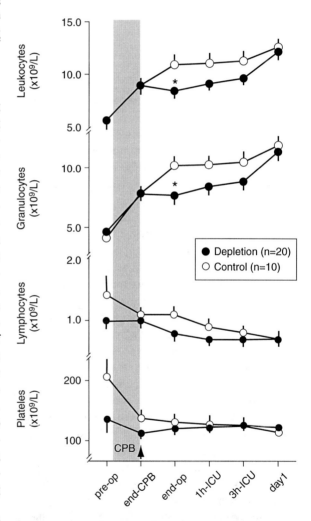

Fig. 26.4 Circulating leukocytes, granulocytes, lymphocytes, and platelets in patients with and without leukocyte depletion of the reinfused heart-lung machine blood after the end of cardiopulmonary bypass (CPB). *Arrow* indicates the start of depletion; *asterisk* represents $p < 0.05$ between the two groups. *pre-op* before operation, *end-op* at end of operation during skin closure, *ICU* intensive care unit. (This figure was published in Gu et al.[26] Copyright 1996, the American Association for Thoracic Surgery)

Table26.1 Inflammatory mediators before and after operation

Parameter	Before CPB	End CPB	End operation	ICU 1 h	ICU 3 h	POD 1
Thromboxane (pg/mL)						
Depletion	ND	48±15	48±9*	33±7	23±29	19±26
Control	ND	62±96	127±63	48±15	59±56	21±34
Interleukin 6(pg/mL)						
Depletion	36±14	126±96	ND	393±116	344±90	125±46
Control	20±24	197±246	ND	208±103	260±38	155±29
Interleukin 2(pg/mL)						
Depletion	UD	UD	ND	UD	UD	UD
Control	UD	UD	ND	UD	UD	UD

Values are expressed as the geometric mean and the standard error of the mean. *CPB* cardiopulmonary bypass, *ICU* intensive care unit, *POD* postoperative day, *ND* not determined, *UD* undetectable (below the lowest detectable level stated by the manufacturer)

*$p < 0.05$ compared with control

This table was published in Gu et al[26] Copyright 1996, The American Association for Thoracic Surgery

Thromboxane A_2 (TXA$_2$) is generated from prostaglandin H2 by thromboxane A synthase, and it is also a major component of blood clots. TXB$_2$ is a metabolite of TXA$_2$ that is known to be highly unstable under physiological conditions. Gu et al.[26] also found that TXB$_2$ levels were significantly decreased in the depletion group at the end of the procedure, and there were no relevant modifications regarding some cytokines, such as IL-6 and IL-2, in both groups (Table 26.1).

We believe that use of leukocyte-depletion filters connected to an arterial line can be useful for minimizing deleterious effects from neutrophilic activity. Nonetheless, we need to keep in mind that this approach can induce reduction of circulating platelets in such a way that hemostasis troubles can occur as well. Ideally, we need to find out which is the most optimal rate of filtration to obtain satisfactory outcomes in terms of less inflammatory response and acceptable hemostatic activity. It is noteworthy that our plan is to filter the blood with no need of massive platelet transfusion postoperatively. That is the challenge we need to deal with in pursuit of modulating neutrophilic activity during heart surgery requiring CPB. Furthermore, other steps can be taken to minimize inflammatory response during heart surgery with CPB (e.g., hemofiltration or ultrafiltration), but discussion of these issues occurs in another chapters. Likewise, the crucial role of heat shock proteins as modulating substances of the inflammatory process and the attention we need to turn to this matter are addressed in subsequent chapters.

References

1. Suzuki T, Fukuda T, Ito T, Inoue Y, Cho Y, Kashima I. Continuous pulmonary perfusion during cardiopulmonary bypass prevents lung injury in infants. *Ann Thorac Surg.* 2000;69(2):602-606.
2. Schlensak C, Doenst T, Preusser S, Wunderlich M, Kleinschmidt M, Beyersdorf F. Bronchial artery perfusion during cardiopulmonary bypass does not prevent ischemia of the lung in piglets: assessment of bronchial artery blood flow with fluorescent microspheres. *Eur J Cardiothorac Surg.* 2001;19(3):326-331. discussion 331–332.
3. Serraf A, Robotin M, Bonnet N, et al. Alteration of the neonatal pulmonary physiology after total cardiopulmonary bypass. *J Thorac Cardiovasc Surg.* 1997;114(6):1061-1069.
4. Kuratani T, Matsuda H, Sawa Y, Kaneko M, Nakano S, Kawashima Y. Experimental study in a rabbit model of ischemia-reperfusion lung injury during cardiopulmonary bypass. *J Thorac Cardiovasc Surg.*1992; 103:564-568.
5. Ege T, Huseyin G, Yalcin O, Us MH, Arar C, Duran E. Importance of pulmonary artery perfusion in cardiac surgery. *J Cardiothorac Vasc Anesth.*2004; 18(2):166-174.
6. Liu Y, Wang Q, Zhu X, et al. Pulmonary artery perfusion with protective solution reduces lung injury after cardiopulmonary bypass. *Ann Thorac Surg.*2000; 69(5):1402-1407.
7. Cai H, Harrison DG. Endothelial dysfunction in cardiovascular diseases: the role of oxidant stress. *Circ Res.* 2000; 87(10):840-844.R eview.
8. Shimamoto A, Pohlman TH, Shomura S, Tarukawa T, Takao M, Shimpo H. Toll-like receptor 4 mediates lung ischemia-reperfusion injury. *Ann Thorac Surg.* 2006;82:2017-2023.
9. Ng CS, Wan S, Yim AP, Arifi AA. Pulmonary dysfunction after cardiac surgery. *Chest.* 2002;121(4):1269-1277. Review.
10. Chong AJ, Shimamoto A, Hampton CR, et al. Toll-like receptor 4 mediates ischemia/reperfusion injury of the heart. *J Thorac Cardiovasc Surg.*2004; 128:170-179.

11. Shimamoto A, Chong AJ, Yada M, et al. Inhibition of toll-like receptor 4 with eritoran attenuates myocardial ischemia-reperfusion injury. *Circulation*. 2006;114(1 suppl): I270-I274.
12. Wei B, Liu YL, Yu CT, Chang YN, Li CH. Pulmonary artery perfusion with hypothermic solution inhibits the apoptosis of lung parenchymal cells during cardiopulmonary bypass. *Zhonghua Wai Ke Za Zhi*.2004; 42(4):227-229.
13. Wei B, Liu Y, Wang Q, Chang Y, Li C. Lung protection by perfusion with hypothermic protective solution to pulmonary artery during total correction of tetralogy of Fallot. *Zhonghua Wai Ke Za Zhi*.2002; 40(9):685-688.
14. Tanita T, Song C, Kubo H, et al. Superoxide anion mediates pulmonary vascular permeability caused by neutrophils in cardiopulmonary bypass. *Surg Today*.1999; 29(8):755-761.
15. Gu YJ, Boonstra PW, Graaff R, Rijnsburger AA, Mungroop H, van Oeveren W. Pressure drop, shear stress, and activation of leukocytes during cardiopulmonary bypass: a comparison between hollow fiber and flat sheet membrane oxygenators. *Artif Organs*.2000; 24(1):43-48.
16. Faymonville ME, Pincemail J, Duchateau J, et al. Myeloperoxidase and elastase as markers of leukocyte activation during cardiopulmonary bypass in humans. *J Thorac Cardiovasc Surg*.1991; 102(2):309-317.
17. Tönz M, Mihaljevic T, von Segesser LK, Fehr J, Schmid ER, Turina MI. Acute lung injury during cardiopulmonary bypass. Are the neutrophils responsible? *Chest*. 1995;108(6): 1551-1556.
18. Martin TR, Pistorese BP, Chi EY, Goodman RB, Matthay MA. Effects of leukotriene B4 in the human lung. Recruitment of neutrophils into the alveolar spaces without a change in protein permeability. *J Clin Invest*. 1989;84(5): 1609-1619.
19. Serraf A, Sellak H, Hervé P, et al. Vascular endothelium viability and function after total cardiopulmonary bypass in neonatal piglets.*Am J Respir Crit Care Med*.1999;159(2):544-551.
20. Goebel U, Siepe M, Mecklenburg A, et al. Reduced pulmonary inflammatory response during cardiopulmonary bypass: effects of combined pulmonary perfusion and carbon monoxide inhalation. *Eur J Cardiothorac Surg*. 2008;34(6):1165-1172. Epub 1 Oct 2008.
21. Friedman M, Sellke FW, Wang SY, Weintraub RM, Johnson RG. Parameters of pulmonary injury after total or partial cardiopulmonary bypass. *Circulation*. 1994;90(5 pt 2):II262-II268.
22. Farivar AS, Krishnadasan B, Naidu BV, Woolley SM, Verrier ED, Mulligan MS. Endogenous interleukin-4 and interleukin-10 regulate experimental lung ischemia reperfusion injury. *Ann Thorac Surg*.2003; 76(1):253-259.
23. Huber TS, Gaines GC, Welborn MB III, Rosenberg JJ, Seeger JM, Moldawer LL. Anticytokine therapies for acute inflammation and the systemic inflammatory response syndrome: IL-10 and ischemia/reperfusion injury as a new paradigm. *Shock*.2000; 13(6):425-434.
24. Fiorentino DF, Zlotnik A, Mosmann TR, Howard M, O'Garra A. IL-10 inhibits cytokine production by activated macrophages. *J Immunol*.1991; 147(11):3815-3822.
25. Hart PH, Vitti GF, Burgess DR, et al. Potential anti-inflammatory effects of interleukin 4: suppression of human monocyte tumor necrosis factor alpha, interleukin one and prostaglandin E2. *Proc Natl Acad Sci U S A*. 1989;86:3803-3807.
26. Gu YJ, deVries AJ, Boonstra PW, van Oeveren W. Leukocyte depletion results in improved lung function and reduced inflammatory response after cardiac surgery. *J Thorac Cardiovasc Surg*.1996; 112:494-500.
27. Bando K, Pillai R, Cameron DE, et al. Leukocyte depletion ameliorates free radical–mediated lung injury after cardiopulmonary bypass. *J Thorac Cardiovasc Surg*. 1990;99:873-877.
28. Al-Ebrahim K, Shafei H. Pall leukocyte depleting filter during cardiopulmonary bypass [letter]. *Ann Thorac Surg*. 1994;58:1560-1561.
29. Solis RT, Noon GP, Beall AC, DeBakey ME. Particulate microembolism during cardiac operation. *Ann Thorac Surg*. 1974;17:332-344.
30. Orr MD, Ferdman AG, Maresh JG. Removal of avitene microfibrillar collagen hemostat by use of suitable transfusion filters. *Ann Thorac Surg*.1994; 57:1007-1011.
31. Joffe SD, Silvay G. The use of microfiltration in cardiopulmonary bypass. *J Cardiothorac Anesth*.1994; 8:685-692.

Cardiopulmonary bypass (CPB), using hypothermia with crystalloid hemodilution, is associated with a capillary leak, which results in an increase in tissue water content, manifested as an increase in total body water after cardiac operation.[1] Also, CPB induces activation of inflammatory cascades, resulting in activation of neutrophils, platelets, and endothelium,[2,3] which release rumor necrosis factor alpha (TNF-α), interleukins (ILs), and other inflammatory mediators.[4] Pulmonary injury, induced by an increase in tissue water and activation of the inflammatory reaction, is one of the complications of CPB with a high incidence. This may adversely affect cardiopulmonary interactions after surgery, delaying extubation and discharge from the intensive care unit (ICU).

A number of strategies may be employed to reduce the accumulation of extravascular water and ameliorate the inflammatory reaction associated with CPB. These strategies include the use of small bypass circuits,[5] the use of high hematocrits at relatively high temperatures, and the use of postoperative peritoneal dialysis. During the 1970s, ultrafiltration (UF), now called conventional ultrafiltration (CUF), was introduced into the management of bypass in adults.[6] Dissatisfied with the effect of CUF in pediatric cases, in 1991 Naik et al[7] set up modified ultrafiltration (MUF). Many studies demonstrated the benefits of UF on organ function recovery by concentrating the blood, decreasing the total body water, and filtering the inflammatory mediators.[8-12]

The purpose of this chapter is to describe the theory and utilities of UF and explain its benefits for the lungs during CPB.

27.1 CardiopulmonaryB ypass and Pulmonary Injury

Pulmonary function in patients after CPB is consistently altered, ranging from microscopic atelectasis of no clinical consequence to fulminant acute respiratory distress syndrome (ARDS). The severity of pulmonary dysfunction is determined by several factors, such as CPB time, fluid needed to be added to the CPB circuit, and lung collapse during CPB. But, it may be difficult to distinguish these from those induced by thoracotomy, pleural resection, and pleural effusions. Decreases in vital capacity, functional residual capacity, lung compliance, and pulmonary function have been shown to persist for more than 3 months after surgery,[13,14] although in several studies the alterations have been considered to have a negligible clinical impact.[15,16]

In one prospective randomized trial of 197 patients undergoing cardiac surgery, off-pump coronary artery bypass (OPCAB) was associated with improved oxygenation and decreased time to tracheal extubation. There were no differences in chest radiographs, spirometry, pneumonia, pleural effusion, pulmonary edema, or mortality between patients undergoing OPCAB and open heart surgery.[17] Airway resistance is consistently increased by CPB and is more pronounced than in patients undergoing OPCAB surgery.[18] There have been a number of reports of fulminant bronchospasm during CPB.[19,20] It is most likely related to contact activation with an idiosyncratic excess activation of human C5a anaphylatoxin, although other causes,

W.W ang (✉)
Department of Pediatric Thoracic and Cardiovascular Surgery, Shanghai Jiaotong University, School of Medicine, Shanghai Children'sM edicalC enter, Shanghai, China
e-mail:w angweicpb@yahoo.com

such as acute cardiogenic pulmonary edema ("cardiac asthma"), should be excluded.[21]

The child with a significant left-to-right shunt compensates for diminished lung compliance by increasing respiratory rate and decreasing spontaneous tidal volume.[22] Although physiologic dead space has been reported to be normal in the context of elevated pulmonary blood flow preoperatively,[22] an increase of 5% up to 15% can occur in these patients during the immediate postoperative period.[23,24]

An increase in total lung resistance, due to either vascular engorgement or pulmonary edema, may be responsible for respiratory failure in the infant with congenital heart defects. The infant will strive to preserve adequate alveolar ventilation at the cost of excessive work imposed by increased resistance. When this load exceeds the infant's compensatory capacity, airflow, and therefore effective tidal volume, diminishes.[25]

27.1.1 Hemodilution

CPB can lead to pulmonary dysfunction manifested by lower pulmonary compliance and poor gas exchange. Sometimes, severe acute dysfunction can lead to death.[1] Hemodilution reduces serum albumin concentration and colloid osmotic pressure and increases the effective capillary filtration pressure. These factors may lead to the accumulation of plasma water in the interstitial space, which will decrease pulmonary compliance and impair gas exchange across the respiratory membrane and increase airway resistance, culminating in respiratory failure.[26,27]

27.1.2 Inflammatory Reaction

Due to exposure of cellular blood elements to nonendothelial surfaces, foreign blood products, and added shear stresses, CPB causes activation of inflammatory cascades, such as complement, kinin-kalliklein, and the coagulation system as well as stimulation of neutrophils, macrophages, platelets, and endothelium.[1-4,28] The alternate (properdin) complement pathway is activated; in fact, the magnitude of postoperative pulmonary dysfunction can be predicted by elevated complement C3a levels determined 3 h postoperatively.[29]

CPB is also associated with increasing levels of bradykinin, C3a, C5a, TNF-α, IL-1, IL-8, eicosanoids, and histamine in blood.[30-32] The systemic inflammatory response contributes to edema formation of the whole body and organ dysfunction and remains a major cause of morbidity and mortality in pediatric open heart surgery. Furthermore, hypothermia, ischemia-reperfusion, and the hemodynamic changes promote the systemic inflammatory response, which can cause further pulmonary damage.[28] It was reported that the levels of proinflammatory cytokines were correlated with duration of CPB, myocardial ischemia, and the development of multiorgan failure, whereas anti-inflammatory cytokines such as IL-10 have a suppressant effect on inflammatory response.[33]

27.1.3 Pulmonary Hypertension

Pulmonary hypertension associated with increased pulmonary vascular resistance (PVR) is a significant cause of morbidity and mortality after the use of CPB for repair of congenital heart defects.[34,35] Although the precise mechanism of pulmonary hypertension after operation for congenital heart disease remains poorly defined, recent evidence suggested that pulmonary vascular tone is regulated by a complex interaction of vasoactive substances that are locally produced by the vascular endothelium,[36,37] which maintains a balance between vasodilators and vasoconstrictors. CPB alters the balance by impairing endothelium-dependent vasodilation and increasing production of vasoconstrictors.[38,39]

Studies have shown that, in patients with preoperative pulmonary hypertension, plasma endothelin 1 (ET-1) levels increase after CPB, resulting in significant postoperative pulmonary hypertension.[40] ET-1 is a 21-amino-acid polypeptide produced by vascular endothelial cells; its potent vasoactive properties have been implicated in the pathophysiology of pulmonary hypertensive disorders.[41] In patients with congenital heart disease and pulmonary hypertension, plasma concentrations of ET-1 increased immediately after CPB and showed a significant correlation to the ratio of pulmonary-systemic arterial pressure.[42] These results suggest that alterations in ET-1 induced during CPB may be responsible in part for the increased PVR and increased vascular reactivity noted in children immediatelya fterc ardiacope rations.[40,42]

27.2 Ultrafiltration

UF is a convective process used during CPB by which the extracorporeal volume passes through a semipermeable (65-kDa) membrane filter, and by means of a transmembrane pressure (TMP) gradient, water, electrolytes, and other substances of small molecular weight are removed.[43,44] UF is different from conventional dialysis, which is diffusion of solutes across a semipermeable membrane into a dialysate bath. UF removes water and plasma concentration of solutes from the blood; the driving force is the pressure gradient across the membrane, so no dialysate on the opposite side of the membrane is required. During UF, all aggregates with a molecular mass less than the membrane pore size are filtered. Dialysis also removes solutes from blood, but the driving force here is the solute gradient between the blood and dialysate bath. When a dialysis patient needs fluid as well as solutes removed, UF is employed either simultaneously or sequentially with dialysis.[45,46]

The ultrafiltrator, sometimes called a hemoconcentrator, can be considered as a tank separated by a semipermeable membrane, commonly manufactured in a hollow-fiber configuration. The hollow fibers are between 180 and 200 μm in diameter, and the pores of the microporous membrane are between 5 and 10 nm.[47,48] Thousands of hollow fibers are configured in a bundle and encased in a polycarbonate shell. During UF, the blood passes through the hollow fibers and creates a positive pressure within the hollow fibers. This results in a pressure differential between the blood side and the atmospheric pressure; sometimes, negative pressure applied on the ultrafiltrate side of the membrane drives water across the membrane. The pressure gradient between the blood path and the ultrafiltrate compartment is called the TMP. The TMP can be expressed by the following formula:

$$TMP = (Pin + Pout) / 2 + NP$$

TMP = Transmembrane pressure
Pin = Blood inlet pressure
Pout = Blood outlet pressure
NP = Negative pressure applied to the effluent side of the ultrafiltrator

The rate of fluid removal depends on the membrane permeability, blood flow, TMP, and hematocrit.[47] The membrane permeability is related to the pore size,

membrane material, and membrane thickness. As the permeability implies, higher TMP and higher blood flow, lower hematocrit levels, and lower plasma protein concentrations will increase the UF rate.

Because the process of UF removes plasma water and diffusible solutes in equal concentration to the plasma water, the overall concentration of the diffusible solutes with low molecular weight are not affected. Dependent on the membrane material and pore size, typically solutes greater than 65-kDa that are not removed by UF will be concentrated.[49]

Some objections for using UF during CPB have been made because some types of dialysis membranes may cause complement activation and a decrease in polymorphonuclear leukocytes.[50] It has been demonstrated that these reactions only occur with membranes made of cuprophan, cellulose acetate, and regenerated cellulose, whereas membranes made of polysullone are not compromised by this.[51]

27.3 CurrentU seo fU ltrafiltration

Experience largely gained in clinical practice has described the use of UF, in relation to CPB, in three main situations.

In 1976, UF, now called conventional CUF was first introduced into clinical use during CPB. This technique has been performed on CPB during the rewarming period to reverse hemodilution. Because the effect of CUF was limited by the level in the reservoir, Naik and Elliott[7] modified the circuit and performed UF for 10–15 min after CPB. It has been shown to effectively reduce body water in pediatric cardiac surgery patients. This is termed MUF.[7] The third method is termed balanced ultrafiltration (BUF) or dilutional ultrafiltration (DUF), in which crystalloid fluid is used to replace the fluid removed by UF.[52] This method is also called "hemofiltration" (details of hemofiltration are provide in Chap. 28).

27.3.1 Conventional Ultrafiltration

In CUF, the ultrafiltrator is positioned in the bypass circuit with its inlet distal to the oxygenator and its outlet positioned into the venous reservoir (Fig. 27.1). UF is carried out during rewarming after the patient's

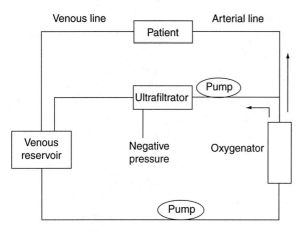

Fig. 27.1 During conventional ultrafiltration, the ultrafiltrator is positioned in the bypass circuit with its inlet distal to the oxygenator and its outlet positioned into the venous reservoir. Ultrafiltration was carried out during rewarming to hemoconcentratethe c ombinedpr ime/bloodv olume

nasopharyngeal temperature reaches 28 °C, thus filtering the patient while on bypass in an attempt to hemoconcentrate the combined prime/blood volume from the on-bypass hematocrit (e.g., 20%) up toward a higher level near the end of bypass.

CUF during CPB reduces the water balance and makes postoperative care easier, and it is more effective in removing proinflammatory cytokines than in adults. It is also more effective in proinflammatory cytokine removal than renal filtration alone.[45,46,53]

Other investigators reported utilizing UF in the extracorporeal circuit and found that removing plasma water during CPB resulted in improvement in a number of aspects of patient care.[54,55] Ramagnoli and coworkers[56] reported using UF in 24 children aged 2–7 years. Filtration was accomplished safely and resulted in an average rise in hematocrit from 21 to 31%.

The process of CUF may potentially lead to hypovolemia, with increased osmolarity in the intravascular volume causing interstitial fluid to slowly shift into the vascular space.[57] CUF may remove excess fluid; however, the amount of fluid removed is limited by the minimal level allowed in the venous reservoir of the extracorporeal circuit. Once the minimum reservoir volume has been achieved, further increases in hematocrit and plasma protein levels may only be accomplished by the addition of homologous red blood cells or albumin. After the addition of the red cells or albumin, UF may continue until a volume equal to the added red cells or albumin is removed.

27.3.2 Modified Ultrafiltration

CUF can remove some of that fluid, but with the limitation of the blood reservoir level, the effect has been inconsistent. In 1991, Naik et al[7] described a procedure in pediatric patients in which, following termination of CPB, the residual contents of the extracorporeal circuits were ultrafiltrated and transfused while the patients were still cannulated and attached to the extracorporeal circuit. They called this procedure modified ultrafiltration or MUF.

In the MUF technique, an identical ultrafiltrator is placed with the inlet connected to the arterial line and the outlet connected to the venous line (Fig. 27.2). The CPB circuit, including the ultrafiltrator, is then primed before CPB. The ultrafiltrator is kept isolated during bypass by clamping the inlet of the ultrafiltrator (Fig. 27.2a). After the patient has been weaned from bypass and is judged hemodynamically stable, the venous line between the cardiotomy reservoir and the outlet of the ultrafiltrator is clamped. The inlet of the ultrafiltrator is unclamped, and UF commenced, with blood flowing from the arterial line through the ultrafiltrator and back through the venous line to the right atrium (Fig. 27.2b). A roller pump is utilized to accelerate blood flow through the filter at a rate of 10–15 mL/min.kg. To compensate for the volume lost from the vascular space of the patient, the arterial pump is simultaneously activated to permit retransfusion of an appropriate volume from the cardiotomy reservoir back through the arterial line via the ultrafiltrator, hence hemoconcentrating the prime prior to delivering the necessary volume to the patient.[7] A constant left atrial pressure is maintained by giving volume from the venous reservoir back to the patient via the ultrafiltrator, thus hemoconcentrating the fluid in the circuit. When the level in the venous reservoir is low, crystalloid is added to the venous reservoir to keep it primed.[8] While the circuit blood continues to be transfused to the patient, it is displaced by the crystalloid solution until almost all the residual blood was transfused to the patient and the circuit is left primed with crystalloid. UF is continued until the patient's hematocrit reached 40% or the bypass circuit is completely emptied of blood. By leaving the circuit lines and the reservoir primed with crystalloid, the bypass circuit is maintained in a state ready for emergency resumption of bypass should this have proved necessary.[7]

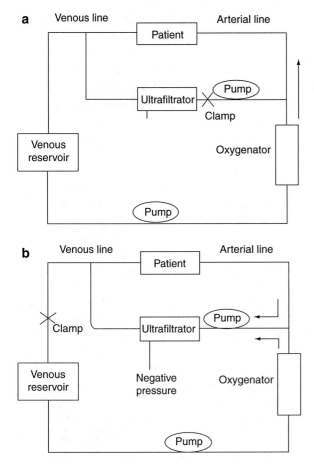

Fig. 27.2 In MUF technique, an ultrafiltrator was placed with the inlet connected to the arterial line and the outlet connected to the venous line. The ultrafiltrator was kept isolated during bypass by clamping the inlet of the ultrafiltrator (**a**). After the patient had been weaned from bypass and was judged haemodynamically stable, the venous line between the cardiotomy reservoir and the outlet of the ultrafiltrator was clamped. The inlet of the ultrafiltrator was unclamped and ultrafiltration was commenced, with blood flowing from the arterial line through the ultrafiltrator and back through the venous line to the right atrium. To compensate the volume lost from the vascular space of the patient, the arterial pump transfused an appropriate volume from the cardiotomy reservoir via the ultrafiltrator, hence haemoconcentrating the prime prior to delivering the necessary volume to the patient (**b**)

In MUF, nearly all of the circuit contents are concentrated and transferred to the patient without the risk of hypovolemia while the circuit remains primed with crystalloid solution. Most studies evaluating the effects of MUF, carried out in the first 10–15 min immediately after bypass, have demonstrated improved patient outcomes in the pediatric heart surgery population.[9,58-60] Specifically, it has been demonstrated markedly and

reproducibly to reduce the accumulation of water associated with bypass and to reduce blood loss and the need for blood transfusion.[9,61-63] Studies have also showed increases in arterial blood pressure[10,58,62,64] and cardiac index,[8,59,62,64,65] improved pulmonary function,[10,62,66-68] decreased PVR,[62] reduced postoperative ventilator requirement,[11,59,63] and fewer days in the ICU.[59] It has also been shown to improve myocardial contractility[64,69] and decrease myocardial edema.[70]

Moreover, studies have demonstrated that some low molecular weight inflammatory mediators can be removed by hemofiltration during CPB.[31,71] After several studies detected inflammatory mediators in the ultrafiltrate, most research efforts have focused on the correlations of blood and ultrafiltrate levels of these mediators and the improved outcomes.[72,73] The results of these studies have been inconclusive, but they suggest that the removal of inflammatory mediators during MUF is at least in part related to the improved outcomes.[74] MUF seems to be most effective in pediatric patients, probably due to the large prime volume relative to the patient's blood volume. A few studies have demonstrated the positive effects of MUF in adult patients, but the effects do not extend past the immediate postoperative period.[75-78] Currently, there is no large prospectively randomized study corroborating clinical outcomes and the removal of inflammatory mediators.[79]

27.3.3 Balanced Ultrafiltration

In BUF, the hemoconcentrator is positioned in the CPB circuit, and plasma water may be removed similar to UF. However, in this technique, sometimes called DUF or hemofiltration, the volume of plasma water removed is replaced by an equal amount of a balanced electrolyte solution.[52,80]

CUF and MUF are processes in which no fluid is replaced after removal of ultrafiltrate, whereas in BUF, crystalloid is continuously added to replace the volume removed by filtration.[52,80] Filtration of low molecular weight substances continues throughout the CPB. Therefore, BUF potentially has the advantage of removing inflammatory mediators more effectively than CUF and MUF because more fluid and dissolved small molecular substances can be removed without hypovolemia or excessive concentration of cellular elements of the blood. Journois et al[52] reported the clinical use of high-volume BUF. They continuously hemofiltrated the blood during the rewarming period, and isovolumic fluid was simultaneously replaced. They demonstrated that the plasma level and TNF-α decreased after hemofiltration, and IL-1, IL-6, and IL-8 were significantly lower at 24 h after operation compared with modified UF. They also suggested that the reduction of several inflammatory mediators might result in a decrease in a subsequent inflammatory reaction and improve the clinical condition of their patients.[52]

BUF during CPB reduced systemic edema formation and reduced the extent of lung dysfunction and depression of cardiac output in neonatal lambs after deep hypothermic circulatory arrest. The beneficial effects of HF did not appear to be due to hemoconcentration. This therapeutic strategy may have a clinical application in preventing systemic edema formation and lung dysfunction after deep hypothermic circulatory arrest.[81]

In a Deep Hypothermic Circulatory Arrest (DHCA) experiment, which included 16 neonatal lambs, Nagashima et al[81] used high-volume BUF (300 mL/kg/h) during cooling and the entire rewarming period. The study showed that BUF ameliorate the increase of PVR and improved lung compliance, alveolar-arterial PO2 difference (AaDO$_2$). Also, malondialdehyde (MDA) in lung tissue was significant lower in the BUF group. In addition, BUF resulted in a trend toward lower lung water content.

UF is a means of removing fluid and low molecular weight molecules from plasma under a pressure gradient. The application of BUF during CPB could attenuate the inflammatory response by filtering the substances that cause acute lung injury.[82] Improvements in postoperative oxygenation and duration of mechanical ventilation have been observed with this technique,[83,84] although it appears to be more effective in pediatric than adult patients.[85]

27.4 Benefits of Ultrafiltration for Pulmonary Function

UF can help attenuate capillary permeability and shifting of fluid to the extravascular space and is therefore an important adjunct to CPB.[86,87] Some studies[8,10,11,66,88] have shown that MUF produced immediate improvement in pulmonary function in children. Naik et al[8] found a respiratory benefit to MUF for a subgroup of patients, those who underwent low-flow, low-temperature CPB. This subgroup had a tendency to earlier extubation and discharge from the ICU and from the hospital if they received MUF vs. control patients. Kameyama et al,[11] observed that MUF improved the respiratory index (RI), which shortened the duration of mechanical ventilation, and MUF did have a significant impact on this improvement. Koutlas et al[60] showed that there was a lower incidence of early postoperative pleural and pericardial effusions in patients who received MUF after the cavopulmonary connection. Meliones et al[89] reported the results of 11 patients in whom MUF contributed to an immediate improvement in dynamic lung compliance compared with that found in a control group. Schlunzen et al[10] reported concerning their large study, which included 138 patients who underwent MUF, and observed that Po$_2$ improved after MUF in a noncontrolled study. In a retrospective study, Onoe et al[88] compared the effect of MUF on AaDO$_2$. All patients had a ventricular septal defect. The control group received no CUF. By the time of postoperative transfer to the ICU, AaDO$_2$ was lower in the MUF group than in the control group, whereas Pao$_2$ was higher in the MUF than in the control group. Their data also indicated that the RI was improved by MUF.[88]

The results of Mahmoud et al[68] also demonstrated that the use of MUF after CPB in patients weighing 5–10 kg can produce an improvement in lung compliance and gas exchange capacity, which may effectively minimize pulmonary dysfunction after biventricular repair of congenital heart disease. However, unlike previous studies,[10,88,89] Mahmoud et al[68] monitored patients beyond the immediate postoperative period and found these improvements were not sustained for the first 6 h postoperatively and did not lead to a decrease in the duration of intubation, ICU stay, or total hospital stay postoperatively. The results agreed with those reported by Keenan et al,[90] who reported on a series of 38 infants for whom MUF after CPB contributed to an immediate improvement in lung compliance, and it had no positive effect on the duration of mechanical ventilation or ICU stay. Thus, it was supposed that the salutary effects of hemoconcentration and removal of water after bypass by MUF are unable to overcome the ongoing effects of capillary leak possibly caused by an activated ongoing inflammatory response.[90]

Most studies with combined BUF and MUF did show a sustained improvement of pulmonary function and shorter ventilatory course and ICU stay. Bando et al[63] studied 100 patients, including neonates and children. They demonstrated that combined BUF and MUF efficiently removes free water and has higher oxygen tension (PO_2) compared with CUF. Moreover, perhaps as a result of the reduced pulmonary arterial pressure/systemic arterial pressure, (Pp/Ps) ratio, patients treated with BUF/MUF did show a marked decrease in postoperative ventilation time and ICU stays postoperatively. Journois et al[52] compared an intervention group who underwent high-volume BUF during rewarming plus post-CPB MUF to a control group who received post-CPB MUF alone. In this study, the intervention group had a significantly shorter time to meet extubation criteria (11 vs. 28 h, $P = 0.02$). Huang et al[91] demonstrated increased pulmonary compliance, decreased airway resistance, and decreased $AaDO_2$ after BUF and MUF. A randomized prospective trial of 192 adult patients undergoing cardiac surgery demonstrated that hemofiltration during CPB is more effective than placebo or steroids in decreasing the time to tracheal extubation.[92] Kiziltepe[78] found that a combination of CUF and MUF could significantly decrease the $A\text{-}aDO_2$ and $a/A\ O_2$ ratio and slightly decrease the duration of intubation, ICU, and postoperative hospital stays. Possibly the technique of BUF followed by MUF will prove to be the most optimal technique for shortening the need for ventilatory support in infants after CPB.

27.5 Mechanism

Pulmonary function is affected both by excess fluid from the hemodilutional effect of bypass and by the systemic inflammatory response. UF, which decreases total body water and removes inflammatory cytokines, results in improvement of pulmonary function.

27.5.1 Lung Edema

Removal of free water and lower transfusion requirements may contribute to improved pulmonary mechanics after CPB and result in significantly lower postoperative Pp/Ps and earlier extubation in BUF/MUF patients. In an animal model, Magilligan and Oyama[45] showed extravascular lung water was significantly less when UF was employed during CPB. Also,

removing lung water using MUF may prevent cardiovascular collapse. MUF can improve delivery of oxygenated blood in the pulmonary circulation, potentially reducing PVR.[66] In addition, the process of UF with increased colloid oncotic pressure in the intravascular volume results in interstitial fluid slowly shifting into the vascular space.[57]

Furthermore, it is possible that the lower level of a variety of low molecular weight bioactive mediators such as cytokines and leukocyte elastase in the pulmonary arterial blood prevents the accumulation of lung tissue water. Therefore, the mechanisms responsible for the elimination of water from the lungs with MUF may involve both direct mechanical and indirect biochemical factors.[66]

27.5.2 Inflammatory Reaction

The systemic inflammatory response syndrome (SIRS) is triggered during heart surgery owing to contact with the artificial surfaces of the CPB circuit, ischemia-reperfusion injury, and operative trauma.[31,93] Respiratory complications are at least partially attributed to SIRS.[94] Most cytokines have a low molecular weight, and numerous studies have demonstrated that, in addition to plasma water, many of these inflammatory mediators are removed during MUF.[84,85,95,96] Both CUF and MUF have been shown to remove inflammatory mediators from the circulation and were more effective than renal filtration alone.[31,95] However, a much greater amount of TNF-α could be removed from the circulation in the modified group, as demonstrated by a greater ultrafiltrate volume and higher removal efficiency compared with the other mediators. Elliott demonstrated marked reductions in serum IL-8 concentration at the end of and after bypass.[62] Watanabe et al[53] showed that UF during CPB should be beneficial in removing IL-6 and IL-8. One study showed a significant reduction of complement activation products by UF.[68] In fact, cytokine elimination has been correlated with the duration of the UF procedure and the amount of fluid removed. Although UF can remove harmful inflammatory mediators during CPB, other mediators or substances with protective effects may also be removed.[97] The anti-inflammatory cytokine IL-10 is also removed by UF, but to a lesser extent than the other proinflammatory mediators owing to its larger molecular weight.[98] However, several studies failed to demonstrate significant reductions in plasma levels despite levels being detected in the ultrafiltrate.[9,99]

Other studies have shown minimal levels of cytokines in the ultrafiltrate but significant reductions in plasma levels. It is supposed that some substances removed from plasma by UF are not necessarily only removed by convection. It has been shown that TNF may be removed from the circulation by adsorbing to the membrane.[100] Many of the synthetic membranes are able to bind complement-regulating proteins such as factor B, factor D, β2m, C3a, and C5a.[80]

It is hypothesized that the beneficial effects of MUF could be attributable to the removal and decreased levels of inflammatory mediators. Currently, no large, prospective, randomized studies have correlated the removal of inflammatory mediators with clinical outcomes.[70] Inconsistent results may be explained by use of various protocols and equipment, different end points, patient type, and measurement techniques.[90,101] Some authors also hypothesized that UF could be removing some mediators, which triggers the production of cytokines.[102]

27.5.3 Pulmonary Hypertension

Pulmonary hypertension is still one of the major complications after CPB. The precise causes for this are unclear; it is possible that increased PVR is somehow related to the generalized inflammatory response and impaired endothelial function.[103]

The plasma ET-1 concentration may play an important role in determining pulmonary vascular tone and may be one of the most important factors after cardiac surgery. The molecular weight of ET-1 is low (2.5 kDa).[104] Bando et al[67] demonstrated that combined BUF and MUF efficiently removed a significant amount of the circulating ET-1 and maintained significantly lower plasma ET-1 levels up to 12 h after operation. Subsequently, the Pp/Ps ratio in the BUF/MUF group was significantly lower compared with the control group for 12 h after operation and resulted in lower ventilator requirements. In addition, 25% of control patients, but none of the BUF/MUF patients, had pulmonary hypertension crises after CPB. Hiramatsu et al[105] reported that BUF and MUF suppress the increase in plasma ET-1 concentration that occurs

immediately after the Fontan procedure and suggested that DUF/MUF may be an effective intervention for maintaining low PVR after the procedure and improving patients' hemodynamics. However, in Kiziltepe's study,[78] ET-1 levels did not show significant differences between the CUF/MUF group and the control group. The peak values were reached just after termination of CPB, and levels decreased quickly.

27.6 Summary

UF can concentrate the blood without the removal of plasma proteins and can be utilized during CPB. Studies have shown that patients who are ultrafiltrated demonstrate decreased lung water, improved oxygenation, attenuated inflammatory reaction, and ameliorated pulmonary hypertension. Although no corroborative results for the effects of UF on pulmonary function exist, it is widely accepted that UF is helpful, more or less, to the recovery of respiratory complications caused by CPB.

References

1. Butler J, Rocker GM, Westaby S. Inflammatory response to cardiopulmonary bypass. *Ann Thorac Surg.* 1993;55: 552-559.
2. Mazer CD, Hornstein A, Freedman J. Platelet activation in warm and cold heart surgery. *Ann Thorac Surg.* 1995;59: 1481-1486.
3. Elliott MJ, Finn AHR. Interaction between neutrophils and endothelium. *Ann Thorac Surg.*1993; 56:1503-1508.
4. Kalfin RE, Engelman RM, Rousou JA, et al. Induction of interleukin-8 expression during cardiopulmonary bypass. *Circulation.*1993; 88:401-406.
5. Elliott MJ. Minimizing the bypass circuit: a rational step in the development of paediatric perfusion. *Perfusion.* 1993;8:81-86.
6. Magilligan DJ. Indication of ultrafiltration in the cardiac surgical patient. *J Thorac Cardiovasc Surg.*1985; 89:183-189.
7. Naik SK, Knight A, Elliott MJ. A successful modification of ultrafiltration for cardiopulmonary bypass in children. *Perfusion.*1991; 6:41-50.
8. Naik SK, Knight A, Elliott M. A prospective randomized study of a modified technique of ultrafiltration during pediatric open-heart surgery. *Circulation.* 1991;84(5 suppl):III422-III431.
9. Wang W, Huang HM, Zhu DM, et al. Modified ultrafiltration in pediatric cardiopulmonary bypass. *Perfusion.* 1998;13:304-311.
10. Schlunzen L, Pedersen J, Hjortholm K, et al. Modified ultrafiltration in pediatric cardiac surgery. *Perfusion.* 1998; 13:105-109.

11. Kameyama T, Ando F, Okamoto F, et al. The effect of modified ultrafiltration in pediatric open-heart surgery. *Ann Thorac Cardiovasc Surg*.2000; 6:19-26.

12. Li CM, Alfieres GM, Walker MJ, et al. Modified venovenous ultrafiltration in infant cardiac surgery [abstract]. *J Am Coll Cardiol*.1995;25:200A .

13. Braun SR, Birnbaum ML, Chopra PS. Pre- and postoperative pulmonary function abnormalities in coronary artery revascularization surgery. *Chest*.1978; 73:316-320.

14. Schenkman Z, Shir Y, Weiss YG, et al. The effects of cardiac surgery on early and late pulmonary functions. *Acta Anaesthesiol Scand*.2000; 44:75-81.

15. Deal C, Osborn J, Miller CJ, et al. Pulmonary compliance in congenital heart disease and its relation to cardiopulmonary bypass. *J Thorac Cardiovasc Surg*.1968; 55:320-327.

16. Karlson K, Saklad M, Paliotta J, et al. Computerized on-line analysis of pulmonary mechanics in patients undergoing cardiopulmonary bypass. *Bull Soc Int Chir*. 1975;2: 121-124.

17. Staton GW, Williams WH, Mahoney EM, et al. Pulmonary outcomes of off-pump vs on-pump coronary artery bypass surgery in a randomized trial. *Chest*.2005; 127:892-901.

18. Babik B, Aszalos T, Petak F, et al. Changes in respiratory mechanics during cardiac surgery. *Anesth Analg*. 2003; 96:1280-1287.

19. Kyosola K, Takkunen O, Maamies T, et al. Bronchospasm during cardiopulmonary bypass: a potential fatal complication of open-heart surgery. *J Thorac Cardiovasc Surg*. 1987;35:375-377.

20. Tuman KJ, Ivankovich AD. Bronchospasm during cardiopulmonary bypass. Etiology and management. *Chest*. 1986;90:635-637.

21. Chenoweth DE. The properties of human C5a anaphylatoxin. The significance of C5a formation during hemodialysis. *Contrib Nephrol*.1987; 59:51-71.

22. Lees MH, Way RC, Ross BB. Ventilation and respiratory gas transfer of infants with increased pulmonary blood flow. *Pediatrics*.1967;40: 259.

23. Downes JJ, Nicodemus HF, Pierce WS, et al. Acute respiratory failure in infants following cardiovascular surgery. *J Thorac Cardiovasc Surg*.1970; 59:21.

24. Yates QP, Lindahl SGE, Hatch DJ. Pulmonary ventilation and gas exchange before and after correction of congenital cardiac malformations. *Br J Anaesth*.1987; 59:170.

25. DiCarlo JV, Steven JM. Respiratory failure in congenital heart disease. *Pediatr Clin North Am*.1994; 41:525-542.

26. Tonz M, Tomislav M, Von Segesser LK, et al. Acute lung injury during cardiopulmonary bypass. *Chest*. 1995;108:1551-1557.

27. DiCarlo JV, Raphaely RC, Steven JM, et al. Pulmonary mechanics in infants after cardiac surgery. *Crit Care Med*. 1992;20:22.

28. Miller BE, Levy JH. The inflammatory response to cardiopulmonary bypass.*J Cardiothorac Vasc Anesth*.1997;11:355-366.

29. Kirklin JK, Westaby S, Blackstone EH, et al. Complement and the damaging effects of cardiopulmonary bypass. *J Thorac Cardiovasc Surg*.1983; 86:845.

30. Pang LM, Stalcup SA, Lipset JS, et al. Increased circulating bradykinin during hypothermia and cardiopulmonary bypass in children. *Circulation*.1979; 60:1503-1507.

31. Millar AB, Armstrong L, van der Linden J, et al. Cytokine production and hemofiltration in children undergoing cardiopulmonary bypass. *Ann Thorac Surg*. 1993;56:1499-1502.

32. Faymonville ME, Deby DG, Larbuisson R, et al. Prostaglandin E2, prostacyclin, and thromboxane changes during nonpulsatile cardiopulmonary bypass in human. *J Thorac Cardiovasc Surg*. 1986;91:858-866.

33. Giomarelli P, Scolletta S, Borrelli E, et al. Myocardial and lung injury after cardiopulmonary bypass: role of interleukin(IL)-10. *Ann Thorac Surg*.2003; 76:117-123.

34. Hopkins RA, Bull C, Haworth SG, et al. Pulmonary hypertension crises during cardiac surgery for congenital heart defects in young children. *Eur J Cardiothorac Surg*. 1991;5:628-634.

35. Bando K, Turrentine MW, Sharp TG, et al. Pulmonary hypertension after operations for congenital heart disease: analysis of risk factors and management. *J Thorac Cardiovasc Surg*. 1996;112:1600-1609.

36. Vane JR, Anggard EE, Botting RM. Regulatory functions of the vascular endothelium. *N Engl J Med*.1990; 323:27-36.

37. Cooper CJ, Landsberg MJ, Anderson TJ, et al. Role of nitric oxide in the local regulation of pulmonary vascular resistance in humans. *Circulation*.1996; 93:266-271.

38. Kirshbom PM, Jacobs MT, Tsui SS, et al. Effects of cardiopulmonary bypass and circulatory arrest on endothelium dependent vasodilation in the lung. *J Thorac Cardiovasc Surg*.1996; 111:1248-1256.

39. Wessel DL, Adatia I, Giglia TM, et al. Use of inhaled nitric oxide and acetylcholine in the evaluation of pulmonary hypertension and endothelial function after cardiopulmonary bypass. *Circulation*.1993; 88:2128-2138.

40. Bando K, Vijayaraghavan P, Turrentine MW, et al. Dynamic changes of endothelin-1, nitric oxide and cyclic GMP in patients with congenital heart disease. *Circulation*. 1997;96(suppl):II346-II351.

41. Yanagisawa M, Kurihara H, Kimura S, et al. A novel potent vasoconstrictor peptide produced by vascular endothelial cells. *Nature*.1988; 332:411-415.

42. Komai H, Adatia IT, Elliot MJ, et al. Increased plasma levels of endothelin-1 after cardiopulmonary bypass in patients with pulmonary hypertension and congenital heart disease. *J Thorac Cardiovasc Surg*.1993; 106:473-478.

43. Graham T. Osmotic force. *Philos Trans R Soc Lond A*.1854; 144:177-228.

44. Peetom F, Gerald PS. A simple and inexpensive method for the concentration of protein solutions by means of ultrafiltration. *Clin Chim Acta*.1964; 10:375-376.

45. Magilligan DJ, Oyama C. Ultrafiltration during cardiopulmonary bypass: laboratory evaluation and initial clinical experience. *Ann Thorac Surg*.1984; 37:33-39.

46. Osipo VP, Lurie MY, Mikhailov Y, et al. Hemoconcentration during open heart operation. *Thorac Cardiovasc Surg*. 1985;33:81-85.

47. Ronco C, Clark W. Hollow-fiber dialyzers: technical and clinical considerations. In: Nissenson A, Fine R, eds. *Clinical Dialysis*. New York: McGraw-Hill; 2005:47-83.

48. Wheeldon D, Bethune D. Haemofiltration during cardiopulmonary bypass. *Perfusion*.1990; 5(suppl):39-51.

49. Ronco C, Ballestri M, Cappelli G. Dialysis membranes in convective treatments [see comment]. *Nephrol Dial Transplant*.2000; 15(suppl2) :31-36.

50. Craddick PR, Fehr J, Brigham KL. Complement and leucocyte-mediated pulmonary dysfunction in hemodialysis. *N Engl J Med*.197 7;296:769-774.

51. Bohler J, Kramer P, Gotze O. Leucocyte counts and complement activation during pump-driven and arteriovenous hemofiltration. In: Krama P, ed. *Arteriovenous Hemofi tration*. Gottingen: Vandenhoek & Ruprecht; 1982:187-192.

52. Journois D, Israel-Biet D, Pouard P, et al. High-volume, zero-balanced hemofiltration to reduce delayed inflammatory response to cardiopulmonary bypass in children. *Anesthesiology*.19 96;85:965-976.

53. Watanabe T, Sakai Y, Mayumi T, et al. Effect of ultrafiltration during cardiopulmonary bypass for pediatric cardiac surgery. *Artif Organs*.1998; 22:1052-1055.

54. Darup J, Bleese N, Kalmar P, et al. Hemofiltration during extracorporeal circulation. *Thorac Cardiovasc Surg*. 1979;27:227.

55. Tamari Y, Nelson R, Levy R, et al. Effects of the hemo-concentrator on blood. *J Extra Corpor Technol*.1984; 16:89-94.

56. Ramagnoli A, Hocker J, Keats A, et al. External hemoconcentration after deliberate hemodilution. *In Abstracts of the Annual Meeting of the American Society of Anesthesiologists*. Park Ridge, IL: American Society of Anesthesiologists; 1975;6:269.

57. Walpoth B, von Albertini B. Ultrafiltration in cardiac surgery. *J Extra Corpor Technol*.1984; 16:68-70.

58. Gaynor JW, Kuypers M, van Rossem M, et al. Haemodynamic changes during modified ultrafiltration immediately following the first stage of the Norwood reconstruction. *Cardiol Young*.2005;15:4-7.

59. Sever K, Tansel T, Basaran M, et al. The benefits of continuous ultrafiltration in pediatric cardiac surgery. *Scand Cardiovasc J*.2004 ;38:307-311.

60. Koutlas TC, Gaynor JW, Nicholson SC, et al. Modified ultrafiltration reduces postoperative morbidity after cavopulmonary connection. *Ann Thorac Surg*.1997; 64:37-42.

61. Draaisma AM, Hazekamp MG, Frank M, et al. Modified ultrafiltration after cardiopulmonary bypass in pediatric cardiac surgery. *Ann Thorac Cardiovasc Surg*. 1997;64:521-525.

62. Elliott MJ. Ultrafiltration and modified ultrafiltration in pediatric open heart operation. *Ann Thorac Surg*. 1993;56:1518-1522.

63. Bando K, Turrentine MW, Vijay P, et al. Effect of modified ultrafiltration in high-risk patients undergoing operations for congenital heart disease. *Ann Thorac Surg*. 1998;66:821-827.

64. Davies MJ, Nguyen K, Gaynor JW, et al. Modified ultrafiltration improves left ventricular systolic function in infants after cardiopulmonary bypass. *J Thorac Cardiovasc Surg*. 1998;115:361-369.

65. Groom RC, Akl BF, Albus RA, et al. Alternative method of ultrafiltration after cardiopulmonary bypass. *Ann Thorac Surg*.1994;58:573- 574.

66. Aeba R, Katogi T, Omoto T, et al. Modified ultrafiltration improves carbon dioxide removal after cardiopulmonary bypass in infants. *Artif Organs*.1999; 24:300-304.

67. Bando K, Vijay P, Turrebtine MW, et al. Dilutional and modified ultrafiltration reduces pulmonary hypertension after operations for congenital heart disease: a prospective randomized study. *J Thorac Cardiovasc Surg*. 1998;115:517-527.

68. Mahmoud AS, Burhani MS, Hannef AA, et al. Effect of modified ultrafiltration on pulmonary function after cardiopulmonary bypass. *Chest*.2005; 128:3447-3453.

69. Chaturvedi RR, Shore DF, White PA, et al. Modified ultrafiltration improves global left ventricular systolic function after open-heart surgery in infants and children. *Eur J Cardiothorac Surg*.1999; 15:742-746.

70. Chew MS, brix-Christensen V, Ravn HB, et al. Effect of modified ultrafiltration on the inflammatory response in paediatric open-heart surgery: a prospective, randomized study. *Perfusion*.2002; 17:327-333.

71. Anderson S, Gothberg S, Berggren H, et al. Hemofiltration modifies complement activation after extracorporeal circulation in infants. *Ann Thorac Surg*.1993; 56:1515-1517.

72. Yndgaard S, Andersen LW, Andersen C, et al. The effect of modified ultrafiltration on the amount of circulating endotoxins in children undergoing cardiopulmonary bypass. *J Cardiothorac Vasc Anesth*.2000; 14:399-401.

73. Myung RJ, Kirshborn PM, Petko M, et al. Modified ultrafiltration may not improve neurologic outcome following deep hypothermic circulatory arrest. *Eur J Cardiothorac Surg*. 2003;24:243-248.

74. Li J, Hoschtitzky A, Allen ML, et al. An analysis of oxygen consumption and oxygen delivery in euthermic infants after cardiopulmonary bypass with modified ultrafiltration. *Ann Thorac Cardiovasc Surg*.2004; 78:1389-1396.

75. Luciani GB, Menon T, Vecchi B, et al. Modified ultrafiltration reduces morbidity after adult cardiac operations: a prospective randomized clinical trial. *Circulation*. 2001;104(12 suppl1) :I253-I259.

76. Boga M, Islamoglu, Badak I, et al. The effects of modified hemofiltration on inflammatory mediators and cardiac performance in coronary artery bypass grafting. *Perfusion*. 2000;15:143-150.

77. Grnnenfelder J, Zund G, Schoeberlein A, et al. Modified ultrafiltration lowers adhesion molecule and cytokine level after cardiopulmonary bypass without clinical relevance in adults. *Eur J Cardiothorac Surg*.2000; 17:77-83.

78. Kiziltepe U, Uysalel A, Corapcioglu T, et al. Effects of combined conventional and modified ultrafiltration in adults patients. *Ann Thorac Surg*.2001; 71:684-693.

79. Chew MS. Does modified ultrafiltration reduce the systemic inflammatory response to cardiac surgery with cardiopulmonary bypass? *Perfusion*.2004; 19(suppl1) :S57-S60.

80. Tassani P, Richter JA, Eising GP, et al. Influence of combined zero-balanced and modified ultrafiltration on the systemic inflammatory response during coronary artery bypass grafting. *J Cardiothorac Vasc Anesth*.1999; 13:285-291.

81. Nagashima M, Shin'oka T, Nollert G, et al. High-volume continuous hemofiltration during cardiopulmonary bypass attenuates pulmonary dysfunction in neonates lambs after deep hypothermic circulatory arrest. *Circulation*. 1998; 98:II378-II384.

82. Schmaldienst S, Horl W. Biocompatibility. In: Nissenson A, Fine R, eds. *Clinical Dialysis*. 4th ed. New York: McGraw-Hill;2005: 101-125.

83. Berdat PA, Eichenberger E, Ebell J, et al. Elimination of proinflammatory cytokines in pediatric cardiac surgery: analysis of ultrafiltration method and filter type. *J Thorac Cardiovasc Surg*.2004; 127:1688-1696.

84. Onoe M, Magara T, Yamamoto Y, et al. Modified ultrafiltration removes serum interleukin-8 in adult cardiac surgery. *Perfusion*.2001;16 :37-42.
85. Teraoka S, Mineshima M, Hoshino T, et al. Can cytokines be removed by hemofiltration or hemoadsorption? *ASAIO*. 2000;46:448-451.
86. Silverstein MEFE, Lysaght MJ, Henderson LW. Treatment of severe fluid overload by ultrafiltration. *N Eng J Med*. 1974;291:747-750.
87. Garup J, Bleese N, Kalmar P, et al. Hemofiltration during extracorporeal circulation. *Thorac Cardiovasc Surg*. 1979;27:227-230.
88. Onoe M, Oku H, Kitayama H. et al Modified ultrafiltration may improve postoperative pulmonary function in children with a ventricular septal defect [abstract]. *Surg Today*. 2001;31:586-590.
89. Meliones J, Gaynor JW, Wilson BG, et al. Modified ultrafiltration reduces airway pressures and improves lung compliance after congenital heart surgery [abstract]. *J Am Coll Cardiol*.1995;25:2 71A.
90. Keenan HT, Thiagarajan R, Stephens KE, et al. Pulmonary function after modified venovenous ultrafiltration in infants: a prospective, randomized trial. *J Thorac Cardiovasc Surg*. 2000;119:501-507.
91. Huang HM, Yao TJ, Wang W, et al. Continuous ultrafiltration attenuates the pulmonary injury that follows open heart surgery with cardiopulmonary bypass. *Ann Thorac Surg*. 2003;76:136-140.
92. Cole L, Bellomo R, Davenport P, et al. The effect of coupled haemofiltration and adsorption on inflammatory cytokines in an ex vivo model. *Nephrol Dial Transplant*. 2002;17:1950-1956.
93. Hauser GJ, Ben-Ari J, Colvin MP, et al. Interleukin-6 levels in serum and lung lavage fluid of children undergoing open heart surgery correlate with postoperative morbidity. *Intensive Card Med*.1998; 24:481-486.
94. Paparella D, Yau TM, Young E. Cardiopulmonary bypass induced inflammation: pathophysiology and treatment. An update. *Eur J Cardiothorac Surg*.2002; 21:232-244.
95. Wang MJ, Chiu IS, Hsu CM, et al. efficacy of ultrafiltration in removing inflammatory mediators during pediatric cardiac operations. *Ann Thorac Surg*.1996; 61:651-656.
96. Hoffmann J, Faist E. Removal of mediators by continuous hemofiltration in septic patients. *World J Surg*. 2001;25: 651-659.
97. Segahaye M, Duchateau J, Bruniaux J, et al. Interleukin-10 release related to cardiopulmonary bypass in infants undergoing cardiac operations. *J Thorac Cardiovasc Surg*. 1996;111:545-553.
98. BaiTera P, Janssen EM, Demacker PN, et al. Removal of interleukin-1 beta and tumor necrosis factor from human plasma by in vitro dialysis with polyacrylonitrile membranes. *Lymphokine Cytokine Res*.1992; 11:99-104.
99. Fujita M, Ishihara M, Kusama Y, et al. Effect of modified ultrafiltration on inflammatory mediators, coagulation factors, and other proteins in blood after an extracorporeal circuit. *Artif Organs*.2004; 28:310-313.
100. Barrera P, Jansosen EM, Demacker PN, et al. Removal of interleukin-1 beta and tumor necrosis factor from human plasma by in vitro dialysis with polyacrylonitrile membrane. *Lymphokine Cytokine Res*.1992; 11:1212-1218.
101. Rubens FD, Mesana T. The inflammatory response to cardiopulmonary bypass: a therapeutic overview. *Perfusion*. 2004;19(suppl1) :S5-S12.
102. Kolff W. First clinical experience with the artificial kidney. *Ann Intern Med*.1965; 62:608-619.
103. Wellel DL, Adatia I, Giglia TM, et al. Use of inhaled nitric oxide and acetylcholine in the evaluation of pulmonary hypertension and endothelial function after cardiopulmonary bypass. *Circulation*.1993; 88:2128-2138.
104. Goto K, Hama H, Kasuya Y. Molecular pharmacology and pathophysiological significance of endothelin. *Jpn J Pharmacol*.1996; 72:261-90.
105. Hiramatsu T, Imai Y, Kurosawa H, et al. Effects of dilutional and modified ultrafiltration in plasma endothelin-1 and pulmonary vascular resistance after the Fontan Procedure. *Ann Thorac Surg*.2002; 73:862-865.

Principles of Pulmonary Protection During Heart Surgery

Benefits of Hemofiltration for Pulmonary Function

Mitsugi Nagashima and Toshiharu Shin'oka

28

28.1 Introduction

Ultrafiltration (UF) is a process of removing excess fluid from the blood through a membrane by exerting pressure and in which no fluid is replaced after removal of ultrafiltrate. The concentration of a solute in a patient's blood is theoretically unchanged before and after UF because the concentration of the solute in the ultrafiltrate and in the patient is the same. UF is not an adequate procedure for blood purification, although it is effective and useful for removal of water. Conventional UF is performed during the rewarming period of cardiopulmonary bypass (CPB) to remove excess water from patients. Modified UF is carried out after weaning from CPB to concentrate the diluted blood.[1] Both conventional UF and modified UF are frequently performed in either pediatric or adult cardiac surgery, and their effects on the postoperative clinical data and organ functions have been assessed.[2-6]

Hemofiltration (HF) involves the removal of plasma water and *simultaneous replacement* with a buffered electrolyte solution. Therefore, the total amount of ultrafiltrate containing inflammatory mediators that can be removed is much more in HF than UF because the amount of ultrafiltrate in UF is practically limited by the extent to which the blood concentration is sufficiently achieved in the CPB circuit. HF could be theoretically more attractive than UF in terms of blood purification and removal of some harmful substances.

M.N agashima(✉)
Department of Surgery, Division of Cardio-Thoracic Surgery
and Regenerative Surgery, Stroke and Cardiovascular Center,
Ehime University School of Medicine, Shitsukawa,
ToonC ity, Japan
e-mail:m itsugi@m.ehime-u.ac.jp

In some old literatures,[7,8] isolated UF without any additional solution added to the CPB system was described as HF. These procedures are not discussed in this chapter. On the other hand, a few different terms, such as "zero balanced or balanced UF,"[9] "dilutional UF,"[10] "continuous UF,"[11] and "washed pump-priming fluid"[12] have often been utilized in the literature. All these terms represent UF with intentional addition of a buffered electrolyte solution to CPB circuits. All these procedures, which are called UF but actually are HF, are also discussed as HF in this chapter.

28.2 Hemofiltration for Prime of Cardiopulmonary Bypass

In adult patients, the prime solution for the CPB circuit is usually a crystalloid solution. In pediatric patients, especially small infants and neonates, the CPB prime is mainly blood, including fresh whole blood or banked concentrated red cells in many institutions to reduce excessive hemodilution. The components of the primed fluid strongly influence the level of metabolites, such as glucose, lactate, and other electrolytes during and even early after CPB in small children because the ratio of pump prime volume to a patient's total amount of blood is much larger than in adult patients.[13,14] Banked blood or even fresh whole blood has high concentrations of potassium and ammonium and can cause severe metabolic acidosis.[14] This undesirable and unphysiologic prime solution might cause postoperative organ dysfunction. In addition, recirculation of blood pump priming within the CPB circuit causes an increase in the concentration of cascade substances of

E.A. Gabriel and T. Salerno (eds.), *Principles of Pulmonary Protection in Heart Surgery*,
DOI: 10.1007/978-1-84996-308-4_28, © Springer-Verlag London Limited 2010

complement, interleukin (IL),[15] and bradykinin.[16] These substances increase microvascular permeability and edema formation of organs. Ridley et al. hemofiltrated primed citrate-phosphate-dextrose stored blood within the CPB circuit to adjust the unphysiologic metabolites and electrolytes before connecting CPB to patients.[12] HF for primed blood successfully decreased the level of ammonium, bradykinin, complement C3a, and thromboxane B2 (TXB_2; TXA_2 inactive metabolite) and improved pH and base excess within the circuit.[16,17] Hemofiltrated pump priming decreased the leukocyte count and the level of some cytokines, including tumor necrosis factor alpha (TNF-α), IL-1β, IL-6, and IL-8 even 1 h after CPB. A prospective, randomized study in pediatric patients revealed HF of primed blood in CPB significantly improved the impaired respiratory index at 3 h after surgery, shortened the duration of ventilator support and intensive care unit (ICU) stay, and reduced inotropic support.[17]

Other observational studies showed the beneficial effects of HF for priming of CPB on postoperative gas exchange ability[16,18] and edema formation[18] in neonates with transposition of the great arteries (Fig. 28.1).

These studies showed the beneficial effect of HF for primed blood on postoperative lung function in pediatric patients. When one uses blood as the pump prime, HF for primed blood may reduce the level of several kinds of inflammatory mediators (bradykinin, complement, TNF-α, and ILs) in the pump circuit. In addition, recirculation of the primed blood in the pump circuit and the hemofilter can make a biocompatible membrane on the surface of the artificial devices. As a result, less initial contact reaction between patient blood and these devices may be expected.

28.3 Hemofiltration During Cardiopulmonary Bypass in Animal Experiments

There is little research on the effect of HF during CPB on postoperative pulmonary function in animal studies. In a study of a lung transplantation model in dogs, continuous HF 20 min before reperfusion to termination of CPB significantly increased arterial oxygenation and alveolar-to arterial-gradient for oxygen ($AaDO_2$) and decreased pulmonary vascular resistance (PVR) after the operation.[19] In this study, the HF dose rate was 600 mL/kg/h, and the total amount of filtrate was 125 mL/kg. Another neonatal lamb model using CPB with 120 min of deep hypothermic circulatory arrest showed that HF for the primed blood followed by continuous high-volume (300 mL/kg/h) HF throughout CPB attenuated pulmonary dysfunction after CPB.[20] In the HF group, there was less rise in PVR at 180 min after CPB, and percentage recovery of pulmonary dynamic compliance and $AaDO_2$ after CPB were preserved significantly at 120 min but not at 180 min after reperfusion (Fig. 28.2). A product of lipid peroxidation in lung tissue was also lower in the HF group. These beneficial effects of HF could be related with less edema formation, which was assessed by measuring total body water using bioimpedance analysis in the HF group. On the other hand, in a pig model using 120 min of CPB with 90 min of aortic cross clamping, HF during 30 min of reperfusion and 30 min after CPB

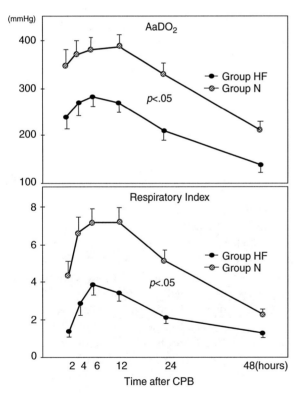

Fig. 28.1 Changes in alveolar-arterial oxygen tension difference (*top*) and respiratory index (*bottom*) after cardiopulmonary bypass in neonates with transpositon of great arteries. *AaDO₂* alveolar-arterial oxygen tension difference, *Group HF* hemofiltrated blood priming group, *Group N* nonhemofiltrated blood priming group, *CPB* cardiopulmonarybypa ss

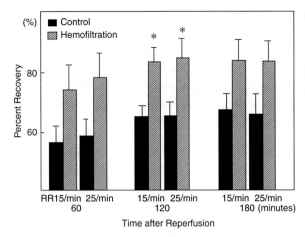

Fig. 28.2 Percentage recovery of lung dynamic compliance after cardiopulmonary bypass (CPB). *$p < 0.05$ compared with control. *RR*re spiratoryra te

was ineffective in improving cardiac performance and reducing inflammatory response by decreasing inflammatory mediators, including TNF-α and IL-8.[21] In this article, unfortunately, there was no information about arterial oxygenation, postoperative lung mechanics, or PVR.

These few animal models may have shown a beneficial effect of high-volume HF during CPB on post-CPB lung dysfunction.

28.4 Hemofiltration During Cardioplmonary Bypass in Pediatric Patients

Journois et al. examined the effect of HF (total filtrate 20–30 mL/kg) during the rewarming period (about 1 h) of CPB in a prospective randomized study with 32 children with tetralogy of Fallot (TOF).[22] In the HF group, there was a significant reduction in postoperative AaDO$_2$, time to extubation, cumulative blood loss, and plasma level of C3a, C5a, and TNF-α compared with patients without HF. In addition, a significant increase in mean arterial pressure was observed in the HF group. Then, their interest was focused on the effect of very-high-volume HF (approximately estimated as 300 mL/kg/h, total amount of filtrate 250 mL/kg) during the rewarming period.[9] They compared clinical data and biological variables between the patients with high-

volume HF during rewarming plus modified UF and the patients with only modified UF. Postoperatively, AaDO$_2$, time to extubation, body temperature, and cumulative blood loss were reduced in the high-volume HF group. They showed that C3a, TNF-α, IL-1β, and IL-6 were also significantly lower, even at 24 h after operation, in the high-volume HF group. They also showed in this study that the plasma level of midazolam and alfentanyl decreased before and after high-volume HF, but not in the group with only modified UF. This finding can be related to an increase in blood pressure after HF. It should be considered that, in the clinical setting, important drugs also may possibly be filtrated and plasma concentration reduced. Further investigation should be required for individual drugs. The group successfully demonstrated the concept that high-volume HF during rewarming has beneficial effect to postoperative clinical course due to an effective removal of inflammatory mediators.

Systemic inflammation theoretically initiates from the beginning of CPB, that is, the time of a contact of the patient's blood with the foreign body surface, although there were some reports that the plasma level of several inflammatory mediators increased during the rewarming period.[23,24] To exert a maximum HF effort for filtrating inflammatory mediators, early application of HF could be theoretically important. In fact, in animal studies with septic shock using administration of endotoxin or pancreatitis shock models, early application of HF was reported to improve survival time[25] and hemodynamics.[26] Bando et al. studied this concept of early application of HF during CPB. They randomly assigned 24 pediatric patients to two groups. One group underwent HF (40–70 mL/kg/h, total filtrate 170 mL/kg) throughout CPB plus modified UF, and the other group underwent conventional UF as a control. In HF through CPB with the modified UF group, significant reductions in the ratio of pulmonary to systemic pressure, duration of ventilation support, requirement for blood products during the first postoperative day, and concentration of endothelin 1(ET-1) after the operation were observed.[10] The levels of cyclic guanosine monophosphate (cGMP, intermediate substance of the nitric oxide pathway) and nitric oxide metabolite were not influenced by this HF procedure.

Hiramatsu et al. assessed 22 patients who underwent the Fontan procedure.[27] They compared semicontinuous HF during CPB followed by modified UF with conventional UF. Plasma ET-1 levels increased significantly after CPB in the control group, but they did not increase immediately after CPB in the continuous HF group. Similarly, PVR increased significantly after CPB in the control group, but it did not increase after CPB in the continuous HF group and remained low at 6 and 24 h after CPB (Fig. 28.3).

Another prospective randomized study in 30 pediatric patients with ventricular septal defect (VSD) or TOF showed that HF throughout CPB with modified UF ameliorated deteriorated pulmonary static compliance, airway resistance, and AaDO$_2$ after CPB.[11] IL-6, TXB$_2$, and ET-1 were measured as inflammatory mediators. HF was effective for reducing the level of IL-6 but failed to reduce TXB$_2$ and ET-1. IL-6 and trivial TXB$_2$, but no ET-1, were in the filtrates.

Williams et al. investigated the clinical outcome after three different strategies of HF or UF.[28] One group of infants received HF throughout CPB (it was called dilutional UF) only, another group of infants received modified UF only, and the third group received both HF throughout CPB and modified UF. They expected the third group would have a better clinical outcome than the other groups. Total amount of filtrate in the

third group was 260 mL/kg, which was much more than two other groups. However, any advantageous effects on clinical data, including duration of mechanical ventilation, duration of ICU stay, and total volume of transfused blood products in the third group. Even for lung functional parameters such as pulmonary compliance and AaDO$_2$, there were no significant differences among the three groups. The authors speculated that one of the negative aspects of their study was that all three groups had HF for the primed, banked, packed red blood cells, which may have reduced severe systemic inflammation. The other factor was that deep hypothermic circulatory arrest, which may cause a large insult on small infant organs, was never used in their study.

In the latter half of 1990s to the early 2000s, most literature showed that HF led to improved postoperative lung dysfunction and reduced many kinds of inflammatory mediators. However, the positive effect of perioperative HF or modified UF has decreased in recent studies. Even in pediatric cardiac surgery, the role of perioperative HF is still controversial. One of the reasons may be that the recent evolution of the CPB system, such as less priming volume because of a miniaturized CPB circuit and increased biocompatibility of the surface of the extracorporeal circulation, may cause less systemic inflammation and edema formation in even small infants and neonates. In addition, avoiding deep hypothermia or circulatory arrest may have a good influence in decreasing systemic inflammation.

28.5 Hemofiltration During Cardiopulmonary Bypass in Adult Patients

A randomized study in 43 adult patients with elective coronary artery bypass grafting (CABG) revealed that HF during the rewarming period plus modified UF (total filtrate 34 mL/kg) shortened the time to extubation[29] and slightly lowered PVR. This study measured perioperative IL-6 and IL-8. However, there was no significant difference between the HF group and the control (without HF), although there were these inflammatory mediators in the filtrate.

A retrospective but large study in 118 adult patients with high-risk cardiac surgery, including repeat operation, valve surgery with CABG, or CPB longer than

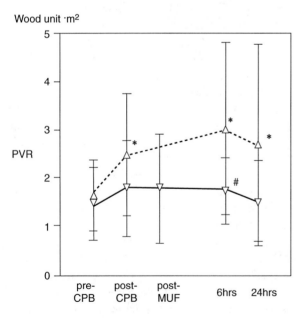

Fig. 28.3 Time course of pulmonary vascular resistance (PVR). *$p<0.05$ versus precardiopulmonary bypass (CPB); # $p<0.05$ versus control. The dashed line represents the control group; the *solid line* represents the HF with modified ultrafiltration (MUF) group. *HF* hemofiltration, *UF* ultrafiltration)

2 h demonstrated higher preservation of platelet counts after CPB and less chest tube drainage after operation in patients with HF throughout CPB (total filtrate 40–45 mL/kg) compared with the other patients without HF.[30] However, this study failed to show a reduced duration of ventilation and hospital stay and amelioration of postoperative cardiac dysfunction.

A large, prospective, randomized, double-blind study in 192 adult patients with standard cardiac surgery, including CABG and valve repair or replacement, showed that HF during CPB (total filtrate 27 mL/kg) led to a shorter duration of mechanical ventilation, less fluid balance, and less mediastinal drainage.[31] This study failed to show that HF reduced the level of complement activation (C3a and C5b-9) after CPB and improved postoperative AaDO$_2$.

Another prospective randomized large study of 79 patients with CABG was reported. This study showed that HF throughout the entire CPB period (total filtrate 15 mL/kg) did not influence the blood concentration levels of IL-6 and IL-10 after CPB. Enzyme-linked immunosorbent assay (ELISA) analysis failed to identify either IL-6 or IL-10 in the filtrate. In addition, incidence of postoperative acute renal failure was slightly higher in the HF group.[32]

HF during CPB in adult surgery generally provided favorable effects on postoperative lung function, such as shorter duration of mechanical ventilation. However, in terms of reduction of inflammatory mediators, most studies failed to demonstrate the advantageous effects ofH F.

28.6 SummaryandPer spective

Most of the reports of perioperative HF in cardiac surgery showed reduced postoperative lung dysfunction and shortened duration of ventilator support. Although its mechanism is unclear, reducing inflammatory mediators and removing excess body water may suppress the accelerated permeability at the level of microvessel circulation. These lead to less edema formation in the lungs. As a result, arterial oxygenation, lung compliance, and even PVR may improve. And, adverse effects of perioperative HF on clinical outcomes were few except for its complicated manipulation, increased costs, and a possible reduction of important drugs due to filtration. Meanwhile, these beneficial effects of HF

may be significant in only transient and subtle parameters, and no advantageous effects may be observed in principle outcomes,[28] such as survival rate and duration of ICU or hospital stay.

The role of HF in reducing inflammatory mediators may be more effective in pediatric patients than adults according to the detailed analysis of the literature. One of the reasons is that the total filtrated volume is much higher in many pediatric patients compared to adults. Actually, approximately a five- to tenfold volume was filtrated in pediatric studies compared to adults. Another reason may be the shorter duration of CPB and small ratio of pump priming volume to patients' blood volume in adult patients. These factors may causes less systemic inflammation during CPB. In fact, in studies of patients who underwent standard cardiac surgery, the advantageous effect of HF, conventional UF, or modified UF on clinical outcomes was very limited.[28,33]

Recent improvements in the CPB system and surgical technique produce less systemic inflammation after cardiac surgery. To clarify the effect of perioperative HF on postoperative morbidity in the recent less invasive CPB system, a powered prospective randomized trial should be required. Especially, HF should be investigated regarding the optimal filtrate volume and rate, optimal contents of the HF solution, timing of initiation, type of membrane, and the HF strategy, including whether performed throughout, during rewarming, or after CPB.

References

1. Naik SK, Knight A, Elliott MJ. A successful modification of ultrafiltration for cardiopulmonary bypass in children. *Perfusion*.1991; 6:41-50.
2. Wang M, Chiu I, Hsu C, et al. Efficacy of ultrafiltration in removing inflammatory mediators during pediatric cardiac operations. *Ann Thorac Surg*.1996; 61:651-656.
3. Bando K, Turrentine MW, Vijay P, et al. Effect of modified ultrafiltration in high-risk patients undergoing operations for congenital heart disease. *Ann Thorac Surg*. 1998;66: 821-828.
4. Boodhwani M, Williams K, Babaev A, Gill G, Saleem N, Rubens FD. Ultrafiltration reduces blood transfusions following cardiac surgery: a meta-analysis. *Eur J Cardiothorac Surg*.2006; 30:892-897.
5. Luciani GB, Menon T, Vecchi B, Auriemma S, Mazzucco A. Modified ultrafiltration reduces morbidity after adult cardiac operations a prospective, randomized clinical trial. *Circulation*2001; 104(supplI):I-253–I-259

6. Myung RJ, Kirshbom PM, Petko M, et al. Modified ultrafiltration may not improve neurologic outcome following deep
   hypothermic circulatory arrest. Eur J Cardiothorac Surg.
   2003;24:243-248.
7. Millar AB, Armstrong L, van der Linden J, et al. Cytokine
   production and hemofiltration in children undergoing cardiopulmonary bypass. Ann Thorac Surg. 1993;56:1499-1502.
8. Boldt J, Kling D, von Bormann B, Scheld HH, Hempelmann
   G. Extravascular lung water and hemofiltration during complicated cardiac surgery. Thorac Cardiovasc Surg. 1987;35:
   161-165.
9. Journois D, Israel-Biet D, Pouard P, et al. High-volume,
   zero-balanced hemofiltration to reduce delayed inflammatory response to cardiopulmonary bypass in children. Anes-
   thesiology.1996;85 :965-976.
10. Bando K, Vijay P, Turrentine MW, et al. Dilutional and mod-
    ified ultrafiltration reduces pulmonary hypertension after
    operations for congenital heart disease: a prospective ran-
    domized study. J Thorac Cardiovasc Surg 1998;115:
    517–525
11. Huang H, Yao T, Wang W, et al. Continuous ultrafiltration
    attenuates the pulmonary injury that follows open heart sur-
    gery with cardiopulmonary bypass. Ann Thorac Surg. 2003;
    76:136-140.
12. Ridley PD, Ratcliffe JM, Alberti KG, Elliott MJ. The meta-
    bolic consequences of a "washed" cardiopulmonary bypass
    pump-priming fluid in children undergoing cardiac opera-
    tions. J Thorac Cardiovasc Surg1990; 100:528–537
13. Ratcliffe JM, Wyse RK, Hunter S, Alberti KG, Elliott MJ.
    The role of the priming fluid in the metabolic response to
    cardiopulmonary bypass in children of less than 15 kg body
    weight undergoing open-heart surgery. Thorac Cardiovasc
    Surg.1988;36:65-7 4.
14. Keidan I, Amir G, Mandel M, Mishali D. The metabolic
    effects of fresh versus old stored blood in the priming of car-
    diopulmonary bypass solution for pediatric patients. J Thorac
    Cardiovasc Surg. 2004;127:949-952.
15. Finn A, Morgan BP, Rebuck N, et al. Effects of inhibition of
    complement activation using recombinant soluble comple-
    ment receptor 1 on neutrophil CD11b/CD18 and L-selectin
    expression and release of interleukin-8 and elastase in simu-
    lated cardiopulmonary bypass. J Thorac Cardiovasc Surg.
    1996;111:451-459.
16. Nagashima M, Imai Y, Seo K, et al. Effect of hemofiltrated
    whole blood pump priming on hemodynamics and respira-
    tory function after the arterial switch operation in neonates.
    Ann Thorac Surg.2 000;70:1901-1906.
17. Shimpo H, Shimamoto A, Sawamura Y, et al. Ultrafiltration
    of the priming blood before cardiopulmonary bypass attenu-
    ates inflammatory response and improves postoperative clin-
    ical course in pediatric patients. Shock. 2001;16(suppl 1):
    51-54.
18. Sakurai H, Maeda M, Sai N, et al. Extended use of hemofil-
    tration and high perfusion flow rate in cardiopulmonary
    bypass improves perioperative fluid balance in neonates and
    infants. Ann Thorac Cardiovasc Surg.1999; 5:94-100.
19. Saitoh M, Tsuchida M, Koike T, et al. Ultrafiltration attenu-
    ates cardiopulmonary bypass-induced acute lung injury in a
    canine model of single-lung transplantation. J Thorac
    Cardiovasc Surg.2 006;132:1447-1454.
20. Nagashima M, Shin'oka T, Nollert G, Shum-Tim D, Rader
    CM, Mayer JE Jr. High-volume continuous hemofiltration
    during cardiopulmonary bypass attenuates pulmonary dys-
    function in neonatal lambs after deep hypothermic circula-
    tory arrest. Circulation 1998;98(suppl):II378–II384
21. Eising GP, Schad H, Heimisch W, et al. Effect of cardiopul-
    monary bypass and hemofiltration on plasma cytokines and
    protein leakage in pigs. Thorac Cardiovasc Surg. 2000;48:
    86-92.
22. Journois D, Pouard P, Greeley WJ, Mauriat P, Vouhé P,
    Safran D. Hemofiltration during cardiopulmonary bypass in
    pediatric cardiac surgery. Effects on hemostasis, cytokines,
    and complement components. Anesthesiology 1994;81:
    1181–1189
23. Andreasson S, Göthberg S, Berggren H, Bengtsson A,
    Eriksson E, Risberg B. Hemofiltration modifies complement
    activation after extracorporeal circulation in infants. Ann
    Thorac Surg.1993; 56:1515-1517.
24. Berdat PA, Eichenberger E, Ebell J, et al. Elimination of
    proinflammatory cytokines in pediatric cardiac surgery:
    analysis of ultrafiltration method and filter type. J Thorac
    Cardiovasc Surg.2004; 127:1688-1696.
25. Yekebas EF, Treede H, Knoefel WT, Bloechle C, Fink E,
    Izbicki JR. Influence of zero-balanced hemofiltration on the
    course of severe experimental pancreatitis in pigs. Ann Surg.
    1999;229:514-522.
26. Mink SN, Li X, Bose D, et al. Early but not delayed continu-
    ous arteriovenous hemofiltration improves cardiovascular
    function in sepsis in dogs. Intensive Care Med. 1999;25:
    733-743.
27. Hiramatsu T, Imai Y, Kurosawa H, et al. Effects of dilutional
    and modified ultrafiltration in plasma endothelin-1 and pul-
    monary vascular resistance after the Fontan procedure. Ann
    Thorac Surg.2002; 73:861-865.
28. Williams GD, Ramamoorthy C, Chu L, et al. Modified and
    conventional ultrafiltration during pediatric cardiac surgery:
    clinical outcomes compared. J Thorac Cardiovasc Surg.
    2006;132:1291-1298.
29. Tassani P, Richter JA, Eising GP, et al. Influence of com-
    bined zero-balanced and modified ultrafiltration on the sys-
    temic inflammatory response during coronary artery bypass
    grafting. J Cardiothorac Vasc Anesth.1999; 13:285-291.
30. Raman JS, Hata M, Bellomo R, Kohchi K, Cheung HL,
    Buxton BF. Hemofiltration during cardiopulmonary bypass
    for high risk adult cardiac surgery. Int J Artif Organs.
    2003;26:753-757.
31. Oliver WC Jr, Nuttall GA, Orszulak TA, et al. Hemofiltration
    but not steroids results in earlier tracheal extubation follow-
    ing cardiopulmonary bypass: a prospective, randomized
    double-blind trial. Anesthesiology.2004; 101:327-339.
32. Musleh GS, Datta SS, Yonan NN, et al. Association of IL6
    and IL10 with renal dysfunction and the use of haemofiltra-
    tion during cardiopulmonary bypass. Eur J Cardiothorac
    Surg2009; 35:511–514
33. Thompson LD, McElhinney DB, Findlay P, et al. A prospec-
    tive randomized study comparing volume-standardized
    modified and conventional ultrafiltration in pediatric cardiac
    surgery. J Thorac Cardiovasc Surg.2001; 122:220-228.

Edmo Atique Gabriel and Tomas Salerno

Gabriel et al.[1] have devised experimental research using 32 male pigs, which were randomly aligned into groups and subgroups as depicted in Table 29.1. It is noteworthy because of the two different strategies of cardiopulmonary bypass (CPB) as well as different types of lung perfusion analyzed in this research.

All the animals were subjected to general anesthesia using sodium pentobarbital (12.5 mg/kg), fentanyl (0.01 mg/kg), and thiopental (1 g). Anesthetic maintenance was achieved using fentanyl (0.01 mg/kg) and thiopental (1 g each 20 min). Prior to the operative procedure, lungs were mechanically ventilated using a pressure-cycled ventilator with 10 mL/kg tidal volume. Hemodynamic monitoring was achieved by insertion of an 8 French catheter into the right internal carotid artery (for measurement of mean artery pressure) and a 7 French Swan-Ganz catheter into right external jugular vein (for measurement of preoperative and postoperative hemodynamic parameters such as mean pulmonary artery pressure). Cardiac output was determined by the thermodilution method considering the mean value of three sequential measurements. Furthermore, urinary output throughout the procedure was evaluated by insertion of a catheter directly into the bladder following a small abdominal incision. The main steps of hemodynamic monitoring are representedinFigs . 29.1–29.4.

In group I animals, CPB was established by cannulating the root of the ascending aorta and both venae cavae, aortic cross clamping, and inducing cardioplegic arrest

and moderate hypothermia. Following aortic cross clamping and the first shot of cardioplegia, the main pulmonary artery was cannulated and lung perfusion performed for 30 min. The left atrium was vented during the period of lung perfusion. The steps for establishing CPB in group II animals was similar; however, the most remarkable difference was that their hearts were allowed to beat at normothermia, while the lungs were perfused for 30 min through cannulation of the main pulmonary artery. Moreover, the right atrium was vented, and both venae cavae remained snared during the lung perfusion in group II. It is noteworthy that mechanical ventilation was discontinued once CPB was established in both groups. The relationship between the great vessels and types of cannulae can seen in Table 29.2.

Our decision regarding the most appropriate lung perfusion pressure for preventing ischemia-reperfusion injury with no additional damage to pulmonary endothelium and parenchyma mandated exhaustive analyses and research. On the assumption that providing lung perfusion under physiologic conditions would be the most adequate strategy for reproduction during heart surgery requiring CPB, we decided to perfuse the main pulmonary artery using physiologic lung perfusion pressure. How could we do it? How could we mostly simulate or reproduce physiologic lung perfusion pressure as well as make this pressure stable during heart surgery with CPB?

That was our great dilemma; our propositions were to use the preoperative mean pulmonary artery pressure taken by Swan-Ganz catheter as the lung perfusion pressure and to connect a digital manometer to the lung perfusion line aiming for stable lung perfusion pressure. It is paramount to let you know that preoperative status can reflect the real cardiopulmonary status under physiologic conditions before midline

E.A.G abriel (✉)
Department of Surgery, Division of Cardiovascular Surgery
FederalU niversityofS aoP aulo, SaoP aulo, Brazil
e-mail:e dag@uol.com.br

E.A. Gabriel and T. Salerno (eds.), *Principles of Pulmonary Protection in Heart Surgery,*
DOI: 10.1007/978-1-84996-308-4_29, © Springer-Verlag London Limited 2010

Table29.1 Experimentalgr oupsa nds ubgroups

| Group I ($n=16$) | | GroupI I($n=16$) | |
Cardioplegia		Beatinge mptyhe art	
Subgroup IA ($n=4$)	Control[a]	IIA($n=4$)	Control[a]
Subgroup IB ($n=6$)	Lung perfusion with arterial blood	IIB($n=6$)	Lung perfusion with arterial blood
Subgroup IC ($n=6$)	Lung perfusion with venous blood	IIC($n=6$)	Lung perfusion with venous blood

[a]Without controlled lung perfusion through inflow cannula

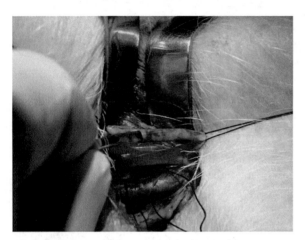

Fig.29.1 Catheterintor ighti nternalc arotida rtery

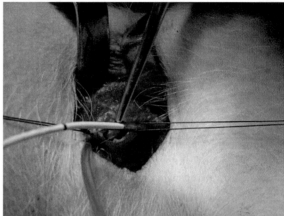

Fig. 29.3 Catheteri ntor ighte xternalj ugularv ein

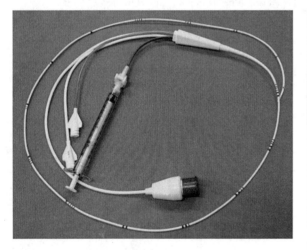

Fig.29.2 Swan-Ganzc atheter

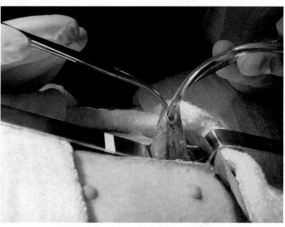

Fig. 29.4 Smalla bdominali ncision:c atheteri ntobl adder

sternotomy as the heart is beating under stable conditions and the lungs are being ventilated and perfused by venous blood from the right chambers. We believe that creating conditions to simulate or reproduce physiologic status can be a safe strategy for lung perfusion.

Furthermore, we believe that there is a need to create protocols and algorithms for lung perfusion; therefore, our propositions can be interesting and effective approaches to optimize postoperative results.

Based on these principles and concepts, mean lung perfusion pressure and mean lung perfusion flow were

Table29.2 Greatv esselsa ndc annulae

Greatv essel	Typeof c annula	Caliber
Aorta	Methal – straight	12 French – 3/16 inch
Superiorv ena cava	Methal – curve	16 French – ¼ inch
Inferiorv ena cava	Methal – curve	16 French – ¼ inch
Mainpul monary artery	Methal–c urve	12 French – 3/16 inch

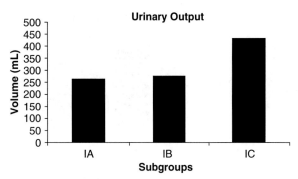

IA – no lung perfusion

IB – lung perfusion with arterial blood

IC – lung perfusion with venous blood

Fig. 29.6 Urinaryout puti ns ubgroupsI A,I B,I C

equivalent to 24.6 mmHg and 200 mL/min, respectively. There were no differences in lung perfusion pressure using arterial or venous blood. Pump flows ranged from 1.2 to 1.4 L/min/m². Average time of CPB ranged from 35 to 40 min. Postoperative hemodynamic measurements were made soon after weaning from CPB, and the animals were then euthanized using potassium intravenously. The results for some hemodynamic parameters in different groups and subgroups are schematicallyre presentedinFigs . 29.5–29.14.

Ultimately, another issue is that our concern should be particularly turned to strictly monitor lung perfusion pressure according to the preoperative measurement. We mean that lung perfusion pressure must remain stable throughout heart surgery with CPB regardless of eventual variations of pulmonary perfusion flow that can result from several intrinsic and extrinsic factors.

Schultz et al.[2] have proposed an experimental study to compare the impact of hypothermic low-flow CPB and circulatory arrest on pulmonary and right ventricular function. For achieving this goal, these authors utilized

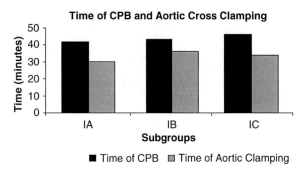

IA – no lung perfusion

IB – lung perfusion with arterial blood

IC – lung perfusion with venous blood

Fig. 29.7 Time of cardiopulmonary bypass (CPB) and aortic crossc lampingi ns ubgroupsI A,I B,I C

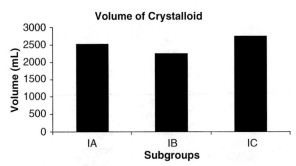

IA – no lung perfusion

IB – lung perfusion with arterial blood

IC – lung perfusion with venous blood

Fig.29.5 Volumeo fc rystalloidsi ns ubgroups IA,I B,I C

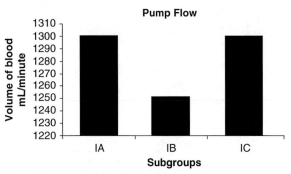

IA – no lung perfusion

IB – lung perfusion with arterial blood

IC – lung perfusion with venous blood

Fig. 29.8 Pumpfl owi ns ubgroupsI A,I B,I C

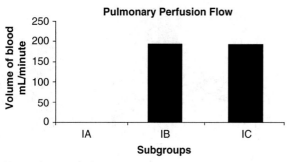

IA – no lung perfusion

IB – lung perfusion with arterial blood

IC – lung perfusion with venous blood

Fig.29.9 Pulmonaryp erfusionfl owi ns ubgroupsI A,I B,I C

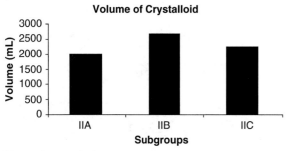

IIA – no lung perfusion

IIB – lung perfusion with arterial blood

IIC – lung perfusion with venous blood

Fig.29.10 Volumeof crystalloidsi ns ubgroupsI IA,I IB,I IC

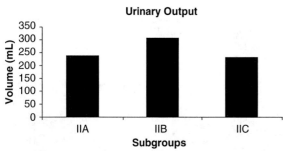

IIA – no lung perfusion

IIB – lung perfusion with arterial blood

IIC – lung perfusion with venous blood

Fig.29.11 Urinaryou tputi ns ubgroupsI IA,I IB,I IC

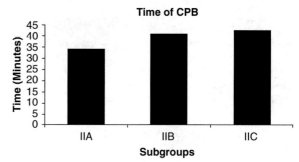

IIA – no lung perfusion

IIB – lung perfusion with arterial blood

IIC – lung perfusion with venous blood

Fig. 29.12 Time of cardiopulmonary bypass (CPB) in subgroupsI IA,I IB,I IC

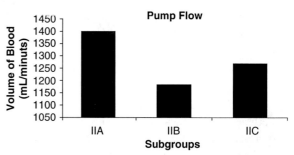

IIA – no lung perfusion

IIB – lung perfusion with arterial blood

IIC – lung perfusion with venous blood

Fig. 29.13 Pumpfl owi ns ubgroupsI IA,I IB,I IC

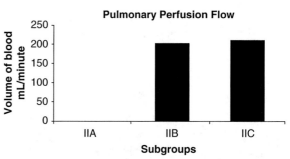

IIA – no lung perfusion

IIB – lung perfusion with arterial blood

IIC – lung perfusion with venous blood

Fig. 29.14 Pulmonary perfusion flow in subgroups IIA, IIB, IIC

some interesting and reproducible approaches aiming to take hemodynamic parameters as predictors of lung function. Following midline sternotomy and heart dissection, an ultrasonic flow probe was placed around the main pulmonary artery to measure right ventricular output. Pulmonary artery pressures were taken using a silicone elastomer catheter, which was inserted into the main pulmonary artery distal to the ultrasonic flow probe. Another silicone elastomer catheter was inserted into the left atrial appendage for measuring left atrial pressure. Furthermore, a system of right ventricle pressure monitoring was created using a third silicone elastomer catheter and a pressure transducer, which were placed through the right ventricle free wall.[2]

Many authors have speculated that there are advantages and limitations of retrograde perfusion of lungs to prevent pulmonary ischemia-reperfusion injury in special situations, like preservation of lungs for transplantation and pulmonary embolism. Clinical and experimental research demonstrated that pulmonary retrograde perfusion can provide some benefits in terms of distribution of perfusate, flushing bronchial circulation, evacuating blood clots and debris, as well as improving oxygenation and decreasing edema formation.[3-11] Based on the principles postulated by Gabriel et al.[1], we think that further investigations to determine optimal values for lung perfusion pressure in case of retrograde perfusion would be considerably relevant so additional damage to the pulmonary endothelium and parenchyma does not occur. Besides, we should always keep in mind that preservation of pulmonary endothelium depends on an adequate balance between perfusion pressure and low resistance of the pulmonary veins.

Some authors have advocated that pulmonary reperfusion injury after a period of aortic cross clamping can be alleviated by controlling the reperfusion pressure. That concept is based on several studies about myocardial preservation that have demonstrated less structural damage using controlled reperfusion techniques.[12-16] Halldorsson et al.[16-18] have demonstrated that pulmonary reperfusion injury can be caused even by pressure levels below normal heart arterial pressure (e.g., 40–50 mmHg); these authors have hypothesized that physiologic pressure levels of 20–30 mmHg can be adequate for lung reperfusion. An experimental model of controlled pulmonary reperfusion was designed as depicted in Fig. 29.15, and animals were equally divided in three groups according to reperfusion strategy. The left main stem bronchus and left pulmonary artery were clamped for 2 h and ventilation adjusted for the right lung. It is noteworthy that the bronchial supply was obliterated by skeletonizing the left bronchus for a length of 1 cm, aiming for complete left lung ischemia. Three methods were adopted for left lung reperfusion: group 1 had *uncontrolled reperfusion*, with the left lung reperfused simply by declamping it and restoring native pulmonary flow; group 2 had *high-pressure controlled reperfusion* by which a modified solution was infused for 10 min distal to the clamp in the left pulmonary artery, keeping reperfusion pressure between 40 and 50 mmHg, and subsequently the left lung was reperfused for an additional 10 min after clamp removal and restoration of native flow; and group 3 had *low-pressure controlled reperfusion low*, with a reperfusion strategy similar to that of group 2 except a modified solution was infused

Fig.29.15 (a)O ur experimental model of controlled pulmonary reperfusion. Blood is taken from the femoral artery and combined with a modified crystalloid solution using a BCD as a mixer and then returned to the pulmonary artery. The pressure in the distal pulmonary artery is constantly measured. (**b**)T he modified reperfusate is given into the left pulmonary artery distal to the clamp and is able to return to the pig through the pulmonary veins. (This figure was published in Halldorsson et al.[16]C opyright 2000, the Society of Thoracic Surgeons)

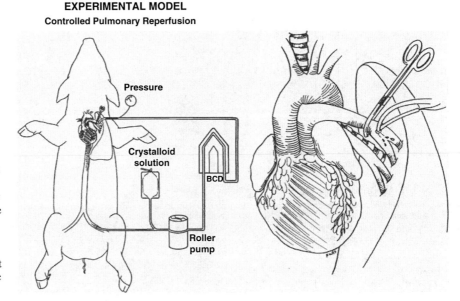

EXPERIMENTAL MODEL
Controlled Pulmonary Reperfusion

Pressure

Crystalloid
solution

BCD

Roller
pump

for 10 min, keeping reperfusion pressure between 20 and 30 mmHg. The benefits of lung reperfusion using low pressure can be confirmed by analyzing Figs. 29.16–29.18a nd Table 29.3[16]

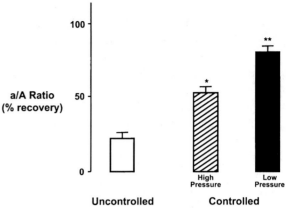

Fig. 29.18 Postreperfusion arterial/alveolar (a/A) ratio measured with the same ventilator settings used to make preischemic measurements. Uncontrolled reperfusion resulted in a very low posttransplant Po_2 (a/A ratio), implying severe alveolar damage in this group. In contrast, the a/A ratio was almost normal in animals receiving low-pressure controlled reperfusion, implying very little alveolar injury, $**p \leq 0.001$. (This figure was published in Halldorsson et al.[16] Copyright 2000, the Society of ThoracicS urgeons)

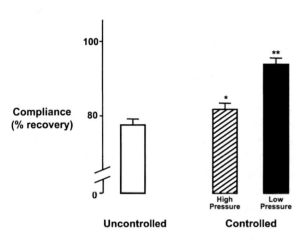

Fig. 29.16 Postreperfusion pulmonary compliance expressed as percentage recovery compared to baseline values. Uncontrolled reperfusion with unmodified blood significantly lowered pulmonary compliance, indicating a reperfusion injury. In contrast, controlled reperfusion using a modified blood solution, given at a low pressure, resulted in almost full recovery of pulmonary compliance, $**p \leq 0.001$. (This figure was published in Halldorsson et al.[16] Copyright 2000, the Society of Thoracic Surgeons)

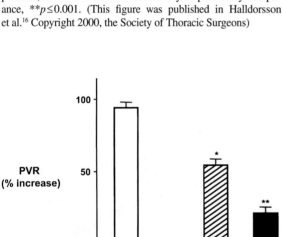

Fig. 29.17 Postreperfusion pulmonary vascular resistance expressed as a percentage increase compared to baseline values. The pulmonary vascular resistance (PVR) increased significantly when the lung was reperfused with unmodified blood in an uncontrolled fashion. Conversely, lungs undergoing controlled reperfusion with a modified reperfusate at a low pressure experienced minimal change in pulmonary vascular resistance, $**p \leq 0.001$. (This figure was published in Halldorsson et al.[16] Copyright2000,t heSo cietyof Thor acicS urgeons)

Table29.3   Postreperfusion left lung functional and tissue results

Reperfusion Method	Compliance (% Recovery)	PVR (% Control)	a/A Ratio (% Recovery)	LungWater	Myeloperoxidase (OD/min/mg Protein)
Uncontrolled (group 1)	77% ± 1%	198% ± 1%	27% ± 2%	84.3% ± 0.2%	0.35 ± .02
Controlledhigh pressure (group 2)	86% ± 1%[a]	154% ± 2%[a]	52% ± 2%[a]	83.5% ± 0.1%[a]	0.23 ± .02[a]
Controlledlo w pressure (group 3)	92% ± 1%[b]	133% ± 2%[b]	76% ± 1%[b]	82.7% ± 0.1%[b]	0.16 ± 0.01[b]
	$F = 106$, $p < 0.001$	$F = 732$, $p < 0.001$	$F = 618$, $p < 0.001$	$F = 58$, $p < 0.0001$	$F = 62$, $p < 0.001$

[a] $p < 0.001$ versus group 1 (uncontrolled reperfusion).

[b] $p < 0.001$ versus group 1 and group 2.

a/A ratio arterial/alveolar ration; *OD* optical density unit; *PVR* pulmonary vascular resistance.

(Thisfi gure was published in Halldorsson et al.[16] Copyright 2000, the Society of Thoracic Surgeons).

References

1. Gabriel EA, Locali RF, Matsuoka PK, et al. Lung perfusion during cardiac surgery with cardiopulmonary bypass: is it necessary? *Interact Cardiovasc Thorac Surg*. 2008;7:1089-1095.
2. Schultz JM, Karamlou T, Swanson J, Shen I, Ungerleider RM. Hypothermic low-flow cardiopulmonary bypass impairs pulmonary and right ventricular function more than circulatory arrest. *Ann Thorac Surg*.2006; 81:474-480.
3. Ferraro P, Martin J, Dery J, et al. Late retrograde perfusion of donor lungs does not decrease the severity of primary graft dysfunction. *Ann Thorac Surg*.2008; 86:1123-1129.
4. Sarsam MAI, Yonan NA, Deiraniya AK, Rahman AN. Retrograde pulmonaryplegia for lung preservation in clinical transplantation: a new technique. *J Heart Lung Transplant*.1993;12: 494-498.
5. Chen CZ, Gallagher RC, Ardery P, Dyckman W, Low HBC. Retrograde versus antegrade flush in canine left lung preservation for six hours. *J Heart Lung Transplant*. 1996;15:395-403.
6. Baretti R, Bitu-Moreno J, Beyersdorf F, Matheis G, Francischetti I, Kreitmayr B. Distribution of lung preservation solutions in parenchyma and airways: influence of atelectasis and route of delivery. *J Heart Lung Transplant*. 1995;14(1 pt 1):91.
7. Kofidis T, Strüber M, Warnecke G, et al. Antegrade versus retrograde perfusion of the donor lung: impact on the early reperfusion phase. *Transpl Int*.2003; 16:801-805.
8. Wittwer T, Franke UFW, Fehrenbach A, et al. Experimental lung transplantation: impact of preservation solution and route of delivery. *J Heart Lung Transplant*. 2005;24:1081-1090.
9. Serrick CJ, Jamjoum A, Reis A, Giaid A, Shennib H. Amelioration of pulmonary allograft injury by administering a second rinse solution. *J Thorac Cardiovasc Surg*. 1996;112:1010-1016.
10. Venuta F, Rendina E, Bufi M, et al. Preimplantation retrograde pneumoplegia in clinical lung transplantation. *J Thorac Cardiovasc Surg*.1999; 118:107-114.
11. Spagnolo S, Grasso MA, Tesler UF. Retrograde pulmonary perfusion improves results in pulmonary embolectomy for massive pulmonary embolism. *Tex Heart Inst J*. 2006; 33(4):473-476.
12. Buckberg GD, Allen BS. Myocardial protection and management in adult cardiac operations. In: Baue AE, Geha AS, Hammond GL, Laks H, Naunheim KS, eds. *Glenn's thoracic and cardiovascular surgery*. 6th ed. Stamford: Appleton and Lange; 1995:1653-1687.
13. Allen BS, Okamoto F, Buckberg GD, Bugyi H, Young H, Leaf J. Studies of controlled reperfusion after ischemia XV. *J Thorac Cardiovasc Surg*.1986; 92:621-625.
14. Allen BS, Buckberg GD, Fontan F, et al. Superiority of controlled surgical reperfusion versus percutaneous transluminal coronary angioplasty in acute coronary occlusion. *J Thorac Cardiovasc Surg*.1993; 105:864-884.
15. Okamoto F, Allen BS, Buckberg GD, Bugyi H, Leaf J. Studies of controlled reperfusion after ischemia. XIV. Reperfusion conditions. *J Thorac Cardiovasc Surg*. 1986;92:613-620.
16. Halldorsson AO, Kronon MT, Allen BS, Rahman S, Wang T. Lowering reperfusion pressure reduces the injury after pulmonary ischemia. *Ann Thorac Surg*.2000; 69:198-203.
17. Halldorsson A, Kronon M, Allen BS, et al. Controlled reperfusion after lung ischemia. *J Thorac Cardiovasc Surg*. 1998;115:415-425.
18. Halldorsson A, Kronon MT, Allen BS, et al. Controlled reperfusion prevents pulmonary injury after 24 hours of lung preservation. *Ann Thorac Surg*.1998; 66:877-885.

Extracorporeal Circuit Pathways for Lung Perfusion

30

Edmo Atique Gabriel and Tomas Salerno

In research carried out by Gabriel et al.,[1] strategies for lung perfusion had to be created so that the compromise conventional pattern of the extracorporeal circuit was not compromised. That was particularly important because it allowed heart surgeon to establish cardiopulmonary bypass (CPB) in a usual manner and perfuse the main pulmonary trunk either intermittently or continuously. For performing experimental procedures, the authors used the UNIQUE cardioplegic system, THYMUS pediatric oxygenator, and the whole extracorporeal circuit manufactured by Nipro Brazil. As pointed out, some adaptations had to be done to create pathways for lung perfusion using either venous blood or arterial blood. All the components of the extracorporeal circuit can be visualized in Figs. 30.1 and 30.2 in detail. Figures 30.3, 30.4, 30.5, and 30.6 demonstrate how lung perfusion happened from the experimental point of view; Fig. 30.7 summarizes all these data simulating the clinical extracorporeal pattern in which employed different strategies of lung perfusion during heart surgery requiring CPB.

Based on all these figures, we propose some recommendations for employing lung perfusion during heart surgery requiring CPB:

1. Creating a bypass line arising from the recirculation line makes a helpful pathway to take arterial blood toward the main pulmonary artery. Other pathways

E.A. Gabriel (✉)

Federal University of Sao Paulo, Sao Paulo, Brazil
e-mail: edag@uol.com.br

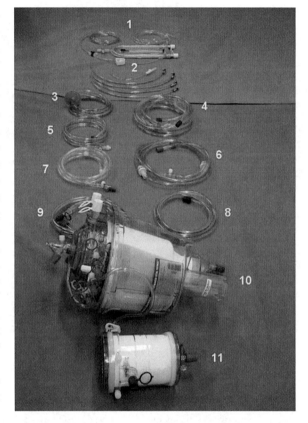

Fig. 30.1 Overview of cardiopulmonary bypass (CPB) components (Nipro Brazil). *1* Blood cardioplegia system *UNIQUE*; *2* arterial, venous, and pulmonary cannulae and vent catheter; *3* oxygen line; *4* suction/aspirator line; *5* vent catheter line; *6* arterial roller line; *7* pulmonary trunk line; *8* arterial line; *9* venous line; *10* venous reservoir; *11* pediatric membrane oxygenator THYMUS. The THYMUS oxygenator is comprised of a cylindrical chamber for gas exchange and a reservoir with a heat permuter. It can operate using blood flows from 0.5 to 4.0 L/min. Its reservoir with the heat permuter can filter air bubbles, increase and decrease blood temperature, as well as filter blood coming throught the suction/aspirator line

E.A. Gabriel and T. Salerno (eds.), *Principles of Pulmonary Protection in Heart Surgery*,
DOI: 10.1007/978-1-84996-308-4_30, © Springer-Verlag London Limited 2010

Fig.30.2 Detailsof
cannulae, UNIQUE
cardioplegia system, and
digital manometer.
1 Aortic cannula,
2 pulmonary trunk cannula,
3 superior vena cava cannula,
4 inferior vena cava cannula,
5 vent catheter, *6*U NIQUE
blood cardioplegia system,
7 digital manometer
connected to pulmonary
trunkline

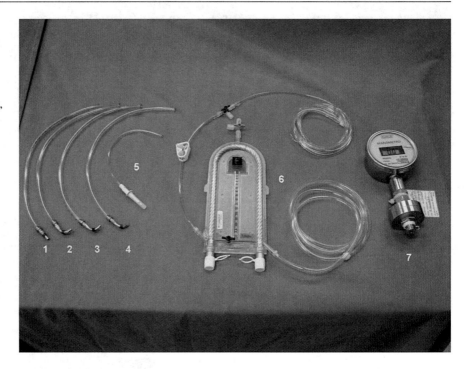

we can consider as feasible for lung perfusion using arterial blood are bypass lines arising either from the cardioplegia line or from the aorta line; however, we do need to bear in mind that flow and pressure modifications may be detected in cardioplegia and systemic parameters.

2. Creating a bypass line coming from the line between the venous reservoir and the oxygenator is a safe pathway to take venous blood toward the main pulmonary artery. It is noteworthy that venous blood should always be taken to the main pulmonary artery after passing through the reservoir filter to prevent trapping air bubbles in the lungs. Furthermore, if venous blood will be taken from the venae cavae line before the venous reservoir, the connection of that line to a filter is of paramount importance to prevent air embolism.

3. Monitoring lung perfusion pressure by a manometer connected to the lung perfusion line is essential to prevent deleterious effects from pulmonary ischemia-reperfusion injury as well as additional damage to pulmonary endothelium and parenchyma.

In addition to the pathways we have proposed for lung perfusion during heart surgery with CPB, we would like to describe some strategies for perfusing lungs when these organs have been harvested along with the heart as a whole block for transplantation.

Wisser et al.[2] created a closed-circuit perfusion model for maintaining continuous circulation of the lung-heart block (Fig. 30.8). The apex of the left ventricle and the main pulmonary artery were cannulated in such a way that blood from the left ventricle was drained by gravity to be pumped into the main pulmonary artery. Likewise, Daggett at al.[3] designed an experimental model using two reservoirs placed at different heights and an ultrasonic flowmeter connected to the lung perfusion line (Fig. 30.9).

Ultimately, we would like to call attention to the extracorporeal lung circuit using a pulsatile roller pump as postulated by some authors.[4-10] Brandes et al.[11] proposed an extracorporeal lung circuit using two roller pumps and two reservoirs (Fig. 30.10). Furthermore, these authors used a flow of 0.3 L/min with a pulse rate of 90/min for lung perfusion.

In summary, we wish to point out that there are different pathways for perfusing lungs during heart surgery with CPB, and the heart surgeon can perfuse lungs either using arterial blood or using venous blood. However, we need to bear in mind that, regardless of pathway, lung perfusion pressure should be adjusted to physiological levels as advocated by some authors.[1,12]

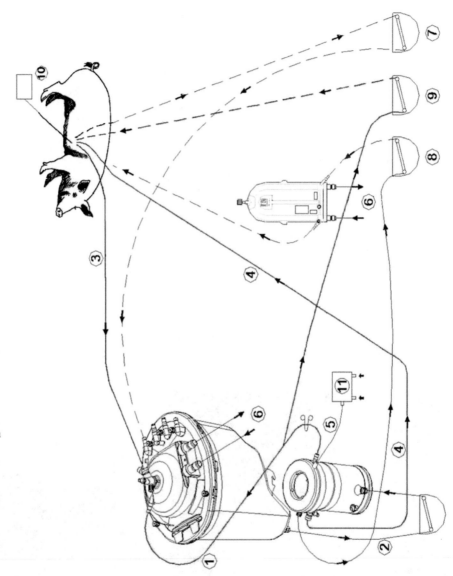

Fig.30.3 Experimental model of lung perfusion with arterial blood. *1* Recirculation line, *2* arterial roller line, *3* venae cavae line, *4* aorta line, *5* gas supply line, *6* water supply line, *7* suction/aspirator line, *8* cardioplegia line, *9* pulmonary trunk perfusion line with arterial blood, *10* pulmonary trunk perfusion pressure (digital manometer), *11* gas blender

Fig.30.4 Experimental model of lung perfusion with venous blood.
1 Recirculation line, *2* arterial roller line, *3* venae cavae line, *4* aorta line, *5*g as supply line, *6* water supply line, *7*s uction/aspirator line, *8* cardioplegia line, *9* pulmonary trunk perfusion line with venous blood, *10* pulmonary trunk perfusion pressure (digital manometer), *11*g asb lender

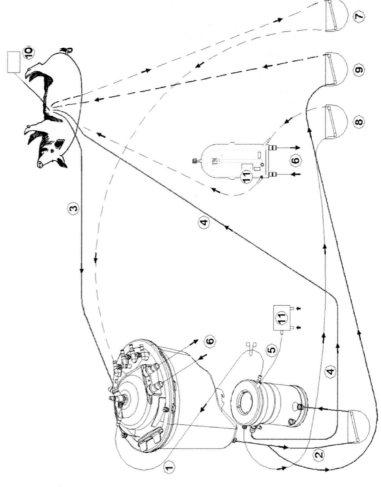

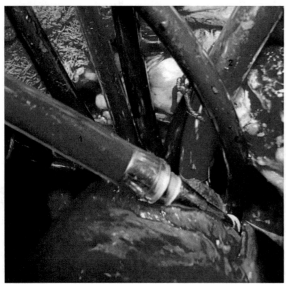

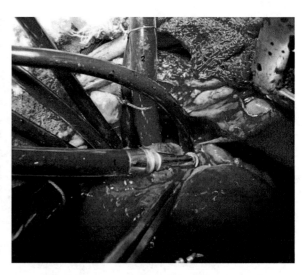

Fig. 30.5 Pulmonary trunk perfusion with arterial blood. *1* Pulmonary trunk cannula with arterial blood, 2a orticc annula

Fig. 30.6 Pulmonary trunk perfusion with venous blood. *1* Pulmonary trunk cannula with venous blood, 2a orticc annula

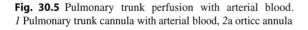

Fig.30.7 Schemeoflu ng perfusion. *1* Vena cava line, *2* arterial roller pump line, *3* aorta line, *4* re circulation line, *5* gas supply line, *6* water supply line, *7* a spirator line, *8* cardioplegia line, *9A* pulmonary trunk perfusion line with arterial blood (*red line*), *9B* pulmonary trunk perfusion line with venous blood (*blue line*), *10* pulmonary trunk perfusion pressure (digital manometer), *11* gas blender. *SVC* s uperior vena cava, *IVC* inferior vena cava, *RA* right atrium, *RV* right ventricle, *AO* aorta, *PT* pulmonary trunk. (Reproduced with permission from Gabriel et al.[1] © 2008 European Association of Cardio-Thoracic Surgery, http://icvts.ctsnetjournals. org/)

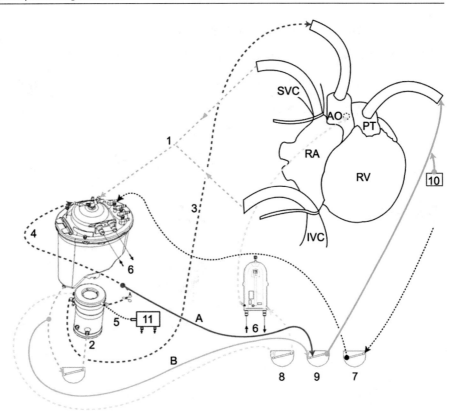

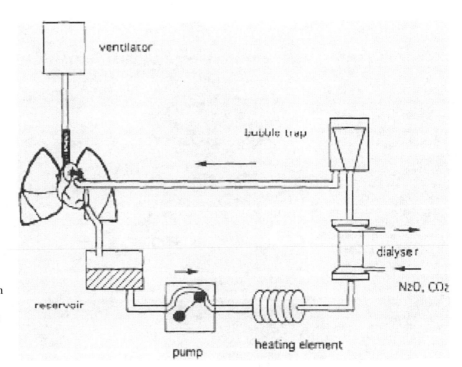

Fig.30.8 Schematicd iagram of closed-circuit perfusion. (This figure was published in Wisser et al.[2] © 1993, European Association of Cardio-ThoracicSur gery)

The Isolated Working Lung Preparation

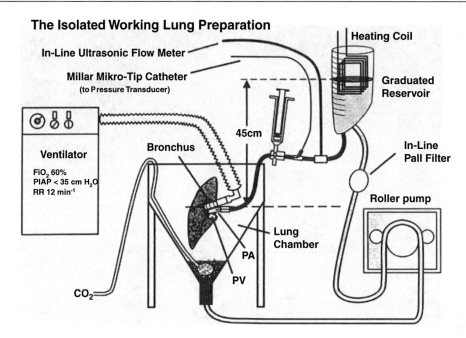

Fig. 30.9 Diagram of isolated working lung apparatus. Plasma enters the pulmonary artery under gravity from the upper reservoir at a height of 45 cm above the pulmonary artery. Plasma is allowed to drain into the lower reservoir, where carbon dioxide is added by a diffuser. The roller pump recirculates the plasma from the lung chamber to the upper reservoir, where it is warmed to 37°C by a heat exchanger. The lung is ventilated with 60% oxygen at a rate of 12 breaths/min. *PA* Pulmonary artery, *PV* pulmonary vein, *RR* respiratory rate, *PIAP* peak inspiratory airway pressure. (This figure was published in Dagget et al.[3] © 1997, t heA mericanA ssociationf orT horacicS urgery)

Fig.30.10 Extracorporeal lung circuit: two reservoirs, two roller pumps to circulate the perfusate, membrane oxygenator (gassed with 95% N_2 and 5% CO_2).Puls atile roller pump or nonpulsatile roller pump for perfusion of the lung. Mechanical room air ventilation with respirator. All vessels water jacketed and temperature controlled by warming pump at 37°C. (This figure was published in Brandes et al.[11] © 2002, S. KargerA G,B asel)

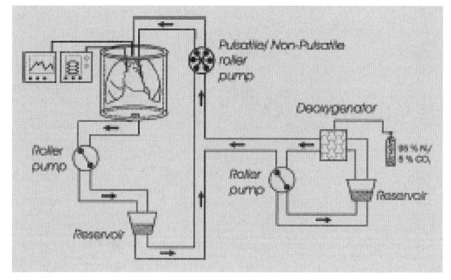

References

1. Gabriel EA, Locali RF, Matsuoka PK, et al. Lung perfusion during cardiac surgery with cardiopulmonary bypass: is it necessary? *Interact Cardiovasc Thorac Surg*. 2008;7:1089-1095.
2. Wisser W, Oturanlar D, Minich R, et al. Closed circuit perfusion of an isolated rabbit lung. A new model for the evaluation of preservation quality of stored lungs. *Eur J Cardiothorac Surg*.1993;7:71-74.
3. Daggett CW, Yeatman M, Lodge AJ, et al. Swine lungs expressing human complement-regulatory proteins are protected against acute pulmonary dysfunction in a human plasma perfusion model. *J Thorac Cardiovasc Surg*. 1997;113:390-398.
4. Schlensak C, Doenst T, Beyersdorf F. Lung ischemia during cardiopulmonary bypass. *Ann Thorac Surg*. 2000;70:337-338.
5. Siepe M, Goebel U, Mecklenburg A, et al. Pulsatile pulmonary perfusion during cardiopulmonary bypass reduces the pulmonary inflammatory response. *Ann Thorac Surg*. 2008; 86:115-122.
6. Steen S. Pulmonary sequelae of prolonged total venoarterial bypass: evaluation with a new experimental model. *Ann Thorac Surg*.1991; 51:794-799.
7. Quaniers JM, Leruth J, Albert A, Limet RR, Defraigne JO. Comparison of inflammatory responses after off-pump and on-pump coronary surgery using surface modifying additives circuit. *Ann Thorac Surg*.2006; 81:1683-1690.
8. Staton GW, Williams WH, Mahoney EM, et al. Pulmonary outcomes of off-pump versus on-pump coronary artery by pass surgery in a randomized trial. *Chest*. 2005;127:892-901.
9. Alghamdi AA, Latter DA. Pulsatile versus nonpulsatile cardiopulmonary bypass flow: an evidence-based approach. *J Card Surg*.2006; 21:347-354.
10. Saito S, Nishinaka T. Chronic nonpulsatile blood flow is compatible with normal end-organ function: implications for LVAD development. *J Artif Organs*.2005; 8:143-148.
11. Brandes H, Albes JM, Conzelmann A, Wehrmann M, Ziemer G. Comparison of pulsatile and nonpulsatile perfusion of the lung in an extracorporeal large animal model. *Eur Surg Res*. 2002;34:321-329.
12. Inokawa H, Sevala M, Funkhouser WK, Egan TM. Ex-vivo perfusion and ventilation of rat lungs from non-heart-beating donors before transplant. *Ann Thorac Surg*. 2006;82:1219-1225.

HemodynamicPer formance

31

Edmo Atique Gabriel and Tomas Salerno

The research carried out by Gabriel et al[1] documented many important findings regarding hemodynamic parameters in group I (cardioplegic arrest – moderate hypothermia) and group II (beating heart and normothermia) cardiopulmonary bypass (CPB) postoperatively. This hemodynamic evaluation was not correlated with lung ventilation as it was discontinued during CPB. Moreover, several comparisons were feasible considering each subgroup itself and its respective preoperative and postoperative period as well as comparisons involving subgroups belonging to same main group. We[1] did not make comparisons between groups I and II and their respective subgroups as the main purpose of the study was to determine benefits and limitations of lung perfusion during heart surgery using two different strategies. Indeed, we believe that the issue of lung perfusion should be embraced by heart surgeons as a useful tool for preventing pulmonary ischemia-reperfusion injury and not as a benchmark regarding whether cardioplegic arrest is a strategy better than the beating heart technique and vice versa. Tables 31.1–31.12 show the impact of lung perfusion on hemodynamic performance in both groups and their respective subgroups. Hemodynamic variables are presented with mean, standard deviation, and significance level. Wilcoxon, Mann–Whitney, and Kruskal–Wallis tests were used to make comparisons among subgroups. A value of $p < 0.05$ adjusted by the Bonferroni correction ($p = 0.0253$) was considered significant.

Our interpretation for the significant reduction of mean artery pressure (MAP) and cardiac output (CO) postoperatively is that this can be induced by the immediate effects of aortic cross declamping on cardiac recovery. Furthermore, we call attention to the relevant elevation of pulmonary vascular resistance (PVR) when the lungs are not perfused in a controlled manner during heart surgery with CPB. On the other hand, perfusing lungs with controlled pressure simulates preoperative and physiological conditions; therefore, postoperative hemodynamic performance tends to be similar to preoperative performance.

Findings in Table 31.5 demonstrate that controlled lung perfusion can be beneficial as it can reduce postoperative PVR, minimizing deleterious effects of pulmonary ischemia-reperfusion injury. We correlate significant findings documented in Table 31.6 with eventual variations in pulmonary perfusion flow when lungs are perfused with either arterial or venous blood.

At this point, it is important to remember that the preoperative status of subgroup IIB is that the lungs are perfused by venous blood while the heart is beating under physiological conditions. When arterial blood is used for controlled lung perfusion during heart surgery with CPB, there are some pulmonary perfusion flow variations that can account for significant findings regarding mean pulmonary artery pressure (MPAP) and PVR. However, another issue that can be raised is that different oxygen contents can justify significant findings regarding MPAP and PVR. As we believe that the impact of different oxygen contents can be greater for the gasometric profile than hemodynamic performance, we prefer advocating the first hypothesis regarding pulmonary perfusion flow variations.

Controlled lung perfusion while the heart was kept beating during CPB was an effective association as it contributed to significantly decrease PVR postoperatively. Additional flow provided by controlled lung

E.A.G abriel (✉)
FederalU niversityofS aoP aulo, SaoP aulo, Brazil
e-mail:e dag@uol.com.br

E.A. Gabriel and T. Salerno (eds.), *Principles of Pulmonary Protection in Heart Surgery*,
DOI: 10.1007/978-1-84996-308-4_31, © Springer-Verlag London Limited 2010

Table31.1 Hemodynamic variables in pre and postoperative times – subgroup IA

| Variables | n | Mean | Standard deviation | Confidencei nterval | | Significance (p) |
				Inferior threshold	Superior threshold	
MAP preop	4	82.5	9.57	73.12	91.88	0.002
MAPpos top	4	58.75	2.5	56.30	61.20	
MPAPpre op	4	26.25	2.5	23.80	28.70	0.854
MPAPpos top	4	26.25	4.79	21.56	30.94	
PCPpr eop	4	17.75	7.14	10.75	24.75	0.854
PCPpos top	4	17	5.03	12.07	21.93	
PVRpr eop	4	38.5	57.68	83.97	493.03	0.009
PVRpos top	4	460	280	185.60	734.40	
COpr eop	4	1.99	0.62	1.38	2.60	0.002
COpos top	4	1.5	0.58	0.93	2.07	

IA cardioplegic arrest with no controlled lung perfusion, *CO* cardiac output, *MAP* mean artery pressure, *MPAP* mean pulmonary artery pressure, *PCP* pulmonary capillary pressure, *PVR* pulmonary vascular resistance

Table31.2 Hemodynamic variables in pre and postoperative times – subgroup IB

| Variables | n | Mean | Standard deviation | Confidencei nterval | | Significance (p) |
				Inferior threshold	Superior threshold	
MAP preop	6	81.67	7.53	75.64	87.70	0.026
MAPpos top	6	59.67	0.82	59.01	60.33	
MPAPpre op	6	22.5	6.12	17.60	27.40	0.039
MPAPpos top	6	18	4.47	14.42	21.58	
PCPpr eop	6	15.33	4.18	11.99	18.67	0.042
PCPpos top	6	12.67	3.56	9.82	15.52	
PVRpr eop	6	311.17	141.9	197.63	424.71	0.172
PVRpos top	6	275.17	96.57	197.90	352.44	
COpr eop	6	1.92	0.33	1.66	2.18	0.026
COpos top	6	1.6	0.28	1.38	1.82	

IB cardioplegic arrest and controlled lung perfusion with arterial blood, *CO* cardiac output, *MAP* mean artery pressure, *MPAP* mean pulmonary artery pressure, *PCP* pulmonary capillary pressure, *PVR* pulmonary vascular resistance

Table31.3 Hemodynamic variables in pre and postoperative times – subgroup IC

| Variables | n | Mean | Standard deviation | Confidence interval | | Significance (p) |
				Inferior threshold	Superior threshold	
MAP preop	6	79.33	8.76	72.32	86.34	0.026
MAPpos top	6	60.83	5.85	56.15	65.51	
MPAPpre op	6	24.17	5.38	19.87	28.47	0.581
MPAPpos top	6	23.33	4.13	20.03	26.63	
PCPpr eop	6	19.5	6.41	14.37	24.63	0.223
PCPpos top	6	18	5.25	13.80	22.20	
PVRpr eop	6	239	155.62	114.48	363.52	0.600
PVRpos top	6	211	104.72	127.21	294.79	
COpr eop	6	2	0.66	1.47	2.53	0.915
COpos top	6	2	0.63	1.50	2.50	

IC cardioplegic arrest and controlled lung perfusion with venous blood, *CO* cardiac output, *MAP* mean artery pressure, *MPAP* mean pulmonary artery pressure, *PCP* pulmonary capillary pressure, *PVR* pulmonary vascular resistance

Table31. 4 Hemodynamic variables in postoperative time – subgroups IA and IB

| Variables | Group | n | Mean | Standard deviation | Confidence interval | | Significance (p) |
					Inferior threshold	Superior threshold	
MAP postop	IA	4	58.75	2.50	56.30	61.20	0.648
	IB	6	59.67	0.82	59.01	60.32	
MPAPpos top	IA	4	26.25	4.79	21.56	30.94	0.038
	IB	6	18.00	4.47	14.42	21.58	
PCPpos top	IA	4	17.00	5.03	12.07	21.93	0.159
	IB	6	12.67	3.56	9.82	15.51	
PVRpos top	IA	4	460.00	280.00	185.61	734.39	0.392
	IB	6	275.17	96.57	197.89	352.44	
COpos top	IA	4	1.50	0.58	0.93	2.07	0.828
	IB	6	1.60	0.28	1.38	1.82	

IA cardioplegic arrest with no controlled lung perfusion, *IB* cardioplegic arrest and controlled lung perfusion with arterial blood, *CO* cardiac output, *MAP* mean artery pressure, *MPAP* mean pulmonary artery pressure, *PCP* pulmonary capillary pressure, *PVR* pulmonary vascular resistance

Table 31.5 Hemodynamic variables in postoperative time – subgroups IA and IC

Variables	Group	n	Mean	Standard deviation	Confidence interval		Significance (p)
					Inferior threshold	Superior threshold	
MAP postop	IA	4	58.75	2.50	56.30	61.20	0.645
	IC	6	60.83	5.85	56.16	65.51	
MPAPpos top	IA	4	26.25	4.79	21.56	30.94	0.232
	IC	6	23.33	4.13	20.03	26.64	
PCPpos top	IA	4	17.00	5.03	12.07	21.93	0.665
	IC	6	18.00	5.25	13.80	22.20	
PVRpos top	IA	4	460.00	280.00	185.61	734.39	0.010
	IC	6	211.00	104.72	127.21	294.79	
COpos top	IA	4	1.50	0.58	0.93	2.07	0.223
	IC	6	2.00	0.63	1.49	2.51	

IA cardioplegic arrest with no controlled lung perfusion, *IC* cardioplegic arrest and controlled lung perfusion with venous blood, *CO* cardiac output, *MAP* mean artery pressure, *MPAP* mean pulmonary artery pressure, *PCP* pulmonary capillary pressure, *PVR* pulmonary vascular resistance

Table 31.6 Hemodynamic variables in postoperative time – subgroups IB and IC

Variables	Group	n	Mean	Standard deviation	Confidence interval		Significance (p)
					Inferior threshold	Superior threshold	
MAP postop	IB	6	59.67	0.82	59.01	60.32	0.858
	IC	6	60.83	5.85	56.16	65.51	
MPAPpo stop	IB	6	18.00	4.47	14.42	21.58	0.126
	IC	6	23.33	4.13	20.03	26.64	
PCPpos top	IB	6	12.67	3.56	9.82	15.51	0.006
	IC	6	18.00	5.25	13.80	22.20	
PVRpos top	IB	6	275.17	96.57	197.89	352.44	0.332
	IC	6	211.00	104.72	127.21	294.79	
COpos top	IB	6	1.60	0.28	1.38	1.82	0.010
	IC	6	2.00	0.63	1.49	2.51	

IB cardioplegic arrest and controlled lung perfusion with arterial blood, *IC* cardioplegic arrest and controlled lung perfusion with venous blood, *CO* cardiac output, *MAP* mean artery pressure, *MPAP* mean pulmonary artery pressure, *PCP* pulmonary capillary pressure, *PVR* pulmonary vascular resistance

Table31.7 Hemodynamic variables in pre and postoperative times – subgroup IIA

Variables	n	Mean	Standard deviation	Confidencei nterval		Significance (p)
				Inferior threshold	Superior threshold	
MAP preop	4	69	8.41	60.76	77.24	0.305
MAPpos top	4	72.5	5	67.60	77.40	
MPAPpre op	4	23.75	2.5	21.30	26.20	0.157
MPAPpos top	4	25	4.08	21.00	29.00	
PCPpr eop	4	15.75	2.87	12.94	18.56	0.157
PCPpos top	4	16.25	3.5	12.82	19.68	
PVRpr eop	4	353.25	121.31	234.37	472.13	0.916
PVRpos top	4	358.75	56.62	303.26	414.24	
COpr eop	4	1.88	0.25	1.64	2.13	0.458
COpos top	4	1.95	0.1	1.85	2.05	

IIA beating heart technique with no controlled lung perfusion, *CO* cardiac output, *MAP* mean artery pressure, *MPAP* mean pulmonary artery pressure, *PCP* pulmonary capillary pressure, *PVR* pulmonary vascular resistance

Table31.8 Hemodynamic variables in pre and postoperative times – subgroup IIB

Variables	n	Mean	Standard deviation	Confidencei nterval		Significance (p)
				Inferior threshold	Superior threshold	
MAP preop	6	73.5	13.03	63.07	83.93	0.719
MAPpos top	6	70	13.7	59.04	80.96	
MPAPpre op	6	25.83	4.92	21.89	29.77	0.021
MPAPpos top	6	23.17	4.49	19.58	26.76	
PCPpr eop	6	17.67	4.59	14.00	21.34	0.294
PCPpos top	6	17.17	5.23	12.99	21.35	
PVRpr eop	6	410	241.62	216.66	603.34	0.012
PVRpos top	6	242.5	55.29	198.26	286.74	
COpr eop	6	1.81	0.55	1.37	2.25	0.386
COpos top	6	1.96	0.22	1.78	2.14	

IIB beating heart technique and controlled lung perfusion with arterial blood, *CO* cardiac output, *MAP* mean artery pressure, *MPAP* mean pulmonary artery pressure, *PCP* pulmonary capillary pressure, *PVR* pulmonary vascular resistance

Table 31.9 Hemodynamic variables in pre and postoperative times – subgroup IIC

Variables	n	Mean	Standard deviation	Confidencei nterval		Significance (p)
				Inferior threshold	Superior threshold	
MAP preop	6	74.17	10.21	66.00	82.34	0.357
MAPpos top	6	70	6.32	64.94	75.06	
MPAPpre op	6	25.83	3.43	23.09	28.57	0.317
MPAPpos top	6	24.17	3.43	21.43	26.91	
PCPpr eop	6	16.5	3.02	14.08	18.92	0.655
PCPpos top	6	16.67	1.86	15.18	18.16	
PVRpr eop	6	407.67	150.93	286.90	528.44	0.043
PVRpos top	6	260.83	66.93	207.27	314.39	
COpr eop	6	1.93	0.58	1.47	2.39	0.043
COpos top	6	2.35	0.59	1.88	2.82	

IIC beating heart technique and controlled lung perfusion with venous blood, *CO* cardiac output, *MAP* mean artery pressure, *MPAP* mean pulmonary artery pressure, *PCP* pulmonary capillary pressure, PVR pulmonary vascular resistance

Table 31.10 Hemodynamic variables in postoperative time – subgroups IIA e IIB

Variables	Group	n	Mean	Standard deviation	Confidencei nterval		Significance (p)
					Inferior threshold	Superior threshold	
MAP postop	IIA	4	72.50	5.00	67.60	77.40	0.581
	IIB	6	70.00	13.70	59.04	80.96	
MPAPpos top	IIA	4	25.00	4.08	21.00	29.00	0.826
	IIB	6	23.17	4.49	19.57	26.76	
PCPpos top	IIA	4	16.25	3.50	12.82	19.68	0.520
	IIB	6	17.17	5.23	12.98	21.35	
PVRpos top	IIA	4	358.75	56.62	303.26	414.24	0.032
	IIB	6	242.50	55.29	198.26	286.74	
COpos top	IIA	4	1.95	0.10	1.85	2.05	0.912
	IIB	6	1.96	0.22	1.79	2.14	

IIA beating heart technique with no controlled lung perfusion, *IIB* beating heart technique and controlled lung perfusion with arterial blood, *CO* cardiac output, *MAP* mean artery pressure, *MPAP* mean pulmonary artery pressure, *PCP* pulmonary capillary pressure, *PVR* pulmonary vascular resistance

Table31.11 Hemodynamic variables in postoperative time – subgroups IIA and IIC

| Variables | Group | n | Mean | Standard deviation | Confidencei nterval | | Significance (p) |
					Inferior threshold	Superior threshold	
MAP postop	IIA	4	72.50	5.00	67.60	77.40	0.510
	IIC	6	70.00	6.32	64.94	75.06	
MPAPpo stop	IIA	4	25.00	4.08	21.00	29.00	0.658
	IIC	6	24.17	3.43	21.42	26.91	
PCPpos top	IIA	4	16.25	3.50	12.82	19.68	0.911
	IIC	6	16.67	1.86	15.18	18.16	
PVRpos top	IIA	4	358.75	56.62	303.26	414.24	0.005
	IIC	6	260.83	66.93	207.28	314.39	
COpos top	IIA	4	1.95	0.10	1.85	2.05	0.007
	IIC	6	2.35	0.59	1.88	2.82	

IIA beating heart technique with no controlled lung perfusion, *IIC* beating heart technique and controlled lung perfusion with venous blood, *CO* cardiac output, *MAP* mean artery pressure, *MPAP* mean pulmonary artery pressure, *PCP* pulmonary capillary pressure, *PVR* pulmonary vascular resistance

Table31.12 Hemodynamic variables in postoperative time – subgroups IIB and IIC

| Variables | Group | n | Mean | Standard deviation | Confidencei nterval | | Significance (p) |
					Inferior threshold	Superior threshold	
MAP postop	IIB	6	70.00	13.70	59.04	80.96	0.738
	IIC	6	70.00	6.32	64.94	75.06	
MPAPpos top	IIB	6	23.17	4.49	19.57	26.76	0.871
	IIC	6	24.17	3.43	21.42	26.91	
PCPpos top	IIB	6	17.17	5.23	12.98	21.35	0.372
	IIC	6	16.67	1.86	15.18	18.16	
PVRpos top	IIB	6	242.50	55.29	198.26	286.74	0.873
	IIC	6	260.83	66.93	207.28	314.39	
COpos top	IIB	6	1.96	0.22	1.79	2.14	0.121
	IIC	6	2.35	0.59	1.88	2.82	

IIB beating heart technique and controlled lung perfusion with arterial blood, *IIC* beating heart technique and controlled lung perfusion with venous blood, *CO* cardiac output, *MAP* mean artery pressure, *MPAP* mcan pulmonary artery pressure, *PCP* pulmonary capillary pressure, *PVR* pulmonary vascular resistance

perfusion could have contributed to greater CO in group IIA than group IIC.

Figure 31.1 summarizes all data regarding hemodynamic performance in groups I and II and respective subgroups.

Friedman et al[2] adopted a different strategy to evaluate the impact of lung perfusion on pulmonary hemodynamic performance. They designed experimental research using sheep in which CPB was established by cannulating the aorta and right atrium, the

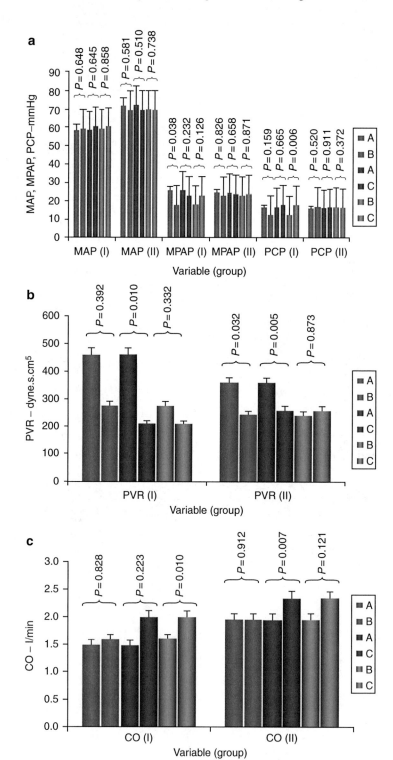

Fig.31.1 Hemodynamic pa rameters in groups I and II postoperatively. (**a**) *MAP* mean artery pressure; *MPAP* m ean pulmonary artery pressure; *PCP* pul monary capillary pressure; (**b**) *PVR* pul monary vascular resistance; (**c**) *CO* cardiac output. *Group I* cardioplegic group, *Group II* beating heart group, *A* no lung perfusion, *B* lung perfusion with arterial blood, *C* l ung perfusion with venous blood. (Reproduced with permission from Gabriel et al.[1] Copyright 2008, European Association of Cardio-ThoracicSur gery, http://icvts. ctsnetjournals.org/)

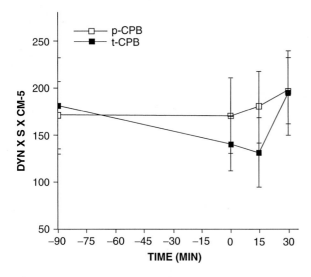

Fig. 31.2 Pulmonary vascular resistance during partial cardiopulmonary bypass (p-CPB) and during total cardiopulmonary bypass (t-CPB). Calculations were done before CPB (time = −90), after separation from CPB (time = 0) then every 15 min until 30 min after separation from CPB (at which time the left atrial balloon inflation obviated physiologic pulmonary vascular resistance). (This figure was published in Friedman et al.[2] Copyright 1995,t heSoc ietyof Thor acicSur geons)

heart was kept beating, and the main pulmonary artery was cannulated only for monitoring pulmonary artery pressure. In seven animals (total CPB), the main pulmonary artery was clamped and mechanical ventilation was stopped in such a way that the entire venous return was diverted to the extracorporeal circuit for 90 min without reaching the pulmonary vasculature. In another seven animals (partial CPB), mechanical ventilation was not halted and the main pulmonary artery was clamped allowing two thirds of the baseline pulmonary arterial flow to pass through the lungs for 90 min. The time course of PVR in both groups is depicted in Fig. 31.2. Despite greater elevation of PVR in the total CPB group postoperatively, no significant difference was detected between the two groups.[2,3]

References

1. Gabriel EA, Locali RF, Matsuoka PK, et al. Lung perfusion during cardiac surgery with cardiopulmonary bypass: is it necessary? *Interact Cardiovasc Thorac Surg*. 2008;7:1089-1095.
2. Friedman M, Wang SY, Sellke FW, Franklin A, Weintraub RM, Johnson RG. Pulmonary injury after total or partial cardiopulmonary bypass with thromboxane synthesis inhibition. *Ann Thorac Surg*.1995; 59:598-603.
3. Friedman M, Sellke FW, Wang SY, et al. Parameters of pulmonary injury after total or partial cardiopulmonary bypass. *Circulation*.1994; 90:II262-II268.

Qualityo fG asExc hange

32

Edmo Atique Gabriel and Tomas Salerno

Gabriel et al.[1] analyzed gasometric parameters in groups I and II cardiopulmonary bypass (CPB) and their respective subgroups. For achieving that goal, we standardized the blood sample withdrawal process as follows:

- Preoperative blood samples were withdrawn from the right pulmonary vein and right internal carotid artery following pericardiotomy.
- Postoperative blood samples were taken from the same sites but because mechanical ventilation might have an influence on gasometric parameters, these were taken on coming off CPB immediately before restoring mechanical ventilation.
- Blood samples taken from the right pulmonary veins were used to determine pulmonary venous oxygen pressure (PvO_2) and pulmonary venous oxygen saturation (SvO_2). Blood samples withdrawn from the right internal carotid artery allowed determination of arterial oxygen pressure (PaO_2), arterial oxygen saturation (SaO_2), and oxygen index (OI). To calculate OI, the following formula was used: $OI = PaO_2/FIO_2$, where FIO_2 is the fraction of inspiredoxyge n.

Tables 32.1–32.12 demonstrate the impact of lung perfusion on the quality of gas exchange in both groups and their respective subgroups. Gasometric variables are presented with mean, standard deviation, and significance level. Wilcoxon, Mann–Whitney, and Kruskal–Wallis tests were used to make comparisons among subgroups. A value of $p < 0.05$ adjusted by the Bonferroni correction ($p = 0.0253$) was considered significant.

When the heart undergoes cardioplegic arrest and the lungs are not perfused in a controlled manner, postoperative gasometric parameters tend to decrease significantly, reflecting some effects of pulmonary ischemia-reperfusion injury on the blood-gas barrier. On the other hand, when the heart is subjected to cardioplegic arrest and the lungs are perfused using a controlled perfusion pressure, few relevant modifications in gasometric variables tend to be detected postoperatively. It is noteworthy that the only significant correlation observed in Table 32.3 could be clarified by the eventual effects of ventilation on the blood-gas barrier.

Despite postoperative elevation of gasometric parameters in subgroups IB and IC compared to IA, these correlations were not significant; therefore, we believe that this finding can be elucidated by the eventual influence of sample size on some outcomes. Furthermore, it is important to emphasize that no relevant differences were detected between subgroups IB and IC.

The data presented in Tables 32.7–32.9 reveal that lack of controlled lung perfusion during beating heart surgery can significantly contribute to decrease gasometric parameters postoperatively. On the other hand, when the heart is beating and the lungs are perfused with arterial blood, no relevant differences were found between pre- and postoperatively, thereby preserving the physiological pattern of gas exchange. Association between beating heart surgery and controlled lung perfusion with venous blood has a particular impact on gas exchange as it causes gasometric parameters to drop postoperatively, as depicted in Table 32.9. This intriguing issue is the subject for another chapter 36 in thisbook .

E.A.G abriel (✉)
Department of Surgery, Division of Cardiovascular Surgery
FederalU niversity ofSa oP aulo, SaoP aulo, Brazil
e-mail:e dag@uol.com.br

E.A. Gabriel and T. Salerno (eds.), *Principles of Pulmonary Protection in Heart Surgery,*
DOI: 10.1007/978-1-84996-308-4_32, © Springer-Verlag London Limited 2010

Table32.1 Gasometric variables in pre- and postoperative times – subgroup IA

Variables	n	Mean	Standard deviation	Confidence interval		Significance (p)
				Inferior threshold	Superior threshold	
PaO$_2$ preop	4	250.5	136.7	116.53	384.47	0.002
PaO$_2$pos top	4	126.25	62.11	65.38	187.12	
SaO$_2$pre op	4	99.5	0.58	98.93	100.07	0.002
SaO$_2$pos top	4	96.43	3.96	92.55	100.31	
PvO$_2$pre op	4	158.25	78.48	81.34	235.16	0.023
PvO$_2$pos top	4	125.5	64.94	61.86	189.14	
SvO$_2$pre op	4	99.35	0.47	98.89	99.81	0.002
SvO$_2$pos top	4	93.88	3.73	90.22	97.54	
OIpre op	4	2.51	1.37	1.17	3.85	0.002
OIpos top	4	1.78	0.87	0.93	2.63	

IA cardioplegic arrest with no controlled lung perfusion, *OI* oxygen index, *PaO2* arterial oxygen pressure, *PvO2* pulmonary venous oxygen pressure, *SvO2* pulmonary venous oxygen saturation

The benefits of controlled lung perfusion with arterial blood when the heart is kept beating become evident in light of the correlation with subgroup IIA and IIC. From a gasometric point of view, we postulate that controlled lung perfusion with venous blood when the heart is kept beating does not provide relevant benefits compared to the subgroup in which the heart is beating and the lungs are not perfused in a controlled manner. As pointed out, there is a special chapter for that topic.

Two issues can be raised by cardiac surgeons regarding the influence of ventilation and temperature on gas exchange during heart surgery with CPB. The issue of ventilation is subject for chapter 37 and issue of temperature is addressed in this current chapter.

We selected interesting and appealing research carried out by Birdi et al.[2] in which pulmonary gas exchange was evaluated using alveolar-arterial oxygen pressure gradients; 45 patients were aligned into three equal groups and underwent myocardial revascularization with CPB at a systemic perfusion temperature of 28°C (hypothermia), 32°C (moderate hypothermia), or 37°C (normothermia). CPB was established by means of ascending aortic and right atrial appendage cannulation, and cardioplegic arrest was induced in all patients. The alveolar-arterial oxygen pressure [P(A–a)O$_2$] gradient was calculated according the formula P(A–a)O$_2$ = PAO$_2$–PaO$_2$, where PAO$_2$ is partial pressure of alveolar oxygen, and PaO$_2$ is the partial pressure of arterial oxygen.[3-5] Main outcomes of this study can be viewed in Table 32.13 and Figs. 32.1 and 32.2. The most striking conclusion was that systemic perfusion temperature did not have a relevant impact on the P(A–a)O$_2$ gradients in the first 12 h following elective myocardial revascularization.

Table32 .2 Gasometric variables in pre- and postoperative times – subgroup IB

Variables	n	Mean	Standard deviation	Confidence interval		Significance (p)
				Inferior threshold	Superior threshold	
PaO$_2$ preop	6	227.67	122.86	129.36	325.98	0.249
PaO$_2$pos top	6	167	137.79	56.75	277.25	
SaO$_2$pre op	6	98.83	2.4	96.91	100.75	0.039
SaO$_2$pos top	6	97.33	3.67	94.39	100.27	
PvO$_2$pre op	6	236.5	119.87	140.58	332.42	0.225
PvO$_2$pos top	6	147.33	88.01	76.91	217.75	
SvO$_2$pre op	6	99.17	1.33	98.11	100.23	0.357
SvO$_2$pos top	6	98.17	1.72	96.79	99.55	
OIpre op	6	2.26	1.21	1.29	3.23	0.752
OIpos top	6	2.37	1.94	0.82	3.92	

IB cardioplegic arrest and controlled lung perfusion with arterial blood, *OI* oxygen index, *PaO$_2$* arterial oxygen pressure, *PvO$_2$* pulmonary venous oxygen pressure, *SvO$_2$* pulmonary venous oxygen saturation

Table32 .3 Gasometric variables in pre- and postoperative times – subgroup IC

Variables	n	Mean	Standard deviation	Confidence interval		Significance (p)
				Inferior threshold	Superior threshold	
PaO$_2$ preop	6	219.5	94.1	144.20	294.80	0.021
PaO$_2$pos top	6	141.83	83.36	75.13	208.53	
SaO$_2$pre op	6	99.7	0.39	99.39	100.01	0.042
SaO$_2$pos top	6	96.1	4.73	92.32	99.88	
PvO$_2$pre op	6	164.17	62.81	113.91	214.43	0.345
PvO$_2$pos top	6	143.83	94	68.61	219.05	
SvO$_2$pre op	6	97.45	3.68	94.51	100.39	0.207
SvO$_2$pos top	6	94.2	6.22	89.22	99.18	
OIpre op	6	2.18	0.95	1.42	2.94	0.463
OIpos top	6	2.01	1.18	1.07	2.95	

IC cardioplegic arrest and controlled lung perfusion with venous blood, *OI* oxygen index, *PaO$_2$* arterial oxygen pressure, *PvO$_2$* pulmonary venous oxygen pressure, *SvO$_2$* pulmonary venous oxygen saturation

---

Table32.4 Gasometric variables in postoperative time – subgroups IA and IB

Variables	Group	n	Mean	Standard deviation	Confidence interval		Significance (p)
					Inferior threshold	Superior threshold	
PaO_2 postop	IA	4	126.25	62.11	65.38	187.12	>0.999
	IB	6	167.00	137.79	56.75	277.25	
SaO_2 postop	IA	4	96.43	3.96	92.55	100.30	0.829
	IB	6	97.33	3.67	94.40	100.27	
PvO_2 postop	IA	4	125.50	64.94	61.86	189.14	0.517
	IB	6	147.33	88.01	76.92	217.75	
SvO_2 postop	IA	4	93.88	3.73	90.22	97.53	0.133
	IB	6	98.17	1.72	96.79	99.54	
OI postop	IA	4	1.78	0.87	0.93	2.63	>0.999
	IB	6	2.37	1.94	0.82	3.92	

IA cardioplegic arrest with no controlled lung perfusion, *IB* cardioplegic arrest and controlled lung perfusion with arterial blood, *OI* oxygen index, *PaO_2* arterial oxygen pressure, *PvO_2* pulmonary venous oxygen pressure, *SvO_2* pulmonary venous oxygen saturation

Table32.5 Gasometric variables in postoperative time – subgroups IA and IC

Variables	Group	n	Mean	Standard deviation	Confidence interval		Significance (p)
					Inferior threshold	Superior threshold	
PaO_2 postop	IA	4	126.25	62.11	65.38	187.12	0.670
	IC	6	141.83	83.36	75.13	208.54	
SaO_2 postop	IA	4	96.43	3.96	92.55	100.30	0.831
	IC	6	96.10	4.73	92.32	99.88	
PvO_2 postop	IA	4	125.50	64.94	61.86	189.14	>0.999
	IC	6	143.83	94.00	68.62	219.04	
SvO_2 postop	IA	4	93.88	3.73	90.22	97.53	0.748
	IC	6	94.20	6.22	89.22	99.18	
OI postop	IA	4	1.78	0.87	0.93	2.63	0.748
	IC	6	2.01	1.18	1.06	2.96	

IA cardioplegic arrest with no controlled lung perfusion, *IC* cardioplegic arrest and controlled lung perfusion with venous blood, *OI* oxygen index, *PaO_2* arterial oxygen pressure, *PvO_2* pulmonary venous oxygen pressure, *SvO_2* pulmonary venous oxygen saturation

Table32 .6 Gasometric variables in postoperative time – subgroups IB and IC

Variables	Group	n	Mean	Standard deviation	Confidence interval		Significance (p)
					Inferior threshold	Superior threshold	
PaO$_2$ postop	IB	6	167.00	137.79	56.75	277.25	0.749
	IC	6	141.83	83.36	75.13	208.54	
SaO$_2$pos top	IB	6	97.33	3.67	94.40	100.27	0.936
	IC	6	96.10	4.73	92.32	99.88	
PvO$_2$pos top	IB	6	147.33	88.01	76.92	217.75	0.519
	IC	6	143.83	94.00	68.62	219.04	
SvO$_2$pos top	IB	6	98.17	1.72	96.79	99.54	0.373
	IC	6	94.20	6.22	89.22	99.18	
OIpos top	IB	6	2.37	1.94	0.82	3.92	0.749
	IC	6	2.01	1.18	1.06	2.96	

IB cardioplegic arrest and controlled lung perfusion with arterial blood, *IC* cardioplegic arrest and controlled lung perfusion with venous blood, *OI* oxygen index, *PaO$_2$* arterial oxygen pressure, *PvO$_2$* pulmonary venous oxygen pressure, *SvO$_2$* pulmonary venous oxygen saturation

Table32 .7 Gasometric variables in pre and postoperative times – subgroup IIA

Variables	n	Mean	Standard deviation	Confidence interval		Significance (p)
				Inferior threshold	Superior threshold	
PaO$_2$ preop	4	174.5	87.41	88.84	260.16	0.011
PaO$_2$pos top	4	82.38	22.44	60.39	104.37	
SaO$_2$pre op	4	97.95	2.73	95.27	100.63	0.011
SaO$_2$pos top	4	92.35	4.06	88.37	96.33	
PvO$_2$pre op	4	189.25	107.11	84.28	294.22	0.011
PvO$_2$pos top	4	43.35	19.89	23.86	62.84	
SvO$_2$pre op	4	99.08	0.9	98.20	99.96	0.011
SvO$_2$pos top	4	62.28	16.39	46.22	78.34	
OIpre op	4	1.75	0.87	0.90	2.60	0.011
OIpos top	4	1.15	0.31	0.85	1.45	

IIA beating heart technique with no controlled lung perfusion, *OI* oxygen index, *PaO$_2$* arterial oxygen pressure, *PvO$_2$* pulmonary venous oxygen pressure, *SvO$_2$* pulmonary venous oxygen saturation

Table32 .8 Gasometric variables in pre and postoperative times – subgroup IIB

| Variables | n | Mean | Standard deviation | Confidence interval | | Significance (p) |
				Inferior threshold	Superior threshold	
PaO$_2$ preop	6	167	64.27	115.57	218.43	0.600
PaO$_2$pos top	6	145.5	64.45	93.93	197.07	
SaO$_2$pre op	6	98.92	1.74	97.53	100.31	0.331
SaO$_2$pos top	6	98.28	1.3	97.24	99.32	
PvO$_2$pre op	6	236.33	149.33	116.84	355.82	0.157
PvO$_2$pos top	6	137.5	39.99	105.50	169.50	
SvO$_2$pre op	6	98.47	1.95	96.91	100.03	0.231
SvO$_2$pos top	6	97.67	1.21	96.70	98.64	
OIpre op	6	1.67	0.64	1.16	2.18	0.345
OIpos top	6	2.07	0.93	1.33	2.81	

IIB beating heart technique and controlled lung perfusion with arterial blood, *OI* oxygen index, *PaO$_2$* arterial oxygen pressure, *PvO$_2$* pulmonary venous oxygen pressure, *SvO$_2$* pulmonary venous oxygen saturation

Table32. 9 Gasometric variables in pre- and postoperative times – subgroup IIC

| Variables | n | Mean | Standard deviation | Confidence interval | | Significance (p) |
				Inferior threshold	Superior threshold	
PaO$_2$ preop	6	232.28	129.44	128.71	335.85	0.028
PaO$_2$pos top	6	55.25	13.27	44.63	65.87	
SaO$_2$pre op	6	99.18	0.79	98.55	99.81	0.028
SaO$_2$pos top	6	80.73	13.12	70.23	91.23	
PvO$_2$pre op	6	187.67	79.02	124.44	250.90	0.028
PvO$_2$pos top	6	34.12	9.12	26.82	41.42	
SvO$_2$pre op	6	99.12	0.82	98.46	99.78	0.028
SvO$_2$pos top	6	53.23	18.74	38.23	68.23	
IO$_2$pre op	6	2.32	1.3	1.28	3.36	0.028
IO$_2$pos top	6	0.78	0.19	0.63	0.93	

IIC beating heart technique and controlled lung perfusion with venous blood, *OI* oxygen index, *PaO$_2$* arterial oxygen pressure, *PvO$_2$* pulmonary venous oxygen pressure, *SvO$_2$* pulmonary venous oxygen saturation

Table32.10 Gasometric variables in postoperative time – subgroups IIA and IIB

Variables	Group	n	Mean	Standard deviation	Confidence interval		Significance (p)
					Inferior threshold	Superior threshold	
PaO₂ postop	IIA	4	82.38	22.44	60.38	104.37	0.033
	IIB	6	145.50	64.45	93.93	197.07	
SaO₂pos top	IIA	4	92.35	4.06	88.37	96.33	0.010
	IIB	6	98.28	1.30	97.25	99.32	
PvO₂pos top	IIA	4	43.35	19.89	23.86	62.84	0.011
	IIB	6	137.50	39.99	105.50	169.50	
SvO₂pos top	IIA	4	62.28	16.39	46.21	78.34	0.010
	IIB	6	97.67	1.21	96.70	98.64	
OIpos top	IIA	4	1.15	0.31	0.85	1.45	0.032
	IIB	6	2.07	0.93	1.33	2.82	

IIA beating heart technique with no controlled lung perfusion, *IIB* beating heart technique and controlled lung perfusion with venous blood, *OI* oxygen index, *PaO₂* arterial oxygen pressure, *PvO₂* pulmonary venous oxygen pressure, *SvO₂* pulmonary venous oxygen saturation

Table32.11 Gasometric variables in postoperative time – subgroups IIA and IIC

Variables	Group	n	Mean	Standard deviation	Confidence interval		Significance (p)
					Inferior threshold	Superior threshold	
PaO₂ postop	IIA	4	82.38	22.44	60.38	104.37	0.033
	IIC	6	55.25	13.27	44.64	65.86	
SaO₂pos top	IIA	4	92.35	4.06	88.37	96.33	0.006
	IIC	6	80.73	13.12	70.23	91.23	
PvO₂pos top	IIA	4	43.35	19.89	23.86	62.84	0.522
	IIC	6	34.12	9.12	26.82	41.42	
SvO₂pos top	IIA	4	62.28	16.39	46.21	78.34	0.394
	IIC	6	53.23	18.74	38.23	68.23	
OIpos top	IIA	4	1.15	0.31	0.85	1.45	0.042
	IIC	6	0.78	0.19	0.63	0.94	

IIA beating heart technique with no controlled lung perfusion, *IIC* beating heart technique and controlled lung perfusion with venous blood, *OI* oxygen index, *PaO₂* arterial oxygen pressure, *PvO₂* pulmonary venous oxygen pressure, *SvO₂* pulmonary venous oxygen saturation

Table32.12 Gasometric variables in postoperative time – subgroups IIB and IIC

Variables	Gv	*n*	Mean	Standard deviation	Confidencei nterval		Significance (*p*)
					Inferior threshold	Superior threshold	
PaO₂ postop	IIB	6	145.50	64.45	93.93	197.07	0.004
	IIC	6	55.25	13.27	44.64	65.86	
SaO₂pos top	IIB	6	98.28	1.30	97.25	99.32	0.004
	IIC	6	80.73	13.12	70.23	91.23	
PvO₂pos top	IIB	6	137.50	39.99	105.50	169.50	0.004
	IIC	6	34.12	9.12	26.82	41.42	
SvO₂pos top	IIB	6	97.67	1.21	96.70	98.64	0.004
	IIC	6	53.23	18.74	38.23	68.23	
OI postop	IIB	6	2.07	0.93	1.33	2.82	0.004
	IIC	6	0.78	0.19	0.63	0.94	

IIB beating heart technique and controlled lung perfusion with arterial blood, *IIC* beating heart technique and controlled lung perfusion with venous blood

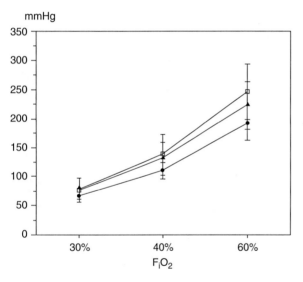

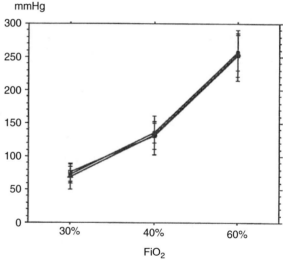

Fig. 32.1 Alveolar-arterial oxygen pressure gradient in the 28°C (*filled circle*), 32°C (*filed rectangle*), and 37°C (*filled triangle*) groups postoperatively during mechanical ventilation (stage 1). F_iO_2 inspired oxygen fraction. (This figure was published in Birdi et al.[2] Copyright 1996, the Society of Thoracic Surgeons)

Fig. 32.2 Alveolar-arterial oxygen pressure gradient in the 28°C (*filled circle*), 32°C (*filled rectangle*), and 37°C (*filled triangle*) groups after extubation (stage 2). F_iO_2 inspired oxygen fraction. (This figure was published in Birdi et al.[2] Copyright 1996,t heS ocietyof T horacicS urgeons)

Table 32.13 Arterial blood gas analysis and alveolar-arterial gradient in the three groups

Variable	28 C Group Air	stage[b] 1	2	32 C Group Air	stage[b] 1	2	37 C Group Air	stage[b] 1	2
PaO$_2$									
Preop	80.5 ± 8.4	…	…	81.8 ± 11.5	…	…	83.9 ± 11.0	…	…
30%	…	97.5 ± 8.3	87.9 ± 10.6	…	89.4 ± 17.3	83.5 ± 10.7	…	88.0 ± 18.1	90.4 ± 16.4
40%	…	125.3 ± 12.0	96.3 ± 14.6	…	96.1 ± 30.8	97.5 ± 17.5	…	107.5 ± 26.9	99.8 ± 24.3
60%	…	185.7 ± 20.7	116.9 ± 24.6	…	130.5 ± 44.9	118.9 ± 36.0	…	159.4 ± 38.6	120.6 ± 29.2
PaCO$_2$									
Preop	35.8 ± 3.3	…	…	34.8 ± 9.9	…	…	36.2 ± 2.1	…	…
30%	…	38.0 ± 7.4	41.3 ± 4.6	…	37.0 ± 6.0	42.1 ± 5.5	…	36.1 ± 3.6	41.9 ± 6.3
40%	…	37.9 ± 8.1	40.7 ± 4.0	…	38.8 ± 7.4	44.0 ± 7.4	…	35.7 ± 4.4	41.4 ± 6.6
60%	…	37.8 ± 8.2	41.8 ± 4.7	…	39.0 ± 8.6	43.4 ± 6.1	…	35.0 ± 5.6	41.7 ± 5.8
P(A–a)O$_2$ gradient									
Preop	24.4 ± 8.2	…	…	24.5 ± 20.4	…	…	20.5 ± 9.5	…	…
30%	…	67.1 ± 12.0	72.4 ± 12.5	…	76.4 ± 20.6	75.7 ± 13.7	…	79.0 ± 18.0	69.1 ± 19.3
40%	…	110.7 ± 14.7	136.1 ± 15.8	…	138.7 ± 34.8	130.5 ± 19.9	…	131.4 ± 28.7	131.6 ± 29.3
60%	…	193.1 ± 30.5	256.6 ± 26.5	…	246.7 ± 47.7	252.7 ± 38.3	…	222.9 ± 40.5	253.1 ± 33.0

[a]Data are shown as the mean ± the standard deviation.

[b]Air is preoperative sampling period with the patient breathing air; stage 1 is 2 to 4 hours postoperatively with the patient on artifical ventilation and stage 2,1 hour after extubation with the patient breathing spontaneously. P(A–a)O$_2$ = alveolar-arterial oxygen pressure; PaCO$_2$ = partial pressure of arterial carbon dioxide; PaO$_2$ = partial pressure of arterial oxygen.

References

1. Gabriel EA, Locali RF, Matsuoka PK, et al. Lung perfusion during cardiac surgery with cardiopulmonary bypass: is it necessary? *Interact Cardiovasc Thorac Surg.* 2008;7:1089-1095.
2. Birdi I, Regragui IA, Izzat MB, et al. Effects of cardiopulmonary bypass temperature on pulmonary gas exchange after coronary artery operations. *Ann Thorac Surg.* 1996; 61:118-123.
3. Parsonnet V, Dean D, Bernstein AD. A method of uniform stratification of risk for evaluating the results of surgery in acquired adult heart disease. *Circulation.* 1989;79(suppl 1): 3-12.
4. Taggart DP, El-Fiky M, Carter R, Bowman A, Wheatley DJ. Respiratory dysfunction after uncomplicated cardiopulmonary bypass. *Ann Thorac Surg.*1993; 56:1123-1128.
5. Carvalho EM, Gabriel EA, Salerno TA. Pulmonary protection during cardiac surgery: systematic literature review. *Asian Cardiovasc Thorac Ann.*2008; 16(6):503-507.

InflammatoryC ellMar kers

33

Edmo Atique Gabriel and Tomas Salerno

As some of our research[1] was marked by a large number of data and issues, some findings still have not been published; these are addressed in this chapter. The influence of cardiopulmonary bypass (CPB) itself on the inflammatory role played by some cell markers as well as the eventual impact of lung perfusion on this kind of inflammatory response were assessed using data obtained from hemograms, arterial blood gas analyses, and pulmonary leukosequestration. The whole hemogram was obtained from blood collected from the external jugular vein, and arterial blood for gas analysis was withdrawn from the internal carotid artery. Pulmonary leukosequestration was expressed as the ratio of the right atrial and left atrial white blood cell counts as postulated in a similar manner by Liu et al.[2] Some authors have postulated that CPB is responsible for the significant rate of leukosequestration postoperatively, particularly in the lungs.[3-5]

CPB and its intrinsic inflammatory process cause endothelial dysfunction and permeability imbalance in such a way that β_2-integrin CD18, a leukocyte adhesion molecule, mediates migration of cell markers, particularly neutrophils, to the lungs, contributing to postoperative pulmonary dysfunction.[6] The significant reduction of cell markers postoperatively is depicted in Tables 33.1–33.3, and this finding can be related to cell migration and tissue sequestration.

Despite significant correlations between preoperative and postoperative times in each cardioplegic arrest subgroup, few significant correlations were found when comparisons between two cardioplegic arrest subgroups focusing on only postoperative time were done, as demonstrated in Tables 33.4–33.6.

Correlations between preoperative and postoperative times in the beating heart subgroups reveal signs of cell migration and tissue sequestration postoperatively. This finding has a valuable impact as inflammatory mechanisms of CPB can cause endothelial permeability disturbances when the heart is arrested as well as when the heart is kept beating (Tables 33.7–33.9).

The postoperative pattern of cell markers in the beating heart subgroups was marked by few significant correlations. However, we have to call attention to the correlation between groups IIA and IIC, in which controlled lung perfusion with venous blood might have contributed to the decreased drop of some cell markers than when controlled lung perfusion was not employed (Tables 33.10–33.12).

There were no significant correlations in the cardioplegic arrest subgroups or the beating heart subgroups regarding leukosequestration and neutrophilic sequestration (Tables 33.13–33.18). We believe that the key issue is the sample size; therefore, further investigation is necessary to precisely determine the impact of controlled lung perfusion on cell sequestration.

In experimental research designed by Liu et al.,[2] the authors perfused lungs using a protective solution of glucose, insulin, Na_2HPO_4, NaH_2PO_4, KCl, mannitol, low molecular weight dextran, anisodamine, L-arginine, and aprotinin. Subsequently, they correlated lung perfusion with pulmonary leukosequestration, as demonstrated in Table 33.19.

E.A.G abriel (✉)
Department of Surgery, Division of Cardiovascular Surgery
FederalU niversityof Sa oP aulo, SaoP aulo, Brazil
e-mail:e dag@uol.com.br

Table33. 1 Preoperative and postoperative cell markers in subgroup IA

Variables	N	Mean	Standard deviation	Confidence interval		Significance (p)
				Inferior threshold	Superior threshold	
Preop total leukocytes	4	7,227.50	4,041.05	3,267.27	11,187.73	0.002
Postopt otall eukocytes	4	2,630.00	1,167.53	1,485.82	3,774.18	
Preopne utrophils	4	3,615.25	1,948.97	1,705.26	5,525.24	0.002
Postopne utrophils	4	1,423.00	438.13	993.63	1,852.37	
Preopl ymphocytes	4	2,881.50	1,298.88	1,608.60	4,154.40	0.002
Postopl ymphocytes	4	1,034.00	661.89	385.35	1,682.65	
Preoppl atelets	4	259,750.00	109,515.22	152,425.08	367,074.92	0.002
Postoppl atelets	4	152,750.00	70,305.88	83,850.24	221,649.76	
Preop right atrial total leukocytes	4	6,687.50	3,903.00	2,862.56	10,512.44	0.002
Postop right atrial total leukocytes	4	3,527.50	2,891.57	693.76	6,361.24	
Preoprighta trialne utrophils	4	4,166.00	2,693.59	1,526.28	6,805.72	0.002
Postoprighta trialne utrophils	4	1,873.00	1,477.04	425.50	3,320.50	
Preop right atrial lymphocytes	4	2,065.00	991.83	1,093.01	3,036.99	0.002
Postop right atrial lymphocytes	4	1,420.00	1,155.89	287.23	2,552.77	
Preoprighta trialpla telets	4	266,000.00	110,066.65	158,134.68	373,865.32	0.002
Postoprighta trialpla telets	4	132,550.00	61,780.34	72,005.27	193,094.73	
Preop left atrial total leukocytes	4	6,162.50	4,068.25	2,175.62	10,149.39	0.002
Postop left atrial total leukocytes	4	3,095.00	3,108.64	48.53	6,141.47	
Preople fta trialne utrophils	4	3,796.00	2,634.09	1,214.59	6,377.41	0.002
Postople fta trialne utrophils	4	1,768.25	1,627.50	173.30	3,363.20	
Preople fta triallymphoc ytes	4	2,151.50	1,560.65	622.06	3,680.94	0.002
Postople fta triallymphoc ytes	4	1,101.50	1,217.52	−91.67	2,294.67	
Preople fta trialpla telets	4	326,500,00	139,648.37	189,644.60	463,355.40	0.002
Postople fta trialpla telets	4	133,500.00	54,249.42	80,335.57	186,664.43	

IA cardioplegic arrest with no controlled lung perfusion

Table33. 2 Preoperative and postoperative cell markers in subgroup IB

Variables	n	Mean	Standard deviation	Confidencei nterval		Significance (p)
				Inferior threshold	Superior threshold	
Preop total leukocytes	6	8,550.00	3,481.24	5,764.43	11,335.57	0.02
Postopt otall eukocytes	6	4,226.67	3,006.91	1,820.64	6,632.70	
Preopne utrophils	6	4,783.00	2,190.34	3,030.36	6,535.64	0.02
Postopne utrophils	6	1,221.83	721.82	644.25	1,799.41	
Preopl ymphocytes	6	2,985.00	1,484.32	1,797.30	4,172.70	0.02
Postopl ymphocytes	6	1,769.83	714.61	1,198.02	2,341.64	
Preoppl atelets	6	259,666.67	98,461.50	180,881.06	338,452.28	0.02
Postoppl atelets	6	130,500.00	38,328.84	99,830.54	161,169.46	
Preop right atrial total leukocytes	6	7,785.00	3,496.82	4,986.96	10,583.04	0.02
Postop right atrial total leukocytes	6	2,365.00	1,121.03	1,467.99	3,262.01	
Preoprighta trialne utrophils	6	4,991.83	2,488.88	3,000.31	6,983.35	0.02
Postoprighta trialne utrophils	6	1,219.67	782.78	593.32	1,846.02	
Preop right atrial lymphocytes	6	2,652.17	1,172.54	1,713.94	3,590.40	0.02
Postop right atrial lymphocytes	6	1,021.17	377.24	719.32	1,323.02	
Preoprighta trialpla telets	6	231,666.67	91,923.16	158,112.82	305,220.52	0.02
Postoprighta trialpla telets	6	133,000.00	26,183.96	112,048.47	153,951.53	
Preop left atrial total leukocytes	6	6,355.00	1,351.00	5,273.97	7,436.03	0.02
Postop left atrial total leukocytes	6	3,388.33	1,614.64	2,096.35	4,680.31	
Preople fta trialne utrophils	6	4,453.67	2,119.58	2,757.65	6,149.69	0.02
Postople fta trialne utrophils	6	1,318.83	1,022.47	500.68	2,136.98	
Preople fta triallymphoc ytes	6	7,366.67	3,236.36	4,777.04	9,956.30	0.02
Postople fta triallymphoc ytes	6	2,468.33	1,430.14	1,323.98	3,612.68	
Preople fta trialpla telets	6	230,500.00	57,999.14	184,091.02	276,908.98	0.02
Postople fta trialpla telets	6	169,333.33	48,305.97	130,680.50	207,986.16	

IB cardioplegic arrest and controlled lung perfusion with arterial blood

Table33 .3 Preoperative and postoperative cell markers in subgroup IC

| Variables | N | Mean | Standard deviation | Confidencei nterval | | Significance (p) |
				Inferior threshold	Superior threshold	
Preop total leukocytes	6	6,741.67	1,505.78	5,536.80	7,946.54	0.02
Postopt otall eukocytes	6	2,570.00	1,296.43	1,532.64	3,607.36	
Preopne utrophils	6	2,949.50	1,117.96	2,054.95	3,844.05	0.02
Postopne utrophils	6	963.33	584.24	495.84	1,430.82	
Preopl ymphocytes	6	3,203.33	1,644.83	1,887.19	4,519.47	0.02
Postopl ymphocytes	6	1,432.67	872.81	734.28	2,131.06	
Preoppl atelets	6	257,166.67	52,916.60	214,824.57	299,508.77	0.02
Postoppl atelets	6	106,750.00	48,659.79	67,814.06	145,685.94	
Preop right atrial total leukocytes	6	6,340.00	1,894.56	4,824.04	7,855.96	0.02
Postop right atrial total leukocytes	6	2,940.00	1,442.87	1,785.46	4,094.54	
Preoprighta trialne utrophils	6	2,582.67	979.93	1,798.56	3,366.78	0.02
Postoprighta trialne utrophils	6	1,215.33	586.9	745.71	1,684.95	
Preop right atrial lymphocytes	6	3,341.50	2,168.11	1,606.65	5,076.35	0.02
Postop right atrial lymphocytes	6	1,426.17	852.57	743.97	2,108.37	
Preoprighta trialpla telets	6	328,500.00	106,088.17	243,611.78	413,388.22	0.02
Postoprighta trialpla telets	6	143,383.33	134,599.71	35,681.13	251,085.53	
Preop left atrial total leukocytes	6	6,355.00	1,351.00	5,273.97	7,436.03	0.02
Postop left atrial total leukocytes	6	3,388.33	1,614.64	2,096.35	4,680.31	
Preople fta trialne utrophils	6	2,543.67	1,087.25	1,673.69	3,413.65	0.02
Postople fta trialne utrophils	6	1,295.17	878.14	592.51	1,997.83	
Preople fta triallymph ocytes	6	3,404.17	1,507.78	2,197.69	4,610.65	0.02
Postople fta triallymp hocytes	6	1,858.67	1,028.58	1,035.63	2,681.71	
Preople fta trialpla telets	6	324,666.67	74,936.42	264,705.05	384,628.29	0.02
Postople fta trialpla telets	6	102,666.67	31,745.91	77,264.65	128,068.69	

IC cardioplegic arrest and controlled lung perfusion with venous blood

Table33. 4 Postoperative correlation of cell markers between subgroups IA and IB

Variables	Group	n	Mean	Standard deviation	Confidencei nterval		Significance (p)
					Inferior threshold	Superior threshold	
Postop total leukocytes	IA	4	2,630.00	1,167.53	1,485.84	3,774.16	0.670
	IB	6	4,226.67	3,006.91	1,820.68	6,632.65	
Postopne utrophils	IA	4	1,423.00	438.13	993.64	1,852.36	0.522
	IB	6	1,221.83	721.82	644.27	1,799.40	
Postoplymphoc ytes	IA	4	1,034.00	661.89	385.36	1,682.64	0.136
	IB	6	1,769.83	714.61	1,198.03	2,341.63	
Postoppla telets	IA	4	152,750.00	70,305.88	83,851.50	221,648.50	0.593
	IB	6	130,500.00	38,328.84	99,831.10	161,168.90	
Postop right atrial total leukocytes	IA	4	3,527.50	2,891.57	693.82	6,361.18	0.522
	IB	6	2,365.00	1,121.03	1,468.01	3,261.99	
Postop right atrial netrophils	IA	4	1,873.00	1,477.04	425.53	3,320.47	0.201
	IB	6	1,219.67	782.78	593.32	1,846.01	
Postop right atrial lymphocytes	IA	4	1,420.00	1,155.89	287.25	2,552.75	0.831
	IB	6	1,021.17	377.24	719.32	1,323.01	
Postoprighta trialpla telets	IA	4	132,550.00	61,780.34	72,006.38	193,093.62	0.831
	IB	6	133,000.00	26,183.96	112,048.85	153,951.15	
Postople fta trialle ukocytes	IA	4	3,095.00	3,108.64	48.59	6,141.41	0.670
	IB	6	2,468.33	1,430.14	1,324.01	3,612.66	
Postop left atrial neutrophils	IA	4	1,768.25	1,627.50	173.33	3,363.17	0.831
	IB	6	1,318.83	1,022.47	500.70	2,136.96	
Postop left atrial lymphocytes	IA	4	1,101.50	1,217.52	91.65	2,294.65	0.286
	IB	6	1,013.00	383.74	705.95	1,320.05	
Postople fta trialpla telets	IA	4	133,500.00	54,249.42	80,336.54	186,663.46	0.286
	IB	6	169,333.33	48,305.97	130,681.22	207,985.45	

IA cardioplegic arrest with no controlled lung perfusion, *IB* cardioplegic arrest and controlled lung perfusion with arterial blood

Table33.5 Postoperative correlation of cell markers between subgroups IA and IC

Variables	Group	n	Mean	Standard deviation	Confidence interval		Significance (p)
					Inferior threshold	Superior threshold	
Postop total leukocytes	IA	4	2,630.00	1,167.53	1,485.84	3,774.16	>0.999
	IC	6	2,570.00	1,296.43	1,532.66	3,607.34	
Postopne utrophils	IA	4	1,423.00	438.13	993.64	1,852.36	0.201
	IC	6	963.33	584.24	495.85	1,430.82	
Postoplymphoc ytes	IA	4	1,034.00	661.89	385.36	1,682.64	0.670
	IC	6	1,432.67	872.81	734.29	2,131.05	
Postoppla telets	IA	4	152,750.00	70,305.88	83,851.50	221,648.50	0.286
	IC	6	106,750.00	48,659.79	67,814.78	145,685.22	
Postop right atrial total leukocytes	IA	4	3,527.50	2,891.57	693.82	6,361.18	>0.999
	IC	6	2,940.00	1,442.87	1,785.48	4,094.52	
Postop right atrial netrophils	IA	4	1,873.00	1,477.04	425.53	3,320.47	0.831
	IC	6	1,215.33	586.90	745.72	1,684.94	
Postop right atrial lymphocytes	IA	4	1,420.00	1,155.89	287.25	2,552.75	0.831
	IC	6	1,426.17	852.57	743.98	2,108.35	
Postoprighta trialpla telets	IA	4	132,550.00	61,780.34	72,006.38	193,093.62	0.522
	IC	6	143,383.33	134,599.71	35,683.11	251,083.55	
Postop left atrial leukocytes	IA	4	3,095.00	3,108.64	48.59	6,141.41	0.394
	IC	6	3,388.33	1,614.64	2,096.38	4,680.29	
Postop left atrial neutrophils	IA	4	1,768.25	1,627.50	173.33	3,363.17	0.670
	IC	6	1,295.17	878.14	592.52	1,997.81	
Postop left atrial lymphocytes.	IA	4	1,101.50	1,217.52	−91.65	2,294.65	0.136
	IC	6	1,858.67	1,028.58	1,035.65	2,681.69	
Postople fta trialpla telets	IA	4	133,500.00	54,249.42	80,336.54	186,663.46	0.454
	IC	6	102,666.67	31,745.91	77,265.12	128,068.22	

IA cardioplegic arrest with no controlled lung perfusion, *IC* cardioplegic arrest and controlled lung perfusion with venous blood

Table33. 6 Postoperative correlation of cell markers between subgroups IB and IC

Variables	Group	n	Mean	Standard deviation	Confidencei nterval		Significance (p)
					Inferior threshold	Superior threshold	
Postop total leukocytes	IB	6	4,226.67	3,006.91	1,820.68	6,632.65	0.262
	IC	6	2,570.00	1,296.43	1,532.66	3,607.34	
Postopne utrophils	IB	6	1,221.83	721.82	644.27	1,799.40	0.522
	IC	6	963.33	584.24	495.85	1,430.82	
Postopl ymphocytes	IB	6	1,769.83	714.61	1,198.03	2,341.63	0.262
	IC	6	1,432.67	872.81	734.29	2,131.05	
Postoppl atelets	IB	6	130,500.00	38,328.84	99,831.10	161,168.90	0.522
	IC	6	106,750.00	48,659.79	67,814.78	145,685.22	
Postop right atrial total leukocytes	IB	6	2,365.00	1,121.03	1,468.01	3,261.99	0.631
	IC	6	2,940.00	1,442.87	1,785.48	4,094.52	
Postop right atrial netrophils	IB	6	1,219.67	782.78	593.32	1,846.01	0.631
	IC	6	1,215.33	586.90	745.72	1,684.94	
Postop right atrial lymphocytes	IB	6	1,021.17	377.24	719.32	1,323.01	0.423
	IC	6	1,426.17	852.57	743.98	2,108.35	
Postopr ighta trialpl atelets	IB	6	133,000.00	26,183.96	112,048.85	153,951.15	0.522
	IC	6	143,383.33	134,599.71	35,683.11	251,083.55	
Postop left atrial leukocytes	IB	6	2,468.33	1,430.14	1,324.01	3,612.66	0.631
	IC	6	3,388.33	1,614.64	2,096.38	4,680.29	
Postop left atrial neutrophils	IB	6	1,318.83	1,022.47	500.70	2,136.96	0.873
	IC	6	1,295.17	878.14	592.52	1,997.81	
Postop left atrial lymphocytes	IB	6	1,013.00	383.74	705.95	1,320.05	0.02
	IC	6	1,858.67	1,028.58	1,035.65	2,681.69	
Postopl efta trialpl atelets	IB	6	169,333.33	48,305.97	130,681.22	207,985.45	0.02
	IC	6	102,666.67	31,745.91	77,265.12	128,068.22	

IB cardioplegic arrest and controlled lung perfusion with arterial blood, *IC* cardioplegic arrest and controlled lung perfusion with venous blood

Table33.7 Preoperative and postoperative cell markers in subgroup IIA

Variables	N	Mean	Standard deviation	Confidencei nterval		Significance (p)
				Inferior threshold	Superior threshold	
Preop total leukocytes	4	10,510.00	772.27	9,753.18	11,266.82	0.011
Postopt otall eukocytes	4	4,385.00	2,093.31	2,333.56	6,436.44	
Preopne utrophils	4	6,314.00	463.69	5,859.58	6,768.42	0.011
Postopne utrophils	4	2,137.50	1,090.00	1,069.30	3,205.70	
Preopl ymphocytes	4	3,483.25	886.93	2,614.06	4,352.44	0.011
Postopl ymphocytes	4	2,037.75	959.9	1,097.05	2,978.45	
Preoppl atelets	4	450,500.00	186,712.79	267,521.47	633,478.53	0.011
Postoppl atelets	4	197,925.00	104,819.00	95,202.38	300,647.62	
Preop right atrial total leukocytes	4	9,787.50	864.46	8,940.33	10,634.67	0.011
Postop right atrial total leukocytes	4	3,912.50	2,170.23	1,785.67	6,039.33	
Preopr ighta trialne utrophils	4	6,084.75	358.25	5,733.67	6,435.84	0.011
Postopr ighta trialne utrophils	4	2,188.00	904.73	1,301.36	3,074.64	
Preop right atrial lymphocytes	4	3,074.75	652.25	2,435.55	3,713.96	0.035
Postop right atrial lymphocytes	4	1,806.00	923.17	901.29	2,710.71	
Preopr ighta trialpl atelets	4	400,500.00	151,777.25	251,758.30	549,241.71	0.011
Postopr ighta trialpl atelets	4	218,000.00	105,555.67	114,555.44	321,444.56	
Preop left atrial total leukocytes	4	9,237.50	2,585.73	6,703.48	11,771.52	0.011
Postop left atrial total leukocytes	4	3,702.50	2,032.43	1,710.72	5,694.28	
Preopl efta trialne utrophils	4	5,708.00	1,170.54	4,560.87	6,855.13	0.011
Postopl efta trialne utrophils	4	2,242.25	916.66	1,343.92	3,140.58	
Preopl efta triall ymphocytes	4	3,095.00	1,386.17	1,736.55	4,453.45	0.035
Postopl efta triall ymphocytes	4	1,432.50	922.47	528.48	2,336.52	
Preopl efta trialpl atelets	4	409,500.00	146,272.58	266,152.87	552,847.13	0.011
Postopl efta trialpl atelets	4	207,225.00	130,419.23	79,414.15	335,035.85	

IIA beating heart technique with no controlled lung perfusion

Table33. 8 Preoperative and postoperative cell markers in subgroup IIB

| Variables | n | Mean | Standard deviation | Confidencei nterval | | Significance (p) |
				Inferior threshold	Superior threshold	
Preop total leukocytes	6	11,556.67	3,207.43	8,990.19	14,123.15	0.002
Postopt otall eukocytes	6	5,315.00	4,505.04	1,710.22	8,919.78	
Preopne utrophils	6	6,097.83	1,956.58	4,532.24	7,663.42	0.002
Postopne utrophils	6	3,082.50	2,917.10	748.33	5,416.67	
Preopl ymphocytes	6	4,794.50	1,630.93	3,489.48	6,099.52	0.002
Postopl ymphocytes	6	1,742.50	1,633.93	435.08	3,049.92	
Preoppl atelets	6	184,500.00	62,468.39	134,514.88	234,485.12	0.012
Postoppl atelets	6	135,333.33	51,364.06	94,233.52	176,433.14	
Preop right atrial total leukocytes	6	11,393.33	3,111.11	8,903.92	13,882.74	0.002
Postop right atrial total leukocytes	6	5,411.67	4,768.44	1,596.12	9,227.22	
Preoprighta trialne utrophils	6	5,598.83	1,765.57	4,186.08	7,011.58	0.002
Postoprighta trialne utrophils	6	3,032.50	2,779.08	808.77	5,256.23	
Preop right atrial lymphocytes	6	5,122.33	1,752.78	3,719.81	6,524.85	0.002
Postop right atrial lymphocytes	6	1,894.67	1,847.00	416.76	3,372.58	
Preoprighta trialpla telets	6	235,500.00	88,199.21	164,925.93	306,074.07	0.012
Postoprighta trialpla telets	6	145,166.67	53,221.86	102,580.31	187,753.03	
Preop left atrial total leukocytes	6	10,416.67	2,985.46	8,027.80	12,805.54	0.002
Postop left atrial total leukocytes	6	5,685.00	4,640.31	1,971.98	9,398.02	
Preople fta trialne utrophils	6	6,143.83	2,272.30	4,325.61	7,962.05	0.002
Postople fta trialne utrophils	6	2,615.17	2,211.57	845.55	4,384.79	
Preople fta triallymphoc ytes	6	3,571.83	1,086.84	2,702.18	4,441.48	0.005
Postople fta triallymphoc ytes	6	1,976.33	2,079.33	312.52	3,640.14	
Preople fta trialpla telets	6	221,500.00	48,023.95	183,072.84	259,927.16	0.002
Postople fta trialpla telets	6	126,166.67	42,508.43	92,152.84	160,180.50	

IIB beating heart technique and controlled lung perfusion with arterial blood

Table33.9 Preoperative and postoperative cell markers in subgroup IIC

Variables	n	Mean	Standard deviation	Confidencei nterval		Significance (p)
				Inferior threshold	Superior threshold	
Preop total leukocytes	6	11,181.67	2,541.42	9,148.11	13,215.23	0.02
Postopt otall eukocytes	6	6,235.00	1,994.46	4,639.10	7,830.90	
Preopne utrophils	6	6,920.50	1,979.22	5,336.79	8,504.21	0.02
Postopne utrophils	6	3,599.83	1,307.17	2,553.88	4,645.78	
Preopl ymphocytes	6	3,492.83	1,083.60	2,625.77	4,359.89	0.02
Postopl ymphocytes	6	2,302.33	954.06	1,538.92	3,065.74	
Preoppl atelets	6	250,000.00	98,185.54	171,435.21	328,564.79	0.02
Postoppl atelets	6	121,683.33	46,793.69	84,240.58	159,126.08	
Preop right atrial total leukocytes	6	10,713.33	2,238.05	8,922.52	12,504.14	0.02
Postop right atrial total leukocytes	6	6,200.00	2,066.90	4,546.14	7,853.86	
Preopr ighta trialne utrophils	6	6,736.00	1,692.17	5,381.98	8,090.02	0.046
Postopr ighta trialne utrophils	6	3,700.00	1,336.56	2,630.53	4,769.47	
Preop right atrial lymphocytes	6	3,301.17	1,171.86	2,363.49	4,238.85	0.02
Postop right atrial lymphocytes	6	2,191.67	919.93	1,455.57	2,927.77	
Preopr ighta trialpl atelets	6	262,383.33	92,066.07	188,715.13	336,051.53	0.02
Postopr ighta trialpl atelets	6	124,916.67	37,146.22	95,193.50	154,639.84	
Preop left atrial total leukocytes	6	10,710.00	2,915.06	8,377.47	13,042.53	0.02
Postop left atrial total leukocytes	6	5,611.67	2,506.27	3,606.24	7,617.10	
Preopl efta trialne utrophils	6	6,917.50	2,868.84	4,621.95	9,213.05	0.046
Postopl efta trialne utrophils	6	3,385.50	1,351.87	2,303.78	4,467.22	
Preopl efta triall ymphocytes	6	3,405.33	1,313.09	2,354.64	4,456.02	0.02
Postopl efta triall ymphocytes	6	1,941.17	1,165.85	1,008.30	2,874.04	
Preopl efta trialpl atelets	6	263,700.00	102,636.35	181,573.82	345,826.18	0.046
Postopl efta trialpl atelets	6	139,116.67	43,936.34	103,960.28	174,273.06	

IIC beating heart technique and controlled lung perfusion with venous blood

Table33 .10 Postoperative correlation of cell markers between subgroups IIA and IIB

Variables	Group	n	Mean	Standard deviation	Confidencei nterval		Significance (p)
					Inferior threshold	Superior threshold	
Postop total leukocytes	IIA	4	4,385.00	2,093.31	2,333.59	6,436.41	0.831
	IIB	6	5,315.00	4,505.04	1,710.28	8,919.72	
Postopne utrophils	IIA	4	2,137.50	1,090.00	1,069.32	3,205.68	0.831
	IIB	6	3,082.50	2,917.10	748.37	5,416.63	
Postoplymphoc ytes	IIA	4	2,037.75	959.90	1,097.06	2,978.44	0.454
	IIB	6	1,742.50	1,633.93	435.11	3,049.89	
Postoppla telets	IIA	4	197,925.00	104,819.00	95,204.27	300,645.73	0.522
	IIB	6	135,333.33	51,364.06	94,234.28	176,432.39	
Postop right atrial total leukocytes	IIA	4	3,912.50	2,170.23	1,785.72	6,039.28	0.831
	IIB	6	5,411.67	4,768.44	1,596.19	9,227.15	
Postop right atrial netrophils	IIA	4	2,188.00	904.73	1,301.38	3,074.62	>0.999
	IIB	6	3,032.50	2,779.08	808.82	5,256.18	
Postop right atrial lymphocytes	IIA	4	1,806.00	923.17	901.31	2,710.69	0.670
	IIB	6	1,894.67	1,847.00	416.78	3,372.55	
Postop right atrial platelets	IIA	4	218,000.00	105,555.67	114,557.34	321,442.66	0.394
	IIB	6	145,166.67	53,221.86	102,581.09	187,752.24	
Postop left atrial leukocytes	IIA	4	3,702.50	2,032.43	1,710.76	5,694.24	>0.999
	IIB	6	5,685.00	4,640.31	1,972.04	9,397.96	
Postop left atrial neutrophils	IIA	4	2,242.25	916.66	1,343.94	3,140.56	0.831
	IIB	6	2,615.17	2,211.57	845.58	4,384.76	
Postop left atrial lymphocytes	IIA	4	1,432.50	922.47	528.49	2,336.51	>0.999
	IIB	6	1,976.33	2,079.33	312.56	3,640.11	
Postop left atrial platelets	IIA	4	207,225.00	130,419.23	79,416.50	335,033.50	0.670
	IIB	6	126,166.67	42,508.43	92,153.46	160,179.87	

IIA beating heart technique with no controlled lung perfusion, *IIB* beating heart technique and controlled lung perfusion with arterial blood

Table 33.11 Postoperative correlation of cell markers between subgroups IIA and IIC

| Variables | Group | n | Mean | Standard deviation | Confidence interval | | Significance (p) |
					Inferior threshold	Superior threshold	
Postop total leukocytes	IIA	4	4,385.00	2,093.31	2,333.59	6,436.41	0.014
	IIC	6	6,235.00	1,994.46	4,639.13	7,830.87	
Postop neutrophils	IIA	4	2,137.50	1,090.00	1,069.32	3,205.68	0.006
	IIC	6	3,599.83	1,307.17	2,553.90	4,645.76	
Postop lymphocytes	IIA	4	2,037.75	959.90	1,097.06	2,978.44	0.522
	IIC	6	2,302.33	954.06	1,538.94	3,065.73	
Postop platelets	IIA	4	197,925.00	104,819.00	95,204.27	300,645.73	0.201
	IIC	6	121,683.33	46,793.69	84,241.27	159,125.40	
Postop right atrial total leukocytes	IIA	4	3,912.50	2,170.23	1,785.72	6,039.28	0.009
	IIC	6	6,200.00	2,066.90	4,546.17	7,853.83	
Postop right atrial netrophils	IIA	4	2,188.00	904.73	1,301.38	3,074.62	0.009
	IIC	6	3,700.00	1,336.56	2,630.55	4,769.45	
Postop right atrial lymphocytes	IIA	4	1,806.00	923.17	901.31	2,710.69	0.522
	IIC	6	2,191.67	919.93	1,455.59	2,927.75	
Postop right atrial platelets	IIA	4	218,000.00	105,555.67	114,557.34	321,442.66	0.011
	IIC	6	124,916.67	37,146.22	95,194.05	154,639.29	
Postop left atrial leukocytes	IIA	4	3,702.50	2,032.43	1,710.76	5,694.24	0.286
	IIC	6	5,611.67	2,506.27	3,606.27	7,617.06	
Postop left atrial neutrophils	IIA	4	2,242.25	916.66	1,343.94	3,140.56	0.014
	IIC	6	3,385.50	1,351.87	2,303.80	4,467.20	
Postop left atrial lymphocytes	IIA	4	1,432.50	922.47	528.49	2,336.51	0.522
	IIC	6	1,941.17	1,165.85	1,008.31	2,874.02	
Postop left atrial platelets	IIA	4	207,225.00	130,419.23	79,416.50	335,033.50	0.394
	IIC	6	139,116.67	43,936.34	103,960.92	174,272.41	

IIA beating heart technique with no controlled lung perfusion, *IIC* beating heart technique and controlled lung perfusion with venous blood

Table33 .12 Postoperative correlation of cell markers between subgroups IIB and IIC

Variables	Group	n	Mean	Standard deviation	Confidencei nterval		Significance (p)
					Inferior threshold	Superior threshold	
Postop total leukocytes	IIB	6	5,315.00	4,505.04	1,710.28	8,919.72	0.522
	IIC	6	6,235.00	1,994.46	4,639.13	7,830.87	
Postopne utrophils	IIB	6	3,082.50	2,917.10	748.37	5,416.63	0.522
	IIC	6	3,599.83	1,307.17	2,553.90	4,645.76	
Postoplymphoc ytes	IIB	6	1,742.50	1,633.93	435.11	3,049.89	0.262
	IIC	6	2,302.33	954.06	1,538.94	3,065.73	
Postoppla telets	IIB	6	135,333.33	51,364.06	94,234.28	176,432.39	0.575
	IIC	6	121,683.33	46,793.69	84,241.27	159,125.40	
Postop right atrial total leukocytes	IIB	6	5,411.67	4,768.44	1,596.19	9,227.15	0.522
	IIC	6	6,200.00	2,066.90	4,546.17	7,853.83	
Postop right atrial netrophils	IIB	6	3,032.50	2,779.08	808.82	5,256.18	0.522
	IIC	6	3,700.00	1,336.56	2,630.55	4,769.45	
Postop right atrial lymphocytes	IIB	6	1,894.67	1,847.00	416.78	3,372.55	0.262
	IIC	6	2,191.67	919.93	1,455.59	2,927.75	
Postop right atrial platelets	IIB	6	145,166.67	53,221.86	102,581.09	187,752.24	0.229
	IIC	6	124,916.67	37,146.22	95,194.05	154,639.29	
Postop left atrial leukocytes	IIB	6	5,685.00	4,640.31	1,972.04	9,397.96	0.631
	IIC	6	5,611.67	2,506.27	3,606.27	7,617.06	
Postop left atrial neutrophils	IIB	6	2,615.17	2,211.57	845.58	4,384.76	0.262
	IIC	6	3,385.50	1,351.87	2,303.80	4,467.20	
Postop left atrial lymphocytes	IIB	6	1,976.33	2,079.33	312.56	3,640.11	0.522
	IIC	6	1,941.17	1,165.85	1,008.31	2,874.02	
Postop left atrial platelets	IIB	6	126,166.67	42,508.43	92,153.46	160,179.87	0.423
	IIC	6	139,116.67	43,936.34	103,960.92	174,272.41	

IIB beating heart technique and controlled lung perfusion with arterial blood, *IIC* beating heart technique and controlled lung perfusion with venous blood

Table33.13 Leukosequestration and neutrophilic sequestration in subgroups IA and IB

Variable	Group	n	Mean	Standard deviation	Confidence interval		Significance (p)
					Inferiort hreshold	Superiort hreshold	
Leucseq	IA	4	1.40	0.57	0.84	1.96	0.201
	IB	6	1.03	0.40	0.71	1.35	
Neutseq	IA	4	1.27	0.53	0.75	1.79	0.394
	IB	6	1.01	0.61	0.52	1.50	

IA cardioplegic arrest without controlled lung perfusion, *IB* cardioplegic arrest and controlled lung perfusion with arterial blood, *Leucseq* leukosequestration (total leukocyte count), *Neutseq* neutrophilic sequestration

Table33.14 Leukosequestration and neutrophilic sequestration in subgroups IA and IC

Variable	Group	n	Mean	Standard deviation	Confidence interval		Significance (p)
					Inferiort hreshold	Superiort hreshold	
Leucseq	IA	4	1.40	0.57	0.84	1.96	0.285
	IC	6	0.89	0.20	0.73	1.05	
Neutseq	IA	4	1.27	0.53	0.75	1.79	0.522
	IC	6	1.03	0.42	0.69	1.37	

IA cardioplegic arrest without controlled lung perfusion, *IC* cardioplegic arrest and controlled lung perfusion with venous blood, *Leucseq* leukosequestration (total leukocyte count), *Neutseq* neutrophilic sequestration

Table33.15 Leukosequestration and neutrophilic sequestration in subgroups IB and IC

Variable	Group	n	Mean	Standard deviation	Confidence interval		Significance (p)
					Inferiort hreshold	Superiort hreshold	
Leucseq	IB	6	1.03	0.40	0.71	1.35	0.630
	IC	6	0.89	0.20	0.73	1.05	
Neutseq	IB	6	1.01	0.61	0.52	1.50	0.522
	IC	6	1.03	0.42	0.69	1.37	

IB cardioplegic arrest and controlled lung perfusion with arterial blood, *IC* cardioplegic arrest and controlled lung perfusion with venous blood, *Leucseq* leukosequestration (total leukocyte count), *Neutseq* neutrophilic sequestration

Table33.16 Leukosequestration and neutrophilic sequestration in subgroups IIA and IIB

Variable	Group	n	Mean	Standard deviation	Confidence interval		Significance (p)
					Inferiort hreshold	Superiort hreshold	
Leucseq	IIA	4	1.09	0.18	0.91	1.27	>0.999
	IIB	6	1.17	0.35	0.89	1.45	
Neutseq	IIA	4	1.03	0.27	0.77	1.29	0.670
	IIB	6	1.05	0.37	0.75	1.35	

IIA beating heart technique without controlled lung perfusion, *IIB* beating heart technique and controlled lung perfusion with arterial blood, *Leucseq* leukosequestration (total leukocyte count), *Neutseq* neutrophilic sequestration

Table33.17 Leukosequestration and neutrophilic sequestration in subgroups IIA and IIC

Variable	Group	n	Mean	Standard deviation	Confidence interval		Significance (p)
					Inferiort hreshold	Superiort hreshold	
Leucseq	IIA	4	1.09	0.18	0.91	1.27	0.831
	IIC	6	1.18	0.25	0.98	1.38	
Neutseq	IIA	4	1.03	0.27	0.77	1.29	0.521
	IIC	6	1.12	0.29	0.89	1.35	

IIA beating heart technique without controlled lung perfusion, *IIC* beating heart technique and controlled lung perfusion with venous blood, *Leucseq* leukosequestration (total leukocyte count), *Neutseq* neutrophilic sequestration

Table33.18 Leukosequestrationa ndne utrophilics equestrationi ns ubgroupsI IBa ndI IC

Variable	Group	n	Mean	Standard deviation	Confidence interval		Significance (p)
					Inferiort hreshold	Superiort hreshold	
Leucseq	IIB	6	1.17	0.35	0.89	1.45	0.936
	IIC	6	1.18	0.25	0.98	1.38	
Neutseq	IIB	6	1.05	0.37	0.75	1.35	0.936
	IIC	6	1.12	0.29	0.89	1.35	

IIB beating heart technique and controlled lung perfusion with arterial blood, *IIC* beating heart technique and controlled lung perfusion with venous blood, *Leucseq* leukosequestration (total leukocyte count), *Neutseq* neutrophilic sequestration

Table 33.19 White blood cell ratios (right atrial/right pulmonary venousc ounts)

Time	Controlgr oup (n=6)	Anti-inflammation group (n=6)
Baseline	1.14±0.12	1.21±0.12
CPB s tart	1.51±0.17	1.57±0.12
X-off 5 min	1.48±0.15	0.89±0.11[a]
30 min	1.38±0.22	0.90±0.14
60 min	1.28±0.16	1.05±0.09
90 min	1.11±0.71	0.97±0.10

CPB cardiopulmonary bypass, *X-off* aortic cross-clamp release

[a]$p<0.05$, anti-inflammation group versus control group. This table was published in Liu et al.[2] Copyright 2000, the Society of Thoracic Surgeons

Friedman et al.[7] also tried to identify significant differences between total CPB and partial CPB regarding the mean ratio of the white blood cell concentration in the right atrium compared to the left atrium as well as the ratio of right atrial to left atrial platelet counts at differenttime points (T ables 33.20–33.21).

Table 33.20 Mean right-atrial-to-left-atrial platelet concentration ratios before cardiopulmonary bypass, at beginning of reperfusion (time=0), and at 15-min intervals after cardiopulmonary bypass for 60 min

Group	BeforeC PB	0m in	+15m in	+30m in	+45m in	+60m in
Partial CPB	0.95±0.03	1.12±0.02	1.16±0.07	1.07±0.10	0.99±0.05	1.08±0.09
TotalC PB	1.01±0.05	1.07±0.08	0.97±0.02	0.99±0.05	1.02±0.04	1.09±0.06
p value (partial vs. total)	NS	NS	NS	NS	NS	NS

CPB cardiopulmonary bypass, *NS* not significant

This table was published in Friedman et al.[7] Copyright 1995, the Society of Thoracic Surgeons

Table 33.21 Mean right-atrial-to-left-atrial white blood cell concentration ratios before cardiopulmonary bypass, at beginning of reperfusion (time=0), and at 15-min intervals after cardiopulmonary bypass for 60 min

Group	BeforeCPB	0m in	+15m in	+30m in	+45m in	+60m in
Partial CPB	1.07±0.06	1.01±0.07	1.09±0.07	0.93±0.05	0.94±0.07	0.93±0.10
Total CPB	0.99±0.04	1.18±0.08	1.00±0.07	0.91±0.07	1.03±0.09	1.01±0.07
p value (partial vs. total)	NS	NS	NS	NS	NS	NS

CPB cardiopulmonary bypass, *NS* not significant
This table was published in Friedman et al.[7] Copyright 1995, the Society of Thoracic Surgeons

References

1. Gabriel EA, Locali RF, Matsuoka PK, et al. Lung perfusion during cardiac surgery with cardiopulmonary bypass: is it necessary? *Interact Cardiovasc Thorac Surg.* 2008;7:1089-1095.
2. Liu Y, Wang Q, Zhu X, et al. Pulmonary artery perfusion with protective solution reduces lung injury after cardiopulmonary bypass. *Ann Thorac Surg.* 2000; 69:1402-1407.
3. Butler J, Rocker GM, Westaby S. Inflammatory response to cardiopulmonary bypass. *Ann Thorac Surg.* 1993;55:552-559.
4. Kirklin JK, Westaby S, Blackstone EH, Kirklin JW, Chenoweth DE, Pacifico AD. Complement and the damaging effects of cardiopulmonary bypass. *J Thorac Cardiovasc Surg.* 1983; 86:845-885.
5. Edmunds LH Jr. Inflammatory response to cardiopulmonary bypass. *Ann Thorac Surg.* 1998; 66:S12-S16.
6. Dreyer WJ, Michael LH, Millman EE, Berens KL, Geske RS. Neutrophil sequestration and pulmonary dysfunction in a canine model of open heart surgery with cardiopulmonary bypass. Evidence for a CD18-dependent mechanism. *Circulation.* 1995;92:2276-2283.
7. Friedman M, Wang SY, Sellke FW, Franklin A, Weintraub RM, Johnson RG. Pulmonary injury after total or partial cardiopulmonary bypass with thromboxane synthesis inhibition. *Ann Thorac Surg.* 1995; 59:598-603.

Cytokines and Cellular Adhesion Molecules

34

Edmo Atique Gabriel and Tomas Salerno

Although we documented data about cytokines and cellular adhesion molecules ,[1] they have not been published yet; we presenting them in this chapter. Preoperative and postoperative pulmonary biopsies were withdrawn from the right inferior lobe of the lung following sternotomy and when ventilation of the lungs was restarted, respectively. Pulmonary specimens were stored at $-80°C$ for sequential analysis, first to determine the amount of total messenger mRNA (mRNA) and second to determine amount of three inflammatory markers: interleukin (IL) 4, tumor necrosis factor alpha (TNF-α), and intercellular adhesion molecule 1 (ICAM-1). We chose these markers because IL-4 has anti-inflammatory properties, whereas TNF-α and ICAM-1 have an inflammatory role in lung injury. Furthermore, ICAM-1 is an adhesion molecule associated with the inflammatory role played by neutrophils in pulmonary ischemia-reperfusion injury.

Following identification of the genetic sequence for TNF-α, ICAM-1, and IL-4, primers were designed for each marker. These primers were used for DNA replication according to principles of real-time polymerase chain reaction (PCR).

Quantification of mean total mRNA in pulmonary samples is demonstrated for each cardioplegic arrest subgroup as well as when comparisons between cardioplegic arrest subgroups were carried out (Tables 34.1–34.6). The most striking finding is that controlled lung perfusion for 30 min did not promote substantial modifications of the amount of total mRNA in the pulmonary specimens. This finding suggests that the quantitative impact of controlled lung perfusion on genetic material of the pulmonary specimens tended to be time dependent. We believe that controlled lung perfusion for a period of time greater than 30 min should be investigated to determine eventual modifications on expression of total mRNA in pulmonary specimens. It is important to bear in mind that a threshold of time for relevant influence of controlled lung perfusion on total mRNA expression in pulmonary tissue needs to be determined more precisely. Theoretically, less expression of total mRNA can be correlated with less expression of inflammatory markers.

Genetic expression was evaluated by the Z test, which took into consideration average values to determine standard deviation and significance level. A value of $P < 0.05$ adjusted by a Bonferroni correction ($P = 0.0253$) was considered significant for levels of TNF-α, IL-4, and ICAM-1 as these were primarily generated as average values of each subgroup. A value of $P < 0.05$ was considered significant for the three markers.

From an analysis of Tables 34.7–34.12, we can postulate that even controlled lung perfusion for 30 min while keeping the heart beating did not promote relevant findings on expression of total mRNA in each beating heart subgroup as well as when beating heart subgroups were correlated with each other. It reinforces the hypothesis that the quantitative impact of controlled lung perfusion on expression of total mRNA in pulmonary tissue tends to be time dependent. Furthermore, we can point out that the role of controlled lung perfusion in preventing expression of inflammatory markers is independent on the cardiopulmonary bypass (CPB) strategy of the beating heart procedure or cardioplegic arrest.

E.A.G abriel (✉)
FederalU niversityof Sa oP aulo, SaoP aulo, Brazil
e-mail:e dag@uol.com.br

E.A. Gabriel and T. Salerno (eds.), *Principles of Pulmonary Protection in Heart Surgery*,
DOI: 10.1007/978-1-84996-308-4_34, © Springer-Verlag London Limited 2010

Table34.1 Amount of preoperative and postoperative mRNA in subgroup IA

| Variables | n | Mean | Standard deviation | Confidencei nterval | | Significance (P) |
				Inferior threshold	Superior threshold	
Preop mRNA	4	0.77	0.65	0.13	1.41	0.715
Postopm RNA	4	0.84	0.29	0.50	1.19	

IA cardioplegic arrest without controlled lung perfusion

Table34. 2 Amount of preoperative and postoperative mRNA in subgroup IB

| Variables | n | Mean | Standard deviation | Confidencei nterval | | Significance (P) |
				Inferior threshold	Superior threshold	
Preop mRNA	6	0.51	0.44	0.09	1.32	0.917
PostopmR NA	6	0.50	0.51	0.00	1.08	

IB cardioplegic arrest and controlled lung perfusion with arterial blood

Table34. 3 Amount of preoperative and postoperative mRNA in subgroup IC

| Variables | n | Mean | Standard deviation | Confidencei nterval | | Significance (P) |
				Inferior threshold	Superior threshold	
Preop mRNA	6	0.88	0.68	0.00	2.00	0.345
PostopmR NA	6	0.60	0.38	0.21	1.26	

IC cardioplegic arrest and controlled lung perfusion with venous blood

Table34. 4 Amount of postoperative mRNA in subgroups IA and IB

| Variable | Group | n | Mean | Standard deviation | Confidencei nterval | | Significance (P) |
					Inferior threshold	Superior threshold	
Postop mRNA	IA	4	0.84	0.29	0.56	1.11	0.285
	IB	6	0.50	0.51	0.09	0.91	

IA cardioplegic arrest without controlled lung perfusion, *IB* cardioplegic arrest and controlled lung perfusion with arterial blood

Table34 .5 Amount of postoperative mRNA in subgroups IA and IC

| Variable | Group | n | Mean | Standard deviation | Confidencei nterval | | Significance (p) |
					Inferior threshold	Superior threshold	
Postop mRNA	IA	4	0.84	0.29	0.56	1.11	0.201
	IC	6	0.60	0.38	0.29	0.90	

IA cardioplegic arrest without controlled lung perfusion, *IC* cardioplegic arrest and controlled lung perfusion with venous blood

Table34. 6 Amount of postoperative RNA in subgroups IB and IC

| Variable | Group | n | Mean | Standard deviation | Confidence nterval | | Significance (P) |
					Inferior threshold	Superior threshold	
Postop mRNA	IB	6	0.50	0.51	0.09	0.91	0.521
	IC	6	0.60	0.38	0.29	0.90	

IB cardioplegic arrest and controlled lung perfusion with arterial blood, *IC* cardioplegic arrest and controlled lung perfusion with venous blood

Table34.7 Amount of preoperative and postoperative mRNA in subgroup IIA

| Variable | Group | n | Mean | Confidence nterval | | Significance (P) |
				Inferior threshold	Superior threshold	
Preop mRNA	4		0.94	0.49	0.36	1.41	0.715
Postopm RNA	4		1.35	1.66	0.45	3.84	

IIA beating heart technique without controlled lung perfusion

Table34.8 Amount of preoperative and postoperative mRNA in subgroup IIB

| Variable | Group | n | Mean | Confidence nterval | | Significance (P) |
				Inferior threshold	Superior threshold	
Preop mRNA	6		0.43	0.49	0.00	1.21	0.753
Postopm RNA	6		0.52	0.65	0.00	1.69	

IIB beating heart technique and controlled lung perfusion with arterial blood

Table34.9 Amount of preoperative and postoperative mRNA in subgroup IIC

| Variable | Group | n | Mean | Confidence nterval | | Significance (P) |
				Inferior threshold	Superior threshold	
Preop mRNA	6		0.39	0.29	0.13	0.88	0.075
Postopm RNA	6		0.68	0.51	0.00	1.33	

IIC beating heart technique and controlled lung perfusion with venous blood

Table34. 10 Amount of postoperative mRNA in subgroups IIA and IIB

| Variable | Group | n | Mean | Standard deviation | Confidence nterval | | Significance (P) |
					Inferior threshold	Superior threshold	
Postop mRNA	IIA	4	1.35	1.66	−0.28	2.98	0.392
	IIB	6	0.52	0.65	0.00	1.04	

IIA beating heart technique without controlled lung perfusion, *IIB* beating heart technique and controlled lung perfusion with arterial blood

Table34.11 Amount of postoperative mRNA in subgroups IIA and IIC

Variable	Group	n	Mean	Standard deviation	Confidence interval Inferior threshold	Superior threshold	Significance (P)
Postop mRNA	IIA	4	1.35	1.66	−0.28	2.98	0.748
	IIC	6	0.68	0.51	0.27	1.09	

IIA beating heart technique without controlled lung perfusion, *IIC* beating heart technique and controlled lung perfusion with venous blood

Table34.12 Amount of postoperative mRNA in subgroups IIB and IIC

Variable	Group	n	Mean	Standard deviation	Confidence interval Inferior threshold	Superior threshold	Significance (P)
Postop mRNA	IIB	6	0.52	0.65	0.00	1.04	0.629
	IIC	6	0.68	0.51	0.27	1.09	

IIB beating heart technique and controlled lung perfusion with arterial blood, *IIC* beating heart technique and controlled lung perfusion with venous blood

The mean value for the amplification threshold of the three markers was correlated with the mean value for the amplification threshold of β-actin (protein found in different cells), and the differential score was calculated according to formula $-\Delta CT = $ Marker CT − β-Actin CT, where CT is the cycle threshold. Subsequently, the value of $2^{-\Delta CT}$ is obtained, determining the score for the genetic differential expression of each inflammatory marker (Table 34.13).[2] All curves of genetic amplification for the three inflammatory markers as well as for β-actin are depicted in Fig. 34.1. Some curve examples were designed just to illustrating the genetic amplification per subgroup (Figs. 34.2–34.5).

Correlations between pre- and postoperative times in all subgroups regarding TNF-α, IL-4, and ICAM-1 are demonstrated in Tables 34.14–34.16, respectively. Comparisons focusing on postoperative time can be viewed in Table 34.17.

We believe that the relationship between time of controlled lung perfusion and levels of the three inflammatory markers is crucial; therefore, a period of 30 min is likely to be insufficient to promote remarkable modifications in the pattern of pulmonary inflammatory response detected by the real-time technique. Moreover, despite some significant findings shown in Tables 34.14–34.17, we prefer not to make ultimate statements about that topic unless further investigations indicate new outcomes.

An experimental model of pulmonary ischemia-reperfusion designed by Farivar et al.[3] was based on clamping the left pulmonary artery for 90 min followed by 4 h of reperfusion. In light of this model, the authors assessed the levels of IL-10 (proinflammatory) and IL-4 (anti-inflammatory) in pulmonary samples by means of the Western blot technique (Figs. 34.6 and 34.7, respectively). A significant increase of these two markers was detected 2 h after starting reperfusion.

We believe that a period of 30 min for controlled lung perfusion is not enough to remarkably change the levels of inflammatory markers in pulmonary tissue. On the other hand, we can hypothesize that there is a threshold time during reperfusion to identify the first relevant modifications in pulmonary inflammatory markers, either following a period of no controlled lung perfusion or following controlled lung perfusion.

Table34.13 Mean value for amplification threshold and ΔCT

Subgroup	Threshold of β-actin	Subgroup	Threshold of markers	ΔCT[a]	Scoref or differential genic expression
Preop β-actin IA	22.85	Preop TNF-α IA	28.63	5.78	0.0182621
Postop β-actinIA	21.16	PostopTN F-αI A	26.80	5.65	0.0199841
Preop β-actinIB	21.19	PreopTN F-αI B	28.30	7.11	0.0072390
Postop β-actinIB	21.86	PostopT NF-αI B	27.02	5.17	0.0278728
Preop β-actinIC	20.43	PreopTN F-αI C	26.52	6.09	0.0146800
Postop β-actinIC	21.10	PostopT NF-αI C	25.95	4.86	0.0345541
Preop β-actinIIA	23.00	PreopTN F-αI IA	27.15	4.15	0.0565237
Postop β-actinIIA	21.81	PostopT NF-αI IA	26.76	4.95	0.0323520
Preop β-actinIIB	22.28	PreopTN F-αI IB	28.08	5.80	0.0179484
Postop β-actinIIB	22.41	PostopT NF-αI IB	27.91	5.50	0.0220971
Preop β-actinIIC	24.55	PreopTN F-αI IC	29.87	5.32	0.0250334
Postop β-actinIIC	23.44	PostopT NF-αI IC	28.67	5.23	0.0267373
Preop β-actinIA	22.85	PreopI L-4I A	31.18	8.33	0.0031184
Postop β-actinIA	21.16	PostopI L-4I A	27.66	6.51	0.0110103
Preop β-actinIB	21.19	PreopI L-4I B	28.06	6.87	0.0085789
Postop β-actinIB	21.86	PostopI L-4I B	27.43	5.58	0.0209777
Preop β-actinIC	20.43	PreopI L-4I C	26.66	6.24	0.0132763
Postop β-actinIC	21.10	PostopI L-4I C	25.98	4.88	0.0339605
Preop β-actinIIA	23.00	PreopI L-4I IA	27.06	4.06	0.0601622
Postop β-actinIIA	21.81	PostopI L-4I IA	26.74	4.94	0.0326902
Preop β-actinIIB	22.28	PreopI L-4I IB	29.12	6.84	0.0087288
Postop β-actinIIB	22.41	PostopI L-4I IB	30.06	7.65	0.0049788
Preop β-actinIIC	24.55	PreopI L-4I IC	29.63	5.09	0.0294620
Postop β-actinIIC	23.44	PostopI L-4I IC	28.01	4.57	0.0421010
Preop β-actinIA	22.85	PreopI CAM-1I A	26.03	3.18	0.1103379
Postop β-actinIA	21.16	PostopI CAM-1I A	24.35	3.19	0.1095757
Preop β-actinIB	21.19	PreopI CAM-1I B	25.00	3.81	0.0715453
Postop β-actinIB	21.86	PostopI CAM-1I B	25.62	3.76	0.0738120
Preop β-actinIC	20.43	PreopI CAM-1I C	23.98	3.56	0.0850821
Postop β-actinIC	21.10	Postop.I CAM-1I C	23.81	2.72	0.1523013
Preop β-actinIIA	23.00	PreopI CAM-1I IA	26.52	3.52	0.0874741
Postop β-actinIIA	21.81	PostopI CAM-1I IA	25.08	3.28	0.1033063
Preop β-actinIIB	22.28	PreopI CAM-1I IB	25.66	3.38	0.0960547
Postop β-actinIIB	22.41	PostopI CAM-1I IB	25.07	2.66	0.1582196

(continued)

Table 34.13 (continued)

Subgroup	Threshold of β-actin	Subgroup	Threshold of markers	ΔCT[a]	Scoref or differential genic expression
Preop β-actinIIC	24.55	PreopI CAM-1I IC	28.17	3.63	0.0810525
Postop β-actinIIC	23.44	PostopI CAM-1I IC	26.80	3.36	0.0977337

IA, IIA no controlled lung perfusion; *IB, IIB* controlled lung perfusion with arterial blood; *IC, IIC* controlled lung perfusion with venous blood; *ICAM-1* intercellular adhesion molecule 1; *IL-4* interleukin 4; *TNF-α* tumor necrosis factor alpha

[a]ΔCT is the mean differential value for the amplification threshold

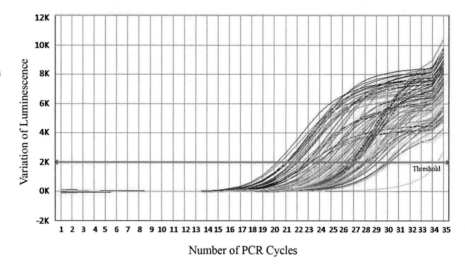

Fig.34.1 Curvesof ge netic amplification for tumor necrosis factor alpha (TNF-α), interleukin 4 (IL-4), intercellular adhesion molecule 1 (ICAM-1), and β-actin in all subgroups pre- and postoperatively. *K* equivalent to 1,000 units of luminescence, *threshold* baseline level of genetic amplification, *PCR*poly-merasec hainr eaction

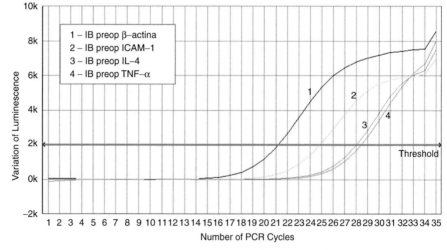

Fig.34.2 Curvesof ge netic amplification for tumor necrosis factor alpha (TNF-α), interleukin 4 (IL-4), intercel-lular adhesion molecule 1 (ICAM-1), and β-actini n subgroup IB preoperatively. *K* equivalent to 1,000 units of luminescence, *threshold* baseline level of genetic amplification, *PCR*pol y-merasec hainre action

Fig.34.3 Curvesof ge netic amplification for tumor necrosis factor alpha (TNF-α), interleukin 4 (IL-4), intercellular adhesion molecule 1 (ICAM-1), and β-actin in subgroup IB postoperatively. *K*e quivalent to 1,000 units of luminescence, *threshold*ba seline level of genetic amplification, *PCR* polymerase chain reaction

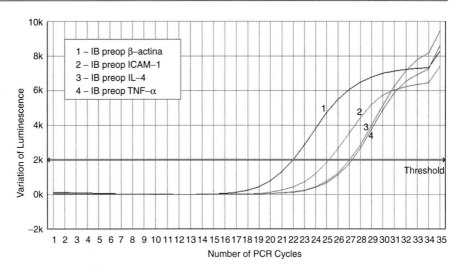

Fig.34.4 Curvesof ge netic amplification for tumor necrosis factor alpha (TNF-α), interleukin 4 (IL-4), intercellular adhesion molecule 1 (ICAM-1), and β-actin in subgroup IIB preoperatively. *K*e quivalent to 1,000 units of luminescence, *threshold*ba seline level of genic amplification, *PCR* polymerase chain reaction

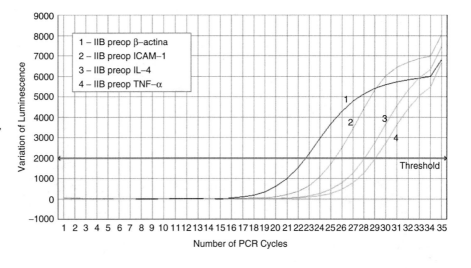

Fig.34.5 Curvesof ge netic amplification for tumor necrosis factor alpha (TNF-α), interleukin 4 (IL-4), intercellular adhesion molecule 1 (ICAM-1), and β-actin in subgroup IIB postoperatively. *K*e quivalent to 1,000 units of luminescence, *threshold*ba seline level of genic amplification, *PCR* polymerase chain reaction

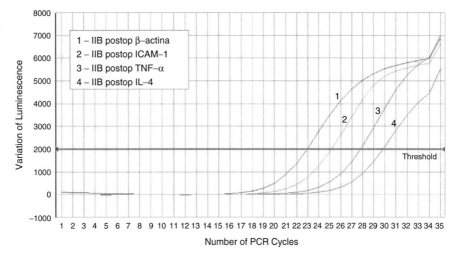

Table 34.14 Pre- and postoperative values of tumor necrosis factor alpha (TNF-α)in gr oupsI a ndI I

Variables	ΔCT[a]	Significance (P)
Preop TNF-α – IA	5.78	0.454
PostopTN F-αIA	5.65	
PreopTN F-αIB	7.11	0.041
PostopTN F-αIB	5.17	
PreopTN F-αIC	6.09	0.134
PostopTN F-αIC	4.86	
PreopTN F-αIIA	4.15	0.841
PostopTN F-αIIA	4.95	
PreopTN F-αIIB	5.80	0.355
PostopTN F-αIIB	5.50	
PreopTN F-αIIC	5.32	0.453
PostopTN F-αIIC	5.23	

IA, IIA no controlled lung perfusion; IB, IIB controlled lung perfusion with arterial blood; IC, IIC controlled lung perfusion with venous blood

[a]ΔCT is the mean differential value for the amplification threshold

Table 34.16 Pre- and postoperative values of the intercellular adhesion molecule 1 (ICAM-1) in groups I and II

Variables	ΔCT[a]	Significance (P)
Preop ICAM-1 IA	3.18	0.504
PostopI CAM-1I A	3.19	
PreopI CAM-1I B	3.81	0.484
PostopI CAM-1I B	3.76	
PreopI CAM-1I C	3.56	0.226
PostopI CAM-1I C	2.72	
PreopI CAM-1I IA	3.52	0.383
PostopI CAM-1I IA	3.28	
PreopI CAM-1I IB	3.38	0.186
PostopI CAM-1I IB	2.66	
PreopI CAM-1I IC	3.63	0.369
PostopI CAM-1I IC	3.36	

IA, IIA no controlled lung perfusion; IB, IIB controlled lung perfusion with arterial blood; IC, IIC controlled lung perfusion with venous blood

[a]ΔCT is the mean differential value for the amplification threshold

Table 34.15 Pre- and postoperative values of interleukin 4 (IL-4) in groups I and II

Variables	ΔCT[a]	Significance (P)
Preop IL-4 IA	8.33	0.052
PostopI L-4I A	6.51	
PreopI L-4I B	6.87	0.124
PostopI L-4I B	5.58	
PreopI L-4I C	6.24	0.112
PostopI L-4I C	4.88	
PreopI L-4I IA	4.06	0.862
PostopI L-4I IA	4.94	
PreopI L-4I IB	6.84	0.842
PostopI L-4I IB	7.65	
PreopI L-4I IC	5.09	0.262
PostopI L-4I IC	4.57	

IA, IIA no controlled lung perfusion; IB, IIB controlled lung perfusion with arterial blood; IC, IIC controlled lung perfusion with venous blood

[a]ΔCT is the mean differential value for the amplification threshold

Table 34.17 Postoperative correlation in all subgroups regarding inflammatorym arkers

Variables	A×B	A×C	B×C
Postop TNF-α, group I	0.334	0.240	0.391
PostopT NF-α,gr oupI I	0.752	0.633	0.367
PostopI L-4,gr oupI	0.289	0.165	0.338
PostopI L-4,gr oupI I	0.914	0.427	0.060
PostopI CAM-1,gr oupI	0.833	0.211	0.039
PostopI CAM-1,gr oupI I	0.099	0.566	0.927

IA, IIA no controlled lung perfusion; IB, IIB controlled lung perfusion with arterial blood; IC, IIC controlled lung perfusion with venous blood; ICAM-1 intercellular adhesion molecule 1; IL-4 interleukin 4; TNF-α tumor necrosis factor alpha

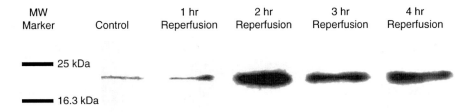

Fig. 34.6 Western blot analysis for interleukin 10. In the far *left lane,* the molecular weight (MW) markers are represented, as referenced from the kaleidoscope marker. There is minimal interleukin 10 protein in negative controls and 1-h reperfused lungs. At 2, 3, and 4 h of reperfusion, there is significantly increased expression of interleukin 10 protein in left lung homogenates. *hr* hour, *kDa* kilodaltons. (This figure was published in Farivar et al.[3] Copyright 2003, the Society of Thoracic Surgeons

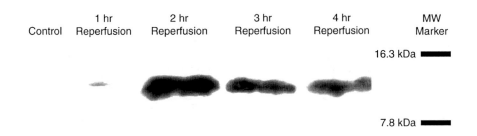

Fig. 34.7 Western blot analysis for interleukin 4. In the far *right lane,* the molecular weight (MW) markers are represented, as referenced from the kaleidoscope marker. There is no detectable interleukin 4 protein in negative controls or 1-h reperfused lungs. At 2, 3, and 4 h of reperfusion, there is significant expression of interleukin 4 protein in left lung homogenates. *hr* hour, *kDa* kilodaltons. (This figure was published in Farivar et al.[3] Copyright2003,t heS ocietyof T horacicS urgeons

References

1. Gabriel EA, Locali RF, Matsuoka PK, et al. Lung perfusion during cardiac surgery with cardiopulmonary bypass: is it necessary? *Interact Cardiovasc Thorac Surg.* 2008;7: 1089-1095.

2. Livak KJ, Schmittgen TD. Analysis of relative gene expression data using real-time quantitative PCR and the 2(-Delta Delta C(T)) method. *Methods.*2001; 25(4):402-408.

3. Farivar AS, Krishnadasan B, Naidu BV, Woolley SM, Verrier ED, Mulligan MS. Endogenous interleukin-4 and interleukin-10 regulate experimental lung ischemia reperfusion injury. *Ann Thorac Surg.*2003; 76:253-259.

MacroscopicalandMi croscopicalFi ndings

35

Edmo Atique Gabriel and Tomas Salerno

In our experimental research,[1] hematoxylin/eosin (HE) and immunohistochemistry (heat shock protein 27 [HSP27] expression) were used for assessing pulmonary extracts. A semiquantitative score for degrees of leukostasis, congested capillaries, alveolar hemorrhage, inflammatory infiltrate within alveoli, and alveolar edema was employed for sequential microscopic fields selected by two blinded pathologists. Each successive field was graded in terms of severity of injury as follows: grade 0, normal tissue; grade 1, mild injury; grade 2, moderate injury; and grade 3, severe injury. The extent of lesions was graded as 0, absent; 1, 1–25% of the slide; 2, 26–50%; and 3, less than 50% of tissue affected. The mean score for successive fields corresponded to the individual score for each pulmonary extract. A value of $p<0.05$ was considered significant.[2]

Absence of controlled lung perfusion during either cardiopulmonary bypass (CPB) with cardioplegic arrest or CPB with the beating heart technique was responsible for a considerable degree of pulmonary injury detected by the HE technique on weaning from CPB (Tables 35.1 and 35.2). On the other hand, when controlled lung perfusion was employed, regardless of type of blood and CPB strategy, there were no additional pulmonary lesions postoperatively (Tables 35.3–35.6).

Concomitant correlation among three cardioplegic subgroups as well as among three beating heart subgroups, focusing on postoperative time, can be viewed in Tables 35.7 and 35.8. Based on these data, subsequent analysis was carried out to differentiate between subgroups within the cardioplegic arrest and beating heart groups (Tables 35.9 and 35.10). The most striking note was that differences between the nonperfused subgroups (no controlled lung perfusion) and perfused subgroups (controlled lung perfusion with arterial or venous blood) were remarkable, whereas there were no relevant findings between subgroups subjected to controlled lung perfusion with arterial or venous blood.

Figure 35.1 illustrates the main pulmonary histologic lesions detected by the HE technique. Note the remarkable differences between lungs subjected to controlled perfusion and those not subjected to controlledpe rfusion.

Hsp27 was used for immunohistochemical assessment as its expression was consistently detected within different kinds of pulmonary cells, and its immunoreactivity appeared to be prominent compared to other heat shock proteins similarly tested. Hsp27 expression was graded separately for intra-acinar arteriole endothelium, alveolar epithelium, and bronchiolar epithelium cells as follows: 0 for absent, 1 for 1–25% cells stained, 2 for 26–50% stained, and 3 for more than 50% tissue stained. A mean score for these three types of pulmonary cell was determined, and a value of $p<0.05$ was considered significant.

Hsp27 usually plays a protective role in light of pulmonary inflammatory response in such a way that its expression tends to be significantly increased in an attempt to modulate tissue injury. There is no doubt that CPB itself is an important etiology for pulmonary injury; consequently, Hsp27 expression in pulmonary tissue is expected to be higher following a period of CPB than before establishing it.[1,3,4] In the vast majority of subgroups, there was higher Hsp27 expression postoperatively, as demonstrated in Table 35.11.

E.A.G abriel(✉)
Department of Surgery, Division of Cardiovascular Surgery
FederalU niversityof Sa oP aulo, SaoP aulo, Brazil
e-mail:e dag@uol.com.br

E.A. Gabriel and T. Salerno (eds.), *Principles of Pulmonary Protection in Heart Surgery,*
DOI: 10.1007/978-1-84996-308-4_35, © Springer-Verlag London Limited 2010

Table 35.1 Pre- and postoperative histologic variables in subgroupIA

IA Variables	Significance (p)
Preop vascular congestion – Postop vascular congestion	0.04
Preop alveolar hemorrhage – Postop alveolar hemorrhage	0.04
Preop alveolar edema – Postop alveolar edema	0.04
Preop leukostasis – Postop leukostasis	0.04
Preop neutrophils in interalveolar septum – Postop neutrophils in interalveolar septum	0.04

IA cardioplegic arrest without controlled lung perfusion

Table 35.4 Pre- and postoperative histologic variables in subgroupI C

ICV ariables	Significance (p)
Preop vascular congestion – Postop vascular congestion	>0.999
Preop alveolar hemorrhage – Postop alveolar hemorrhage	>0.999
Preop alveolar edema – Postop alveolar edema	>0.999
Preop leukostasis – Postop leukostasis	>0.999
Preop neutrophils in interalveolar septum – Postop neutrophils in interalveolar septum	>0.999

IC cardioplegic arrest and controlled lung perfusion with venous blood

Table 35.2 Pre- and postoperative histologic variables in subgroupIIA

IIAV ariables	Significance (p)
Preop vascular congestion – Postop vascular congestion	0.04
Preop alveolar hemorrhage – Postop alveolar hemorrhage	0.04
Preop alveolar edema – Postop alveolar edema	0.04
Preop leukostasis – Postop leukostasis	0.04
Preop neutrophils in interalveolar septum – Postop neutrophils in interalveolar septum	0.04

IIA beating heart technique without controlled lung perfusion

Table 35.5 Pre- and postoperative histologic variables in subgroupI IB

IIBV ariables	Significance (p)
Preop vascular congestion – Postop vascular congestion	>0.999
Preop alveolar hemorrhage – Postop alveolar hemorrhage	>0.999
Preop alveolar edema – Postop alveolar edema	>0.999
Preop leukostasis – Postop leukostasis	>0.999
Preop neutrophils in interalveolar septum – Postop neutrophils in interalveolar septum	>0.999

IIB beating heart technique and controlled lung perfusion with arterial blood

Table 35.3 Pre- and postoperative histologic variables in subgroupIB

IB Variables	Significance (p)
Preop vascular congestion – Postop vascular congestion	>0.999
Preop alveolar hemorrhage – Postop alveolar hemorrhage	>0.999
Preop alveolar edema – Postop alveolar edema	>0.999
Preop leukostasis – Postop leukostasis	>0.999
Preop neutrophils in interalveolar septum – Postop neutrophils in interalveolar septum	>0.999

IB cardioplegic arrest and controlled lung perfusion with arterial blood

Table 35.6 Pre- and postoperative histologic variables in subgroupI IC

IICV ariables	Significance (p)
Preop vascular congestion – Postop vascular congestion	>0.999
Preop alveolar hemorrhage – Postop alveolar hemorrhage	>0.999
Preop alveolar edema – Postop alveolar edema	>0.999
Preop leukostasis – Postop leukostasis	>0.999
Preop neutrophils in interalveolar septum – Postop neutrophils in interalveolar septum	>0.999

IIC beating heart technique and controlled lung perfusion with venous blood

Table 35.7 Concomitant analysis of pulmonary histologic variables within group I

IA × IB × IC	Significance (p)
Postop vascular congestion	0.001
Postopa lveolarhe morrhage	0.001
Postopa lveolare dema	0.001
Postopl eukostasis	0.001
Postop neutrophils in interalveolar septum	0.001

IA cardioplegic arrest without controlled lung perfusion, *IB* cardioplegic arrest and controlled lung perfusion with arterial blood, *IC* cardioplegic arrest and controlled lung perfusion with venous blood

Table 35.8 Concomitant analysis of pulmonary histologic variables within group II

IIA × IIB × IIC	Significance (p)
Postop vascular congestion	0.001
Postopa lveolarhe morrhage	0.001
Postopa lveolare dema	0.001
Postopl eukostasis	0.001
Postop neutrophils in interalveolar septum	0.001

IIA beating heart technique without controlled lung perfusion, *IIB* beating heart technique and controlled lung perfusion with arterial blood, *IIC* beating heart technique and controlled lung perfusion with venous blood

Table 35.9 Analysis of pulmonary histologic variables between twoc ardioplegica rrests ubgroups

Variable	IA × IB	IA × IC	IB × IC
Postop vascular congestion	0.003	0.003	>0.999
Postopa lveolar hemorrhage	0.003	0.003	>0.999
Postopa lveolare dema	0.003	0.003	>0.999
Postople ukostasis	0.003	0.003	>0.999
Postop neutrophils in interalveolar septum	0.003	0.003	>0.999

IA cardioplegic arrest without controlled lung perfusion, *IB* cardioplegic arrest and controlled lung perfusion with arterial blood, *IC* cardioplegic arrest and controlled lung perfusion with venous blood

Table 35.10 Analysis of pulmonary histologic variables between two beating heart subgroups

Variable	IIA × IIB	IIA × IIC	IIB × IIC
Postop vascular congestion	0.003	0.003	>0.999
Postopa lveolar hemorrhage	0.003	0.003	>0.999
Postopa lveolar edema	0.003	0.003	>0.999
Postop leukostasis	0.003	0.003	>0.999
Postopne utrophils in interalveolar septum	0.003	0.003	>0.999

IIA beating heart technique without controlled lung perfusion, *IIB* beating heart technique and controlled lung perfusion with arterial blood, *IIC* beating heart technique and controlled lung perfusion with venous blood

Concomitant immunohistochemical assessment focusing on postoperative time revealed that there were relevant differences among three cardioplegic subgroups regarding Hsp27 expression in intra-acinar arteriole, pneumocyte, and bronchiole, whereas the only difference among the beating heart subgroups was regarding Hsp27 expression in the intra-acinar arteriole (Table 35.12). Correlations between two subgroups within the cardioplegic arrest or beating heart group are depicted in Figs. 35.2–35.4.

Figure 35.5 illustrates relevant findings in lungs subjected to controlled perfusion with venous blood in group I comparing to lungs not subjected to controlled perfusion.

From a macroscopic point of view, we selected some images to demonstrate interesting differences between lungs subjected to controlled perfusion and those not subjected to controlled perfusion. We did not identify important features to macroscopically differentiate lungs subjected to controlled perfusion with arterial blood from those subjected to controlled perfusion using venous blood (Figs. 35.6–35.8). Furthermore, we obtained computed tomographic images in an attempt to make pulmonary parenchyma assessment complete. In a general way, we observed that lungs subjected to controlled perfusion had tomographic features that looked like normal lungs, whereas the tomographic features of lungs not subjected to controlled perfusion had remarkable distortions (Figs. 35.9 and 35.10). It is crucial to emphasize that all macroscopic findings were assessed by subjective criteria; therefore, overall impact of these data is limited in such a way that further macroscopic investigations will be warranted.

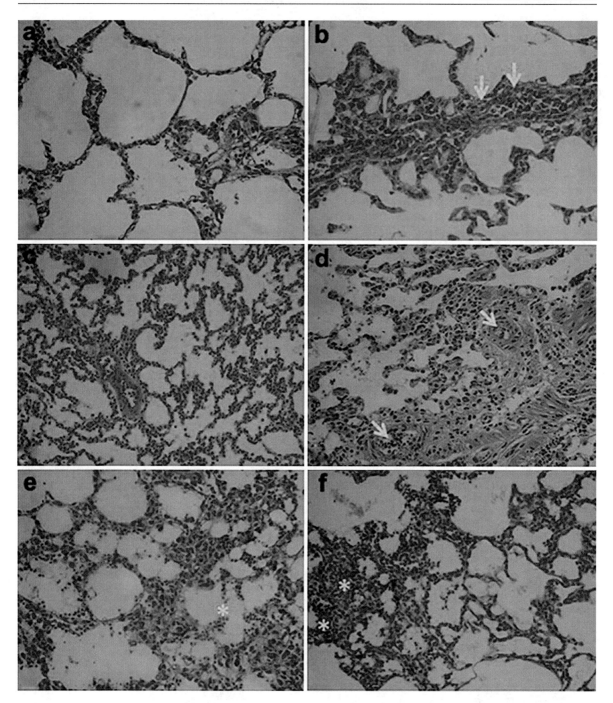

Fig. 35.1 Histological evaluation through hematoxylin-eosin (HE). (**a**) Histological section of the lung. Normal histoarchitecture of lungs with pulmonary trunk perfusion. (**b**) Nonperfused lung. Histological section showing leukostasis accumulation of inflammatory cells within intra-acinar arterioles (*arrows*). HE ×400. (**c**) Histological section of the lung. Normal histoarchitecture with pulmonary trunk perfusion. (**d**) Nonperfused lung. Histological section showing dilated, tortuous, and congested capillaries (*arrows*). HE ×400. (**e**) Histological section of the lung. Histoarchitecture of lungs with pulmonary trunk perfusion, showing a lesser degree of intra-alveolar hemorrhage (*asterisk*). (**f**) Nonperfused lung. Histological section showing extensive areas of hemorrhage within the alveoli (*asterisks*). HE ×400. (**g**) Histological section of the lung. Normal histoarchitecture of lungs with pulmonary trunk perfusion. (**h**) Nonperfused lung. Histological section showing infiltrate of inflammatory cells (neutrophils and lymphocytes) within the alveoli (*arrows*). HE ×400. (**i**) Histological section of the lung. Normal histoarchitecture of lungs with pulmonary trunk perfusion. (**j**) Nonperfused lung. Histological section showing an accumulation of amorphous protein material (edema) within the alveoli (*asterisks*). HE ×400. (Reproduced with permission from Gabriel et al.[1] Copyright 2008, European Association of Cardio-Thoracic Surgery, http://icvts.ctsnetjournals.org/)

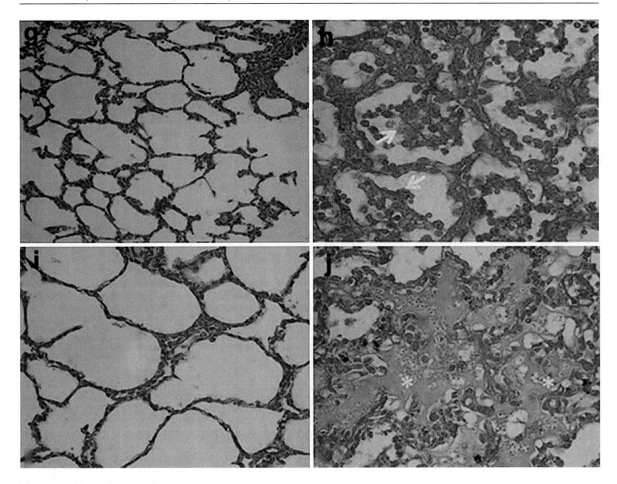

Fig. 35.1 continued

Table 35.11 Pre-a ndpos toperativei mmunohistochemicala nalysispe rs ubgroup

Variable	IA	IB	IC	IIA	IIB	IIC
Postop arteriole – Preop arteriole	0.014	0.010	0.414	0.046	0.003	0.008
Postop pneumocyte – Preop pneumocyte	0.010	0.004	0.046	0.010	0.004	0.010
Postop bronchiole – Preop bronchiole	0.005	0.002	>0.999	0.008	0.004	0.008

IA, IIA no controlled lung perfusion; *IB, IIB* controlled lung perfusion with arterial blood; *IC, IIC* controlled lung perfusion with venous blood

Table 35.12 Postoperative immunohistochemical analysis within groups I and II

Variable	IA × IB × IC	IIA × IIB × IIC
Postop arteriole	0.009	0.034
Postoppne umocyte	0.001	0.377
Postopbr onchiole	<0.001	0.190

IA, IIA no controlled lung perfusion, *IB, IIB* controlled lung perfusion with arterial blood, *IC, IIC* controlled lung perfusion with venous blood

As addendum to this chapter, we would like to show cardiac histologic assessment done in specimens withdrawn from the right ventricle. The purpose of this analysis was to demonstrate the inflammatory effects of CPB on myocardium. In our point of view, use of controlled lung perfusion could have an impact on the degree of cardiac injury during CPB. However, it is difficult to make statements or conclusions in this regard. We decided not to make comparisons

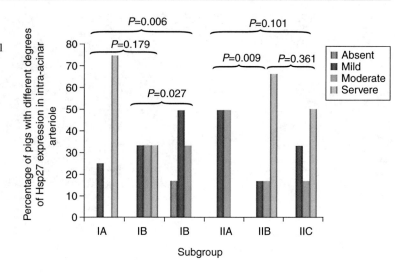

Fig.35.2 Hsp27e xpressioni n intra-acinar-arteriolee ndothelium (Reproduced with permission from Gabriel et al.[1] Copyright 2008, European Association of Cardio-Thoracic Surgery, http://icvts.ctsnetjournals.org/)

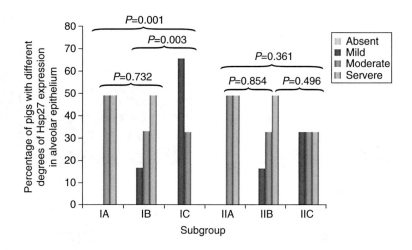

Fig.35.3 Hsp27 expression in alveolar epithelium (Reproduced with permission from Gabriel et al.[1] Copyright 2008, European Association of Cardio-Thoracic Surgery, http://icvts.ctsnetjournals.org/)

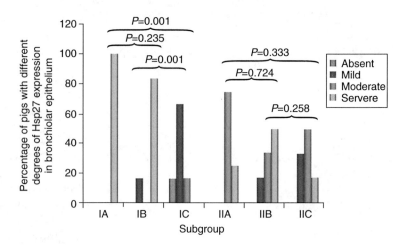

Fig.35.4 Hsp27 expression in bronchiolar epithelium (Reproduced with permission from Gabriel et al.[1] Copyright 2008, European Association of Cardio-Thoracic Surgery, http://icvts.ctsnetjournals.org/)

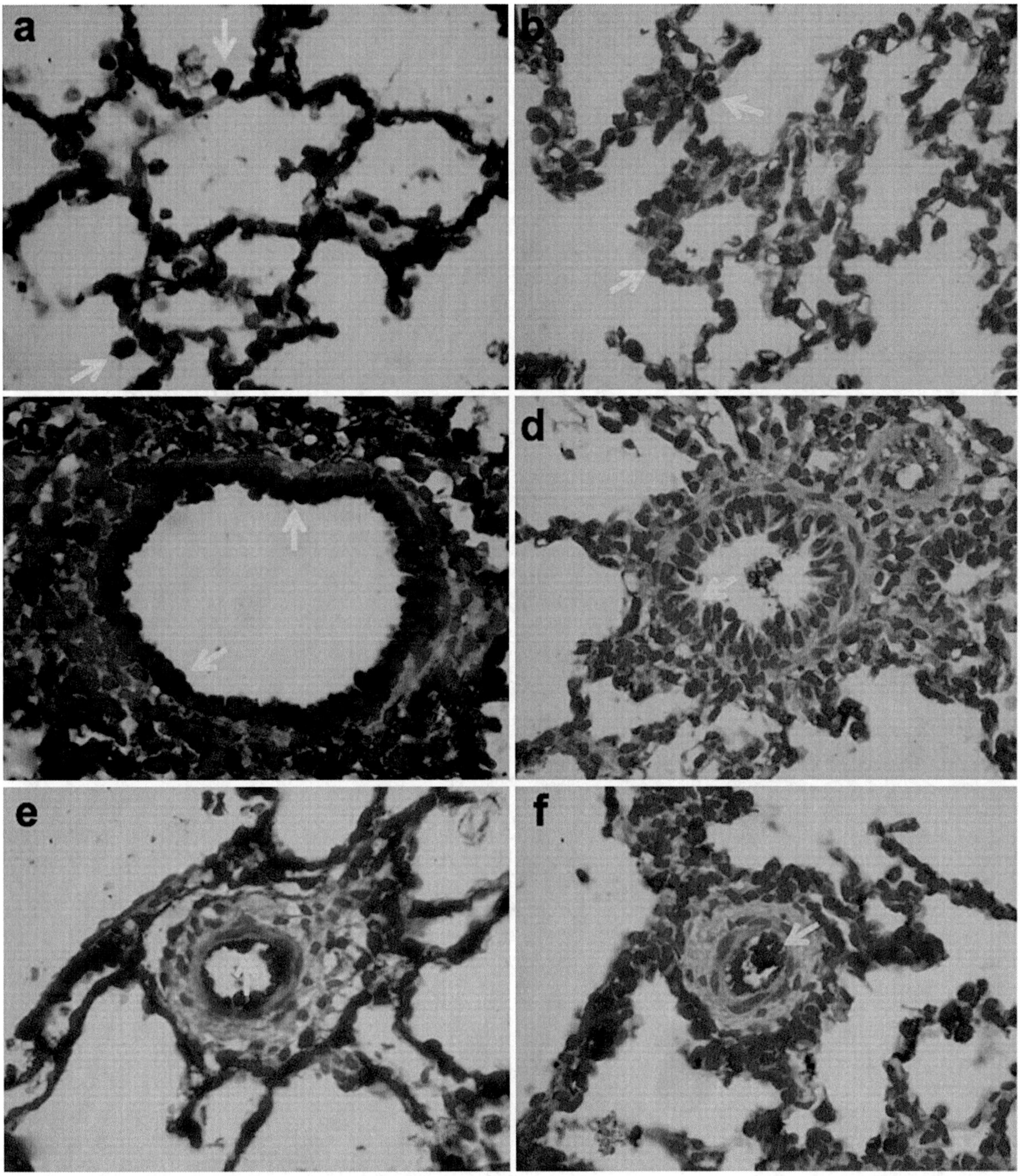

Fig. 35.5 Heat shock protein 27 (Hsp27) expression in nonperfused lungs and perfused lungs with venous blood in group I. (**a**) Histological section of the lung – alveolar epithelium. Nonperfused lung. Hsp27 expression by type II pneumocytes (*arrows*). (**b**) Perfused lung with venous blood. Note a decreased Hsp27 expression by type II pneumocytes (*arrows*). Immunohistochemistry ×400. (**c**) Histological section of the lung – bronchiolar epithelium. Nonperfused lung. Hsp27 expression by respiratory epithelium (*arrows*). (**d**) Perfused lung with venous blood. Note a decreased Hsp27 expression by respiratory epithelium (*arrow*). Immunohistochemistry ×200. (**e**) Histological section of the lung – intra-acinar arteriole. Nonperfused lung. Hsp27 expression by endothelial cells (*arrow*). (**f**) Perfused lung with venous blood. Note a decreased Hsp27 expression by endothelial cells (*arrow*). Immunohistochemistry ×200. (Reproduced with permission from Gabriel et al.[1] Copyright 2008, European Association of Cardio-Thoracic Surgery, http://icvts.ctsnetjournals.org/)

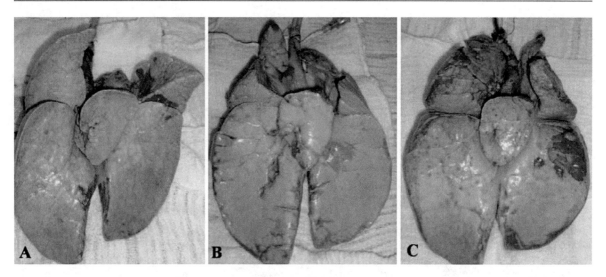

Fig. 35.6 Macroscopical view of the lungs (**a**) Normal lung in preoperative period. Note reddish aspect of pulmonary parenchyma; (**b**) Non-perfused lung. Note pale aspect of pulmonary parenchyma; (**c**) Perfused lung. Note pinkish aspect of pulmonary parenchyma

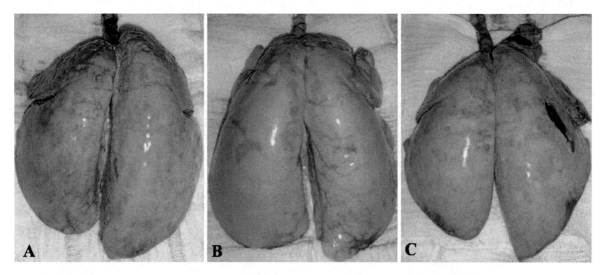

Fig. 35.7 Macroscopical view of the lungs (**a**) Normal lung in preoperative period. Note reddish aspect of pulmonary parenchyma; (**b**) Non-perfused lung. Note pale aspect of pulmonary parenchyma; (**c**) Perfused lung. Note pinkish aspect of pulmonary parenchyma

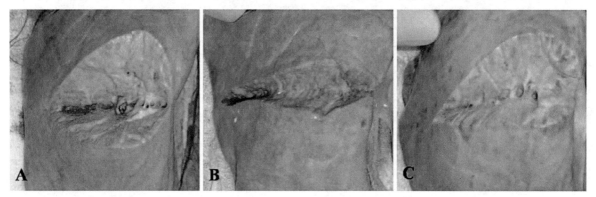

Fig. 35.8 Macroscopical view of the lungs and section of inferoposterior portion of right lower lobe (**a**) Normal lung in preoperative period. Note reddish and homogenous aspect of pulmonary parenchyma; (**b**) Non-perfused lung. Note heterogeneous aspect of pulmonary parenchyma; (**c**) Perfused lung. Note homogeneous aspect of pulmonary parenchyma.

Fig. 35.9 Tomography of
lungs (**a**) Normal lung during
the preoperative period. Sparse
gravity-dependent opacities
(attributed to the decubitus and
anesthetic procedure); (**b**) Nonperfused lung. Note presence
of multiple striae and
ground-glass opacities, septum
thickening and other linear
diffuse bilateral opacities
affecting specially lower lobes.

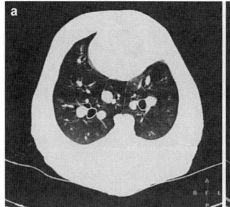 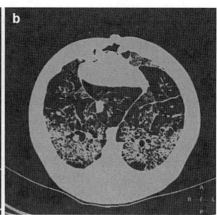

Fig. 35.10 Tomography of
lungs (**a**) Normal lung during
the preoperative period. Sparse
gravity-dependent opacities
(attributed to the decubitus and
anesthetic procedure);
(**b**) Perfused lung. There are no
significant parenchymal
lesions.

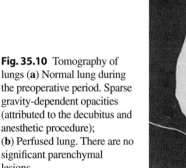 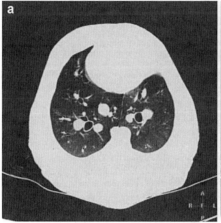 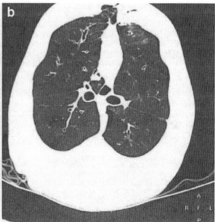

between degree of cardiac injury and controlled lung
perfusion.

Different types of inflammatory lesions were identified in the main three layers of the heart: pericardium,
myocardium, and endocardium (Tables 35.13–35.18).

All subgroups were marked by at least one relevant
inflammatory lesion postoperatively. As pointed out previously, we attributed cardiac injury to intrinsic mechanisms related to CPB. Some examples of inflammatory
cardiac lesion are depicted in Figs. 35.11–35.13.

Table 35.13 Pre- and postoperative cardiac histologic variables ins ubgroupI A

IA Variables	Significance (p)
Preop interstitial edema – Postop interstitial edema	0.157
Preop interstitial hemorrhage – Postop interstitial hemorrhage	0.046
Preop myocardial infiltrate – Postop myocardial infiltrate	>0.999
Preop myocardial contraction bands – Postop myocardial contraction bands	>0.999
Preop myocardial necrosis – Postop myocardial necrosis	0.157
Preop myocardial hypertrophy – Postop myocardial hypertrophy	>0.999
Preop endocardial and pericardial infiltrate – Postop endocardial and pericardial infiltrate	0.414
Preop endocardial and pericardial edema – Postop endocardial and pericardial edema	0.234
Preop endocardial and pericardial hemorrhage – Postop endocardial and pericardial hemorrhage	0.458
Preop endocardial and pericardial fibrin – Postop endocardial and pericardial fibrin	0.157

IA cardioplegic arrest without controlled lung perfusion

Table 35.14 Pre- and postoperative cardiac histologic variables ins ubgroupI B

IB Variables	Significance (p)
Preop interstitial edema – Postop interstitial edema	>0.999
Preop interstitial hemorrhage – Postop interstitial hemorrhage	0.014
Preop myocardial infiltrate – Postop myocardial infiltrate	0.157
Preop myocardial contraction bands – Postop myocardial contraction bands	0.023
Preop myocardial necrosis – Postop myocardial necrosis	0.014
Preop myocardial hypertrophy – Postop myocardial hypertrophy	>0.999
Preop endocardial and pericardial infiltrate – Postop endocardial and pericardial infiltrate	0.063
Preop endocardial and pericardial edema – Postop endocardial and pericardial edema	0.305
Preop endocardial and pericardial hemorrhage – Postop endocardial and pericardial hemorrhage	>0.999
Preop endocardial and pericardial fibrin – Postop endocardial and pericardial fibrin	0.157

IB cardioplegic arrest and controlled lung perfusion with arterial blood

Table 35.15 Pre- and postoperative cardiac histologic variables ins ubgroupI C

IC Variables	Significance (*p*)
Preop interstitial edema – Postop interstitial edema	0.414
Preop interstitial hemorrhage – Postop interstitial hemorrhage	0.414
Preop myocardial infiltrate – Postop myocardial infiltrate	>0.999
Preop myocardial contraction bands – Postop myocardial contraction bands	0.046
Preop myocardial necrosis – Postop myocardial necrosis	>0.999
Preop myocardial hypertrophy – Postop myocardial hypertrophy	>0.999
Preop endocardial and pericardial infiltrate – Postop endocardial and pericardial infiltrate	0.046
Preop endocardial and pericardial edema – Postop endocardial and pericardial edema	0.046
Preop endocardial and pericardial hemorrhage – Postop endocardial and pericardial hemorrhage	0.157
Preop endocardial and pericardial fibrin – Postop endocardial and pericardial fibrin	0.157

IC cardioplegic arrest and controlled lung perfusion with venous blood

Table 35.16 Pre- and postoperative cardiac histologic variables ins ubgroupI IA

IIA Variables	Significance (*p*)
Preop interstitial edema – Postop interstitial edema	>0.999
Preop interstitial hemorrhage – Postop interstitial hemorrhage	0.157
Preop myocardial infiltrate – Postop myocardial infiltrate	>0.999
Preop myocardial contraction bands – Postop myocardial contraction bands	0.557
Preop myocardial necrosis – Postop myocardial necrosis	0.046
Preop myocardial hypertrophy – Postop myocardial hypertrophy	>0.999
Preop endocardial and pericardial infiltrate – Postop endocardial and pericardial infiltrate	0.458
Preop endocardial and pericardial edema – Postop endocardial and pericardial edema	0.157
Preop endocardial and pericardial hemorrhage – Postop endocardial and pericardial hemorrhage	0.157
Preop endocardial and pericardial fibrin – Postop endocardial and pericardial fibrin	0.063

IIA beating heart technique without controlled lung perfusion

Table 35.17 Pre- and postoperative cardiac histologic variables ins ubgroupI IB

IIBV ariables	Significance (p)
Preop interstitial edema – Postop interstitial edema	0.058
Preop interstitial hemorrhage – Postop interstitial hemorrhage	0.107
Preop myocardial infiltrate – Postop myocardial infiltrate	0.157
Preop myocardial contraction bands – Postop myocardial contraction bands	0.088
Preop myocardial necrosis – Postop myocardial necrosis	>0.999
Preop myocardial hypertrophy – Postop myocardial hypertrophy	>0.999
Preop endocardial and pericardial infiltrate – Postop endocardial and pericardial infiltrate	0.014
Preop endocardial and pericardial edema – Postop endocardial and pericardial edema	0.473
Preop endocardial and pericardial hemorrhage – Postop endocardial and pericardial hemorrhage	>0.999
Preop endocardial and pericardial fibrin – Postop endocardial and pericardial fibrin	>0.999

IIB beating heart technique and controlled lung perfusion with arterial blood

Table 35.18 Pre- and postoperative cardiac histologic variables ins ubgroupI IC

IICV ariables	Significance (p)
Preop interstitial edema – Postop interstitial edema	0.414
Preop interstitial hemorrhage – Postop interstitial hemorrhage	0.058
Preop myocardial infiltrate – Postop myocardial infiltrate	0.014
Preop myocardial contraction bands – Postop myocardial contraction bands	0.414
Preop myocardial necrosis – Postop myocardial necrosis	0.002
Preop myocardial hypertrophy – Postop myocardial hypertrophy	0.157
Preop endocardial and pericardial infiltrate – Postop endocardial and pericardial infiltrate	0.107
Preop endocardial and pericardial edema – Postop endocardial and pericardial edema	0.062
Preop endocardial and pericardial hemorrhage – Postop endocardial and pericardial hemorrhage	0.473
Preop endocardial and pericardial fibrin – Postop endocardial and pericardial fibrin	>0.999

IIC beating heart technique and controlled lung perfusion with venous blood

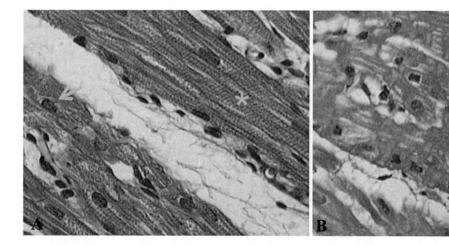

Fig. 35.11 (a) Normal cardiac miocytes (*arrow*) and myocardial fibers (*asterisk*). (b) Hypercontraction of cardiac miocytes with transverse contraction bands (*arrow*). HE × 400.

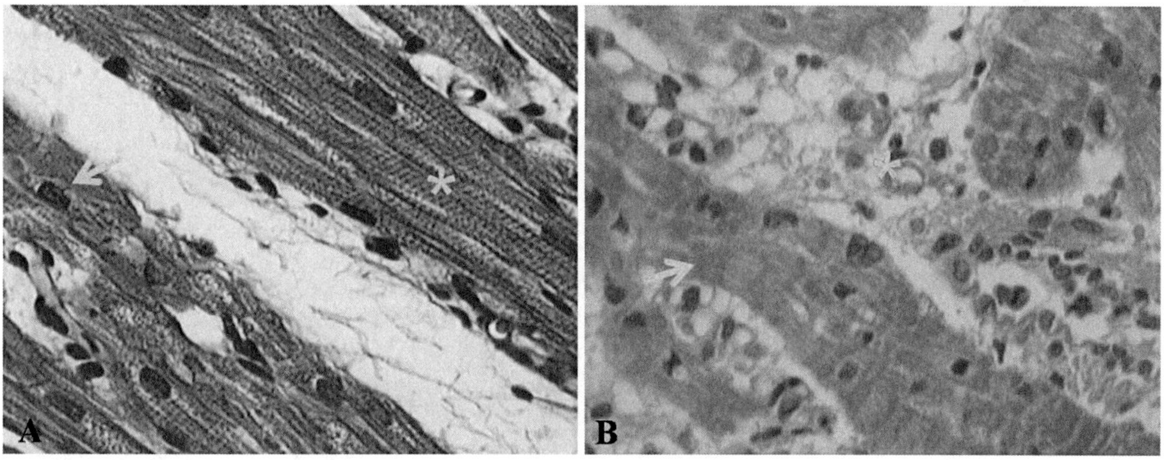

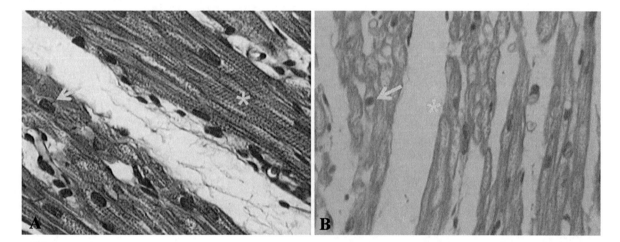

Fig. 35.12 (**a**) Normal cardiac miocytes (*arrow*) and myocardial fibers (*asterisk*). (**b**) Myocardial interstitial response marked by hemorrhage, edema, moderate tumefaction of endothelium and leukocyte margination (*asterisk*). Presence of multiples transverse contraction bands in adjacent cardiac miocytes (*arrow*). HE × 400

Fig. 35.13 (**a**) Normal cardiac miocytes (*arrow*) and myocardial fibers (*asterisk*). (**b**) Myocardial cytolysis marked by intense cytoplasmic vacuolization of cardiac miocytes (*arrows*). Absence of inflammatory interstitial response (*asterisk*). HE × 400

References

1. Gabriel EA, Locali RF, Matsuoka PK, et al. Lung perfusion during cardiac surgery with cardiopulmonary bypass: is it necessary? *Interact Cardiovasc Thorac Surg*. 2008;7:1089-1095.
2. Gutierrez EB, Zanetta DM, Saldiva PH, Capelozzi VL. Autopsy-proven determinants of death in HIV-infected patients treated for pulmonary tuberculosis in Sao Paulo. *Pathol Res Pract*.2002; 198(5):339-346.
3. Szerafin T, Hoetzenecker K, Hacker S, et al. Heat shock proteins 27, 60, 70, 90, and 20S proteasome in on-pump versus off-pump coronary artery bypass graft patients. *Ann Thorac Surg*.2008; 85:80-87.
4. Vaage J, Valen G. Preconditioning and cardiac surgery. *Ann Thorac Surg*.2003; 75:S709-S714.

Continuous or Intermittent Lung Perfusion with Arterial or Venous Blood

36

Edmo Atique Gabriel and Tomas Salerno

The first issue to be addressed in this chapter is to try to determine if there are relevant differences between lung perfusion using arterial blood and lung perfusion using venous blood. Based on our data[1], controlled lung perfusion with venous blood had, on one hand, hemodynamic and inflammatory benefits; on the other hand, postoperative gasometric performance was not marked by optimal parameters. Before making another consideration, we would like to point out that venous blood itself is not deleterious for lung tissue as normal pulmonary physiology is characterized by lung perfusion exactly with venous blood pumped by the right ventricle into the main pulmonary artery. The real limitation is that controlled lung perfusion using venous blood is not capable of ensuring optimal gasometric parameters postoperatively, especially if the heart is kept beating in cardiopulmonary bypass (CPB).[1]

We think that there are some interesting alternatives and solutions that may be employed during heart surgery with CPB to improve gasometric performance when controlled lung perfusion with venous blood is used. At some point, we believe that controlled lung perfusion can be useful, especially for children with cyanotic cardiac diseases in which high levels of oxygen are not attractive from a physiological point of view.[1]

The proposition of alternative approaches for minimizing gasometric limitations of controlled lung perfusion using venous blood warrants meticulous investigation. Keep in mind the following:

1. There can be an association between controlled lung perfusion using venous blood and mechanical ventilation, probably low-frequency mechanical ventilation, throughout CPB.
2. The main pulmonary artery can be perfused with venous blood during CPB, but the perfusionist should keep the inspired oxygen fraction at high levels.
3. While lungs are perfused with venous blood, the perfusionist should increase the pump flow as much as possible.
4. Approaches 2 and 3 can be employed in a concomitant manner during CPB.

We would like to reinforce that these strategies must be investigated to obtain consistent results and to draw conclusions.

Friedman et al.[2] obtained good results in animals subjected to lung perfusion using venous blood (partial CPB) with lung ventilation. The authors demonstrated that there is higher expression of thromboxane A_2 when lungs are deprived of blood flow.[2] Likewise, Massoudy et al.[4] demonstrated that association between lung perfusion using venous blood and ventilation, according to principles of the Drew technique, can be useful as it can mitigate an increase in extravascular pulmonary fluid.[4]

In addition to the controversies on lung perfusion using arterial or venous blood, the issue of perfusing lungs in a continuous or intermittent fashion during CPB needs to be addressed.

First, heart surgeons are reminded that there are the following well-known methods for coronary perfusion:

1. Intermittently each 15–20 min by ostial cannula
2. Retrograde coronary perfusion (continuous or intermittent fashion)

E.A. Gabriel (✉)
Federal University of São Paulo, San Paulo, Brazil
e-mail: edag@uol.com.br

E.A. Gabriel and T. Salerno (eds.), *Principles of Pulmonary Protection in Heart Surgery*,
DOI: 10.1007/978-1-84996-308-4_36, © Springer-Verlag London Limited 2010

3. Continuous coronary perfusion by keeping the heart beating during CPB
4. Coronary perfusion according to the principles of a dual system: antegrade plus retrograde perfusion

In an attempt to create a parallel line with coronary perfusion, we can enumerate the following strategies for lung perfusion during CPB:

1. Intermittently by main pulmonary artery cannula (it can be called *pneumoplegia*)
2. Retrogradepulm onarype rfusion5
3. Continuous lung perfusion by keeping the heart beating during CPB
4. Duallungpe rfusion:a ntegradeplus re trograde

In contrast to coronary perfusion, meticulous investigations focusing on different strategies for lung perfusion are missing. Furthermore, there is no consistent evidence in the literature regarding whether lung perfusion should be done intermittently or during the entire CPB procedure. Based on concepts about coronary perfusion, we believe that the most important undertaking is to try to prevent pulmonary ischemia-reperfusion injury during CPB. It can be done providing some flow other than bronchial flow to the lungs throughout CPB. Moreover, we must bear in mind that postoperative lung dysfunction can be minimized by perfusing lungs either intermittently or continuously during CPB as long as lung perfusion pressure is strictly controlled to prevent additional pulmonary tissue damage.[1]

References

1. Gabriel EA, Locali RF, Matsuoka PK, et al. Lung perfusion during cardiac surgery with cardiopulmonary bypass: is it necessary? *Interact Cardiovasc Thorac Surg.* 2008;7:1089-1095.
2. Friedman M, Sellke FW, Wang SY, Weintraub RM, Johnson RG. Parameters of pulmonary injury after total or partial cardiopulmonary bypass. *Circulation.* 1994;90(5 pt 2):II262-II268.
3. Friedman M, Wang SY, Sellke FW, Franklin A, Weintraub RM, Johnson RG. Pulmonary injury after total or partial cardiopulmonary bypass with thromboxane synthesis inhibition. *Ann Thorac Surg.*1995; 59:598-603.
4. Massoudy P, Piotrowski JA, van de Wal HCJM, et al. Perfusing and ventilating the patient's lungs during bypass ameliorates the increase in extravascular thermal volume after coronary bypass grafting. *Ann Thorac Surg.* 2003; 76:516-521.
5. Spagnolo S, Grasso MA, Tesler UF. Retrograde pulmonary perfusion improves results in pulmonary embolectomy for massive pulmonary embolism. *Tex Heart Inst J.* 2006; 33(4):473-476.

Lung Perfusion and Mechanical Ventilation

37

Edmo Atique Gabriel and Tomas Salerno

Imagine what it is like to encourage heart surgeons to use controlled lung perfusion without ceasing mechanical ventilation for all cardiac surgeries requiring cardiopulmonary bypass (CPB). We have no doubt that it will be a harsh challenge, and it will be necessary to blaze a steep trail to reach that goal. At this time, lung perfusion associated with mechanical ventilation is not a usual concept in heart surgery concept; however, we believe that ongoing studies will bring additional information to allow both approaches to run together through the pathway of progress in heart surgery with CPB.

Before making comments about some experimental and clinical research, we need to keep in mind that there is a physiologic relationship between pulmonary volume and pulmonary vascular resistance. Inspiration and expiration are events that can modify the pattern of vascular distensibility in the lungs as they promote conformational alterations in alveolar vessels and extra-alveolar vessels in different manners.[1]

During normal inspiration, pulmonary volume tends to increase, and alveoli become expanded. Furthermore, alveolar vessels (pulmonary capillaries) become distended as alveoli expand continuously in such a way that resistance of these vessels increases in proportion to the degree of pulmonary capillary distension. Therefore, if the lungs will be mechanically ventilated using high volumes, alveolar vessel resistance will increase considerably. By contrast, low pulmonary volumes will be associated with lower alveolar vessel resistance.[1]

Another cluster of vessels – the extra-alveolar vessels – is subjected to different intensities of intrapleural pressure. During inspiration, intrapleural pressure becomes negative as the pulmonary volume increases. On the other hand, intrapleural pressure becomes positive as the pulmonary volume decreases throughout progressive expiration. The functional behavior of extra-alveolar vessels is opposite that of alveolar vessels. Extra-alveolar vessels are expected to distend when high pulmonary volumes are used, and interestingly, the resistance of these vessels tends to decrease. In light of low pulmonary volumes, extra-alveolar vessels will be compressed in such a way that their resistance will increase. Alveolar vessel resistance and extra-alveolar vessel resistance contribute to generate total pulmonary vascular resistance.[1]

Use of positive end-expiratory pressure during mechanical ventilation can cause elevation of alveolar and intrapleural pressures; consequently, alveolar and extra-alveolar vessels will be compressed, and pulmonary vascular resistance will increase. Therefore, it is important to bear in mind that high levels of positive end-expiratory pressure can contribute to cardiac output reduction.[1] Bayindir et al.[2] advocated that pulmonary ventilation during CPB can make the surgical view difficult and may cause bronchoconstriction secondary to alveolar hypocapnia.

Taking into consideration all these comments, we introduce some experiences of different cardiac centers worldwide regarding the benefits of ventilation during heart surgery with CPB. Actually, these authors have proposed the use of lung ventilation during CPB as a protective adjunct in an attempt to minimize postoperative pulmonary dysfunction.

E.A.G abriel (✉)
Department of Surgery, Division of Cardiovascular Surgery
FederalU niversity ofSa oP aulo, SaoP aulo, Brazil
e-mail:e dag@uol.com.br

Lamarche et al.[3] performed experimental research in which 30 pigs were allocated to six groups as follows:

Group1 :C ontrolgroup

Group 2: Sham without CPB – atrial appendage and the right femoral artery cannulated

Group 3: CPB for 150 min with no reperfusion, mechanical ventilation stopped during CPB, heart left beating during CPB, and no aortic cross clampinge mployed

Group 4: CPB for 150 min, reperfusion for 60 min, and mechanical ventilation discontinued throughoutC PB

Group 5: CPB 150 min, mechanical ventilation during the entire experiment, reperfusion for 60 min

Group 6: CPB for 150 min, mechanical ventilation during the entire experiment, nitric oxide (NO) inhalation, and 60 min of reperfusion

It is crucial to emphasize that when mechanical ventilation was not discontinued during CPB, there was an association between lung ventilation and no controlled lung perfusion (partial CPB). Benefits of ventilation were predominantly related to gasometric performance as it increased arterial oxygen pressure at 30 min and an hour following cessation of CPB (Fig. 37.1 and Tables 37.1–37.3).

There were no additional benefits of association between ventilation and NO inhalation regarding relaxation

Table 37.1 Pulmonary artery pressure before, during, and after cardiopulmonarybypa ssi ns wine

Time	PAP(mmHg)		
	Pre-CPB	30 post-CPB	60 post-CPB
Ventilated	9.7±3.1	27.7±1.5	26.0±3.0
Nonventilated	12.7±2.3	22.0±2.6	23.3±2.5

$P>0.05$

CPB cardiopulmonary bypass, *PAP* pulmonary artery pressure
This table was published in Lamarche et al.[3] Copyright 2004, European Association for Cardio-Thoracic Surgery

of pulmonary arteries, but there was decreased sensitivity to contractile substances.[3]

Different strategies of lung ventilation can be considered for use during heart surgery with CPB. The decision about should be made after discussion involving the cardiac surgeon and anesthesiologist. These two professionals should analyze advantages and disadvantages of ventilatory techniques, such as continuous positive airway pressure (CPAP); high-frequency, low-volume ventilation; different inspired oxygen concentrations; and bilateral extracorporeal circulation using the lungs to oxygenate blood.

For the Drew technique, Vohra et al.[4] performed meticulous literature search for the best evidences on the topic (Table 37.3). Despite several key results, there was no consensus about the benefits of using lung ventilation

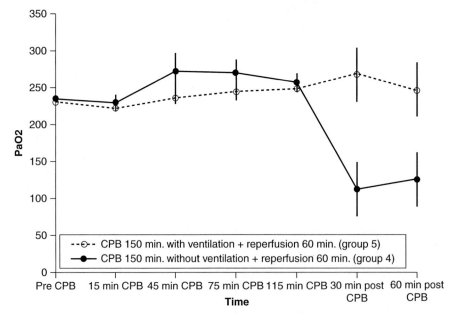

Fig.37.1 Arterialoxy gen pressure before, during 150 min of cardiopulmonary bypass (CPB), and after CPB. *X-axis* time of the surgery, *Y-axis* arterial oxygen pressure, *solid line* non ventilated group (group 4), *dashed line* ventilated group (group 5). Difference in the two groups: 30 min post-CPB: $P=0.0003$, 60 min post-CPB: $P=0.0033$. (This fi gure was published in Lamarche et al.[3] Copyright 2004, European Association for Cardio-ThoracicSur gery)

Table37.2 Cardiac output before, during, and after cardiopulmonary bypass in swine

Time	Pre	Cardiac output (L/min)					
		15 per CPB	45 per CPB	75 per CPB	115 per CPB	30 post-CPB	60 post-CPB
Ventilated	2.9±0.6	3.0±0.5	3.0±0.5	3.1±0.6	3.3±0.6	3.4±0.5	3.5±0.6
Nonventilated	3.8±1.2	2.8±0.2	2.8±0.2	2.8±0.2	2.8±0.1	4.3±2.6	4.6±3.8

$P>0.05$

CPB cardiopulmonary bypass

This table was published in Lamarche et al.[3] Copyright 2004, European Association for Cardio-Thoracic Surgery

Table37.3 Best-evidencea rticles

Author	Patientgroup	Studytype	Outcome	Keyre sults	Comments
Lamarche et al.[3]	Six groups (*n*=5) of 30 Landrace swine: Control WithoutC PB CPB 150 min with no reperfusion CPB 150 min with reperfusion 60 min	Experimental study (level 5)	Endothelial function	Endothelium-dependent relaxations to acetylcholine is prevented by ventilation during CPB. Ventilation and NO inhalation during CPB has the same effect on endothelium as ventilation alone	No cross clamping of the aorta. No cardioplegia used
	CPB 150 min with ventilation with reperfusion 60 min CPB 150 min with NOinha lation+ventilation with 60 min of reperfusion		Pao$_2$	Nonventilateda nimals had a decrease in the Pao$_2$follo wing separation from CPB, with the Pao$_2$/Fio$_2$ as low as 166. In the ventilation group, this ratio was never lower than 330	
Magnusson et al.[6]	In six pigs, CPAP with 5 cm H$_2$O pressure was applied during CPB In another six pigs, the lungs were open to the atmosphere during CPB	Experimental study (level 5)	V-Qdis tribution	Intrapulmonarys hunt increased and Pao$_2$ decreased after CPB in both groups	
			Postop atelectasis by CT scan	14.5±5.5% in the CPAP group and 18.7±5.2% in the controls (*P*=0.20)	
Massoudy et al.[7]	34 consecutive patients undergoing CABG	Cohorts tudy (level 3b)	Extravascular thermal volume	Increasefrom 4.8±0.2 mL/kg to 6.7±0.4 ml/kg w ith conventional CPB but remained unchanged with bilateral ECC	Authorsc oncluded that using the patient's lungs as an oxygenator during bypass mitigates the increase in extravascular pulmonary fluid

(continued)

Table 37.3 (continued)

Author	Patientgroup	Studytype	Outcome	Keyre sults	Comments
	Group 1 ECC: 24 patients had CPB using bilateral ECC (additional cannulation of pulmonary artery and left atrium and lungs perfused and ventilated during bypass)				
			Hemodynamic parameters	Nos ignificant differences in Cardiac Index, PApre ssure,orSV R1 4 h post-operatively	Only transient and clinically small improvement in Pao_2/Fio_2 ratio was found
	Group 2 CPB: 10 were operated using conventional CPB.		Intraopfl uid balance	+1,955±233 mL in group 1 vs. +2,654±210 mL ($P<0.05$) in group 2	
			Inflammatory cytokines	Nodif ference	
Gilbert et al.[8]	18 patients undergoing elective CABG with CPB	Cohortstudy (level 3b)	Lungre sistance and elastance	Increased equally after CPB in both groups. The increase was relatively less with intact pleurae or net negative fluid balance	
	Group 1: CPAP applied to 9 patients during CPB				
	Group 2: no CPAP applied to 9 patients during CPB				
Loeckinger et al.[9]	14 patients undergoing elective cardiac surgery	PRCT(le vel2b)	V/Qdis tribution	Morepe rfusionoflung areas with a normal V/Q distribution and less shunt in CPAP group	No difference in postoperative outcome found, although study was too small to find any clinical outcome differences
	Group 1: 7 patients received CPAP at 10 cm H_2O during CPB				
	Group 2: In 7 patients, the lungs were open to the atmosphere		Pao_2 4 h postsurgery	Controls:P ao$_2$ 99±9 mmH g, CPAP Pao_2 123 ±23 mmH g, $P<0.05$	
			Shunt fraction	Controls: 8.1±3.7, CPAP: 14.1±46, $P<0.05$	
			Hemodynamic variables	CI,SV RI,C VP,M APa ll similar between groups	

Table 37.3 (continued)

Author	Patient group	Study type	Outcome	Key results	Comments
Cogliati et al.[10]	30 patients undergoing elective CABG	PRCT (level 2b)	PaO_2, $P(A-a)O_2$, Qs/Qt, and Cstat	Minor impairment of gas exchange in the third group of patients. Lung inflation with air effectively preserved respiratory system mechanics	
	Group 1 ($n=101$): lungs deflated				
	Group 2 ($n=10$): $PEEP=5 cm H_2O$ and $FIO_2=1.0$				
	Group 3 ($n=10$): $PEEP=5 cm H_2O$ and $FIO_2=0.21$				
Berry et al.[11]	61 patients undergoing elective CABG	PRCT (level 2b)	$P(A-a)O_2$ measured at 30 min	Group 1: 43.3 kPa Group 2: 35.5 kPa Group 3: 36.8 kPa, $P=0.036$	No sample size calculations given to support the null hypothesis that there is no difference between groups
	Group 1 ($N=17$) no CPAP during CPB				
	Group 2 ($N=22$): 5 cm H_2O CPAP (FIO_2 0.21)				
	Group 3 ($N=22$): 5 cm H_2O CPAP (FIO_2 1.0)		$P(A-a)O_2$ measured at 4 h	Group 1: 28.7 kPa Group 2: 35.5 kPa Group 3: 28.3 kPa, $P=0.32$	There were several occasions when the surgeon requested lung deflation due to difficult surgical access
			Time to extubation	Not affected by the use of CPAP	
Zabeeda et al.[12]	75 patients undergoing CABG (15 patients in each group)	Single blind PRCT (level 2b)	Compliance and mean airway pressures	No difference	Number of grafts and aortic cross-clamping times significantly shorter in groups 1 and 5
	Group 1: high-frequency, low-volume ventilation with FIO_2 1.0, frequency 100 breaths per min				
			PaO_2 and $P(A-a)O_2$	Group 3 had higher PaO_2 and lower $P(A-a)O_2$ 5 min after weaning from CPB, but this became nonsignificant after chest closure	
	Group 2: high-frequency, low-volume ventilation with FIO_2 0.21				

(continued)

Table 37.3 (continued)

Author	Patient group	Study type	Outcome	Key results	Comments
	Group 3: 5 cm H_2O CPAP with F_{IO_2} 1.0				
	Group 4: 5 cm H_2O CPAP with F_{IO_2} 0.21				
	Group 5: disconnected from ventilator		Extubation time	Similar in all groups	
Boldt et al.[13]	90 patients undergoing CABG (15 patients in each group)	Single blind PRCT (level 2b)	Extravascular lung water	Group 4 had an increase of 35% and Group 5 had an increase of 45% in extravascular lung water compared to other groups. This remained higher at 5 h postsurgery	
	Group 1: lungs collapsed				
	Group 2: CPAP with PEEP 5 cm H_2O and F_{IO_2} 1.0				
	Group 3: CPAP with PEEP 5 cm H_2O and F_{IO_2} 0.21				
			Pao_2	Greatest decrease in groups 4 (−109 mmHg) and 5 (−130 mmHg). It was least pronounced in group 3 (−33 mmHg)	
	Group 4: CPAP with PEEP 15 cm H_2O and F_{IO_2} 1.0				
	Group 5: CPAP with PEEP 15 cm H_2O and F_{IO_2} 0.21				
	Group 6: mechanical ventilation PEEP 5 cm H_2O and F_{IO_2} 1.0				

CABG coronary artery bypass grafting, *CI* cardiac index, *CPAP* continuous positive airway pressure, *CPB* cardiopulmonary bypass, *CT* computed tomography, *CVP* central venous pressure, *ECC* extracorporeal circulation, *MAP* mean arterial pressure, *NO* nitric oxide, *PA* pulmonary artery, *PEEP* positive end-expiratory pressure, *PRCT* prospective randomized controlled trial, *SVRI* systemic vascular resistance index Reproduced with permission from Vohra et al.[4] Copyright 2005, doi: 10.1510/icvts.2005.114710. European Association of Cardio-Thoracic Surgery http://icvts.ctsnetjournals.org/

during heart surgery requiring CPB. However, that was an additional encouraging reason to keep performing new trials and investigations to find out how lung ventilation could be used during heart surgery with CPB in a physiological manner. Imura et al.[5] have performed new experiments concerning the use of low-frequency mechanical ventilation during heart surgery with CPB, and this is addressed in a chapter of this book.

References

1. Levitzky MG. *Pulmonary physiology*, Lange Physiology Series. 7th ed. New York: McGraw-Hill; 2007.
2. Bayindir O, Akpinar B, Özbek U, et al. The hazardous effects of alveolar hypocapnia on lung mechanics during weaning from cardiopulmonary bypass. *Perfusion*. 2000;15:27-31.
3. Lamarche Y, Gagnon J, Malo O, Blaise G, Carrier M, Perrault LP. Ventilation prevents pulmonary endothelial dysfunction and improves oxygenation after cardiopulmonary bypass without aortic cross-clamping. *Eur J Cardiothorac Surg*.2004;26:554-563.
4. Vohra HA, Levine A, Dunning J. Can ventilation while on cardiopulmonary bypass improve post-operative lung function for patients undergoing cardiac surgery? *Interact Cardiovasc Thorac Surg*. 2005;4:442-446.
5. Imura H, Caputo M, Lim K, et al. Pulmonary injury after cardiopulmonary bypass: beneficial effects of low-frequency mechanical ventilation. *J Thorac Cardiovasc Surg*. 2009;137:1530-1537.
6. Magnusson L, Zemgulis V, Wicky S, Tydén H, Hedenstierna G. Effect of CPAP during cardiopulmonary bypass on postoperative lung function. An experimental study. *Acta Anaesthesiol Scand*.1 998;42(10):1133-8.
7. Massoudy P, Piotrowski JA, van de Wal HCJM, Giebler R, Marggraf G, Peters J, Jakob HG. Perfusing and Ventilating the patient's lungs during bypass ameliorates the increase in extravascular thermal volume after coronary bypass grafting. *Ann Thorac Surg*2 003;76:516-522.
8. Gilbert TB, Barnas GM, Sequeira AJ. Impact of pleurotomy, continuous positive airway pressure, and fluid balance during cardiopulmonary bypass on lung mechanics and oxygenation. *J Cardiothorac Vasc Anesth*.1 996;10(7):844-9.
9. Loeckinger A, Kleinsasser A, Lindner KH, Margreiter J, Keller C, Hoermann C. Continuous positive airway pressure at 10 cm H2O during cardiopulmonary bypass improves postoperative gas exchange. *Anesth Analg*. 2000;91(3):522-7.
10. Cogliati AA, Menichetti A, Tritapede L, Conti G. Effects of three techniques of lung management on pulmonary function during cardiopulmonary bypass. *Acta Anaesthesiol Belg*.1 996;47(2):73-80.
11. Berry CB, Butler PJ, Myles PS. Lung management during cardiopulmonary bypass: is continuous positive airways pressure beneficial? *Br J Anaesth*.1 993;71(6):864-8.
12. Zabeeda D, Gefen R, Medalion B, Khazin V, Shachner A, Ezri T. The effect of high-frequency ventilation of the lungs on postbypass oxygenation: A comparison with other ventilation methods applied during cardiopulmonary bypass. *J Cardiothorac Vasc Anesth*.2 003;17(1):40-4.
13. Boldt J, King D, Scheld HH, Hempelmann G. Lung management during cardiopulmonary bypass: influence on extravascular lung water. *J Cardiothorac Anesth*. 1990 Feb;4(1):73-9.

Edmo Atique Gabriel and Tomas Salerno

The topic of this chapter is quite appealing and interesting as eventual correlation between natriuretic peptides and controlled lung perfusion is discussed. In our proposed experimental research,[1] this matter was addressed particularly for the relationship between brain natriuretic peptide (BNP) and controlled lung perfusion. These data have not yet been published.

Cardiac specimens of animals were withdrawn from the right ventricle as we know that most synthesis of this peptide takes place in the ventricular myocardium, differently from synthesis of atrial natriuretic peptide (ANP). The same molecular biology methods employed for pulmonary specimens were used for cardiac extracts. We just focused on the postoperative time (Tables 38.1 and 38.2) because BNP expression was extremely low preoperatively, and it made sense as the increase of BNP expression usually is related to right ventricular overload. All curves of genic amplification for β-actin and BNP are depicted in Fig. 38.1.

Why would we correlate BNP expression or natriuretic peptides in a general way with use of controlled lung perfusion during cardiopulmonary bypass (CPB)? First, bear in mind that BNP is used in clinical practice as a marker for heart failure. particularly indicating a certain degree of ventricular overload.[2–9] Second, if controlled lung perfusion during CPB can be hemodynamically beneficial in reducing pulmonary vascular resistance and mean pulmonary artery pressure,

then we can hypothesize that the intensity of BNP expression by myocardial cells will tend to be lower when controlled lung perfusion is employed. However, we[1] did not find out relevant outcomes postoperatively regarding BNP expression when controlled lung perfusion was employed. The main reason for this is believed to be the sample. Furthermore, looking at the sample size of all subgroups in Tables 38.1 and 38.2, note that the number of elements in each subgroup became lower than the original sample size, caused by too low or almost undetectable BNP in some animals. We think that the issue of BNP expression versus controlled lung perfusion warrants further attention, and it should not be overlooked.

Nagaya et al.[10] advocated that BNP should be used as a noninvasive marker for heart failure, particularly in light of right ventricular overload due to pulmonary hypertension. Moreover, these authors postulated that BNP levels should be used to assess the efficacy of pulmonary thromboendarterectomy. Thirty-four patients with chronic thromboembolic pulmonary hypertension were studied before and 1 month following pulmonary thromboendarterectomy. The main results of this research demonstrated the benefits of BNP as a noninvasive marker for right ventricular overload (Figs. 38.2–38.5).

Ultimately, we would like to make some comments about experimental research designed and published by Aoyama et al.[11] These authors studied three groups of rats in which a cannula was inserted into the main pulmonary artery through a right ventricular incision, and another cannula was put inside the left atrium by means of a left ventricular incision. Lung perfusion was carried out in

E.A.G abriel (✉)
FederalU niversityof Sa oP aulo, SaoP aulo, Brazil
e-mail:e dag@uol.com.br

E.A. Gabriel and T. Salerno (eds.), *Principles of Pulmonary Protection in Heart Surgery*,
DOI: 10.1007/978-1-84996-308-4_38, © Springer-Verlag London Limited 2010

three groups, as demonstrated in Fig. 38.6, with particular interest to lung perfusion using synthetic ANP (carperitide). The main results of this research are depicted in Figs. 38.7 and 38.9; the most striking conclusion was the likely ability of ANP to increase levels of lung tissue cyclic guanosine monophosphate (cGMP), alleviating deleterious effects from warm ischemia-reperfusion injury at the onset of reperfusion.[11]

Table38.1 Postoperative brain natriuretic peptide (BNP) expression in cardioplegic arrest subgroups

Variable	Subgroup	N	Mean	Standard deviation	Minimum	Maximum	Significance (p)
Postop BNP	IA	3	9.09	0.46	8.78	9.69	0.228
	IB	5	9.12	1.42	7.01	11.05	
	IC	4	8.29	1.08	7.16	9.79	
	Total	12	8.83	1.16	7.01	11.05	

IA cardioplegic arrest without controlled lung perfusion, *IB* cardioplegic arrest and controlled lung perfusion with arterial blood, *IC* cardioplegic arrest and controlled lung perfusion with venous blood

Table38.2 Postoperative brain natriuretic peptide (BNP) expression in beating heart subgroups

Variable	Subgroup	N	Mean	Standard deviation	Minimum	Maximum	Significance (p)
Postop BNP	IIA	4	6.68	2.41	3.05	8.78	0.325
	IIB	3	8.36	2.06	5.77	10.19	
	IIC	3	7.94	0.11	7.80	8.02	
	Total	10	7.56	1.96	3.05	10.19	

IIA beating heart technique without controlled lung perfusion, *IIB* beating heart technique and controlled lung perfusion with arterial blood, *IIC* beating heart technique and controlled lung perfusion with venous blood

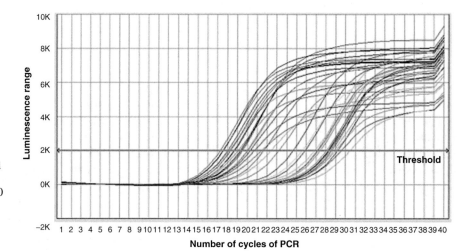

Fig.38.1 Curvesof ge nic amplification for β-actina nd brain natriuretic peptide (BNP). *K* equivalent to 1,000 units of luminescence, *Threshold* baseline level for genic amplification, *PCR* polymerasec hainr eaction

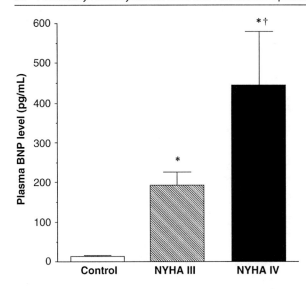

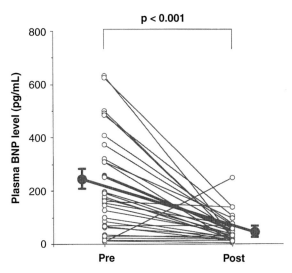

Fig. 38.2 Preoperative plasma brain natriuretic peptide (BNP) levels in patients with chronic thromboembolic pulmonary hypertension according to New York Heart Association (NYHA) functional classes. *p less than 0.05 versus controls, †p less than 0.05 versus NYHA functional class III. (This figure was published in Nagaya et al.[10] Copyright 2002, the Society of Thoracic Surgeons)

Fig. 38.4 Change in plasma brain natriuretic peptide (BNP) level by pulmonary thromboendarterectomy. *Post* postoperative, *Pre* preoperative. (This figure was published in Nagaya et al.[10] Copyright2002,t heS ocietyof T horacicS urgeons)

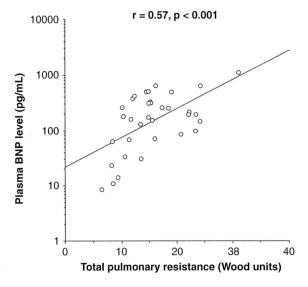

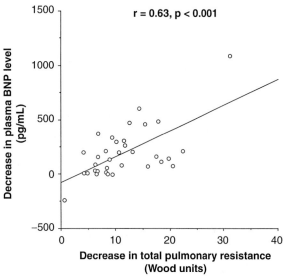

Fig. 38.3 Relationship between preoperative plasma brain natriuretic peptide (BNP) level and total pulmonary resistance in patients with chronic thromboembolic pulmonary hypertension. (This figure was published in Nagaya et al.[10] Copyright 2002, the SocietyofThora cicSur geons)

Fig. 38.5 Relationship between change in plasma brain natriuretic peptide (BNP) level and change in total pulmonary resistance by pulmonary thromboendarterectomy. (This figure was published in Nagaya et al.[10] Copyright 2002, the Society of ThoracicS urgeons)

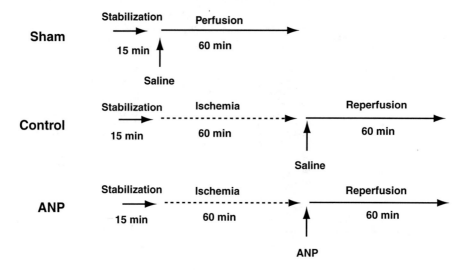

Fig. 38.6 Experimental protocols. In the sham group, the lungs were continuously perfused, and saline was added to the perfusate after the period of stabilization. In the control and atrial natriuretic peptide (ANP) groups, 60-min warm ischemia was initiated by interrupting the perfusion after 15 min for stabilization. The lungs were then reperfused. In the control group, saline was added to the perfusate at the onset of reperfusion. In the ANP group, synthetic ANP was added to the perfusate at the onset of reperfusion. (This figure was published in Aoyama et al.[11] Copyright 2009, International Society for Heart and Lung Transplantation.E lsevier)

Fig.38.7 (**a**)Pulmona ry vascular resistance, (**b**)l ung weight gain, and (**c**)pu lmo-nary shunt fraction compari-sons between the sham (*open circles*), control (*filled squares*), and atrial natriuretic peptide (ANP) (*filled circles*) groups. Values are expressed as mean ± standard error of the mean (SEM). **$p<0.01$ between the ANP group and the control group; ++$p<0.01$ between the sham group and the control group; ##$p<0.01$ between the ANP and the sham group. *BL*ba seline. (This figure was published in Aoyama et al.[11]C opyright 2009, International Society for Heart and Lung Transplantation.El sevier)

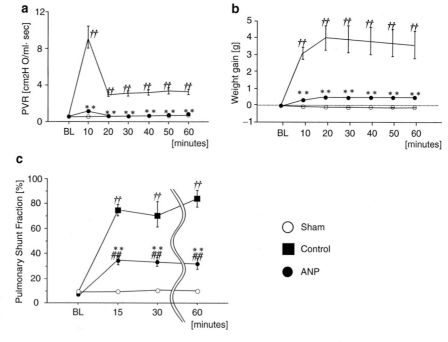

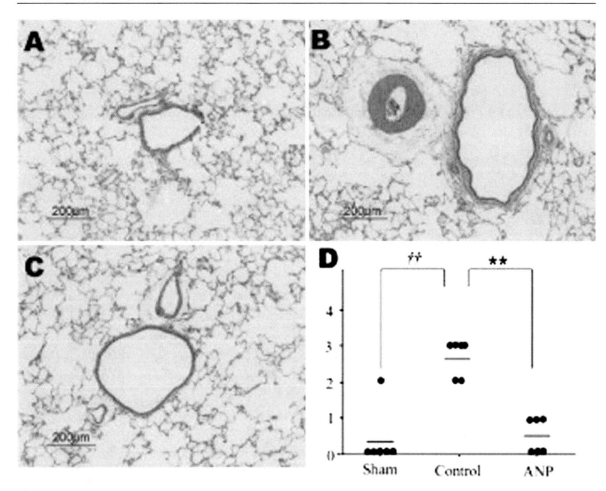

Fig. 38.8 Histologic evaluation of reperfused lungs. Representative figures of the sham (**a**), control (**b**), and atrial natriuretic peptide (ANP) (**c**) groups. Hematoxylin-eosin staining; original magnification ×200. (**d**) Scatterplots of the score of the grade of lung injury in each group. **$p<0.01$ between the ANP group and the control group; ++$p<0.01$ between the sham group and the control group. (This figure was published in Aoyama et al.[11] Copyright 2009, International Society for Heart and Lung Transplantation.E lsevier)

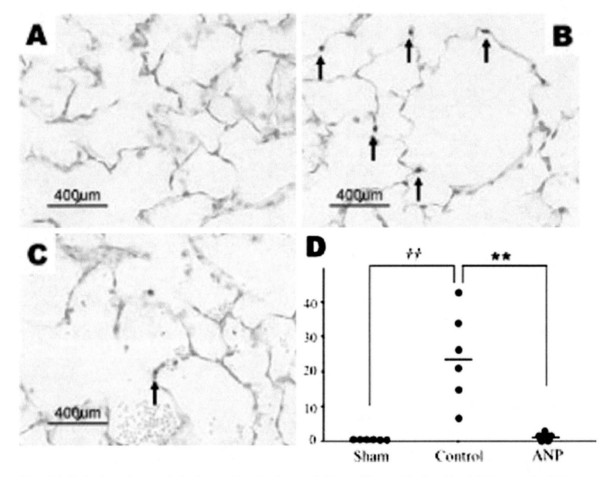

Fig. 38.9 Evaluation of apoptosis by immunohistochemistry. Representative results of immunohistochemistry for single-stranded DNA (ssDNA) in the sham (**a**), control (**b**), and atrial natriuretic peptide (ANP) (**c**) groups. *Arrows* indicate immunoreactive nuclei for the anti-ssDNA antibody. (**d**) Scatterplots of the number of ssDNA-positive cells in 10 randomly chosen fields at ×400 magnification. **p < 0.01 between the ANP group and the control group; ++*p* < 0.01 between the sham group and the control group. (This figure was published in Aoyama et al.[11] Copyright 2009, International Society for Heart and Lung Transplantation. Elsevier)

References

1. Gabriel EA, Locali RF, Matsuoka PK, et al. Lung perfusion during cardiac surgery with cardiopulmonary bypass: is it necessary? *Interact Cardiovasc Thorac Surg.* 2008;7:1089-1095.
2. Krishnaswamy P, Lubien E, Clopton P, et al. Utility of B-natriuretic peptide levels in identifying patients with left ventricular systolic or diastolic dysfunction. *Am J Med.* 2001;111(4):274-279.
3. Omland T, Aakvaag A, Bonarjee VV, et al. Plasma brain natriuretic peptide as an indicator of left ventricular systolic function and long-term survival after acute myocardial infarction. Comparison with plasma atrial natriuretic peptide and N-terminal proatrial natriuretic peptide. *Circulation.* 1996;93(11):1963-1969.
4. Yasue H, Yoshimura M, Sumida H, et al. Localization and mechanism of secretion of B-type natriuretic peptide in comparison with those of A-type natriuretic peptide in normal subjects and patients with heart failure. *Circulation.* 1994;90(1):195-203.
5. Kohno M, Horio T, Yokokawa K, et al. Brain natriuretic peptide as a cardiac hormone in essential hypertension. *Am J Med.*1992; 92(1):29-34.
6. Nishikimi T, Yoshihara F, Morimoto A, et al. Relationship between left ventricular geometry and natriuretic peptide levels in essential hypertension. *Hypertension.* 1996;28(1): 22-30.
7. Jensen KT, Carstens J, Ivarsen P, Pedersen EB. A new, fast and reliable radioimmunoassay of brain natriuretic peptide in human plasma. Reference values in healthy subjects and in patients with different diseases. *Scand J Clin Lab Invest.* 1997;57(6):529-540.

8. Wallen T, Landahl S, Hedner T, Saito Y, Masuda I, Nakao K. Brain natriuretic peptide in an elderly population. *J Intern Med*.1997;242(4):307- 311.

9. Nagaya N, Nishikimi T, Okano Y, et al. Plasma brain natriuretic peptide levels increase in proportion to the extent of right ventricular dysfunction in pulmonary hypertension. *J Am Coll Cardiol*.1998; 31(1):202-208.

10. Nagaya N, Ando M, Oya H, et al. Plasma brain natriuretic peptide as a noninvasive marker for efficacy of pulmonary thromboendarterectomy. *Ann Thorac Surg*. 2002;74:180-184.

11. Aoyama A, Chen F, Fujinaga T, et al. Post-ischemic infusion of atrial natriuretic peptide attenuates warm ischemia–reperfusion injury in rat lung. *J Heart Lung Transplant*. 2009; 28(6):628-634.

Low-Frequency Mechanical Ventilation DuringC ardiopulmonaryB ypass

39

Hajime Imura, Raimondo Ascione, and Gianni D Angelini

39.1 Introduction

Pulmonary dysfunction during cardiac surgery may range from subclinical changes up to acute lung injury and acute respiratory distress syndrome. Causative factors include inflammation, pulmonary ischemia and reperfusion-related injury, blood contact with the surface of cardiopulmonary bypass (CPB) machinery, endotoxemia, surgical trauma, blood loss, and transfusion. Strikingly thin, the laminated, tripartite construction of the blood–gas barrier promotes gas exchange by passive diffusion. Considering its exceptional thinness, the blood–gas barrier is strikingly strong, allowing it to tolerate prevailing stresses and maintain structural integrity under physiological conditions of operation. This equilibrium is markedly altered by the iatrogenic, prolonged lung collapse/atelectasis induced during CPB when lungs are left open to air and the ischemia related to cardiopulmonary blood supply diversion. This iatrogenic condition determines very poor alveolar blood supply with high potential for marked alveolar ischemia, triggering hypoxic pulmonary vasoconstriction, and has been associated with marked ischemia-reperfusion injury and inflammatory response, leading to subsystem organ dysfunction, in-hospital mortality, and morbidity.

Atelectasis is regarded as a main cause for post-CPB lung injury, and a correlation between the degree of atelectasis and intrapulmonary shunt has been reported. It has been suggested that ventilation or even keeping air in the alveoli during CPB might protect the lungs from ischemic damage. Previous studies have shown that oxygen in the alveolar space helps keep tissue adenine nucleotides level and prevents histopathological damage in the lungs during ischemia.

The issue of myocardial ischemia and reperfusion injury has been addressed by developing effective cardioplegic techniques. By contrast, the issue of lung ischemia and related reperfusion injury remains a major concern. Current surgical practice includes no strategy of active lung protection because following institution of CPB the lungs are disconnected from the mechanical ventilator and are left collapsed for the entire CPB duration. Our group has evaluated in an established experimental pig model the efficacy of low-frequency ventilation (LFV) during CPB to reduce post-CPB lung injury. Our study suggested that the use of LFV is associated with significantly better pulmonary gas exchange, higher adenine nucleotide levels, lower lactate levels, and reduced histological damage.

39.2 Mechanismo fPul monaryI njury During Cardiac Surgery

Pulmonary dysfunction is a substantial problem for patients undergoing cardiac surgery using CPB.[1] This dysfunction may range from subclinical and unnoticed functional changes up to prolonged postoperative ventilation, acute lung injury, and acute respiratory distress syndrome.[2] Causative factors for pulmonary inflammation are the pulmonary ischemia and related reperfusion injury, blood contact with the surface of CPB machinery, endotoxemia, surgical trauma, blood loss, and transfusion.[3,4] These factors have been associated with in-hospital mortality, morbidity, and hospital costs.[5–7]

H.I mura(✉)
Department of Surgery, Division of Cardiovascular Surgery,
NipponM edicalSc hool, Tokyo, Japan
e-mail:hi mura@nms.ac.jp

E.A. Gabriel and T. Salerno (eds.), *Principles of Pulmonary Protection in Heart Surgery*,
DOI: 10.1007/978-1-84996-308-4_39, © Springer-Verlag London Limited 2010

39.2.1 Inflammatory Response

Inflammatory activation and cytokine release have been correlated with outcome after cardiac surgery.[8] Suppression of activation of inflammatory mediators during CPB correlates with reduction of pulmonary dysfunction.[9] Pulmonary function 24 h after bypass is inversely correlated with plasma interleukin (IL) 10 concentrations.[10] Furthermore, mechanical ventilation with abnormal shear stress may be responsible for eliciting cytokine release from the lung.[11] The inflammatory response from the lung during CPB and mechanical ventilation originates at the alveolar membrane as a result of ischemia, reperfusion injury, and mechanical stress.[11–13] This detrimental effect still persists despite advances in anesthetic techniques, including maintenance of hemodynamic stability and examination and validation of pharmacological and immunomodulatory agents in clinical studies.[14] Current clinical practice includes no specific strategies of lung protection during cardiac surgery as once on CPB both lungs are disconnected from the ventilator, are left open to air, and therefore are fully collapsed and poorly perfused for the entire CPB period.

39.2.2 Ischemia-Reperfusion Injury

Compared with other organs, the lung possesses certain unique structural and functional attributes. It is the only organ in the body that receives the total cardiac output, a quantity that increases several-fold between rest and exercise[15] and contains air and blood, fluid media that substantially differ in specific densities. The lung counters challenges of maintaining structural integrity under forces such as surface tension, intramural blood pressures, and the very weight of the blood that it contains.[16] In the air capillaries and alveoli of the terminal respiratory units, the blood–gas barrier is comprises of a thin (squamous) epithelial cell facing the air space and intervening intercellular matrix, and an endothelial cell that fronts the vascular space. Strikingly thin, the laminated, tripartite construction of the blood–gas barrier promotes gas exchange by passive diffusion. Considering its exceptional thinness, the blood–gas barrier is strikingly strong, allowing it to tolerate prevailing stresses and maintain structural integrity under physiological conditions of operation.[17–19] This equilibrium is dramatically altered by the iatrogenic, prolonged lung collapse/atelectasis induced during CPB.[20] This condition may affect the gas exchange by passive diffusion at the blood–gas barrier.[12,15–2012,15–20] It may also determine poor alveolar blood supply with high potential for marked alveolar ischemia, triggering hypoxic pulmonary vasoconstriction mediated by arachidonic acid metabolites and endothelin.[21] Nitric oxide (NO) synthases originate from cells lining the airways and alveoli.[22] Therefore, alveolar ischemia may also affect NO production and postoperative pulmonary vascular resistance.[22]

39.2.3 Atelectasis and Mucin Accumulation

Atelectasis is regarded as a main cause for post-CPB lung injury and a correlation between the degree of atelectasis and intrapulmonary shunt has been reported.[12,20] It is known that ventilation or even keeping air in the alveoli protects the lungs from ischemic damage. Previous studies have shown that oxygen in the alveolar space helps keep tissue adenine nucleotides level and prevents histopathological damage in the lungs during ischemia.[23–26] A report has shown benefits of maintaining ventilation during CPB on post-CPB oxygenation and shorter mechanical ventilation, although its mechanism remained unclear.[27]

Mucin, which is known as a key component of the mucosal defensive barrier of the airway and the ability of the host to resist lung injury, increases in the respiratory tract during CPB and correlates with pulmonary abnormalities and respiratory complications in pediatric cardiac surgery.[28] Mucin accumulation can cause atelectasis by occupying alveolar space and disturbing gas exchange in the lungs.[29,30] Previous work by our group in pediatric cardiac surgery showed that the increase in mucin in BAL (bronchoalveolar lavage) correlates with higher $AaDO_2$ (alveolar-to-arterial gradient for oxygen) and PCO_2 during CPB (Fig. 39.1). Alveolar DNA increase during CPB also correlates with duration of CPB (Fig. 39.2). Although the underlying mechanism of mucin increase is still unclear, we speculate that mucin can be released from disrupted epithelial cells

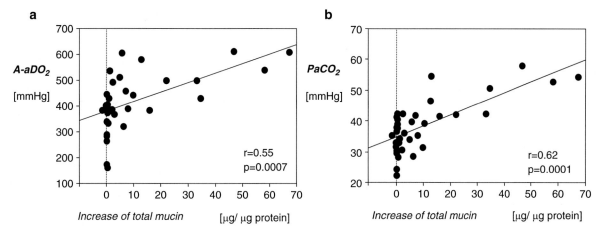

Fig. 39.1 Mucin increase and pulmonary dysfunction after cardiopulmonary bypass (CPB) in pediatric cardiac surgery. Relationships between alveolar mucin increase during CPB and alveolar-arterial oxygen difference (AaDO$_2$) (**a**) and Paco$_2$

(**b**) immediately after CPB were investigated. There were positive correlations between them. *ADP* adenosine diphosphate, *AMP* adenosine monophosphate, *ATP* adenosine triphosphate (Reproduced with permission[28])

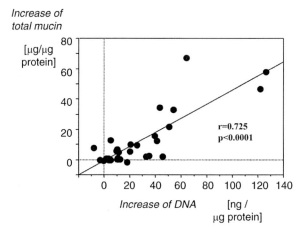

Fig. 39.2 Mucin increase and ischemia reperfusion injury of the lung after cardiopulmonary bypass (CPB) in pediatric cardiac surgery. There was a positive correlation between mucin increase and DNA in airway lavage during CPB. (Reproduced with permission[28])

and also stimulated by cytokine- or neutrophil elastase-mediated reaction[31–34] in response to CPB.

39.3 Low-FrequencyV entilation in an Experimental Model

Our group has evaluated in an established experimental pig model the efficacy of both LFV and continuous positive airway pressure (CPAP) during CPB to

reduce post-CPB lung injury.[35] The rationale of this experimental study was to maintain some degree of ventilation during CPB to prevent persisting lung collapse and complete loss of gas exchange by passive diffusion at the blood–gas barrier. A similar concept was used by Miranda et al.,[36] who, in a small clinical study with a ventilation strategy initiated soon after anesthetic induction, observed an attenuation of the reduction in functional residual capacity and the occurrence of hypoxemia and lower levels of IL-10 and IL-8 release.

Our experimental study was conducted in 18 Yorkshire pigs subjected to 120 min of CPB (1 h of cardioplegic arrest) followed by 90 min of recovery prior to sacrifice. Six animals served as control with the endotracheal tube open to atmosphere during CPB. The remaining animals were divided into two groups of six; one group received CPAP of 5 cm H$_2$O and the other LFV (5 min) with air (21% oxygen) at a tidal volume of about 8–10 mL/kg during CPB. Lung tissue biopsy and BAL samples were obtained serially for measurement of adenine nucleotides (adenine triphosphate [ATP], adenine diphosphate [ADP], adenine monophosphate [AMP]), lactate, DNA levels, and histology. Hemodynamic data and arterial blood gases were also collected throughout the study. This study strongly suggested that the use of LFV is associated with significantly better Po$_2$ and AaDO$_2$, higher adenine nucleotide levels, lower lactate levels, and reduced histological damage in lung

370

H. Imura et al.

biopsy as well as lower DNA levels in BAL compared to the control group. The CPAP group showed only significantly reduced lactate levels compared to the control group.

39.3.1 Improvement in Arterial Blood Gas Analysis

There was an improvement in arterial blood gas analysis (Fig. 39.3). Pigs receiving LFV had fewer pulmonary abnormalities than the CPAP and control groups. They showed no significant deterioration in Pao_2, $Paco_2$, and $AaDO_2$ after 120 min of CPB, and this was maintained for the subsequent 90-min recovery. The CPAP group did not show significant deterioration in Pco_2 after CPB ($p=0.08$), although the Po_2 level was similar to the control group.

39.3.2 Reduction of Ischemia-Reperfusion Injury

1. DNAinB AL(Fig. 39.4)

The increase of the DNA level in BAL has been used by our group previously as a parameter of ischemic damage of the lungs during CPB.[28] We showed that it correlated with CPB time and pulmonary abnormalities in blood gas analysis after CPB. In the present study, DNA levels in BAL samples were significantly increased in the control and CPAP groups during CPB but not in the LFV-treated group.

2. Tissuea deninenuc leotides(Fig. 39.5)

Total adenine nucleotides (ATP+ADP+AMP) and ATP/ADP ratio were decreased after CPB in the control group and to a lesser extent in the CPAP group.

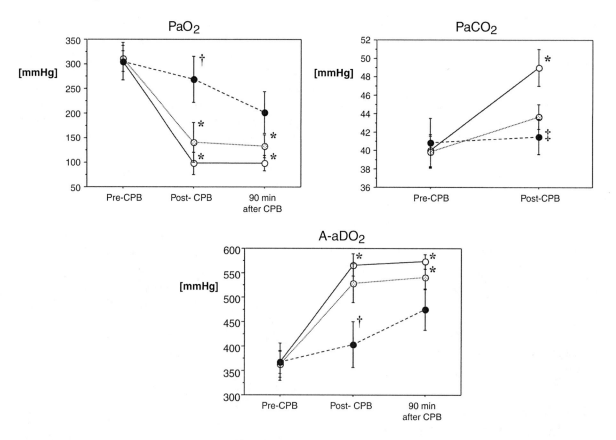

Fig. 39.3 Changes in arterial blood gas analysis in pig model. Only the low-frequency ventilation (LFV) group showed no significant deterioration in Pao_2, $Paco_2$, and $AaDO_2$ during cardiopulmonary bypass (CPB), and this was maintained throughout the post-CPB period. The LFV group showed significant improvements in Po_2 and $AaDO_2$ over the control group imme- diately after CPB. *Open circles* control group, *closed black circles* LFV group, *small dotted circles* CPAP group. *Circles* represent average, and *lines* represent standard deviation. * $p<0.05$ in Friedman test and $P<0.1$ versus pre-CPB value; † $p<0.05$ versus control group; ‡ $p<0.05$ in Kruskal–Wallis test and $P<0.1$ versus control. (Reproduced with permission[35])

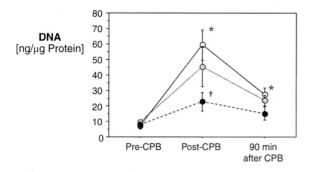

Fig. 39.4 DNA level in bronchoalveolar lavage sample. DNA level in BAL was increased during CPB in control and CPAP groups ($P < 0.005$ and < 0.01 respectively in Friedman test). Two hours after CPB, mean values were still 2–4-folds higher but not statistically significant. The LFV group did not show significant increase ($p > 0.1$ in Friedman test) after CPB and showed significantly less DNA level than control but not CPAP group at the end of CPB. *Open circles* = control group, *closed black circles* = LFV group and *small dots circles* = CPAP group. *Circles* represent average and *line* represents standard deviation. *CPB* cardiopulmonary bypass; * $p < 0.05$ in Friedman test and $P < 0.1$ vs. pre-CPB value; † $p < 0.05$ vs. control group. Reproduced with permission[35]

In contrast, the LFV group showed a higher adenine nucleotide level and ATP/ADP ratio after CPB and subsequent recovery.

3. Tissuela ctate(Fig. 39.6)

Tissue lactate contents were increased during CPB in all groups. However, the increase was significantly less in the LFV group. The CPAP group showed less lactatea ccumulationtha nthe c ontrolgroup.

39.3.3 Histopathological Examinations

Regarding histopathological examinations (Figs. 39.7 and 39.8 and Table 39.1), lung injury was summarized as atelectasia and pulmonary edema in light microscopy and type I cell edema and microvilli diminutions of type II cells in electronic microscopy. The LFV group showed significantly less derangement than the control group during and after CPB in all pathological examinations (Fig. 39.7b, c and Fig. 39.8c, Table 39.1). The CPAP group also showed improvements, although the benefits were less than for the LFV group (Fig. 39.8d, e, Table 39.1). Atelectasis was the most prominent change during CPB, and the protective effect of LFV was largely attributed to a significant reduction in this group of animals.

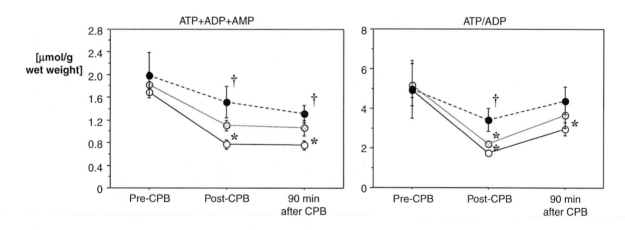

Fig. 39.5 Changes in adenine nucleotides in lung tissue. Total adenine nucleotides (ATP + ADP + AMP) and ATP/ADP ratio were decreased after cardiopulmonary bypass (CPB) in the control ($p = 0.01$ and 0.006 in Friedman test) group, whereas no significant changes in these parameters were seen in the low-frequency ventilation (LFV) group. The continuous positive airway pressure (CPAP) group also showed a decrease in ATP/ADP ratio at the end of CPB ($p = 0.03$ in Friedman test; Fig. 39.4). The LFV group showed higher adenine nucleotide levels and ATP/ADP ratio after CPB over the control group. The CPAP group showed higher total adenine nucleotide levels than the control group, but this did not reach statistical significance. *Open circles* control group, *closed black circles* LFV group, *small dotted circles* CPAP group. *Circles* represent average, and *lines* represent standard deviation. * $p < 0.05$ in Friedman test and $P < 0.1$ versus pre-CPB value; † $p < 0.05$ versus control group. *ADP* adenosine diphosphate, *AMP* adenosine monophosphate, *ATP* adenosine triphosphate (Reproduced with permission[35])

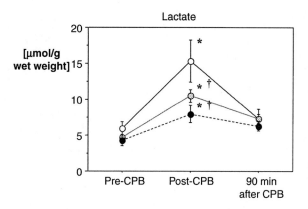

Fig. 39.6 Changes in lactate in lung tissue. Tissue lactate contents were increased during cardiopulmonary bypass (CPB) in each group (control $P = 0.009$, continuous positive airway pressure [CPAP] $p = 0.006$, and low-frequency ventilation [LFV] $p = 0.018$ in Friedman test). The increase was significantly less in the LFV than in control group. *Open circles* control group, *closed black circles* LFV group, *small dotted circles* CPAP group. *Circles* represent average, and *lines* represent standard deviation. * $p < 0.05$ in Friedman test and $P < 0.1$ versus pre-CPB value; † $p < 0.05$ versus control group. (Reproduced with permission[35])

39.4 Limitation and Controversy for Mechanical Ventilation During CPB

A study of neonatal piglets in which mechanical ventilation was used during CPB reported significant metabolic damage and deficiency of oxygenation attributed to ischemia and reperfusion injury.[37] This may be related to the difference between matured and immature pig lungs concerning the behavior of bronchial arterial blood flow during CPB, which is thought to be important to decrease ischemia damage during CPB. In matured piglets, a significant deterioration in pulmonary functions after CPB has been observed following ligation of bronchial arteries before CPB is instituted.[38] There is also evidence that bronchial arterial blood flow is extremely decreased during CPB in the neonatal piglet.[39] Mucin increases in the respiratory tract during CPB, and a positive correlation with postoperative pulmonary dysfunction has been shown only in pediatric surgery and not in adult cardiac surgery.[28]

The evidence regarding the effect of LFV or mechanical ventilation during CPB is now being accumulated; however, most experimental studies, including ours, only focused on the first 1 or 2 h after CPB. Furthermore, the ideal frequency of ventilation is still not known.

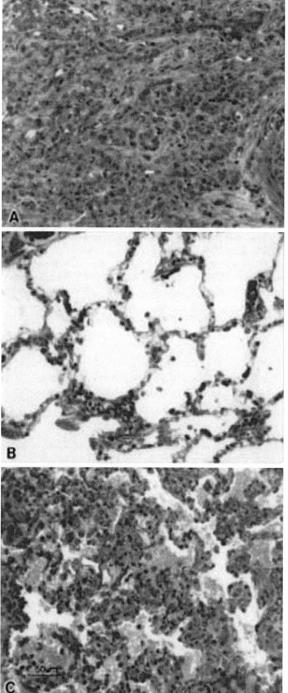

Fig. 39.7 Light micrographs showing alveoli 90 min after cardiopulmonary bypass. (a) Control group showing many atelectases and tissue pulmonary edema. (b) Low-frequency ventilation (LFV) group showing normal lung tissue. (c) Continuous positive airway pressure (CPAP) group showing amorphous material field in alveolar space. (Reproduced with permission[35])

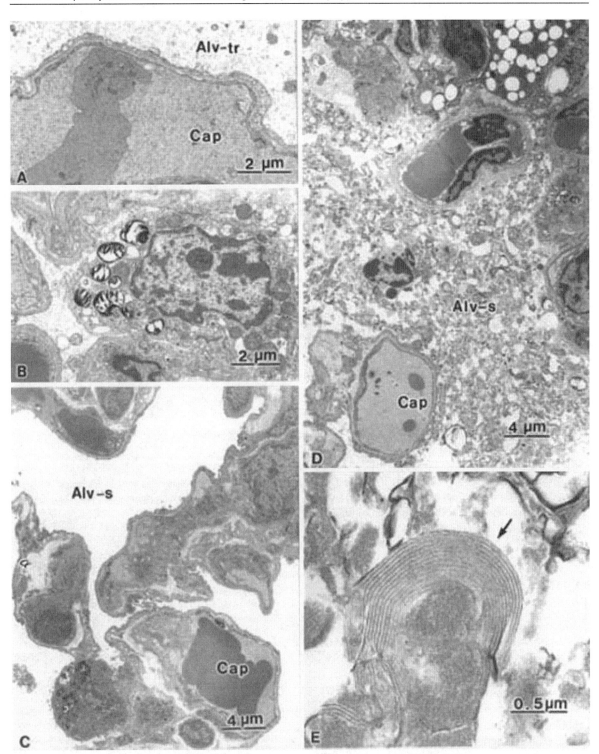

Fig. 39.8 Electron micrographs showing alveoli 90 min after cardiopulmonary bypass. (**a**) Cell edema is seen in type I alveolar epithelial cells (control group). (**b**) Degenerated microvilli are seen in type II alveolar epithelial cells (control group). (**c**) Low-frequency ventilation (LFV) showing no damages. (**d**) Surfactant materials filed in alveolar space (continuous positive airway pressure [CPAP] group). (**e**) Lamellar structures and onion-like surfactant material structures (*arrow*) (CPAP group). *Alv-s* alveolar space, *Alv-tr* alveolar transudate, *Cap* capillary. (Reproduced with permission[35])

Table39 .1 Semiquantification of histopathological changes in lung tissues evaluated by light and electron microscopy

		Atelectasis	Pulmonary edema	Edema of type I cells	Disappearanceof microvilli in type II cells
Before CPB	LFV	±	±	−	−
	CPAP	±	−	−	−
	Control	±	±	−	−
Endof C PB	LFV	±**	±**	−**	−**
	CPAP	+*,**	−**	+	−**
	Control	++*	+*	+*	+*
90 mina fterC PB	LFV	±**	±**	−**	−**
	CPAP	+*	±*	−***	−
	Control	++*	+*	+*	±

CPB cardiopulmonary bypass, *LFV* low-frequency ventilation, *CPAP* continuous positive airway pressure

Control group showed significant atelectasis and pulmonary edema 90 min after cardiopulmonary bypass. Control group also showed edema of type I cells and disappearance of microvilli of type II cells. LFV and CPAP groups showed less damage; however, the CPAP group showed proteinosis 90 min after cardiopulmonary bypass

Statistical analysis was applied by converting the grading to ordinal numbers: grade (−)=0, (±)=1, (+)=2, (++)=3. The final grading results were determined from the median value of all observations in each respective group

*$p<0.05$ in Friedman test and $P<0.1$ versus pre-CPB value

**$p<0.05$ versus control group

***$p<0.05$ in Kruskal–Wallis test and $P<0.1$ versus control. Reproduced with permission[35]

In clinical practice, the technique can create visualization problems during inflation of the lungs or due to increased blood flow return, particularly in mitral valve surgery. Prospective, randomized studies will be necessary to determine whether the experimental findings can be translated into routine clinical practice.

39.5 Conclusion

In summary, LFV during CPB reduced tissue metabolic and histopathological damages in the lungs and was associated with improved postoperative gas exchange in an experimental pig model. The mode of action of this technique is probably due to reduction in ischemic changes and prevention of atelectasis. The technique to decrease ischemic damage in our experimental model is based on ventilation and does not influence pulmonary flow. These findings might have important clinical implications since many cardiac surgeons believe that maintaining ventilation is more practicable than keeping blood flow to the lungs during cardiac operations. LFV did not reduce visualization of the surgical fieldi nourpigC PBmode l.

References

1. Grover FL. The Society of Thoracic Surgeons National Database: current status and future directions. *Ann Thorac Surg*.1999; 68:367-373.
2. Hall RI, Smith MS, Rocker G. The systemic inflammatory response to cardiopulmonary bypass: pathophysiological, therapeutic, and pharmacological considerations. *Anesth Anal*.1997; 85:766-782.
3. Gao D, Grunwald GK, Rumsfeld JS, et al. Variation in mortality risk factors with time after coronary artery bypass operations. *Ann Thorac Surg*.2003; 75:74-81.
4. Ascione R, Clinton TL, Underwood MJ, et al. Inflammatory response after coronary revascularisation with or without cardiopulmonary bypass. *Ann Thorac Surg*. 2000;69:1198-1204.
5. Rothenburger M, Soeparwata R, Deng MC, et al. Prediction of clinical outcome after cardiac surgery: the role of cytokines, endotoxin, and anti-endotoxin core antibodies. *Shock*. 2001;16(suppl1) :44-50.
6. Ascione R, Lloyd CT, Underwood MJ, Lotto AA, Pitsis AA, Angelini GD. Economic outcome of off-pump coronary artery bypass surgery: a prospective randomized study. *Ann Thorac Surg*.1999; 68(6):2237-2242.
7. Johnson D, Thomson D, Hurst TBM, et al. Neutrophilmediated acute lung injury after extracorporeal perfusion. *J Thorac Cardiovasc Surg*.1994; 107:1193-1202.
8. Ranieri VM, Suter PM, Tortorella C, et al. Effect of mechanical ventilation on inflammatory mediators in patients with acute respiratory distress syndrome: a randomized controlled trial. *JAMA*.1999; 282:54-61.

9. Asimokopoulos G, Smith PLC, et al. Lung injury and acute respiratory distress syndrome after cardiopulmonary bypass. *Ann Thorac Surg*.1999; 68:1107-1115.

10. Seghaye M, Duchateau J, Bruniaux J, et al. Interleukin-10 release related to cardiopulmonary bypass in infants undergoing cardiac operations. *J Thorac Cardiovasc Surg*. 1996; 111:545-553.

11. Pinhu L, Whitehead T, Evans T, Griffiths M. Ventilator-associated lung injury. *Lancet*.2003; 361:332-340.

12. Magnusson L, Zemgulis V, Wicky S, Tyden H, Thelin S, Hedenstierna G. Atelectasis is a major cause of hypoxemia and shunt after cardiopulmonary bypass. An experimental study. *Anesthesiology*.1996; 87:1153-1163.

13. Goebel U, Siepe M, Mecklenburg A, et al. Reduced pulmonary inflammatory response during cardiopulmonary bypass: effects of combined pulmonary perfusion and carbon monoxide inhalation. *Eur J Cardiothorac Surg*. 2008;34:1165-1172.

14. Borgermann J, Flohe S, et al. Regulation of cytokine synthesis in cardiac surgery: role of extracorporeal circuit and humoral mediators in vivo and in vitro. *Inflamm Res*. 2007;56:126-132.

15. Constantinopol M, Jones JH, Weibel ER, Hoppelar H, Lidholm A, Karas RH. Oxygen transport during exercise in large mammals. II. Oxygen uptake by the pulmonary gas exchanger. *J Appl Physiol*.1989; 67:871-878.

16. West JB, Mathews FL. Stresses, strains, and surface pressures in the lung caused by weight. *J Appl Physiol*. 1987; 32:332-345.

17. West JB, Mathieu-Costello O. Strength of the pulmonary blood–gas barrier. *Respir Physiol*.1992; 88:141-148.

18. West JB, Mathieu-Costello O. Structure, strength, failure, and remodeling of the pulmonary blood–gas barrier. *Annu Rev Physiol*.1999;61: 543-572.

19. West JB. Cellular responses to mechanical stress: pulmonary capillary stress failure. *J Appl Physiol*. 2000;89: 2483-2489.

20. Verheiji J, van Lingen A, Raijmakers PG, et al. Pulmonary abnormalities after cardiac surgery are better explained by atelectasis than increased permeability oedema. *Acta Anaesthesiol Scand*.2005; 49:1302-1310.

21. Liu X-L, Sato S, Dai W, Yamanaka N. The protective effect of hepatocyte growth-promoting factor (pHGF) against hydrogen peroxide-induced acute lung injury in rats. *Med Electron Microsc*.2001; 34:92-102.

22. Ovechkin AV, Lominadze D, Sedoris KC, Robinson TW, Tyagi SC, Roberts AM. Lung ischemia-reperfusion injury: implication of oxidative stress and platelet-arteriolar wall interactions. *Arch Physiol Biochem*. 2007;113:1-12.

23. Mordy DL, Chiu C-J, Hinchey EJ. The roles of ventilation and perfusion in lung metabolism. *J Thorac Cardiovasc Surg*. 1977;74:275-285.

24. Hamvas A, Park C-K, Palazzo R, Liptay M, Cooper J, Schuster DP. Modified pulmonary ischemia-reperfusion injury by altering ventilatory strategies during ischemia. *J Appl Physiol*.1992; 73:2112-2119.

25. De Leyn PRJ, Lerut TE, Schreinemmakers HHJ, Van Raemdonck DEM, Mubagwa K, Flameng W. Effect of infla-

tion on adenosine triphosphate catabolism and lactate production during normothermic lung ischemia. *Ann Thorac Surg*.1993; 55:1073-1079.

26. Bishop MJ, Holman RG, Guidotti SM, Alberts MK, Chi EY. Pulmonary artery occlusion and lung collapse depletes rabbit lung adenosine triphosphate. *Anesthesiology*. 1994; 80:611-617.

27. John LCH, Ervine IM. A study assessing the potential benefit of continued ventilation during cardiopulmonary bypass. *Interact Cardiovasc Thorac Surg*.2008; 7:14-17.

28. Imura H, Duncan P, Corfield P, et al. Increased airway mucin after cardiopulmonary bypass associated with postoperative respiratory complications in children. *J Thorac Cardiovasc Surg*.2004; 127:963-969.

29. Aikawa T, Shimura H, Sasaki H, et al. Marked goblet cell hyperplasia with mucus accumulation in the airway of patients who died of severe acute asthmatic attacks. *Chest*. 1992;101:916-921.

30. Bernstein JM, Reddy M. Bacteria-mucin interaction in the upper aerodigestive tract shows striking heterogeneity: Implications in otitis media, rhinosinusitis, and pneumonia. *Otolaryngol Head Neck Surg*.2000; 122:514-520.

31. Louahed J, Toda M, Jen J, et al. Interleukin-9 upregulates mucus expression in the airways. *Am J Respir Cell Mol Biol*. 2000;22(6):649-656.

32. Amitani R, Wilson R, Rutman A, et al. Effects of human neutrophil elastase and Pseudomonas aeruginosa proteinases on human respiratory epithelium. *Am J Respir Cell Mol Biol*. 1991;4:26-32.

33. Breuer R, Christensen TG, Lucey EC, et al. An ultrastructural morphometric analysis of elastase-treated hamster bronchi shows discharge followed by progressive accumulation of secretory granules. *Am Rev Respir Dis*.1987; 136:698-703.

34. Voynow JA, Young LR, Wang Y, et al. Neutrophil elastase increase MUC5AC mRNA and protein expression in respiratory epithelial cells. *Am J Physiol*.1999; 276:L835-L843.

35. Imura H, Caputo M, Lim K, et al. Pulmonary injury after cardiopulmonary bypass: beneficial effects of low frequency mechanical ventilation. *J Thorac Cardiovasc Surg*. 2009; 137(6):1530-1537.

36. Miranda DR, Gommers D, Papadakos J, Lachmann B. Mechanical ventilation affects pulmonary inflammation in cardiac surgery patients: the role of the open-lung concept. *J Cardiothorac Vasc Anesth*.2007; 21:279-284.

37. Serraf A, Robotin M, Bonnet N, et al. Alteration of the neonatal pulmonary physiology after total cardiopulmonary bypass. *J Thorac Cardiovasc Surg*.1997; 114:1061-1069.

38. Dodd-o JM, Welsh LE, Salazar JD, et al. Effect of bronchial artery blood flow on cardiopulmonary bypass-induced lung injury. *Am J Physiol Heart Circ Physiol*. 2004; 286: H693-H700.

39. Schlensak C, Doenst T, Preußer S, Wunderlich M, Kleinschmidt M, Beyersdorf F. Cardiopulmonary bypass reduction of bronchial blood flow: A potential mechanism for lung injury in a neonatal pig model. *J Thorac Cardiovasc Surg*. 2002;123:1199-1205.

40

Inhaled Carbon Monoxide as an Experimental Therapeutic Strategy of Lung Protection During CardiopulmonaryB ypass

Torsten Loop, Ulrich Goebel, Friedhelm Beyersdorf, and Christian Schlensak

Pulmonary dysfunction in patients after cardiac surgery using cardiopulmonary bypass (CPB) is associated with an increase in morbidity and mortality.[1,2] Pulmonary impairment and dysfunction may range in severity from subclinical functional changes and prolonged postoperative ventilation to acute lung injury and acute respiratory distress syndrome.[3] Acute respiratory distress syndrome occurs in about 2% of all cases after CPB and has an associated mortality of more than 60%.[4] Causative factors for the inflammatory response are, among others, the pulmonary ischemia during bypass and reperfusion injury after declamping, blood contact with the surface of the extracorporeal circulation unit, endotoxemia, surgical trauma, and blood loss.

This chapter describes experimental evidence of the pharmacological strategy of carbon monoxide inhalation adopted or under investigation to reduce pulmonary dysfunction.

The gaseous molecule carbon monoxide has anti-inflammatory and antiapoptotic properties.[5,6] At low concentrations of carbon monoxide (250 ppm), it has been demonstrated to suppress inflammation and reduce apoptosis in numerous in vitro and in vivo studies.[6–9] The limited toxicity of carbon monoxide is underscored by the observation that carbon monoxide is also generated endogenously via the inducible heme oxygenase enzyme I. Previous studies reported a significant reduction in renal cytokine expression due to carbon monoxide administration in various ischemia and reperfusion models.[6,8] In a previous study, we tested the hypothesis that inhaled carbon monoxide before initiation of CPB would reduce the inflammatory response in the lungs.[10]

Our findings support the hypothesis that inhaled carbon monoxide provides pulmonary anti-inflammatory and antiapoptotic effects during CPB.[10] In addition, and of greater importance, these effects occurred when carbon monoxide was administered only as a pretreatment, with the advantage of short exposure time, which results in limited binding to hemoglobin since the extent of carbon monoxide hemoglobin formation depends on the dose and the time of application.[11] The effect had the following characteristics: (1) Systemic inflammation and adverse effects on extrapulmonary organs seemed to be less important since cytokine messenger RNA (mRNA) expression in mononuclear blood cells was not detectable, and serum markers of hepatic, cardiac, or renal injury were also not detectable. (2) Carbon monoxide inhalation suppressed the CPB-induced pulmonary expression of the proinflammatory cytokines tumor necrosis factor alpha (TNF-α) and interleukin (IL) 1β. (3) Carbon monoxide inhalation significantly induced pulmonary IL-10 protein levels during the whole experiment. (4) Analysis of mRNA cytokine transcripts suggested a transcriptional regulation due to carbon monoxide-mediated effects. (5) Apoptosis in the lung was attenuated since carbon monoxide inhalation inhibited effector caspase activity in lung tissue during CPB.

T. Loop(✉)
Department of Anesthesiology and Critical Care Medicine, UniversityM edicalC enter, Freiburg, Germany
e-mail:t orsten.loop@uniklinik-freiburg.de

E.A. Gabriel and T. Salerno (eds.), *Principles of Pulmonary Protection in Heart Surgery*,
DOI: 10.1007/978-1-84996-308-4_40, © Springer-Verlag London Limited 2010

Our data suggest that the anti-inflammatory and antiapoptotic properties of carbon monoxide may confer cytoprotection in a pig model of CPB-induced pulmonary inflammation and dysfunction (see Fig. 40.1).[10]

In a similar study, Lavitrano et al. reported that inhaled carbon monoxide may also improve cardiac bioenergetics and attenuate myocardial apoptosis after CPB.[12]

The protective effects of carbon monoxide involve an increased heat shock response, demonstrated by expression of the inducible heat shock protein 70 (HSP70) in murine lung endothelial cells and fibroblasts.[13] The cytoprotective capacity of heat shock proteins may be partly related to their ability to stabilize intracellular protein structures, which allows cells and organisms facing life-threatening insults resumption of normal cellular and physiological activities.[14,15]

The aim of our next study was to elucidate the mechanism by which inhaled carbon monoxide may exert its protective effects during CPB. We hypothesized that the protective effects of inhaled carbon monoxide may be mediated via an increased expression of heat shock proteins.

The main findings of our randomized experimental in vivo study in pigs can be summarized as follows: Inhalation of carbon monoxide before CPB (1) induced pulmonary Hsp70 and Hsp90 gene and protein expression, (2) induced Heat Shock Factor-1 (HSF-1) DNA binding activity, (3) prevented CPB-associated increases in pulmonary IL-6 mRNA and protein concentration, (4) prevented CPB-associated histological findings of lung injury, and (5) inhibited CPB-associated alveolar macrophage infiltration. Intravenous administration of quercetin before pretreatment with inhaled carbon monoxide antagonized the analyzed carbon monoxide-induced changes; it (1) abolished expression of pulmonary heat shock proteins, (2) inhibited activation of HSF-1, (3) prevented suppression of increases in IL-6 protein concentration, (4) abolished suppression of histopathological lung injury, and (5) attenuated the carbon monoxide-related inhibition of macrophage infiltration.[16]

These findings support our hypothesis that inhaled carbon monoxide before CPB mediates its pulmonary anti-inflammatory and cytoprotective effects via increased expression of heat shock proteins (see Figs. 40.2a nd 40.3).[16]

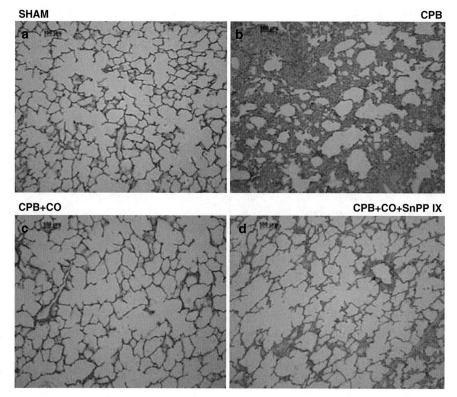

SHAM **CPB**

CPB+CO **CPB+CO+SnPP IX**

Fig.40.1 Microscopic images of the pig's lung at 120 min after CPB. Representative lung sections of animals treated with SHAM (**a**), CPB (**b**), CPB + CO (**c**),a nd CPB + CO + SnPP IX (**d**)a fter hematoxylin and eosin staining. Original magnification ×40 (**a**–**d**). *SHAM* control group, *CPB*c ardiopulmonary bypass, *CO* carbon monoxide, *SnPP IX* tin protoporphyrineI X[10]

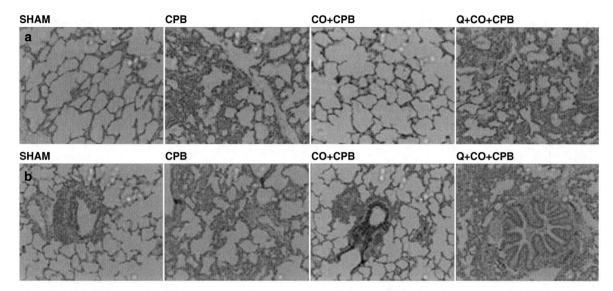

Fig. 40.2 Representative histological lung sections at 120 min after cardiopulmonary bypass (CPB). Lung sections (×40) in SHAM (control) and following CPB, pretreatment with inhaled carbon monoxide (CO+CPB), and administration of quercetin (Q) before pretreatment with inhaled carbon monoxide (Q+CO+CPB) after heat shock protein 70 (Hsp70) (**a**) and Hsp90 staining (**b**). The brown staining reflects Hsp expression[16]

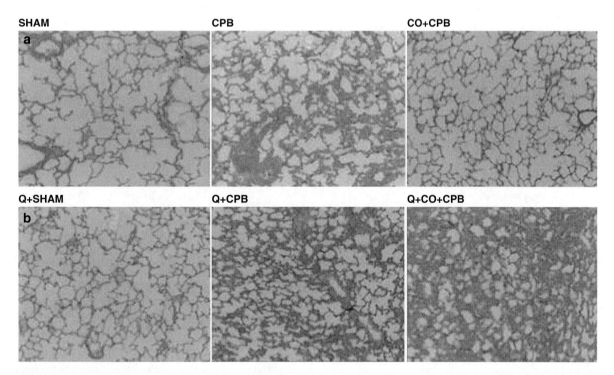

Fig. 40.3 Representative histological lung sections at 120 min after cardiopulmonary bypass (CPB). Lung sections (hematoxylin and eosin staining, ×40) in SHAM (control) and following CPB alone, pretreatment with inhaled carbon monoxide (CO+CPB), pretreatment of SHAM controls with quercetin (Q+SHAM), pretreatment of CPB group with quercetin (Q+CPB), and administration of quercetin before pretreatment with inhaled carbon monoxide (Q+CO+CPB)[16]

Since use of CPB may be associated with extrapulmonary organ dysfunction as hepatic or kidney injury, we hypothesized that pretreatment with inhaled carbon monoxide prevents CPB-associated acute kidney injury.

The main findings of the unpublished data in the same pig model can be summarized as follows: CPB was associated with renal (1) inflammatory response, (2) cellular injury, and (3) apoptosis. Pretreatment with inhaled carbon monoxide was associated with a renal (1) anti-inflammatory effect, (2) protective effect, (3) antiapoptotic effect, and (4) activation of the heat shock response. Pretreatment with quercetin counteracted the carbon monoxide-associated (1) anti-inflammatory effect, (2) protective effect, (3) antiapoptotic effect, and it counteracted (4) the activation of the heat shock response.

These findings are suggestive of renal anti-inflammatory and antiapoptotic effects and renoprotection by inhaled carbon monoxide administered before CPB. They further supported our hypothesis that the renoprotective effect of inhaled carbon monoxide is mediated by activation of the heat shock response, in particular by the increased renal expression of Hsp70.

On the basis of the results presented here in animal studies, we cannot propose that carbon monoxide might possibly used as an anti-inflammatory agent in human cardiac surgery with CPB because controlled human studies correlating carboxyhemoglobin to organ function do not exist. The use of a gas normally considered toxic must be carefully weighed. We used lower concentrations compared to the few human studies, which examined the effects of continuous carbon monoxide inhalation on carboxyhemoglobin levels.[17–19] A clinical study by Mayr et al. showed no clinical signs of carbon monoxide toxicity after exposure of 250 and 500 ppm in healthy humans.[20] Modest increases in carboxyhemoglobin levels equivalent to that resulting from cigarette smoking do not have any appreciable acute sympathetic and hemodynamic effects in healthy humans.[19] Furthermore, the concentrations used here were lower than the levels used in humans (0.2%) during measurement of lung diffusion capacity for carbon monoxide lung diffusion capacity for carbon monoxide. Defined in the text and well known lung function test (DLCO), a standard pulmonary function test.[21]

In conclusion, the findings of carbon monoxide treatment prior to CPB supported the theories that inhaled carbon monoxide provides pulmonary and renal protective effects during CPB. The upregulation of heat shock proteins may be an important mediator of the protective effects of inhaled carbon monoxide. Based on the observations of our work, it is tempting to speculate that inhaled carbon monoxide could represent a potential new therapeutic modality for counteractingC PB-inducedlunginjury .

References

1. Butler J, Baigrie RJ, Parker D, et al. Systemic inflammatory responses to cardiopulmonary bypass: a pilot study of the effects of pentoxifylline. Respir Med.1993; 87:285-288.
2. Laffey JG, Boylan JF, Cheng DC. The systemic inflammatory response to cardiac surgery: implications for the anesthesiologist. Anesthesiology.2002; 97:215-252.
3. Weissman C. Pulmonary function after cardiac and thoracic surgery. Anesth Analg.1999; 88:1272-1279.
4. Milot J, Perron J, Lacasse Y, Letourneau L, Cartier PC, Maltais F. Incidence and predictors of ARDS after cardiac surgery. Chest.2001; 119:884-888.
5. Zhang B, Tang C, Du J. Changes of heme oxygenase-carbon monoxide system in vascular calcification in rats. Life Sci. 2003;72:1027-1037.
6. Otterbein LE, Bach FH, Alam J, et al. Carbon monoxide has anti-inflammatory effects involving the mitogen-activated protein kinase pathway. Nat Med.2000; 6:422-428.
7. Dolinay T, Szilasi M, Liu M, Choi AM. Inhaled carbon monoxide confers antiinflammatory effects against ventilator-induced lung injury. Am J Respir Crit Care Med. 2004;170:613-620.
8. Song R, Kubo M, Morse D, et al. Carbon monoxide induces cytoprotection in rat orthotopic lung transplantation via anti-inflammatory and anti-apoptotic effects. Am J Pathol. 2003;163:231-242.
9. Liu XM, Chapman GB, Peyton KJ, Schafer AI, Durante W. Carbon monoxide inhibits apoptosis in vascular smooth muscle cells. Cardiovasc Res.2002; 55:396-405.
10. Goebel U, Siepe M, Mecklenburg A, et al. Carbon monoxide inhalation reduces pulmonary inflammatory response during cardiopulmonary bypass in pigs. Anesthesiology. 2008;108:102536.
11. Hoetzel A, Dolinay T, Schmidt R, Choi AM, Ryter SW. Carbon monoxide in sepsis. Antioxid Redox Signal. 2007;9:2013-2026.
12. Lavitrano M, Smolenski RT, Musumeci A, et al. Carbon monoxide improves cardiac energetics and safeguards the heart during reperfusion after cardiopulmonary bypass in pigs. FASEB J.2004; 18:1093-1095.
13. Kim HP, Wang X, Zhang J, et al. Heat shock protein-70 mediates the cytoprotective effect of carbon monoxide: involvement of p38 beta MAPK and heat shock factor-1. J Immunol.2005; 175:2622-2629.
14. Wong HR. Heat shock proteins. Facts, thoughts, and dreams. A. De Maio. Shock 11:1–12, 1999. Shock. 1999;12:323-325.
15. Cobb JP, Hotchkiss RS, Karl IE, Buchman TG. Mechanisms of cell injury and death. Br J Anaesth.1996; 77:3-10.
16. Goebel U, Mecklenburg A, Siepe M, et al. Protective effects of inhaled carbon monoxide in pig lungs during cardiopul-

monary bypass are mediated via an induction of the heat shock response. *Br J Anaesth*.2009; 103:173-184.

17. Takeuchi A, Vesely A, Rucker J, et al. A simple "new" method to accelerate clearance of carbon monoxide. *Am J Respir Crit Care Med*.2000; 161:1816-1819.

18. Hausberg M, Mark AL, Winniford MD, Brown RE, Somers VK. Sympathetic and vascular effects of short-term passive smoke exposure in healthy nonsmokers. *Circulation*. 1997; 96:282-287.

19. Hausberg M, Somers VK. Neural circulatory responses to carbon monoxide in healthy humans. *Hypertension*. 1997;29:1114-1118.

20. Mayr FB, Spiel A, Leitner J, et al. Effects of carbon monoxide inhalation during experimental endotoxemia in humans. *Am J Respir Crit Care Med*.2005; 171:354-360.

21. Graham BL, Mink JT, Cotton DJ. Effects of increasing carboxyhemoglobin on the single breath carbon monoxide diffusing capacity. *Am J Respir Crit Care Med*. 2002;165:1504-1510.

Lung Perfusion and Coronary Artery BypassG rafting

41

Parwis Massoudy and Heinz Jakob

41.1 PhysiologicalC onsiderations

If there is no shunt defect, the total blood volume entering the right heart is thereafter ejected into the lungs. Apart from the blood entering the lungs over the right heart, the lungs are perfused via bronchial arteries that are branches of the descending aorta. The bronchial arteries primarily have nutritive function and are thought not to contribute to the oxygenation of the circulating blood. The contribution of bronchial arteries to the perfusion of the lungs may be as low as 1–3%.[1,2] Bronchial venous blood is collected in the right and, mainly, left atrium.

41.2 CardiopulmonaryB ypass and Lung Function

Routine cardiac surgery, conducted with cardiopulmonary bypass (CPB), is performed by draining blood from the right atrium and thereby excluding the lungs from the circulation. When atrial drainage is complete, only the nutritive blood supply to the lungs via the bronchial arteries remains. During CPB, the relative contribution of the bronchial and pulmonary arteries in delivering oxygen to maintain lung tissue viability is unclear.[3]

In cardiac surgery using CPB, pulmonary ischemia is always of longer duration than is cardiac ischemia. After release of the aortic cross clamp, cardiac reperfusion on

CPB begins and is performed according to the duration of prior cardiac ischemia. Meanwhile, lung ischemia continues until termination of CPB. Nevertheless, with regard to a critical duration of organ ischemia, the heart is always in the focus of the discussion, whereas recovery of the lungs is taken for granted. This is explained with the longer ischemic tolerance of the lungs compared with the heart, but it may also be associated with a certain rest perfusion of the lungs via the nutritive circulation over the bronchial arteries as mentioned here. However, with the beginning of CPB, bronchial arterial blood flow also seems to decrease and remain decreased until termination of CPB. Sixty minutes after the end of CPB, it was described to return to baseline levels.[4]

In patients undergoing CPB, postoperative pulmonary dysfunction remains a significant clinical problem. The observed changes range from subclinical functional changes to severe and life-threatening complications, such as adult acute respiratory distress syndrome (ARDS), which was reported to occur in about 2% of cases after CPB.[3]

41.3 Pathophysiologyo f Cardiopulmonary Bypass

Accordingly, postoperative pulmonary dysfunction after cardiac surgery using CPB may lead to prolonged periods of mechanical ventilation or reduced pulmonary blood gas levels before or after extubation. Some authors even described long-standing deterioration in pulmonary function up to 3.5 months after cardiac surgery.[5] Pulmonary dysfunction may, however, not be as overt and thus only be quantified using more sophisticated measures. Pulmonary neutrophil entrapment and resultant oxidative injury are thought to be primary

P.M assoudy (✉)
Departmentof C ardiacSur gery,
KlinikumP assau, Germany
e-mail:P arwis.Massoudy@klinikum-passau.de

E.A. Gabriel and T. Salerno (eds.), *Principles of Pulmonary Protection in Heart Surgery*,
DOI: 10.1007/978-1-84996-308-4_41, © Springer-Verlag London Limited 2010

mechanisms of CPB-induced lung injury.[6] We determined the levels of leukocytes and platelets in the blood of the right atrium and pulmonary vein during CPB.[7] Leukocyte counts in the pulmonary vein were 85% of leukocyte counts in the right atrium. Homonymous results were obtained for platelet counts, polymorphonuclear cell counts, and monocyte counts, indicating retention of the respective blood cells in the lungs under CPB conditions.[7] On CPB, inflammatory cytokines such as interleukin (IL) 6 and IL-8 have been found to be produced in the lungs.[8] Aprotinin was found to reduce neutrophil accumulation in the lungs post-CPB, namely by a reduction of IL-8 production.[6] Accordingly, the application of a monoclonal antibody against IL-8 prevented neutrophil infiltration in the reperfused lung.[9] Sequestration of neutrophils into post-CPB lung tissue was found to be mediated by CD18, a leukocyte adhesion molecule.[10] Cardiopulmonary bypass was also shown to increase endothelin 1 (ET-1) production and ET-1 receptor expression in the lung,[11] indicating an impairment of the balance between endothelium-dependent vasodilation and vasoconstrictor production, favoring pulmonary hypertension. Thromboxane A_2, another potent vasoconstrictor, was also found to be produced in the lungs of patients undergoing CPB.[12] Reduction of pulmonary perfusion, largely entire in cases of total CPB, was shown to yield significant alterations of endothelium-dependent pulmonary microvascular responses.[13]

Thus, inflammatory mediators are produced by the ischemic and reperfused pulmonary tissues, leading to activation and retention of circulating blood cells, which again may release inflammatory mediators and thereby aggravate the initial inflammatory reaction.

Findings have demonstrated the prominent role of the endothelial glycocalyx in the regulation of inflammation and vascular permeability.[14] The endothelial glycocalyx is astonishingly thick (>300 nm) and seems to constitute an exclusion zone for circulating blood cells. Ischemia and reperfusion seem to promote shedding of the endothelial glycocalyx, thus exposing the underlying endothelial cells and thereby enabling the much shorter adhesion molecules (<10 nm) to make contact with circulating cells.[14] This may then lead to the described release of inflammatory mediators (Fig. 41.1) and retention of circulating blood cells during pulmonary passage.[8]

Another factor contributing to the proinflammatory status of CPB is the large extracorporeal surface of the heart-lung machine. It consists not only of the tubing system but also and to a large extent, of the external oxygenator with a surface area of over 3 m[2].[15] The direct blood-gas interface further induces contact activation of circulating blood cells.[16] Furthermore, although high-dose heparin is applied to prevent coagulation, the generation of thrombin by activation of the coagulation cascade cannot be completely inhibited.[17] Thrombin is again involved in the activation of leukocytes and platelets and acts on the endothelium to release a variety of vasoactive and inflammatory mediators.[18]

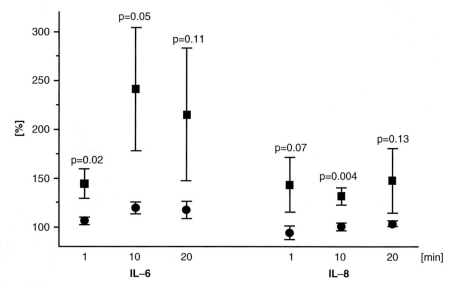

Fig.41.1 Pulmonaryv enous levels of interleukin (IL) 6 and 8 in percentage of right atrial values at 1, 10, and 20 min after the release of the aortic cross clamp in patients undergoing coronary artery bypass grafting (CABG). Conventional cardiopulmonary bypass (CPB) (*boxes*) and bilateral extracorporeal circulation (ECC) (*circles*). Mean ± SEM; be tween-group significance levels are placed above error bars. (From Massoudy et al.[16])

41.4 Perfusion and Ventilation of the Lungs During Extracorporeal Circulation (Bilateral Extracorporeal Circulation)

The early days of the heart-lung machine in the 1950s were associated with considerable morbidity and mortality, for which the external oxygenator was mainly made responsible.[19] In those days, Charles Drew, a cardiac surgeon from London, devised an extracorporeal circulatory support system in which the patient's own lungs functioned as an oxygenator (bilateral extracorporeal circulation [ECC]), thus making the external oxygenator and its large artificial surface unnecessary.[19] He used this technique for 22 years.[20]

Even today, with modern systems for ECC that allow performance of routine cardiac surgery at a very low level of mortality,[21] a significant number of our patients develop postoperative pulmonary dysfunction.[3] In part, this problem is attributed to the blood-synthetic surface interface experienced in the extracorporeal circuit. The inflammatory response described is initiated here, which may escalate to an overt systemic inflammatory response syndrome (SIRS) promoting multiple organ dysfunction.[22,23]

In the late 1990s, a number of studies were published concerning bilateral ECC without the use of an external oxygenator. It is called bilateral because the left and the right sides of the heart are cannulated, and the systemic circulation and the lungs are perfused separately. In the bilateral ECC technique, two additional cannula are placed in the left atrium and the pulmonary artery. The left atrium is cannulated via either the left atrial appendage or the right superior pulmonary vein. During ECC, blood is thus drained from the right atrium into an external reservoir and is thereafter pumped into the pulmonary artery to perfuse the ventilated lungs in an antegrade fashion. After oxygenation in the lungs, pulmonary venous blood is drained from the left atrium into a second reservoir and pumped into the ascending aorta; from there, it is distributed to all other organs in the conventional fashion. Inspiratory oxygen fraction (FIO_2) is set to achieve a target arterial partial pressure of oxygen (PaO_2) of at least 200 mmHg.[7] For the perfusionist, this technique is much more demanding because two circuits have controlled separately.

In a prospective randomized controlled study, 15 patients undergoing elective coronary artery bypass grafting (CABG) were operated with routine CPB, another 15 patients were operated using bilateral ECC.[24] The peak values of proinflammatory IL-6 and IL-8 were significantly lower in patients operated with the bilateral ECC technique. Postoperative treatment was standardized in all 30 patients, thus making their postoperative lung function comparable. The respiratory indices were significantly lower and the partial pressures of oxygen were significantly higher in the patients in the bilateral ECC group, indicating better postoperative lung function. Alveolar-arterial oxygen tension difference and intrapulmonary right-to-left shunting were significantly less in the bilateral ECC group. Along with the described improvement of respiratory parameters, time to extubation was significantly reduced from 9.5 ± 1.2 h in the control group to 5.2 ± 0.4 h in the bilateral ECC group.[24]

Despite the considerably greater prime volume in the bilateral ECC group (2,200 vs. 1,600 mL in the control group) and a more positive fluid balance, extravascular thermal volume did not change in the bilateral ECC group, while it significantly increased in the conventional group. Thus, using the patient's lungs as an oxygenator during ECC was shown to mitigate the increase in extravascular pulmonary fluid observed in conventional CPB,[15] which can easily explain the observed improved respiratory function.

In 18 patients, randomly assigned to either conventional CPB or bilateral ECC, the extent of intraoperative inflammatory response was investigated.[16] Levels of proinflammatory IL-6 and IL-8 and the levels of the adhesion molecules CD11b on monocytes, CD11b on polymorphonuclear neutrophils (PMNs), and CD41 on monocytes were investigated drawing samples of blood from the right atrium and pulmonary vein. In the bilateral ECC patients, levels of both ILs were more or less equal in the right atrial and in the pulmonary venous blood. In the conventional CPB patients, levels in pulmonary venous blood were significantly increased compared with levels in the right atrial blood at various time points (Fig. 41.1), indicating a pulmonary inflammatory reaction in these patients.

In addition, there was a retention of activated leukocytes and platelet-leukocyte coaggregates. The latter changes speak for increased contact between activated blood cells and the pulmonary vascular endothelium.[16] The cellular origin of the increased cytokine levels after pulmonary passage remains unclear. IL-6 and IL-8 have been shown to be released by a variety of leukocyte subsets. On the other hand, lung tissue itself could be the origin of the increased cytokine levels. IL-8 is known to be localized, preformed, in vascular endothelial cells, from where it can be released on stimulation.[25]

Thus, the bilateral ECC technique showed some advantages in a clinical setting. However, all patients investigated were at relatively low risk. These patients typically have an uneventful postoperative recovery after conventional CABG.

41.5 OtherC linicalandExp erimental Models of Perfusion of the Lungs During Extracorporeal Circulation

In a population of children with congenital heart defects and pulmonary hypertension, Suzuki et al. performed cardiopulmonary bypass with an external oxygenator and concomitant perfusion of the lungs at a flow rate of 30 mL/min via a cardioplegic cannula inserted into the pulmonary artery.[26] When compared with a group of children operated under a conventional CPB regimen, the ratio of Pao_2/Fio_2 was higher in the perfused group than in the control group, with the difference persisting throughout the observation period from 3 to 24 h after termination of CPB. Duration of postoperative ventilatory support was significantly less in the perfused group.[26] In an adult cardiac surgical patient population, cardiopulmonary bypass was supplemented by pulmonary artery perfusion with 1 L/min of arterial blood from the CPB circuit, cooled to 15°C by a separate heat exchanger. Perfusion was maintained for 10 min.[27] After termination of CPB, alveolar-arterial oxygen difference ($AaDO_2$) was significantly higher in the control group than in the perfusion group. The effect was further improved when ultrafiltration was applied.[28]

In an experimental model, piglets (mean weight 5.0 ± 0.5 kg) were subjected to 120 min of total CPB, and controlled lung perfusion was performed via the pulmonary artery. Oxygenated, normothermic autologous blood was perfused at a maximum pressure of 20 mmHg, which was equivalent to a blood flow of 100–150 mL/min.[4] An increase in alveolar thickness and significant accumulations of albumin, lactate dehydrogenase, neutrophils, and elastase in the bronchoalveolar lavage,

observed under control conditions, could all be significantly attenuated under controlled pulmonary perfusion.[4] The same group also demonstrated a reduced pulmonary inflammatory response during CPB when the lungs were perfused, and the vasodilator carbon monoxide was inhaled.[27] In another experimental model, CPB was performed in mongrel dogs. The right lungs were perfused with either lactated Ringer's solution or a protective solution, enriched with glucose, insulin, low molecular weight dextran, L-arginine, and aprotinin. The left lungs of both groups remained unperfused. Histologic examination revealed that the left lungs from both groups had marked intra-alveolar edema and abundant intra-alveolar neutrophils. The right lungs in the group perfused with lactated Ringer's solution showed only moderate injury, while the group perfused with the protective solution showed normal parenchyma.[29]

41.6 CardiacSur geryW ithout Cardiopulmonary Bypass

In off-pump coronary artery bypass (OPCAB) grafting, lung perfusion and ventilation are maintained during the surgical procedure, thus preventing ischemia-reperfusion injury of the lungs. The OPCAB technique was revived at the end of the 1990s and now constitutes 10–40% of the total amount of CABG procedures worldwide, with considerable differences in international comparison.[30] With the advent of refined retractors and stabilizers, exposition, not only of the anterior but also of the anterolateral and posterior wall of the heart, became possible, so that complete coronary revascularization can be performed without CPB. In a randomized controlled study performed with 200 patients, 100 patients were assigned CABG with CPB, and 100 patients were assigned CABG without CPB.[31] At the end of surgery, 46% of the OPCAB patients but only 32% of the control patients could be extubated. Within 4 h after surgery, 77% of OPCAB patients but only 53% of the control patients could be extubated. All OPCAB patients were extubated within 24 h after surgery, whereas 5% of the control patients did not meet the extubation criteria until more than 24 h after surgery.[31] In patients with a preoperative EuroScore of 5 or higher, who were considered to be at higher risk during subsequent CABG, 42% of an OPCAB subpopulation could be weaned from the ventilator within 24 h after surgery, while only 20% of the patients operated with CPB could be weaned from the ventilator within the same time interval.[32] Patients, however, who are repeatedly shown to be at very high risk when undergoing a cardiac surgical procedure with CPB, are patients with chronic obstructive pulmonary disease (COPD) who are old and who are taking steroids at the same time.[33] An advantage of the OPCAB technique in this population with severe COPD has not yet been described.

As mentioned, circulating leukocytes overexpress adhesion molecules and signaling factors after contact with the artificial surface of CPB, which may facilitate their trapping (e.g., in the lungs) and may promote a subsequent tissue-associated inflammatory response.[34] But the concept may be oversimplified that CPB triggers a short-lasting and reversible inflammatory reaction caused by the activation of circulating blood cells after their contact with nonphysiological surfaces of the different CPB components, while deliberate avoidance of CPB in OPCAB patients prevents this reaction. Indeed, in samples of pericardial fluid, hemolysis, inflammatory mediator release, and coagulation activation were much more pronounced than in blood from the ventricular cavity to which suction forces of the CPB circuit had been applied.[35] The surgical trauma itself was found to be an important trigger for the release of inflammatory mediators. Interestingly, minithoracotomy procedures – with or without the use of CPB – were even shown to be related to higher maximum IL-6 levels when compared to sternotomy procedures with or without the use of CPB.[36] Thus, OPCAB or other less-invasive procedures may reduce an inflammatory reaction but, since other factors such as surgical trauma, manipulation of the heart, pericardial suction, and so on are still there, do not prevent it.[37]

41.7   Treatment Op tionsf orOver t Postoperative Respiratory Failure

In the following paragraph, we discuss treatment options in the case of the development of respiratory failure in post-CPB patients on an intensive care unit. First, steroid treatment, with its anti-inflammatory and vasodilating effects, may improve perfusion of the

lungs and reduce the need for ventilatory support.[38] Steroids have been used in cardiac surgery for many years and still have a role in the treatment of respiratory failure. Second, a reduction of pulmonary resistance with substances like nitric oxide, cyclosporin analoga, or inhibitors of phosphodiesterase have significantly helped to improve pulmonary perfusion in cases of severe pulmonary hypertension. Third, controlled mechanical ventilation itself – as opposed to spontaneous breathing – can induce dysfunction of the diaphragm.[39] Therefore, protective ventilation with a tidal volume of about 6 mL/kg body weight and a peak pressure less than 30 mbar, along with a positive endexpiratory pressure high enough to prevent alveolar collapse, is applied. In addition to protective ventilation, percutaneous tracheostomy has become a valuable tool to facilitate weaning from ventilatory support. Meanwhile, the technique is easily applicable and has dramatically improved mobilization of and communication with patients who need prolonged postoperative ventilation. Moreover, ventilation of the patient in the prone position, especially in combination with percutaneous tracheostomy, can recruit pulmonary tissue that does not take part in the overall gas exchange of the lungs when the patient is in permanent supine position. When these conservative measures do not help, temporary treatment with extracorporeal gas exchange systems, such as extracorporeal membrane oxygenation (ECMO, which is operated with a centrifugal pump) or extracorporeal lung assist (ECLA, which is operated without a pump) have significantly contributed to better survival in patients with severe ARDS.[40]

41.8   Conclusion

During cardiac surgery with CPB, lung perfusion is dramatically reduced so that the lungs are basically ischemic. Although the clinical course is uneventful in the vast majority of cases, ischemia and reperfusion induce a number of processes that include injury to the endothelium, release of inflammatory mediators, expression of adhesion molecules, activation of circulating blood cells, and others. This inflammatory cascade may contribute to postoperative complications, such as transient respiratory failure and even ARDS. To date, techniques like bilateral ECC, CPB with additional lung perfusion, the off-pump technique, and others have promised improvements with respect to the inflammatory reaction and even duration of postoperative ventilatory support. However, the high-risk, old-age patients with COPD and additional steroid treatment were not addressed in the respective studies. In these patients, significant progress in conservative ventilatory support techniques and intensive care treatment have improved postoperative outcome. With respect to the respiratory system, however, these patients remain to constitute the biggest challenge withinthe c ardiacs urgicalpa tientpopula tion.

References

1. Ng CSH, Wan S, Yim APC, Arifi AA. Pulmonary dysfunction after cardiac surgery. *Chest*.2002; 121:1269-1277.
2. Ungerleider RM. Lung ischemia during cardiopulmonary bypass. Letter to the editor. Reply. *Ann Thorac Surg*. 2000;70:337-338.
3. Calvin SH, Wan S, Yim APC, Arifi AA. Pulmonary dysfunction after cardiac surgery. *Chest*.2002; 121:1269-1277.
4. Schlensak C, Doenst T, Preußer S, Wunderlich M, Kleinschmidt M, Beyersdorf F. Cardiopulmonary bypass reduction of bronchial blood flow: a potential mechanism for lung injury in a neonatal pig model. *J Thorac Cardiovasc Surg*.2002;123:119 9-1205.
5. Shenkman Z, Shir Y, Weiss YG, Bleiberg B, Gross D. The effects of cardiac surgery on early and late pulmonary functions. *Acta Anaesthesiol Scand*.1997; 41:1193-1199.
6. Hill GE, Pohorecki R, Alonso A, Rennard SI, Robbins RA. Aprotinin reduces interleukin-8 production and lung neutrophil accumulation after cardiopulmonary bypass. *Anesth Analg*.1996;83:696- 700.
7. Massoudy P, Zahler S, Becker BF, et al. Significant leukocyte and platelet retention during pulmonary passage after declamping of the aorta in CABG patients. *Eur J Med Res*. 1999;4:178-182.
8. Massoudy P, Zahler S, Becker BF, Braun SL, Barankay A, Meisner H. Evidence for inflammatory responses during coronary artery bypass grafting with cardiopulmonary bypass. *Chest*.2001 ;119:31-36.
9. Sekido N, Mukaida N, Harada A, Nakanishi I, Watanabe Y, Matsushima K. Prevention of lung reperfusion injury in rabbits by a monoclonal antibody against interleukin-8. *Nature*. 1993;365:654-657.
10. Dreyer WJ, Michael LH, Millman EE, Berens KL, Geske RS. Neutrophil sequestration and pulmonary dysfunction in a canine model of open heart surgery with cardiopulmonary bypass. Evidence for a CD-18 dependent mechanism. *Circulation*.1995;92: 2276-2283.
11. Kirshbom PM, Page SO, Jacobs MT, et al. Cardiopulmonary bypass and circulatory arrest increase endothelin-1 production and receptor expression in the lung. *J Thorac Cardiovasc Surg*.1997;113:777- 783.
12. Erez E, Erman A, Snir E, et al. Thromboxane production in human lung during cardiopulmonary bypass: beneficial effect of aspirin? *Ann Thorac Surg*.1998; 65:101-106.
13. Shafique T, Johnson RG, Dai HB, Weintraub RM, Seke FW. Altered pulmonary microvascular reactivity after total cardiopulmonary bypass. *J Thorac Cardiovasc Surg*. 1993; 106:479-486.
14. Rehm M, Bruegger D, Christ F, et al. Shedding of the endothelial glycocalyx in patients undergoing major vascular surgery with global and regional ischemia. *Circulation*. 2007;116:1896-1906.
15. Massoudy P, Piotrowski JA, van de Wal HCJM, et al. Perfusing and ventilating the patient's lungs during bypass ameliorates the increase in extravascular thermal volume after coronary bypass grafting. *Ann Thorac Surg*. 2003;76:516-522.
16. Massoudy P, Zahler S, Tassani P, et al. Reduction of proinflammatory cytokine levels and cellular adhesion in CABG procedures with separated pulmonary and systemic extracorporeal circulation without an oxygenator. *Eur J Cardiothorac Surg*.2000; 17:729-736.
17. Cardigan RA, Hamilton-Davies C, McDonals S, et al. Hemostatic changes in the pulmonary blood during cardiopulmonary bypass. *Blood Coagul Fibrinolysis*. 1996;7:567-577.
18. Cicala C, Cirino G. Linkage between inflammation and coagulation: an update on the molecular basis of the crosstalk. *Life Sci*.1998; 62:1817-1824.
19. Drew CE, Anderson IM. Profound hypothermia in cardiac surgery. Report of three cases. *Lancet*.1959; 1:748-750.
20. Dobell ARC, Bailey JS. Charles Drew and the origins of deep hypothermic circulatory arrest. *Ann Thorac Surg*. 1997;63:1193-1199.
21. Edmunds LH. Why cardiopulmonary bypass makes patients sick: strategies to control the blood synthetic surface interface. *Adv Cardiac Surg*.1995; 6:131-167.
22. Cameron D. Initiation of white cell activation during cardiopulmonary bypass: cytokines and receptors. *J Cardiovasc Pharmacol*.1996; 27(suppl1) :S1-S5.
23. Morse DS, Adams D, Magnani B. Platelet and neutrophil activation during cardiac surgical procedures: impact of cardiopulmonary bypass. *Ann Thorac Surg*.1998; 65:691-695.
24. Richter JA, Meisner H, Tassani P, Barankay A, Dietrich W, Braun SL. Drew-Anderson technique attenuates systemic inflammatory response syndrome and improves respiratory function after coronary artery bypass grafting. *Ann Thorac Surg*.1999; 69:77-83.
25. Utgaard JO, Jahnsen FL, Bakka A, Brandtzaeg P, Haraldsen G. Rapid secretion of prestored interleukin 8 from Weibel palade bodies of microvascular endothelial cells. *J Exp Med*. 1998;188:1751-1756.
26. Suzuki T, Fukuda T, Ito T, Inoue Y, Cho Y, Kashima I. Continuous pulmonary perfusion during cardiopulmonary bypass prevents lung injury in infants. *Ann Thorac Surg*. 2000;69:602-606.
27. Goebel U, Siepe M, Mecklenburg A, et al. Reduced inflammatory response during cardiopulmonary bypass: effects of a combined pulmonary perfusion and carbon monoxide inhalation. *Eur J Cardiothorac Surg*.2008; 34:1165-1172.
28. Sievers H-H, Freund-Kaas C, Eleftheriadis S, et al. Lung protection during total cardiopulmonary bypass by isolated

lung perfusion: preliminary results of a novel perfusion strategy. *Ann Thorac Surg*.2002; 74:1167-1172.

29. Liu Y, Wang Q, Zhu X, et al. Pulmonary artery perfusion with protective solution reduces lung injury after cardiopulmonary bypass. *Ann Thorac Surg*.2000; 69:1402-1407.

30. Gummert JF, Funkat A, Beckmann A, et al. Cardiac surgery in Germany during 2007: A report on behalf of the German Society for Thoracic and Cardiovascular Surgery. *Thorac Cardiovasc Surg*.2 008;56:328-336.

31. Puskas JD, Wiliams WH, Duke PG, et al. Off-pump coronary artery bypass grafting provides complete revascularisation with reduced myocardial injury, transfusion requirements, and length of stay: a prospective randomised comparison of two hundred unselected patients undergoing off-pump versus conventional coronary artery bypass grafting. *J Thorac Cardiovasc Surg*.2003; 125:797-808.

32. Al-Ruzzeh S, Nakamura K, Athanasiou T, et al. Does off-pump coronary artery bypass (OPCAB) surgery improve the outcome in high-risk patients? A comparative study of 1398 high-risk patients. *Eur J Cardiothorac Surg*. 2003;23:50-55.

33. Samuel LE, Kaufmann MS, Morris RJ, Promisloff R, Brockmann SK. Coronary artery bypass grafting in patients with COPD. *Chest*.1998; 113:878-882.

34. Tomic V, Russwurm S, Möller E, et al. Transcriptomic and proteomic patterns of systemic inflammation in on-pump and off-pump coronary artery bypass grafting. *Circulation*. 2005;112:2912-2920.

35. Fabre O, Vincentelli A, Corseaux D, et al. Comparison of blood activation in the wound, active vent, and cardiopulmonary bypass circuit. *Ann Thorac Surg*.2008; 86:537-542.

36. Gulielmos V, Menschikowski M, Dill H-M, et al. Interleukin-1, interleukin-6 and myocardial enzyme response after coronary artery bypass grafting – a prospective randomised comparison of the conventional and three minimally invasive surgical techniques. *Eur J Cardiothorac Surg*. 2000;18:594-601.

37. Raja SG, Berg GA. Impact of off-pump coronary artery bypass surgery on systemic inflammation: current best available evidence. *J Card Surg*.2007; 22:445-455.

38. Wan S, Le Clerc JL, Vincent JL. Inflammatory response to cardiopulmonary bypass. Mechanisms involved and possible therapeutic strategies. *Chest*1997; 112:676–692

39. Vassilakopoulos T, Zakynthinos S. When mechanical ventilation mimics nature. *Crit Care Med*.2008; 36:818-827.

40. Beiderlinden M, Eikermann M, Boes T, Breitfeld C, Peters J. Treatment of severe acute respiratory distress syndrome: role of extracorporeal gas exchange. *Intensive Care Med*. 2006;32:1627-1631.

Edmo Atique Gabriel and Tomas Salerno

When we surveyed the medical literature, we noted that there is little material addressing the use of lung perfusion during clinical mitral valve surgery. In light of this reality, we would like to point out that pulmonary hypertension is seen frequently in mitral valve disease, and it can effectively contribute to a patient's prognosis. We think that heart surgeons should turn their attention to this issue as well as keep in mind that the use of controlled lung perfusion during mitral valve surgery can be a useful approach for minimizing the deleterious effects of underlying pulmonary hypertension. If the patient having mitral valve surgery does not present clinical or echocardiographic signs of pulmonary hypertension at the time of operation, we believe that controlled lung perfusion can play a prophylactic role. On the other hand, if the clinical status of such a patient is really marked by pulmonary hypertension, we advocate that the use of controlled lung perfusion can prevent serious additional damage to lung tissue.

In this chapter, two experiences from Chinese cardiac centers are discussed to demonstrate the benefits of lung perfusion as a protective adjunct for mitral valve operation.

Song et al.[1] designed clinical research to assess the impact of main pulmonary artery perfusion using hypothermic washed red blood cell solution (4°C) during a mitral valve operation. Thirty patients for mitral valve surgery were studied, and all presented with pulmonary hypertension at the time of operation. Hemodynamic, gasometric, respiratory, and inflammatory parameters were evaluated in the control group ($n=15$) and the perfusion group ($n=15$), as demonstrated in Figs. 42.1–42.4, respectively. Results indicated that pulmonary artery perfusion can contribute to postoperative optimal performance in patients with pulmonary hypertension undergoing mitral valve surgery.

Another interesting clinical research study was carried out by Liu et al.[2] to assess effects of continuous pulmonary artery perfusion with oxygenated blood during mitral valve surgery with cardiopulmonary bypass (CPB). Thirty patients were divided into two equal groups: a control group and a perfusion group (continuous lung perfusion with oxygenated blood). Gasometric, respiratory, and histologic variables were evaluated in both groups preoperatively, immediately after coming off CPB, and 6 h after surgery. In a general way, results confirmed that pulmonary artery perfusion can alleviate the degree of postoperative pulmonary injury by means of higher oxygen index, shorter time of mechanical ventilation and intensive care unit (ICU) stay, as well as few remarkable pathological findings.

E.A.G abriel(✉)
Federal University of Sao Paulo, Sao Paulo, Brazil
e-mail:e dag@uol.com.br

E.A. Gabriel and T. Salerno (eds.), *Principles of Pulmonary Protection in Heart Surgery,*
DOI: 10.1007/978-1-84996-308-4_42, © Springer-Verlag London Limited 2010

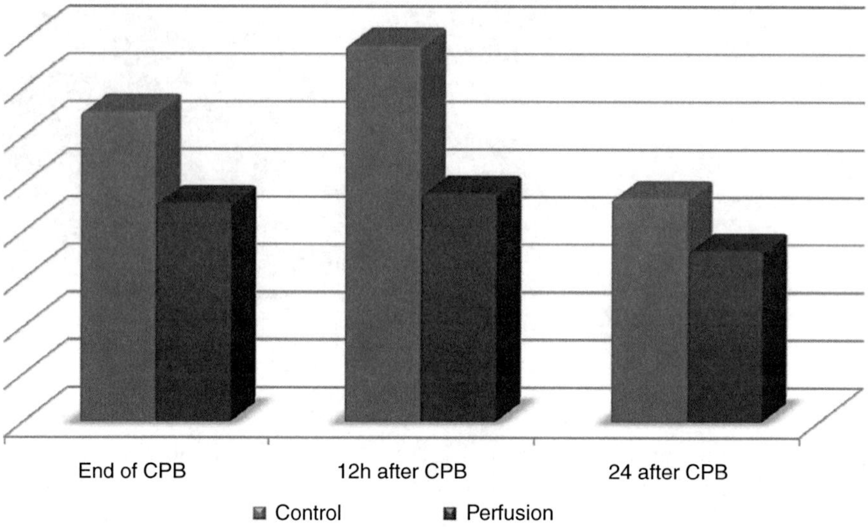

Fig. 42.1 Pulmonary vascular resistance (PVR), $p<0.05$. *CPB* cardiopulmonary bypass

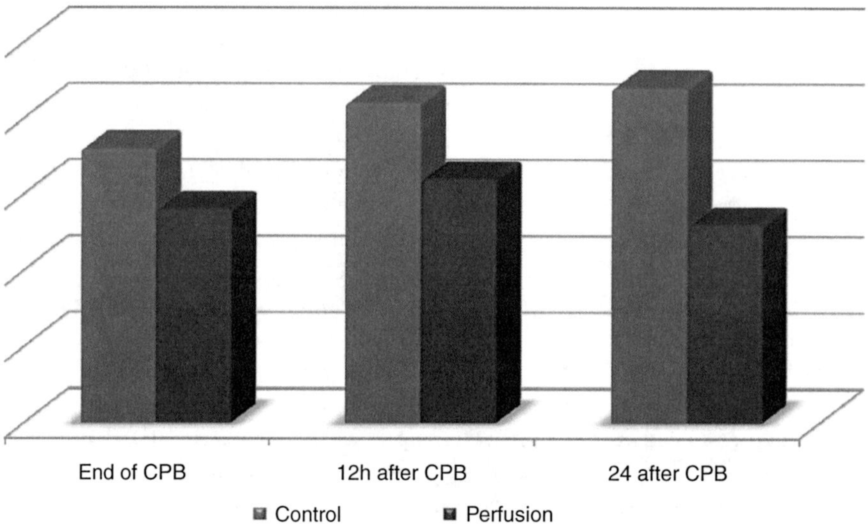

Fig. 42.2 Malondialdehyde (MDA), $p<0.05$. *CPB* cardiopulmonary bypass

Fig. 42.3 Oxygeninde x (OI), $p < 0.05$. *CPB*c ardio-pulmonarybypa ss

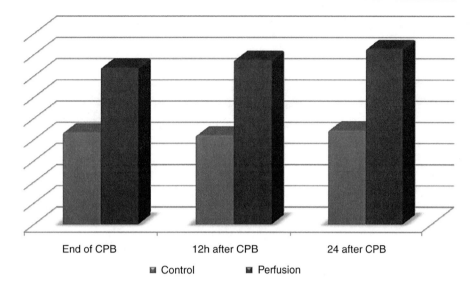

References

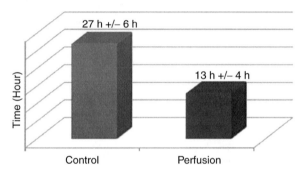

Fig. 42.4   Time of mechanical ventilation, $p < 0.01$

1. Song Y, Gong XJ, Gu XH, Li R, Zhang G, Zhang XQ. Influence of pulmonary artery perfusion with solution of washed red blood cells on lung injury after cardiopulmonary bypass. *Zhonghua Yi Xue Za Zhi*. 2006;86(20): 1421-1424.
2. Liu LM, Hu JG, Yin BL, et al. Lung protection of continuous pulmonary artery perfusion with oxygenated blood during cardiopulmonary bypass. *Zhong Nan Da Xue Xue Bao Yi Xue Ban*. 2005;30(4):413-416.

LungPer fusioni nC linicalA orticSur gery

43

Luca Salvatore De Santo

Despite several developments in surgical, anesthetic, and perfusion strategies, clinical outcomes of acute type A aortic dissection (AAAD) remain unchanged. Indeed, in-hospital mortality according to the report from the International Registry of Acute Aortic Dissection still averages 23.9%.[1]

Operative strategies are usually based on hypothermic circulatory arrest (HCA) since it allows repair using an open distal anastomosis technique, which eliminates the need to clamp a fragile aorta and prevents false lumen pressurization. A number of technical implementations to HCA have been developed, such as antegrade selective cerebral perfusion (SCP) and retrograde cerebral perfusion (RCP), to help prevent its inherent neurologic consequences. But, the use of HCA also implies significant nonneurologic morbidity, such as increased perioperative hemorrhage and postoperative renal and pulmonary dysfunction.[2]

Again, on a mere clinical ground, need for prolonged mechanical ventilation (PMV) after surgery for AAAD is frequent (up to 36%) and potentially lethal. Preoperative hemodynamic instability, organ malperfusion, and prolonged cardiopulmonary bypass (CPB) along with high rates of reexploration for bleeding and neurologic deficits, which are common perioperative features of this patient subset, may individually and synergistically contribute to PMV.[3]

CPB has long been known to cause acute lung injury. This injury is characterized by decreased gas exchange and decreased lung compliance associated with increased pulmonary vascular resistance (PVR), permeability, and edema. The mechanisms behind these abnormalities are poorly understood but are thought to result from the injurious effects of both cellular and humoral mediators within the pulmonary circulation.[4,5] These include toxic products of sequestered neutrophils as well as prostanoids, cytokines, and reactive oxygen species. The observation that with less deprivation of blood flow in the pulmonary artery (PA) there is less-severe subsequent lung injury, as evidenced both by the preservation of postoperative lung gas exchange function and by a reduced length of mechanical ventilation, suggests that PA ischemia-reperfusion (I/R) plays a significant role. Indeed, it exacerbates functional and structural damage of the endothelium and promotes extensive neutrophil sequestration in the lung. Bronchial artery (BA) blood flow may influence the effect of pulmonary I/R on subsequent lung dysfunction. Another determinant of the postoperative need for PMV may be related to the acute aortic dissection process per se. Pathological studies of acute aortic dissections showed the infiltration of macrophages and leukocytes and higher cytokine expression (interleukin [IL] 6 and IL-8) in dissected aorta. These findings suggest that local aortic insult can be the source of humoral factors, which pass through the pulmonary vasculature and activate both resident leukocytes and the pulmonary vascular endothelium. Thus, it is possible that the powerful assault of intimal rupture and propagation of the dissection into the media may provoke activation of the cellular and humoral inflammatory systems, including leukocytes, macrophages, and various cytokines, and subsequently lead to insufficiency of pulmonary gas exchange.[6,7] C-reactive protein (CRP) is a clinically useful nonspecific marker of inflammation and is produced in the liver by stimulation of proinflammatory cytokines

L.S.D eSa nto
Department of Cardiovascular Surgery and Transplant,
V.M onaldiH ospital, Naples, Italya nd
Departmentof C ardiacSur gery, Universityof F oggia,
Foggia, Italy
e-mail:l uca.desanto@ospedalemonaldi.it

E.A. Gabriel and T. Salerno (eds.), *Principles of Pulmonary Protection in Heart Surgery*,
DOI: 10.1007/978-1-84996-308-4_43, © Springer-Verlag London Limited 2010

(predominantly IL-6). Focus has been on serum CRP levels as a marker of disease progression in patients with vascular diseases. Schillinger et al. reported that elevated CRP levels on admission were independently associated with higher mortality in patients with acute aortic diseases.[8] Notably, CRP is highly dependent on the elapsed time from the onset.

All in all, the complete definition of the pathophysiology of PMV following AAAD surgery is still under way, and experimental studies of preventive measures are scarce, with limited sample size and above all usually targeted to account just some of the several basic mechanisms actually involved in the genesis of the unfavorable clinical outcomes.

The Department of Cardiovascular Surgery and Transplant of the V. Monaldi Hospital in Naples, Italy, is a university-affiliated tertiary care center with a high caseload of aortic arch surgery. We have performed four clinical studies that might add some knowledge to this delicate topic.

43.1 FourC linicalExp eriences in a Single Tertiary Care Center

43.1.1 First Experiment: Pulmonary Perfusion in Patients Referred for Type A Acute Aortic Dissection

In 2001, we prospectively evaluated the effect of continuous pulmonary perfusion during RCP on lung function. Twenty-two patients referred for AAAD, who were free from preoperative respiratory dysfunction,

were assigned prospectively and alternately to one of two treatment groups. The conventional Ueda technique was applied in group A, whereas pulmonary perfusion was performed during RCP in group B. Continuous pulmonary perfusion was accomplished with the oxygenated blood at a flow rate of 300 mL m^{-2} min^{-1}. The perfusate was infused into the pulmonary trunk through a 24-French cannula and was drained away from the left atrium through an 18-French vent circuit to secure a bloodless field. During perfusion, mechanical ventilation was arrested with positive end-expiratory pressure (PEEP) at 10 cm H_2O. Lung function was evaluated on the basis of intubation time, scoring of chest radiographs at 12 h after CPB, and Pao$_2$/fraction of inspired oxygen ratio assessed from immediately before the operation to 72 h after termination of CPB. Study groups were homogeneous for age, sex, interval between symptom onset and surgical operation, previous aortic surgery, preoperative ejection fraction and pulmonary gas exchange function, extent of aortic repair, and concomitant procedures. CPB time, length of RCP, operation time, need for blood substitutes, and surgical revision for bleeding did not differ between treatment groups. Postoperative Pao$_2$/fraction of inspired oxygen ratios were higher in group B than in group A, and the difference remained statistically significant throughout the study period (Fig. 43.1). The incidence of prolonged ventilator support (>72 h) and the severity of the radiographic pulmonary infiltrate score were lower in the perfused group (18.2 vs. 72.7% [$p = 0.015$] and 0.81 ± 0.75 vs. 1.8 ± 0.78 [$p = 0.028$], respectively). Continuous pulmonary perfusion provided better preservation of lung function in patients operated on with deep systemic hypothermia.[9]

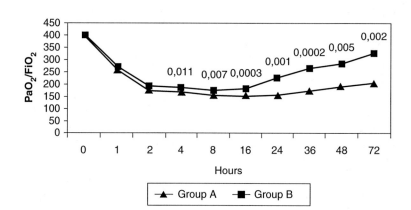

Fig.43.1 Pao$_2$/Fio$_2$ra tiot rends

43.1.2 Second Experiment: Effectiveness of Kazui Technique in Protecting Both Brain and Pulmonary Function During Treatment of Acute Type A Aortic Dissection

In a prospective fashion, we subsequently aimed to assess the effectiveness of SCP (Kazui technique) in protecting both brain and pulmonary function during surgical treatment of AAAD. Between January 1997 and January 2001, alternating assignments of 114 patients free from preoperative neurological and respiratory dysfunction were made to one of three protocols of brain protection: group A HCA, group B RCP, and group C Kazui technique. Cerebral injury was evaluated by neurological examination and S-100 serum release, while lung function was evaluated by intubation time, arterial/alveolar oxygen ratios, and serum levels of IL-1, tumor necrosis factor alpha (TNF-α), IL-6, and IL-8 at nine intervals in the first 72 h. Group C patients experienced significantly better outcomes regarding stroke rate ($p=0.025$), incidence of prolonged ventilator support ($p=0.017$), and mean arterial/alveolar oxygen ratios ($p=0.026$) (Tables 43.1 and 43.2). Consistently, increases in postoperative serum S-100, IL-1, TNF-α, IL-6, and IL-8 levels were significantly higher ($p=0.034$ and 0.025, respectively) in group A and B (Table 43.3). Notably, hospital mortality was significantly lower in group C (group A 17.8%, group B 23.7%, vs. 5.3%). The Kazui technique proved superior in reducing both brain and pulmonary dysfunction.[10]

43.1.3 Third Experiment: Pulmonary Artery Flushing with a Protective Solution During Treatment of Acute Type A Aortic Dissection

From January 2002 to December 2002, we undertook a pilot prospective study to evaluate the effect of PA flushing with a protective solution on lung function during SCP. Twenty patients referred for AAAD, who were free from preoperative respiratory dysfunction, were assigned prospectively and alternately to two

Table43. 1 Outcomesa ndope rativev ariables

Variables	GroupA (DHCA)	Group B (RCP)	Group C (SCP)	Total	p
Hospital mortality	7 (17.8)	9 (23.7)	2 (5.3)	18 (15.8)	0.03[a]
Permanentne urological dysfunction	9(23.7)	5(13.2)	1(2.6)	15(13.2)	0.025
Transientne urological dysfunction	9(23.7)	8(21.1)	3(7.9)	20(17.5)	NS
Brain pr otection t ime	49.8±15.2	52.4±17.77	47.8±21.4	52±3.5	NS
	51±4.4	52±3.1	53±2.5		
CPB t ime	182.1±41.9	179.6±46.5	174.1±48.8		NS
	51±4.4	52±3.1	53±2.5		NS
Operation t ime	457±44.3	490±58.2	380±60		<0.001
	51±4.4	52±3.1	53±2.5		
Units of blood substitute required	10.15±5.6	9.02±6.2	4.03±8.4	8.01±7.1	0.02
	51±4.4	52±3.1	53±2.5		
Surgical revision of bleeding	2(5.3)	3(7.9)	1(2.6)	6(5.26)	NS
Pulmonarydys function	12(31.6)	14(36.8)	5(13.2)	31(27.2)	0.017[a]

[a]Group C vs. groups A+B
CPB cardiopulmonary bypass, *NS* not significant, *RCP* retrograde cerebral perfusion, *SCP* selective cerebral perfusion
DHCA Deep Hypothermic Circulatory Arrest

Table 43.2 Pulmonary gas exchange evaluation by means of the Pao_2/PAo_2

$Pao_2/$ PAo_2 (h)	GroupA	GroupB	GroupC	p
1	0.44±0.1	0.43±0.11	0.63±0.13	<0.0001
2	0.37±0.05	0.4±0.07	0.53±0.15	<0.0001
4	0.39±0.05	0.4±0.04	0.59±0.12	<0.0001
8	0.38±0.04	0.4±0.06	0.56±0.14	<0.0001
16	0.49±0.07	0.51±0.09	0.6±0.13	0.0008
24	0.47±0.1	0.45±0.08	0.62±0.2	<0.0001
36	0.51±0.08	0.5±0.06	0.61±0.15	0.001
48	0.49±0.05	0.5±0.04	0.61±0.17	0.0005
72	0.48±0.06	0.47±0.07	0.61±0.2	0.0003

Table43. 3 Cytokinequa ntifications

Hours	GroupA	GroupB	GroupC	p
IL-6(pg/mL)				
1	410±56	395±65	390±53	0.3
2	820±65	805±85	530±60	0.005
4	1,758±317	1,754±333	723±111	0.007
8	1,255±152	1,238±165	554±72	0.0001
16	596±98	581±115	260±60	0.004
24	404±89	394±101	185±50	0.03
36	201±85	186±94	96±43	0.052
48	99±45	93±60	40±22	0.063
72	0	0	0	–
IL-1(pg/mL)				
1	0.45±0.15	0.43±0.18	0.25±0.12	0.0001
2	0.90±0.16	0.88±0.2	0.5±0.14	<0.0001
4	1.8±0.3	1.7±0.35	0.3±0.2	<0.0001
8	1.0±0.15	0.98±0.19	0.1±0.08	<0.0001
16	0.2±0.07	0.17±0.09	0	<0.0001
24	0	0	0	–
36	0	0	0	–
48	0	0	0	–
72	0	0	0	–
IL-8(pg/mL)				
1	28±6.3	26±8.5	16±3.4	0.009

(*continued*)

Table 43.3   (continued)

2	56±9	54±11	31±6.8	0.006
4	50±9.2	48±10.2	20±5.5	0.008
8	32±5	30±6.4	13±3.1	0.01
16	18±2.5	17±3.7	8±1.5	0.02
24	12±2.5	11±3.4	7.5±2.2	0.024
36	10±2.5	·10±2.8	7±1.5	0.04
48	9±2.3	8.5±2.9	8±2.8	0.062
72	8±1.5	8.3±1.3	7±2.4	0.094
TNF-α(pg/mL)				
1	39±14	37±18	4.5±1.7	0.007
2	78±28	74±18	9±3.7	0.001
4	8±2.8	8.5±3	8±2.3	0.054
8	4±2.3	4±2.5	3±2.5	0.066
16	0	0	0	–
24	0	0	0	–
36	0	0	0	–
48	0	0	0	–
72	0	0	0	–

IL interleukin, *TNF-α* tumor necrosis factor alpha

treatment groups. Pulmonary flushing was performed during SCP in group P, while the conventional Kazui technique was applied in group N. Lung perfusion consisted of single-shot hypothermic (5°C) PA flush with Celsior solution after prostaglandin E1 (PGE1) intrapulmonary bolus. The perfusate was infused into the pulmonary trunk through a 24-French cannula and was drained away from the left atrium through an 18-French vent circuit to secure a bloodless field. The mechanical ventilation was arrested in both groups with PEEP at 10 cm H_2O. Lung function was evaluated by intubation time, scoring of chest radiograms at 12 h after CPB, and Pao_2/Fio_2 assessed from immediately before surgery to 72 h after termination of CPB. Incidence of pre-, intra-, and postoperative determinants of lung dysfunction proved homogeneous in both groups. Lung oxygenation function showed a marked postoperative decline followed by a slow improvement in both groups. Analysis of respiratory ratios did not disclose significant differences even though the all patients in the flushed group had better performance. The incidence of prolonged ventilator support (longer than 72 h) (30% vs. 20%, p=NS [not significant]) and severity of X-ray pulmonary infiltrate score were comparable (mean score 1.7 ± 0.71 vs. 1.6 ± 0.68, p=NS). PA flushing with Celsior solution did not provide effective preservation of lung function.[11]

43.1.4 The Fourth Experiment: Thoracoabdominal Perfusion

In 2005, we tested the hypothesis that thoracoabdominal aorta perfusion (TAP) may protect end organs during HCA with cerebral perfusion in aortic arch procedures. Two hundred two arch procedures performed with moderate hypothermia (22–26°C) and antegrade cerebral perfusion (ACP) were the objects of retrospective investigation. Acute type A dissection was the indication in 164 patients, aortic aneurysm in 38. In 80 patients, during ACP the thoracoabdominal aorta was perfused in either an antegrade fashion through proximal descending aorta endoluminal cannulation (in 62 dissections) or retrograde through femoral artery cannulation with proximal descending aorta endoluminal occlusion (in 18 aneurysms) (Fig. 43.2). Hospital mortality and morbidity rates were compared between the two treatments (group A: ACP only, 122 patients; group B: ACP plus TAP, 80 patients), and the underlying

aortic disease (dissection/aneurysm) was stratified. Cerebral perfusion (p=0.008) and CPB times (p=0.035) were significantly longer in group B. No complication related to the TAP technique was observed in group B. Overall hospital mortality was 12.9%, without significant difference between groups. No differences were found in terms of permanent neurological dysfunction between groups A (9.3%) and B (9.1%; p=0.58). Group B patients showed lower rates of respiratory failure (18.2% vs. 30.5% group A; p=0.038), shorter mechanical ventilation times (18.1 ± 26 h vs. 57.9 ± 70.1; $p<0.001$), and lower incidence of acute renal failure (6.5% vs. 18.6%; p=0.012). Shorter intensive care and hospital stays were observed in group B (p=0.02). The adjunction of TAP to ACP was associated with lower rates of end-organ complications, even in more extensive and time-consuming procedures.[12]

43.2 AnOver view

The studies discussed simply reflect the great efforts spent since 1997 to develop newer strategies for the treatment of AAAD to reduce the inherent relevant neurologic and end-organ morbidity. Some peculiarities are inherent to this surgical setting as far as lung

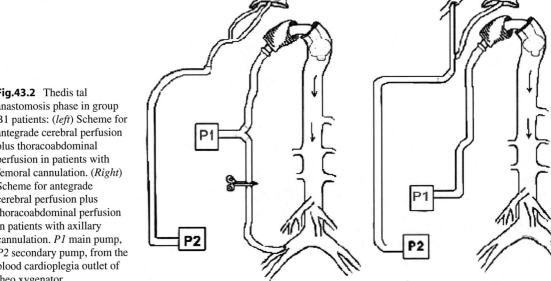

Fig.43.2 Thedis tal anastomosis phase in group B1 patients: (*left*) Scheme for antegrade cerebral perfusion plus thoracoabdominal perfusion in patients with femoral cannulation. (*Right*) Scheme for antegrade cerebral perfusion plus thoracoabdominal perfusion in patients with axillary cannulation. *P1* main pump, *P2* secondary pump, from the blood cardioplegia outlet of theo xygenator

function preservation is concerned. As mentioned, the lungs have a bimodal blood supply from the pulmonary arteries and the BAs, with extensive anastomotic connections. The bronchial circulation originates from the descending aorta and intercostal arteries. It supplies the airways, pleura, lymph nodes, nerves, and pulmonary vascular vasa vasorum before draining into the pulmonary circulation through bronchopulmonary anastomoses. BA perfusion during CPB has been considered by some investigators to be problematic, possibly contributing to pulmonary vascular congestion and systemic hypotension. Others have hypothesized that BA blood flow is a possible ameliorating factor in CPB-induced lung injury. The relative contribution of the BAs and PAs and of alveolar ventilation in delivering oxygen to maintain lung tissue viability is still unclear.[13] In aortic dissection surgery, HCA prevents both BA and PA flow, thus determining complete lung ischemia. The metabolism of lung tissue is still active during HCA, and oxygen consumption is high. When blood perfusion resumes, there is a further I/R injury from the oxygen free radicals, calcium paradox, and abnormal energy metabolism. The second distinctive feature is that BAs arising from the inner curvature of the aortic arch might be affected both by the dissecting process and by the surgical procedure (distal aortic wall reinforcement), so lungs might become completely dependent on PA flow.

RCP, as developed by Ueda et al., rapidly gained a certain popularity in the surgical community.[14] We incorporated such implementation for HCA in our surgical strategies and tested the effectiveness of combined RCP plus pulmonary perfusion in the reduction of postoperative lung morbidity.[9] To the best of our knowledge, we demonstrated for the first time that continuous pulmonary perfusion favorably affects postoperative lung function, as supported by better preserved postoperative lung gas exchange (Pao_2/Fio_2 ratio), reduced ventilator support, and better chest radiographic scoring. These patterns were almost comparable with those reported by Suzuki et al., who assessed the effect of continuous pulmonary perfusion with oxygenated blood during total CPB in infants with congenital heart disease. They demonstrated superior preservation of lung gas exchange function and a significantly reduced length of mechanical ventilation as the effect of continuous pulmonary perfusion during total CPB in humans.[15,16] Optimal flow rates and temperature for the continuous pulmonary perfusion

are still under investigation. There is experimental evidence that flow rates exceeding 25% of the systemic blood flow result in less-severe pulmonary dysfunction. Other studies suggested 35 mL kg^{-1} min^{-1} as the protective amount of blood support, whereas the studies discussed here in human subjects were performed with 30 mL kg^{-1} min^{-1} blood support.[17,18] Pulmonary perfusion in our study was performed at 300 mL/m^2 and 18°C. Two different factors influenced the choice of such a perfusion protocol: core cooling on CPB and need for a perfusate temperature associated with a lower PVR to exert a more uniform washout of the pulmonary vasculature and to avoid risk of injury to the alveolo-capillary membrane.

There has been a significant trend toward widespread adoption of SCP in arch procedures since it significantly contributed in reducing adverse neurologic outcomes, even in more complex and time-consuming procedures. This strategy implies a lesser degree of hypothermia. Although hypothermia per se seems not to cause a significant increase in respiratory failure, the lower the temperature, the longer the extracorporeal circulation time needed for rewarming, and therefore the more severe the systemic inflammatory response. In a prospective randomized study, we assessed the effectiveness of SCP according to the Kazui protocol.[10] SCP proved superior to deep HCA and RCP both in protecting brain function and in reducing the incidence of blood loss and pulmonary dysfunction. Cytokines are critical mediators of the whole-body inflammatory response elicited by CPB. Because high levels of cytokines can be detected during CPB, these humoral agents may be used as markers for ongoing tissue damage. Tepid or normothermic CPB has been reported to reduce inflammatory reactions and blood loss compared with deep hypothermic CPB. Cytokine quantification in our study groups strictly followed this pattern. Intriguingly, lower levels of proinflammatory cytokines resulted in reduced blood loss and transfusion requirements. Consistent with cytokine activation, the rate of pulmonary impairment in our study was higher in patients in deep hypothermia than in those in the Kazui group, in 34.2% and 13.2%, respectively. These results favorably compare with those reported by Svenson et al.[19] on Deep Hypothermic Circulatory Arrest (DHCA) patients and those forwarded by Coselli et al.[20] on an RCP series. However, in a study on total arch replacement Kazui et al. reported an incidence as high as 32.7% of pulmonary failure requiring a respirator for more than 5 days after surgery.[21] This apparent discordance may be explained by the greater extent of surgical repair requiring longer bypass time and by higher mean age in Kazui et al.'s series and by the selection criteria of the present trial. Finally, advantages of cold blood ACP in conjunction with those deriving from a temperature management shifting toward even more tepid systemic conditions have given great impulse to the development of a new surgical strategy, namely, the so-called cool head–warm body perfusion. Encouraging results in terms of equal cerebral protectiveness and reduction of CPB drawbacks are in fact emerging from small nonrandomized series.[22]

But, temperature management during SCP is not a panacea but more realistically a double-edged sword. Indeed, on one side end organs may benefit from the avoidance of deep hypothermia; on the other hand, complex and time-consuming distal aortic procedures may require lengthy "warm" circulatory arrest periods that in turn exacerbate the risk of nonneurologic complications.

Liu and associates proved the protective effect of pulmonary perfusion with hypothermic anti-inflammatory solution on lung function after CPB in a canine model. This anti-inflammatory solution consisted of anisonamide, L-arginine, aprotinine, glucose-insulin potassium, and phosphate buffer.[23] In 2002, we tested the effectiveness of pulmonary perfusion with a preservation solution as an adjunct to SCP.[11] This prospective study failed to demonstrate any significant beneficial effect of pulmonary flushing with Celsior solution. The chemical composition of the extracellular solution Celsior accounts for the basic principles of graft protection during harvesting for solid organ transplantation. Indeed, the impermeants mannitol and lactobionate reduce cell swelling. Reduced glutathione, histidine, and mannitol decrease the formation of damaging superoxide anions from oxygen. The energy substrate glutamate enhances energy production. Calcium overload is limited by high magnesium content, a low ionized calcium content, and maintenance of slight acidosis (pH 7.3). The effectiveness of Celsior for preservation of a lung allograft before clinical transplantation has been supported by several studies.[24] Nevertheless, Celsior flushing did not exert any significant beneficial effect on lung performance. Such unexpected lack of protective effect may be multifactorial. On one side, work by Andrade et al. disclosed that microvascular permeability may be, at least transiently, affected by hypothermic PA flushing.[25] On the other,

experimental studies of pulmonary preservation in minipigs demonstrated that even though Celsior solution provides distinct improvements in postischemic pulmonary function, it does not preserve surfactant function, which is a major determinant of lung performance.[26] Finally, route of solution administration (pressure and temperature) may have played an important role. The ideal temperature of the flush solution is still under debate.[27] Rapid cooling of the pulmonary graft with a hypothermic solution (4–8°C) after a bolus of a potent vasodilator is still the golden standard in lung preservation. Nevertheless, lower PVR during flushing and hence more uniform washout of the pulmonary vasculature are associated with a flush temperature of 23°C. As far as flushing pressure is concerned, it should be kept between 10 and 15 mmHg to prevent hydrostatic pulmonary edema. In this study, infusion was driven by gravity and pulmonary vasodilation, but no pressure monitoring device was inserted on the pulmonary infusion cannula.

Another possible strategy to protect end organs during HCA with SCP may consist of concomitant TAP, as suggested by several articles. In our experience, with the TAP adjunct, the time of circulatory arrest to the body is reduced to less than 3 min overall, even in total arch replacement procedures, without excessively increasing SCP duration and surgical complexity.[12] Continuing body perfusion proved a safe procedure, and it was associated with significantly lower rates of postoperative respiratory dysfunction along with lower rates of acute kidney injury. The perfusion of the BAs through the descending aorta and the intercostal arteries has certainly a primary role in this strategy. As derived from authoritative experimental studies, by providing oxygen, antioxidants, or nutrients to the ischemic lung, BA anastomotic blood flow during PA ischemia may prevent both the PA endothelial barrier dysfunction caused by ischemia alone and the separate injury that occurs at the time of reperfusion. Consistent with this hypothesis, BA blood flow, as estimated by anastomotic flow during CPB for congenital heart disease repair was shown to inversely correlate with postoperative alveolar-to-arterial oxygen gradient and morphometrically determined interstitial edema and epithelial injury. Notably, in several studies in adults, BA blood flow was shown to vary over a wide range despite similar pump flow levels, suggesting significant differences in bronchial vascular resistance. This variability may perhaps be related to either differing amounts of atherosclerotic vascular obstruction or decreased aortic branch perfusion pressure. Such phenomena could contribute to the excessive incidence of respiratory failure complicating CPB for descending aortic aneurysm repair as well as for AAAD.[13] Although our study design prevented more physiopathologic insights, other possible factors should be considered to explain the amelioration of pulmonary performance in the TAP group. Indeed, the expected limitation of systemic inflammatory reaction by prevention of the I/R phenomenon in the lower body, and the lower number of transient neurologic disorders, a possible cause of ventilatory dysfunction or airway clearance impairment may have contributed as well.

43.3 The Clinical Bottom Line

In addition to neurologic outcomes, reduction of pulmonary and other end-organ morbidity is a main goal of AAAD surgery. Several implementations have gained clinical acceptance, and newly developed strategies for end-organ perfusion and temperature management certainly proved effective. Isolated pulmonary perfusion in this respect, although selectively effective, may not suffice for a whole-body protection strategy. A relevant body of knowledge is accumulating on pharmacological agents that may further broaden the armamentarium. An article by Morimoto and coworkers demonstrated that prophylactic administration of sivelestat sodium hydrate, a synthetic, specific, and low molecular weight neutrophil elastase inhibitor, at the initiation of CPB results in better postoperative pulmonary function, leading to earlier extubation time after total arch replacement under deep hypothermia.[28] A critical review of possible therapeutic interventions is beyond the scope of this chapter, but the evidence is certainly for the development of global preventive strategies that rely not only on continued CPB equipment refinement or implementation of newer perfusion strategy but also incorporation of state-of-the-art perioperative medical treatment. But, the basics of lung damage pathophysiology allow for another consideration. If the severity of the dissecting process per se may be a powerful determinant of a systemic inflammatory response long before and beyond CPB, then timing of surgical referral is a critical determinant of postoperative morbidity. This should lead to a profound reprisal of

this topic and the development of multidisciplinary treatment algorithms that include correct diagnosis, timely referral, and combined medical and surgical state-of-the-art strategies. Lack of such algorithms, besides changing patients' profiles, is the main reason for the relatively unchanged clinical outcomes.

References

1. Rampoldi V, Trimarchi S, Eagle KA, et al. Simple risk models to predict surgical mortality in acute type A aortic dissection: the International Registry of Acute Aortic Dissection score. *Ann Thorac Surg*.2007; 83:55-61.
2. Harrington DK, Lilley JP, Rooney SJ, Bonser RS. Nonneurologic morbidity and profound hypothermia in aortic surgery. *Ann Thorac Surg*.2004; 78:596-601.
3. Kimura N, Tanaka M, Kawahito K, et al. Risk factors for prolonged mechanical ventilation following surgery for acute type A aortic dissection. *Circ J*.2008; 72:1751-1757.
4. Ng CSH, Wan S, Yim APC, Ahmed A. Pulmonary dysfunction after cardiac surgery. *Chest*.2002; 121:1269-1277.
5. Asimakopoulos G, Smith PLC, Ratnatunga CP, Taylor KM. Lung injury and acute respiratory distress syndrome after cardiopulmonary bypass. *Ann Thorac Surg*. 1999;68:1107-1115.
6. Hasegawa Y, Ishikawa S, Ohtaki A, et al. Impaired lung oxygenation in acute aortic dissection. *J Cardiovasc Surg (Torino)*.1999; 40:191-195.
7. Muller BT, Modlich O, Prisack HB, et al. Gene expression profiles in the acutely dissected human aorta. *Eur J Vasc Endovasc Surg*.2002; 24:356-364.
8. Schillinger M, Domanovits H, Bayegan K, et al. C-reactive protein and mortality in patients with acute aortic disease. *Intensive Care Med*.2002; 28:740-745.
9. De Santo LS, Romano G, Amarelli C, et al. Surgical repair of acute type A aortic dissection: continuous pulmonary perfusion during retrograde cerebral perfusion prevents lung injury in a pilot study. *J Thorac Cardiovasc Surg*. 2003;126:826-831.
10. Cotrufo M, Renzulli A, De Santo LS, et al. Neurological and Pulmonary Protection During Surgical Treatment of Type A Acute Aortic Dissection abstract no 39 In: 2001 AATS Meeting Program at http://www.aats.org/annualmeeting/Program-Books/2001/Tuesday-Afternoon.html.
11. De Santo LS, Romano G, Amarelli C, et al. Pilot study on prevention of lung injury during surgery for type A acute aortic dissection: no evident improvements with Celsior flushing through the pulmonary artery. *Int J Artif Organs*. 2003;26:1032-1038.
12. Della Corte A, Scardone M, Romano G, et al. Aortic arch surgery: thoracoabdominal perfusion during antegrade cerebral perfusion may reduce postoperative morbidity. *Ann Thorac Surg*.2006; 81:1358-1364.
13. Dodd-o JM, Welsh LE, Salazar JS, et al. Effect of bronchial artery blood flow on cardiopulmonary bypass-induced lung injury. *Am J Physiol Heart Circ Physiol*. 2004;286: 693-700.

14. Ueda Y, Miki S, Kusuhara K, Okita Y, Tahata T, Yamanaka K. Surgical treatment of aneurysm or dissection involving the ascending aorta and aortic arch, utilizing circulatory arrest and retrograde cerebral perfusion. *J Cardiovasc Surg.* 1990;31:553-558.

15. Suzuki T, Fukuda T, Ito T, Inoue Y, Cho Y, Kashima I. Continuous pulmonary perfusion during cardiopulmonary bypass prevents lung injury in infants. *Ann Thorac Surg.* 2000;69:602-606.

16. Suzuki T, Ito T, Kashima I, Teruya K, Fukuda T. Continuous perfusion of pulmonary arteries during total cardiopulmonary bypass favorably affects levels of circulating adhesion molecules and lung function. *J Thorac Cardiovasc Surg.* 2001;122:242-248.

17. Serraf A, Robotin M, Bonnet N, et al. Alteration of the neonatal pulmonary physiology after total cardiopulmonary bypass. *J Thorac Cardiovasc Surg.* 1997;114: 1061-1069.

18. Kuratani T, Sawa Y, Shimazaki Y, Kadoba K, Matsuada H. Ultrastructural assessment of postoperative lung injury: the effect of bronchial blood flow during cardiopulmonary bypass. *J Jpn Assoc Thorac Surg.*1994; 42:1132-1136.

19. Svenson LG, Crawford ES, Hess KR, Coselli JS, Raskin S, Shenach SA. Deep hypothermia with circulatory arrest: determinants of stroke and early mortality in 656 patients. *J Thorac Cardiovasc Surg.*1993; 106:19-31.

20. Coselli JS, Bueket S, Djukanovic B. Aortic arch surgery: current treatment and results. *Ann Thorac Surg.* 1995;59:19-27.

21. Kazui T, Washiyama N, Muhammad BAH, Terada H, Yamashita K, et al. Extended total arch replacement for acute type A aortic dissection: experience with seventy patients. *J Thorac Cardiovasc Surg.*2000; 119:558-565.

22. Boston US, Sungurtekin H, McGregor CGA, Macoviak JA, Cook DJ. Differential perfusion: a new technique for isolated brain cooling during cardiopulmonary bypass. *Ann Thorac Surg.*2000; 69:1346-1350.

23. Liu Y, Wang Q, Zhu X, et al. Pulmonary artery perfusion with protective solution reduces lung injury after cardiopulmonary bypass. *Ann Thorac Surg.*2000; 69:1402-1407.

24. Baron O, Fabre S, Haloun A, et al. Retrospective clinical comparison of Celsior solution to modified blood Wallwork solution in lung transplantation for cystic fibrosis. *Prog Transplant.*2002; 12:176-180.

25. Andrade RS, Wangesteen OD, Jo JK, Tsai MY, Bolman RM. Effect of hypothermic pulmonary artery flushing on capillary filtration coefficient. *Transplantation.* 2000;70:267-271.

26. Van Raemdonck D. The best preservation solution for then worst graft. In: Postgraduate Programme 2002 Book of Proceedings, 16th Annual Meeting of the European Association for Cardiothoracic Surgery. Monaco, 22–25 September 2002; pp. 89–99.

27. Görler A, Haverich A. Adequate lung preservation for clinical lung transplantation: an important condition for satisfactory graft function. J Card Surg. 2000;15:141–148.

28. Morimoto N, Morimoto K, Morimoto Y et al. Sivelestat attenuates postoperative pulmonary dysfunction after total arch replacement under deep hypothermia. Eur J Cardiothorac Surg.2008; 34:798–804

Lung Perfusion in Clinical Heart–Lung Surgery:C ongenitalHear tDi seaseSur gery

44

Takaaki Suzuki

44.1 Background

Although the technical refinement of cardiopulmonary bypass (CPB) has progressively improved the surgical outcomes of heart diseases, postoperative CPB-induced lung dysfunction still remains a serious complication that could lead to a life-threatening problem, particularly for infants with congenital heart disease.[1] An infant's immature lung is more vulnerable to CPB.[2,3] CPB provokes a cytokine-mediated inflammatory reaction that is initiated by neutrophil adhesion to endothelial cells. The interaction between neutrophils and endothelial cells is enhanced under endothelial cell injury that occurs as a result of free radical activation during CPB. These pathogenic processes can be augmented in the morphologically and functionally abnormal pulmonary endothelium in pulmonary hypertensive infants.

The pathogenic relation between CPB and cytokine-induced inflammation has been clearly elucidated. A number of reports have emphasized that direct contact of blood with the synthetic surface of the CPB circuit provokes systemic inflammatory response,[4] which induces inflammatory cytokines and progressive accumulation of neutrophils in the pulmonary circulatory system,[5] which are presently known to result in tissue injury mediated by oxygen-derived free radicals.[6,7] The inflammatory cytokines exert activating stimuli on pulmonary endothelial cells.[8,9] The activated endothelial cells promote widespread expression of a variety of adhesion molecules, which facilitates the adhesion of complement-activated neutrophils to endothelial cell surfaces and causes neutrophil migration into the extravascular spaces.[10-12]

In addition, ischemic and reperfusion insults play a critical role in the development of CPB-derived lung damage. The lung is at risk for ischemic insults during total CPB because lung perfusion is maintained solely by the bronchial arterial system. Schlensak et al. demonstrated that CPB lessens even bronchial arterial blood flow in a neonatal pig model.[13] Several reports demonstrated that reperfusion following the cessation of blood flow of pulmonary arteries further aggravates structural and functional abnormalities of pulmonary endothelial cells.[14] Neutrophil sequestration in the lung tissue that occurs during CPB is particularly prominent at the moment of lung reperfusion.[15-17] The endothelial injury and neutrophil sequestration induced by ischemia and reperfusion fall into the class of cytokine-mediated lung injury.

Accordingly, it is postulated that controlled pulmonary perfusion could alleviate CPB-induced lung injury. Several experimental studies exhibited that the lung injury was much less severe with less deprivation of the flow of blood in the pulmonary arteries during CPB.[18,19] Kuratani et al. demonstrated that total CPB decreases pulmonary regional blood flow to 11% and adenosine triphosphate (ATP) in the lung tissue to 50% compared with those of the prebypass status, while partial CPB reduces blood flow only to 41% and does not alter ATP in the experimental model.[20] It is highly probable that continued pulmonary circulation throughout the period of CPB may minimize ischemic insult and eventually can prevent lung injury.

T.Suz uki
Department of Pediatric Cardiac Surgery, Saitama International Medical Center and Saitama Medical University,
Yamane, Hidaka-City, Saitama, Japan
e-mail:t ksuzuki@saitama-med.ac.jp

E.A. Gabriel and T. Salerno (eds.), *Principles of Pulmonary Protection in Heart Surgery,*
DOI: 10.1007/978-1-84996-308-4_44, © Springer-Verlag London Limited 2010

44.2 History

Drew and Anderson formulated the first trial of CPB with continuous pulmonary perfusion in 1959.[21] They introduced biventricular bypass using patients' own lungs as the oxygenator because the use of the artificial lung was not well established yet. The technique had a theoretical advantage of eliminating direct contact between blood and the synthetic surface of the oxygenator. At that time, however, the procedure deservedly failed to show any biochemical and clinical benefits for prevention of CPB-induced lung injury. Since then, this work had gone unrecognized. In the late 1990s, Drew and Anderson's method was revisited by several investigators, who drew attention to its potential benefit, and they showed that it has significant biochemical and clinical benefits for prevention of CPB-induced lung injury; yet, the drawback is that the technique is applicable only to closed-heart procedures, such as with uncomplicated coronary surgery.[22-24]

On the other hand, Serraf and associates reported an experimental work of a neonatal piglet model in 1997, which first showed the potential capability of supplementary pulmonary perfusion to alleviate CPB-induced lung injury. They showed that additional low-flow continuous perfusion of the lung during total CPB resulted in better preservation of tissue ATP stores and arterial oxygen tension.[25] They also developed the single-dose pulmonary artery perfusion with protective solution as pneumoplegia during total CPB and showed that the procedure prevented hemodynamic alteration after CPB. The advantage of the additional lung perfusion technique is applicable to any sort of open heart surgery.

Since then, the clinical application of the additional lung perfusion has begun with promising results in the practice of cardiac surgery. Jaggers and associates drew particular attention to ischemic lung damage due to extracorporeal membrane oxygenation (ECMO) therapy in the management of congenital heart diseases.[26] They demonstrated that patent aortopulmonary shunt during ECMO to maintain pulmonary blood flow support enhances the outcome of patients with single-ventricle physiology. Wei and associates reported on clinical and experimental works in that lung perfusion with protective solution as pneumoplegia yields a favorable outcome in surgical correction for patients with tetralogy of Fallot.[27,28] These experiences suggested that additional lung perfusion during CPB is promising in pediatric cardiac surgery. In this context, we first reported in 2000 our experiences that continuous lung perfusion was able to reduce postoperative lung injury in children with congenital heart diseases.[29] Clinical and experimental works have consistently shown protective effects of supplementary lung perfusion on CPB-induced lung injury.[30,31]

44.3 Technique

44.3.1 Continuous Lung Perfusion During Total CPB

During conventional total CPB, the lung is perfused solely by the bronchial arterial system. Therefore, we assumed that additional lung perfusion prevents ischemic lung injury more efficaciously in noncyanotic patients than in cyanotic patients because the former group develops bronchial collateral flow to the pulmonary artery to a lesser degree. Accordingly, we applied our continuous lung perfusion technique during CPB mostly to noncyanotic patients with pulmonary hypertension. The technical details are discussed next.

The CPB circuit was comprised of a roller pump and membrane oxygenator. The circuit was primed with lactated Ringer's solution, albumin, mannitol, and leukocyte-depleted packed red blood cells. Nonpulsatile flow of 2.8–3.0 L/m²/min was maintained throughout CPB. Patients were cooled to moderate hypothermia ranging from 30 °C to 34 °C. The temperature selection depended on operative methods. Cardiac arrest was accomplished by aortic cross clamping coupled with infusion of high-potassium (20 mEq/L) blood cardioplegic solution (20 mL/kg) through the aortic root. The same solution was repeatedly infused in 30-min intervals (10 mL/kg) during the cross clamping. Blood gas management during CPB was directed toward maintenance of pH at 7.35–7.40 and arterial carbon dioxide tension ($Paco_2$) at 35–40 mmHg. Arterial oxygen tension (Pao_2) was sustained higher than 200 mmHg. Continuous hemofiltration of the perfusate using the hemoconcentrator with or without supplemental transfusion of leukocyte-depleted packed red cells was performed to keep the hematocrit level greater than 25–30 %. The patients underwent continuous perfusion of oxygenated blood to the pulmonary arteries with a nonpulsatile flow of 30 mL/kg/min using another separate roller pump during total CPB. The perfusate was infused into the main pulmonary trunk through an 18-gauge pediatric cardioplegia cannula (DLP, Grand Rapids, MI, USA), and it was drained from the left atrium through a vent circuit to secure a bloodless field. Modified ultrafiltration was also routinely utilized for 15 min using arterial and venous cannulae after cessation of CPB. Anesthetic management consisted of weight-related doses of morphine sulfate (50–100 μg/kg/h) and incremental doses of pancuronium bromide (0.2 mg/kg) as needed. During total CPB, the mechanical ventilation was arrested at a positive end-expiratory pressure (PEEP) of 5 cm H_2O.

We demonstrated that our method gives rise to well-preserved Pao_2/Fio_2 ratio (Fig. 44.1) and reduces the duration of postoperative mechanical ventilation. Furthermore, this procedure lessened the elevation of plasma levels of circulating adhesion molecules, including intercellular adhesion molecule 1 (ICAM-1) (Fig. 44.2) and soluble granule membrane protein 140 (Fig. 44.3) after cessation of CPB.[32] These results suggest that continuous pulmonary perfusion during total CPB minimizes ischemic insult and inhibits intrapulmonary neutrophil sequestration by minimizing

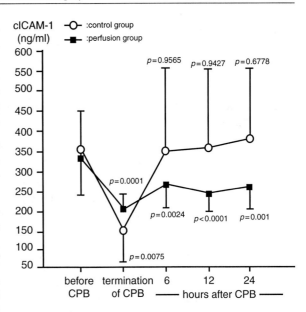

Fig. 44.2 Perioperative trends of the plasma levels of cICAM-1 in the perfusion ($n=8$) and control ($n=6$) groups. A p value represents a result compared with the prebypass value. *CPB* cardiopulmonary bypass, *cICAM-1* circulating intercellular adhesion molecule 1. (Reprinted from Suzuki et al.,[33] p. 244, with permissionf romE lsevier)

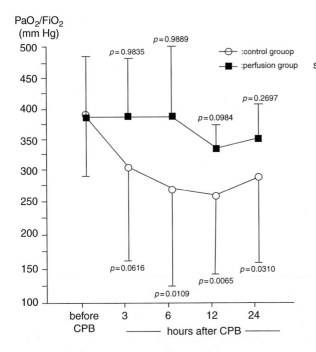

Fig. 44.1 Postoperative trends of Pao_2/Fio_2 ratios in the perfusion ($n=8$) and control ($n=6$) groups. A p value represents a result compared with the prebypass value within each group. *CPB* cardiopulmonary bypass, Pao_2/Fio_2 *ratios* ratio of arterial oxygen tension to inspired oxygen fraction. (Reprinted from Suzuki et al.,[33]p.245,w ithpe rmissionf romEl sevier)

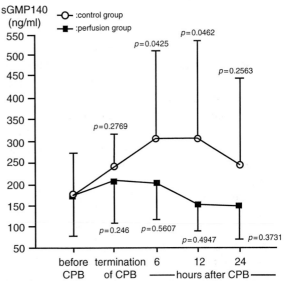

Fig. 44.3 Perioperative trends of the plasma levels of sGMP140 in the perfusion ($n=8$) and control ($n=6$) groups. A p value represents a result compared with the prebypass value within each group. *CPB* cardiopulmonary bypass, *sGMP140* soluble granule membrane protein 140. (Reprinted from Suzuki et al.,[33] p. 244, withpe rmissionf romE lsevier)

neutrophil–endothelial interaction mediated by adhesion molecules in the pulmonary microvessels.

44.3.2 Intermittent Lung Perfusion with the Protective Solution

The other method of additional lung perfusion in congenital heart diseases was formulated by Wei and associates.[27] They demonstrated that lung perfusion with hypothermic protective solution during CPB is advantageous to relieve lung injury in corrections of tetralogy of Fallot. Their procedure is composed of a single dose of lung perfusion with cold (4°C) protective solution following aortic cross clamping. The solution (20 mL/kg) is infused through a cannula inserted into the main pulmonary artery with flow rates ranging between 70 and 80 mL/min. The perfusion is repeated when the cross-clamping time is longer than 70 min. The solution is comprised of a basic solution of dextran 40 (7–8 mL/kg) with additives of anisodamine (1 mg/kg), L-arginine (0.2 g/kg), aprotine (50,000 KIU/kg), 5% sodium hydrogen carbonate (1 mL/kg), and methylprednisolone (30 mL/kg). The amount of all additives is 20–30 mL. Oxygenated blood (10 mL/kg) is added to the solution. The proportion of oxygenated blood to the solution is 1:1. The total amount of protective solution is 20 mL/kg.

Wei and associates[27] showed that the oxygen index and alveolar-arterial O_2 gradient were better preserved in children who underwent the procedure compared with those in the control group. The duration of mechanical ventilation and stay in the intensive care unit were shorter as well. The method suppressed plasma levels of the tumor necrosis factor alpha, malondialdehyde, von Willebrand factor, and endothelin. The concentrations of interleukin 6 and interleukin 8 in bronchoalveolar lavage fluid were also reduced. Histopathological examination revealed no capillary hyperemia or hemorrhage, intra-alveolar edema, leukocyte accumulation, mitochondria swelling or vacuolation, or gas-blood barrier broadening. Histochemical examination showed suppression of ICAM-1 in lung vascular endothelial cells. They concluded that the procedure prohibited vascular endothelial cell injury in the lung and relieved CPB-induced lung injury.

44.4 CurrentSi tuation and Future Perspective

Despite the general esteem for lung protection with pulmonary artery perfusion during total CPB, it remains controversial whether the procedure provides significant clinical benefits in adult cardiac surgery. Sievers et al. showed that it yields no differences in postoperative pulmonary artery pressure, weaning time from respiratory support, or duration of stay in the intensive care unit.[30] On the contrary, the advantageous effects on postoperative lung function of additional lung perfusion have been definitively proven in pediatric cardiac surgery. However, there remains a question whether the continuous perfusion technique with oxygenated blood would protect the lung better than the intermittent perfusion technique with protective solution. The cause of CPB-derived lung injury is multifactorial. In this context, it is tempting to assume that the physiologic disposition of the continuous pulmonary perfusion technique is more promising to preserve lung function than the intermittent pulmonary perfusion technique.

Another question is what flow rate in the continuous perfusion technique is appropriate for lung protection. In normal individuals, the bronchial blood flow is nearly 8–10% of systemic blood flow. Kuratani and associates demonstrated that impairment of postoperative pulmonary function and ultrastructural derangement of lung tissue was less severe in patients whose bronchial blood flow exceeded 25% of systemic blood flow.[20] The experience implied that more than normal bronchial blood flow was the prerequisite to protect the lung during CPB. We employed a flow rate of 30 mL/kg/min in our technique. An experimental work of continuous pulmonary perfusion using neonatal piglets reported by Serraf et al. deserves particular attention because this animal study was aimed at its application to neonatal heart diseases in humans.[25] The lung was perfused with venous blood during CPB using an independent pump at a flow rate of 35 mL/min. Mean perfusion pressure was 14 mmHg. The method resulted in significantly lower pulmonary vascular resistance and PA-aO_2.

Recent experimental reports have implied another future possibility of refinement of supplementary lung perfusion techniques. Experimental work of Siepe and associates exhibited that active pulmonary perfusion reduces conventional CPB-related inflammatory response and apoptosis in the lung, and this alleviating effect is greatest in the continuous pulmonary perfusion using a pulsatile flow of 20% of systemic circulation.[33] They also reported that adjunctive inhalation of carbon monoxide provided an additive alleviating effect on CPB-mediated pulmonary inflammation and pulmonary apoptosis. Rahman and colleagues reported that usage of aprotinin resulted in less increase of lung tissue levels of malondialdehyde, which is a biological marker of ischemia-reperfusion lung injury after pulmonary artery clamping.[34] These refinements would provide further benefits in the surgical management for congenital heart diseases in the near future. Finally, we draw special attention to the work of Badellino et al., which demonstrated that continuous ventilation during the period of lung ischemia reduced lung injury.[35] The lung is uniquely oxygenated through alveolar diffusion and vascular perfusion; thus, ventilation during total CPB may be helpful for lung protection, as is lung perfusion.

References

1. Komai H, Haworth SG. The effect of cardiopulmonary bypass on the lung. In: Jonas RA, Elliott MJ, eds. *Cardiopulmonary bypass in neonates, infants, and young children.* Oxford: Butterworth-Heinemann; 1994:242-262.
2. McGowan FX Jr, Ikegami M, del Nido PJ, et al. Cardiopulmonary bypass significantly reduces surfactant activity in children. *J Thorac Cardiovasc Surg.* 1993;106:68-77.
3. Komai H, Yamamoto F, Tanaka K, et al. Increased lung injury in pulmonary hypertensive patients during open heart operation. *Ann Thorac Surg.*1993; 55:1147-1152.
4. Kirklin JK, Westaby S, Blackstone EH, Kirklin JW, Chenoweth DE, Pacifico AD. Complement and the damaging effects of cardiopulmonary bypass. *J Thorac Cardiovasc Surg.*1983;86:845- 857.
5. Howard RJ, Crain C, Franzini DA, Hood CI, Hugli TE. Effects of cardiopulmonary bypass on pulmonary leukostasis and complement activation. *Arch Surg.* 1988;123:1496-1501.
6. Martin WJ II. Neutrophils kill pulmonary endothelial cells by a hydrogen-peroxide-dependent pathway. *Am Rev Respir Dis.*1984;130:209-213.
7. Harlan JM. Leukocyte-endothelial interactions. *Blood.* 1985;65:513-525.
8. Frering B, Philip I, Dehoux M, Rolland C, Langlois JM, Desmonts JM. Circulating cytokines in patients undergoing normothermic cardiopulmonary bypass.*J Thorac Cardiovasc Surg.*1994;108:636- 641.
9. Finn A, Naik S, Klein N, Levinsky RJ, Strobel S, Elliott M. Interleukin-8 release and neutrophil degranulation after pediatric cardiopulmonary bypass. *J Thorac Cardiovasc Surg.*1993;105:234- 241.
10. Springer TA. Adhesion receptors of the immune system. *Nature.*1990; 346:425-434.
11. Smith CW, Marlin SD, Rothlein R, Toman C, Anderson DC. Cooperative interactions of LFA-1 and Mac-1 with intercellular adhesion molecule-1 in facilitating adherence and transendothelial migration of human neutrophils in vitro. *J Clin Invest.*1989; 83:2008-2017.
12. Gillinov AM, Redmond JM, Zehr KJ, et al. Inhibition of neutrophil adhesion during cardiopulmonary bypass. *Ann Thorac Surg.*1994; 57:126-133.
13. Schlensak C, Doenst T, Preusser S, Wunderlich M, Kleinschmidt M, Beyersdorf F. Cardiopulmonary bypass reduction of bronchial blood flow: a potential mechanism for lung injury in a neonatal pig model. *J Thorac Cardiovasc Surg.*2002; 123:1199-1205.
14. Horgan MJ, Wright SD, Malik AB. Antibody against leukocyte integrin (CD18) prevents reperfusion-induced lung vascular injury. *Am J Physiol.*1990; 259:L315-L319.
15. Chenoweth DE, Cooper SW, Hugli TE, Stewart RW, Blackstone EH, Kirklin JW. Complement activation during cardiopulmonary bypass – evidence for generation of C3a and C5a anaphylatoxins. *N Engl J Med.* 1981;304:497-503.
16. Royston D, Fleming JS, Desai JB, Westaby S, Taylor KM. Increased production of peroxidation products associated with cardiac operations – evidence for free radical generation. *J Thorac Cardiovasc Surg.*1986; 91:759-766.
17. Gu YJ, Wang YS, Chiang BY, Gao XD, Ye CX, Wildevuur CRH. Membrane oxygenator prevents lung reperfusion injury in canine cardiopulmonary bypass. *Ann Thorac Surg.* 1991;51:573-578.
18. Friedman M, Sellke FW, Wang SY, Weintraub RM, Johnson RG. Parameters of pulmonary injury after total or partial cardiopulmonary bypass. *Circulation.*1994; 90:II-262-II-268.
19. Chai PJ, Williamson JA, Lodge AJ, et al. Effects of ischemia on pulmonary dysfunction after cardiopulmonary bypass. *Ann Thorac Surg.*1999; 67:731-735.
20. Kuratani T, Matsuda H, Sawa Y, Kaneko M, Nakano S, Kawashima Y. Experimental study in a rabbit model of ischemia-reperfusion lung injury during cardiopulmonary bypass. *J Thorac Cardiovasc Surg.*1992; 103:564-568.
21. Drew CE, Anderson IM. Profound hypothermia in cardiac surgery. Report of three cases. *Lancet.*1959; 1:748-750.
22. Glenvile B, Ross D. Coronary artery surgery with patient's lungs as oxygenator. *Lancet.*1986; 4:1005-1006.
23. Richter JA, Meisner H, Tassani P, Barankay A, Dietrich W, Braun SL. Drew-Anderson technique attenuates systemic inflammatory response syndrome and improves respiratory function after coronary artery bypass grafting. *Ann Thorac Surg.*1999; 69:77-83.
24. Mendler N, Heimisch W, Schad H. Pulmonary function after biventricular bypass for autologous lung oxygenation. *Eur J Cardiothorac Surg.*2000; 17:325-330.
25. Serraf A, Robotin M, Bonnet N, et al. Alteration of the neonatal pulmonary physiology after total cardiopulmonary bypass. *J Thorac Cardiovasc Surg.*1997; 114:1061-1069.
26. Jaggers JJ, Forbess JM, Shah AS, et al. Extracorporeal membrane oxygenation for infant postcardiotomy support: significance of shunt management. *Ann Thorac Surg.* 2000;69:1476-1483.

27. Wei B, Liu Y, Wang Q, et al. Lung perfusion with protective solution relieves lung injury in corrections of tetralogy of Fallot. *Ann Thorac Surg*.2004; 77:918-924.

28. Liu Y, Wang Q, Zhu X, et al. Pulmonary artery perfusion with protective solution reduces lung injury after cardiopulmonary bypass. *Ann Thorac Surg*.2000; 69:1402-1407.

29. Suzuki T, Fukuda T, Ito T, Inoue Y, Cho Y, Kashima I. Continuous pulmonary perfusion during cardiopulmonary bypass prevents lung injury in infants. *Ann Thorac Surg*. 2000;69:602-606.

30. Sievers H, Freund-Kaas C, Eleftheriadis S, et al. Lung protection during total cardiopulmonary bypass by isolated perfusion: preliminary results of a novel perfusion strategy. *Ann Thorac Surg*.2002; 74:1167-1172.

31. Gabriel EA, Locali RF, Matsuoka PK, et al. Lung perfusion during cardiac surgery with cardiopulmonary bypass: is it necessary? *Interact Cardiovasc Thorac Surg*. 2008;7:1089-1095.

32. Suzuki T, Ito T, Kashima I, Teruya K, Fukuda T. Continuous perfusion of pulmonary arteries during total cardiopulmonary bypass favorably affects levels of circulating adhesion molecules and lung perfusion. *J Thorac Cardiovasc Surg*. 2001;122:242-248.

33. Siepe M, Goebel U, Mecklenburg A, et al. Pulsatile pulmonary perfusion during cardiopulmonary bypass reduces the pulmonary inflammatory response. *Ann Thorac Surg*. 2008;86:115-122.

34. Rahman A, Ustunda B, Burma O, Ozercan IH, Cekirdekci A, Bayar MK. Does aprotinin reduce lung reperfusion damage after cardiopulmonary bypass? *Eur Cardiothorac Surg*. 2000;18:583-588.

35. Badellino MM, Morganroth ML, Grum CM, Lynch MJ, Bolling SF, Deeb GM. Hypothermia or continuous ventilation decreases ischemia-reperfusion injury in an ex vivo rat lung model. *Surgery*.1989; 105:752-760.

Retrograde Pulmonary Perfusion forPul monaryT hromboembolism

Salvatore Spagnolo, Maria Antonia Grasso,
Paata Kalandadze, and Ugo Filippo Tesler

45.1 Defectso fC onventional Pulmonary Embolectomy

Options for the treatment of pulmonary embolism include medical management using thrombolytics, invasive procedures such as catheter pulmonary embolectomy, and surgical embolectomy with or without cardiopulmonary bypass. The common view was that surgical pulmonary embolectomy should be reserved for those patients who are hemodynamically compromised but for whom thrombolytic treatment is contraindicated and for those who are so severely affected that the time required attempting medical management is unacceptable.[1,2]

The major argument against surgical embolectomy was the mortality associated with the procedure.

The recently observed improvement in the results of surgical pulmonary embolectomy for massive pulmonary embolism has largely been credited to judicious selection of patients, rapid diagnosis, and early surgery performed on hemodynamically stable patients.[3-7] Reports stated that results of open pulmonary embolectomy have improved, with mortality ranging from 8% to 27%.[3-5] However, these series consisted primarily of patients who were not in critical condition at the time of surgery. Mortality rates remain high, ranging from 30% to 45% when embolectomy for massive pulmonary embolism is performed on critically ill patients,[3,8-10] reaching 60% when those patients have experienced cardiac arrest before the procedure.[8,9]

The causes of death in patients who undergo pulmonary embolectomy have been attributed to right heart failure secondary to persistent pulmonary hypertension, intra-alveolar and interstitial pulmonary edema with normal left-sided pressures, and massive parenchymal and intrabronchial hemorrhage. The common pathologic finding is pulmonary hemorrhagic infarction.[8,11-13]

The extraction of clots from the distal branches of the pulmonary artery is commonly performed through an extended pulmonary arteriotomy by suction and the use of standard or gallbladder-stone forceps, Fogarty catheters, or similar instruments, along with manual compression of the lungs as advocated in the original report by Cooley et al.[14]

Mechanical injury to the pulmonary arterial wall by these means is thought to be responsible for the parenchymal and endobronchial bleeding.[6,15,16] The danger of injury to distal vessels has prompted recommendations to avoid blind instrumentation and to limit extraction to visible clots.

Incomplete removal of thrombotic material lodged in the distal pulmonary arterial tree is considered an important cause of persistent pulmonary hypertension.[17-19] Embolectomy performed through the main pulmonary artery may not be complete. There are reports of intraoperative pulmonary angioscopy carried out after embolectomy where residual thrombi were detected.[20] The same has been seen in our patients during operation.

Surgical embolectomy in the patients who require resuscitation before surgical embolectomy or who are massaged onto cardiopulmonary bypass may be unsatisfactory because cardiac massage has displaced significant amounts of embolic material into the distal pulmonary arterial tree, where it may be inaccessible from a central pulmonary arteriotomy.

S.S pagnolo(✉)
Department of Cardiac Surgery, Policlinico di Monza,
Monza, Italy
e-mail:s alvatore.spagnolo@policlinicodimonza.it

E.A. Gabriel and T. Salerno (eds.), *Principles of Pulmonary Protection in Heart Surgery*,
DOI: 10.1007/978-1-84996-308-4_45, © Springer-Verlag London Limited 2010

Scant attention has been devoted to the role of air embolism in causing these adverse, often fatal, effects during pulmonary embolectomy. We have seen during intraoperative pulmonary angioscopy that peripheral pulmonary arteries are open during conventional pulmonary embolectomy, and entrapped air remains in the peripheral arterial branches (Fig. 45.1). Experimental[21,22] and clinical[23-27] evidence indicates that pulmonary air embolism, release of endothelium-derived cytokines, damaging and occluding the microvasculature, with consequent pulmonary hypertension, pulmonary edema, and injury to the lung parenchyma. These findings are strikingly similar to those presented by critically ill patients who undergo pulmonary embolectomy. We believe that pulmonary air embolism can be considered a contributor to the negative outcomes in these patients.

Therefore, conventional pulmonary embolectomy fails to optimally evacuate thrombi and air from the peripheral pulmonary arteries and thus impedes recovery to preoperational pulmonary artery pressure. The severity of the obstructive syndrome depends on the quantity of entrapped air, which in turn depends on the ratio between the volume of air that has entered the pulmonary arterial system and the capability of the lungs to dissipate it through the alveoli. This renders more vulnerable those patients in whom there is a combination of negative factors: massive air embolism, peripheral migration of thrombotic material, right ventricular failure, and critical preoperative condition.

45.2 Surgical Technique of Retrograde Pulmonary Perfusion

The first clinical use of retrograde pulmonary embolectomy was reported in 1965[28]; however, it has been used in a few isolated cases.[29-32] Its absence from the literature suggests its use and potential benefits have not become widely known. The first report in which retrograde pulmonary perfusion was used as an adjunct to standard pulmonary embolectomy in a consecutive series of patients was published by our group.[19]

The retrograde pulmonary perfusion technique uses standard normothermic cardiopulmonary bypass with bicaval cannulation. The arterial line is connected to a Y connector (Fig. 45.2). One branch of the connector is joined to the arterial cannula, which is inserted into the ascending aorta. The other branch of the connector is joined to a 20-French clamped plastic cannula, which is inserted into the left atrium through a purse-string suture placed on the right upper pulmonary vein. After institution of cardiopulmonary bypass, cross clamping of the aorta, and infusion of the cardioplegic solution, a longitudinal incision is made in the pulmonary artery trunk distal to the pulmonary valve and is extended into the proximal right and left pulmonary artery branches. The thrombotic material is extracted by forceps and suction. The right atrium and ventricle are then explored if necessary, and all visible clots are removed. Then, while the pulmonary artery is still

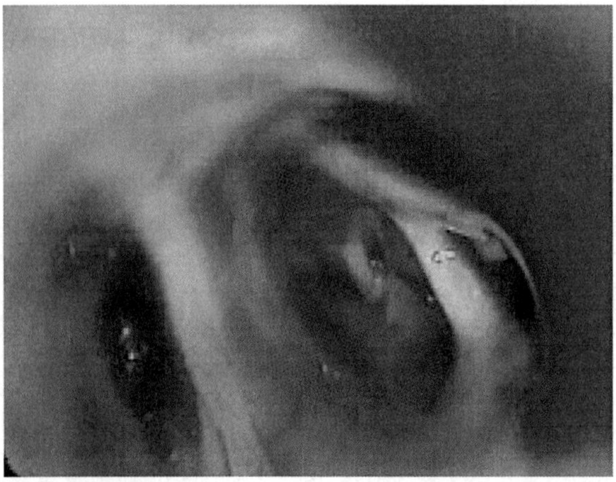

Fig. 45.1 Pulmonary angioscopy performed during operation: peripheral pulmonary arteries remain open during conventional pulmonary embolectomy

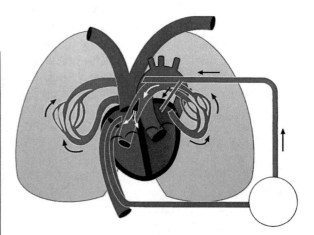

Fig. 45.2 The arterial line is connected to a Y connector. One branch of the connector is joined to the arterial cannula, which is inserted into the ascending aorta. The other branch of the connector is joined to a 20-French clamped plastic cannula, which is inserted into the left atrium through a purse-string suture placed on the right upper pulmonary vein

open, the clamp on the left atrial cannula is released. Blood fills the left atrium, and after a few seconds the blood begins flowing into the pulmonary artery in a retrograde fashion. The mean pressure on the line is 20 mmHg. During reperfusion, the left ventricle is compressed manually to avoid flow from the left atrium to the left ventricle. We continue retrograde perfusion for from 5 to 7 min. At the end of retrograde perfusion, lungs are repeatedly inflated to mobilize any residual fragment of thrombotic material that may be lodged in the distal branches of the pulmonary artery and to facilitate the elimination of residual air bubbles. The clots are aspirated, and all air is progressively eliminated from the pulmonary circulation. The pulmonary arteriotomy is then closed, and the left atrial cannula is disconnected from the arterial line and is used as a vent. The aorta is declamped, and the patient is weaned from cardiopulmonary bypass by the standard method.

In our series, 25 consecutive patients with massive pulmonary embolism underwent pulmonary embolectomy by retrograde pulmonary embolectomy. There were six critically ill patients who experienced cardiac arrest before or during operation. There were no in-hospital deaths. All patients were discharged from the hospital on anticoagulant therapy.

45.3 Goalso fR etrograde Pulmonary Perfusion

During conventional pulmonary embolectomy, pulmonary arterial branches are held open by the elastic parenchyma of the lung itself. On discontinuation of cardiopulmonary bypass and restoration of normal blood flow, the entrapped air is driven into the peripheral arterial branches, where it forms microbubbles that contribute to the obstruction of the circulation. Blood flow is obstructed further by the persistence of peripheral thrombi between the air bubbles and the alveolo-capillary barrier. This thrombotic obstruction in turn impedes the air from reaching the alveoli, where it could be dissipated.

Retrograde pulmonary perfusion performed as an adjunct to pulmonary embolectomy appears to confer two benefits: It helps to flush out residual thrombotic material lodged in the distal pulmonary arterial branches and prevents air embolism within

the pulmonary artery. The technique is simple, and it appears effective in reducing the morbidity and death thatha vea ccompaniedpulmona rye mbolectomy.

References

1. Meyer G, Tamisier D, Sors H, et al. Pulmonary embolectomy: a 20-year experience at one centre. *Ann Thorac Surg.* 1991;51:232-236.
2. Gray HH, Miller GAH. Pulmonary embolectomy is still appropriate for a minority of patients with acute massive pulmonary embolism. *Br J Hosp Med.*1989; 41:467-468.
3. Aklog L, Williams CS, Byrne JG, et al. Acute pulmonary embolectomy: a contemporary approach. *Circulation.* 2002; 105:1416-1419.
4. Yalamanchili K, Fleisher AG, Lehrman SG, et al. Open pulmonary embolectomy for treatment of major pulmonary embolism. *Ann Thorac Surg.*2004; 77:819-823.
5. Dauphine C, Omari B. Pulmonary embolectomy for acute massive pulmonary embolism. *Ann Thorac Surg.* 2005; 79:1240-1244.
6. Kucher N, Goldhaber SZ. Management of massive pulmonary embolism. *Circulation.*2005; 112:28-32.
7. Leacche M, Unic D, Goldhaber SZ, et al. Modern surgical treatment of massive pulmonary embolism: results in 47 consecutive patients after rapid diagnosis and aggressive surgical approach. *J Thorac Cardiovasc Surg.* 2005;129:1018-1023.
8. Schmid C, Zietlow S, Wagner TO, et al. Fulminant pulmonary embolism: symptoms, diagnostics, operative technique, and results. *Ann Thorac Surg.*1991; 52:1102-1107.
9. Ullmann M, Hemmer W, Hannekum A. The urgent pulmonary embolectomy: mechanical resuscitation in the operating theatre determines the outcome. *Thorac Cardiovasc Surg.*1999; 47:5-8.
10. Doerge H, Schoendube FA, Voss M, et al. Surgical therapy of fulminant pulmonary embolism: early and late results. *Thorac Cardiovasc Surg.*1999; 47:9-13.
11. Jakob H, Vahl C, Lange R, et al. Modified surgical concept for fulminant pulmonary embolism. *Eur J Cardiothorac Surg.*1995; 9:557-561.
12. Meyns B, Sergeant P, Flameng W, et al. Surgery for massive pulmonary embolism. *Acta Cardiol.*1992; 47:487-493.
13. Stulz P, Schlapfer R, Feer R, et al. Decision making in the surgical treatment of massive pulmonary embolism. *Eur J Cardiothorac Surg.*1994; 8:188-193.
14. Cooley DA, Beall AC Jr, Alexander JK. Acute massive pulmonary embolism. Successful surgical treatment using temporary cardiopulmonary bypass. *JAMA.*1961; 177:283-286.
15. Shimokawa S, Uehara K, Toyohira H, et al. Massive endobronchial hemorrhage after pulmonary embolectomy. *Ann Thorac Surg.*1996; 61:1241-1242.
16. Shimokawa S, Watanabe S, Kobayashi A. Exsanguinating hemoptysis after pulmonary embolectomy. *Ann Thorac Surg.*1999; 68:2385-2386.
17. Stein PD, Alnas M, Beemath A, et al. Outcome of pulmonary embolectomy. *Am J Cardiol.*2007; 99:421-423.

18. Zarrabi Kh, Mollazadeh R, Ostovan MA, et al. Retrograde pulmonary embolectomy in 11 patients. *Ann Thorac Surg.* 2008;85(4):1471-1472.

19. Spagnolo S, Grasso M, Tesler UF. Retrograde pulmonary perfusion improves results in pulmonary embolectomy. *Tex Heart Inst J.*2006; 33:473-476.

20. Morshuis WJ, Jansen EW, Vincent JG, Heystraten FJ, Lacquet LK. Intraoperative fiberoptic angioscopy to evaluate the completeness of pulmonary embolectomy. *J Cardiovasc Surg.*1989;30:630- 634.

21. Wang D, Li MH, Hsu K, et al. Air embolism induced lung injury in isolated rat lungs. *J Appl Physiol.* 1992;72:1235-1242.

22. Huang KL, Lin YC. Activation of complement and neutrophils increases vascular permeability during air embolism. *Aviat Space Environ Med.*1997; 68:300-305.

23. Kuhn M, Fitting JW, Leuenberger P. Acute pulmonary edema caused by venous air embolism after removal of a subclavian catheter. *Chest.*1987; 92:364-365.

24. Fitcher A, Fitzpatrick AP. Central venous air embolism causing pulmonary edema mimicking left ventricular failure. *BMJ.*1998;316: 604-606.

25. Boer WH, Hene RJ. Lethal air embolism following removal of a double lumen jugular vein catheter. *Nephrol Dial Transplant.*1999;14: 1850-1852.

26. Kapoor T, Gutierrez G. Air embolism as a cause of the systemic inflammatory response syndrome: a case report. *Crit Care.*2003; 7:R98-R100.

27. Couves CM, Nakai SS, Sterns LP, et al. Hemorrhagic lung syndrome. Hemorrhagic lung infarction following pulmonary embolectomy. *Ann Thorac Surg.*1973; 15:187-195.

28. Gahagan T, Manzor A. Preliminary report: pulmonary embolectomy utilizing retrograde flushing of the pulmonary veins. *Henry Ford Hosp Med Bull.*1965; 13:87-90.

29. Gahagan T, Manzor A, Mathur AN, et al. Removal of impacted pulmonary emboli by retrograde injection of fibrinolysin into the pulmonary veins. Report of three cases and experimental studies. *Ann Surg.*1966; 164:315-320.

30. Sistino JJ, Blackwell M, Crumbley AJ. Transport on emergency bypass for pulmonary embolism followed by surgical repair using retrograde pulmonary perfusion: a case report. *Perfusion.*2004; 19:385-387.

31. Zarrabi K, Yarmohammadi H, Ostovan MA. Retrograde pulmonary embolectomy in massive pulmonary embolism. *Eur J Cardiothorac Surg.*2005; 28:897-899.

32. John LC, Awad WI, Anderson DR. Retrograde pulmonary embolectomy by fleshing of the pulmonary veins. *Ann Thorac Surg.*1995; 60:1404-1406.

Lung Perfusion in Clinical Heart–Lung Transplantation

46

Bernhard Gohrbandt and Axel Haverich

46.1 History

The initial steps of cardiac transplantation were conducted more than 100 years ago by Carerel and Guthrie in 1905, employing an acute model with anastomosis of the neck vessels to cardiac structures.[1] Reports of the cardiac function do not exist. In 1933, Mann, Pristley, and Markowitz published on donor hearts being connected to the neck vessels of dogs in various different ways. None of them allowed an active support of the cardiac graft to the recipient's circulation. The functional status of the grafts remains unknown. The animals survived not longer than 8 days.[1,2] In 1940, Demikhov initialized experiments with hearts transplanted into the inguinal position and concluded from his recent and other former results that the heart can only function actively if it would be transplanted into the chest due to its anatomical and physiological features. When it would be transplanted to vessels of the neck or inguinal region, it remained completely dependent on the recipient's blood without any active movement of the blood.[2]

On February 26, 1946, Demikhov performed the first successful heterotopic heart transplantation into the chest, followed by the first worldwide heterotopic heart–lung transplantation on June 30, 1946. Until 1955, Demikhov conducted more than 250 experimental transplantations of thoracic organs, developing more than 40 different techniques not using any kind of recipient support, such as hypothermia or use of a

pump oxygenator. One animal survived 141 days after heterotopic heart–lung transplantation with an active support of the cardiac graft to the recipient's organism. Demikhov's experiments included several techniques to preserve the combined graft, mainly by its own closed-circuit circulation (autoperfusion) using the blood from the left ventricle pumped into the aorta, through the coronary arteries supplying the myocardium to the right atrium and ventricle into the lungs, from where oxygenated blood was returned to the left atrium. Demikhov did not make any contributions to the immunology of transplantation.[1,2]

In 1953, Neptune and colleagues conducted the first heart–lung transplantation in a dog under hypothermia with circulatory arrest.[3] Within the next two decades, several experiments were performed by numerous groups to establish surgical techniques and research in the field of physiology.

Hypothermia decreases the rate at which intracellular enzymes degrade essential cellular components for organ viability but does not stop metabolism. After investigations of elective cardiac arrest by normothermic potassium solution following the 1883 observation by Sydney Ringer about potassium arresting the beating heart, clinical results were not satisfying. Alternatively, cooling below 10°C without potassium enabled the heart to tolerate 1 h of anoxia. To further investigate this effect, the model of orthotopic heart transplantation became frequently used, and soon up to 7 h of anoxia was tolerated by the heart. In 1959, cardiac transplantation altered from theory to reality. Heart-transplanted canines were alive several days after orthotopic transplantation.[4]

Physiologic parameters of the heart reflecting the periods of retrieval, ischemia, and transplantation were investigated. The transplanted heart tolerated denervation

B.G ohrbandt (✉)
Department of Cardiothoracic, Transplantation and Vascular Surgery, Hannover MedicalSc hool, Hannover, Germany
e-mail:gohr bandt.bernhard@mh-hannover.de

E.A. Gabriel and T. Salerno (eds.), *Principles of Pulmonary Protection in Heart Surgery,*
DOI: 10.1007/978-1-84996-308-4_46, © Springer-Verlag London Limited 2010

and lymphatic interruption. Immunological consequences of allotransplantation were addressed by the effort to suppress the response of the recipient, adopting existing protocols from renal transplantation.[5] 6-Mercaptopurine was identified in rabbits to suppress the antibody response to an administered antigen.[6] Lower et al. observed prolonged cardiac graft survival in transplanted dogs treated with immunosuppressant drugs.[7]

In contrast to cardiac transplantation, no specific experimental work was accomplished for pulmonary graft preservation prior to its clinical application. After pulmonary denervation in dogs, regular respiratory control was not detectable, and bronchial clearance was diminished. Attempts at weaning dogs from mechanical ventilation failed after heart–lung transplantation. Contrarily to dogs, primates as study animals achieved normal posttransplant respiratory function. These results enabled surgeons to ensure a physiological pulmonary function after transplantation.[8]

The first human lung transplantation by Hardy and colleagues on June 11, 1963, at the University of Mississippi employed a cold, heparinized glucose solution as the perfusion solution for the pulmonary artery followed by immersion of the deflated lung in hypothermic saline. The single-lung recipient died from complications after renal failure 18 days after transplantation. Retrospectively, there was an ABO mismatch between the donor (type B) and the recipient (type A), but no histologic evidence of allograft rejection.[9]

Results after lung transplantation in the following two decades were disappointing. Survival of the recipients mostly did not exceed weeks. Major reasons for the fatal course were infection, rejection, graft dysfunction (described as pulmonary graft response), and airway complications. Preservation of the grafts varied considerably. Lung perfusion was performed in 50% of the certain cases using different preservation solutions. Hypothermia had not been employed regularly, either in the donor or for graft storage. The lung grafts were obtained by living related donation, by non-heart-beating donation, and from brain dead donors.[10,11] Corticosteroids and azathioprine were predominantly employed for the immunosuppressive therapy. Besides development of surgical techniques to improve the bronchial healing, corticosteroids were found to contribute to the airway complications after lung transplantation in a dog model of autotransplantation.[12]

Due to the intention to keep ischemic graft times short, donor and recipient were at the same hospital. For the operating procedures, both recipient and donor were often operated in adjoining theaters, starting simultaneously with the recipient operation and organ procurement. To procure the heart and lung grafts and, sometimes, additional organs, the donor bodies were cooled by extracorporeal bypass to body temperatures of 25°C or less before also perfusing the thoracic organs or without perfusion. The heart–lung block had been excised and the donor organ, immersed in cold solution, transferred to the recipient's operating theater.

On December 3, 1967, Barnard carried out the first human heart transplantation. He transplanted the heart of a young girl who died after fatal brain injury from a car accident into a 54-year-old man suffering from ischemic cardiomyopathy. On the 18th day, the patient died from intractable pneumonia (by *Klebsiella* and *Pseudomonas aeruginosa*) and consecutive hypoxia. On January 2, 1968, Barnard performed the second cardiac transplantation into a 57-year-old dentist with ischemic cardiomyopathy.[13]

The first combined heart–lung transplantation was performed by Cooley on September 15, 1968, in a 2.5-year-old girl, who died 14 h later after reexploration for hemorrhage. Lillehei and colleagues transplanted a 43-year-old man with a combined heart–lung graft for the diagnosis of end-stage emphysema and pulmonary hypertension on December 25, 1969. After an uneventful course, the patient died from respiratory failure only 8 days after the operation. It was again Barnard in 1971 who transplanted the third recipient of a heart–lung graft. The 49-year-old man suffered from chronic obstructive lung disease (COPD) and survived only 23 days.[14]

Numerous experiments were carried out to improve the physiological understanding of lung preservation, long-term preservation, and surgical techniques. The progress of gaining advantages in these fields was slow compared to those for other organs. Lung parenchyma seems obviously more sensitive to the procurement process, including retrieval, preservation, and ischemia-reperfusion (I/R). Long-term preservation was achieved in experiments, and the precondition of sufficient lung preservation was basically defined.[15-18]

Since the initial experimental reports on cyclosporine A as an antilymphocytic agent in mice skin graft rejection in 1976, it has been investigated in several experimental settings of solid organ transplantations. The renal allograft survival in rabbits was extensively prolonged for more than 6 months, even after initial short-time administration for only 28 days, but only in contrast to recipients without immunosuppressant therapy or controls receiving olive oil instead.[19]

Calne proved prolonged survival of mismatched cardiac allografts in pigs treated with cyclosporine continuously or initially after transplantation only in comparison to the regular immunosuppressant regimen of those days, which consisted of methylprednisolone and azathioprine.[20]

The advent of cyclosporine A and its transfer to clinical employment in thoracic organ transplantation enabled transplant centers to conduct thoracic allografting with beneficial perspectives. Encouraged by initial results reflecting safe and sufficient immunosuppression in cardiac allograft recipients since 1980 and the achieved knowledge in the fields of thoracic organ transplantation, Reitz performed the first successful heart–lung transplantation in 1981 at Stanford University. The heart–lung graft was procured from an on-site donor after flush perfusion of the pulmonary artery with a cardioplegic solution.[21]

A large variety of models was developed in small and large animals or isolated organs to investigate beneficial options of graft preservation and storage. In the mid-1980s, Haverich and colleagues reviewed the progress in the field of lung preservation in the prior decades. Many unanswered problems were discussed, intending to implicate new investigational research, especially to improve pulmonary preservation to allow for distant procurement prospectively.[22] The basic instrument of sufficient organ preservation remains hypothermia, which has to be delivered to the entire graft. To ensure profound cooling of the graft equally and rapidly, several different options were at hand that had been developed and established throughout the decades. In addition, specific rinse solutions were intended to further enhance posttransplant graft function by improving organ preservation, thus reducing the grade of I/R injury.

46.2 Clinical Status of Heart–Lung Transplantation

Since the first successful combined heart–lung transplantation at Stanford University in March 1981, there have been 3,272 heart–lung transplantations reported to the registry of the International Society of Heart and Lung Transplantation (ISHLT) by 146 centers worldwide

until June 2007. Starting in 1981, a rapid increase of heart–lung transplants occurred until 1990, with nearly 250 heart–lung transplants performed per year. From 1990, a continuous decline of the procedures performed per year was evident until 2006, when 70 transplants were counted.[23] In the early years, patients originally with pulmonary diseases also underwent combined heart–lung transplantation due to a beneficial prognosis compared to lung transplantation only. Since intriguing reports after the first successful single-lung transplant in 1983 and bilateral pulmonary allografting in 1986 by Cooper and colleagues in Toronto, the solitary-lung transplantation revealed a sufficient alternative,[11,24,] and the spectrum of indications altered.

Now, the major indication for combined thoracic transplantation in Europe is congenital heart disease, followed by idiopathic pulmonary arterial hypertension, other indications (as COPD; emphysema, including α_1-antitrypsin deficiency; or bronchiectasis), cystic fibrosis, idiopathic pulmonary fibrosis, and acquired heart diseases.

There is no consensus on the short- and long-term immunosuppressant regimen of heart–lung transplant recipients. More than 60% of the recipients received any kind of induction therapy of immunosuppression in recent years. While the employment of polyclonal anti-thymocyte/anti-lymphocyte antibodies decreased from 58% to 15% since 2000, the use of interleukin (IL) 2 receptor antagonists increased and was applied for every third recipient in 2006. Immunosuppressant maintenance therapy is commonly conducted by calcineurin inhibitors in combination with a purine synthesis antagonist and corticosteroids. Sirolimus or everolimus as growth factor-driven blockers of cell proliferation are more often used in immunosuppression in recent years.[23,25]

The ISHLT registry report of 2008 cited a high 1-year mortality of 36% following heart–lung transplantation in the overall adult population since 1982 compared to 29.3% in the latest period between January 2000 and June 2006. The survival rate of the recipients at 3, 5, and 10 years was 50.1%, 43.6%, and 29.5%, respectively. In the most recent era between January 2000 and June 2006, the survival rate at 1, 3, and 5 years after transplantation of 70.7%, 58.4%, and 51.6% indicates a significant improvement of survival after combined transplantation compared to the previous eras. Survival has been shown to diverge noticeably in dependency on the underlying indication for combined transplantation. Patients with Eisenmenger's syndrome or idiopathic pulmonary arterial hypertension had better survival compared to patients with other congenital anomalies.[23]

While graft failure, technical complications, and non-cytomegalovirus (CMV) infections contributed most to the 30-day mortality after combined heart–lung transplantation between January 1992 and June 2007, non-CMV infections and bronchiolitis obliterans syndrome (BOS) remained major reasons for mortality beyond the first year to beyond the fifth year.

The onset of specific long-term pathologies as a mostly immunologic response to the combined allograft significantly differs for the lungs and the heart. Freedom from coronary artery vasculopathy (CAV) 3 and 7 years after transplantation, respectively, was 98% and 96.8% compared to only 71.6% and 48.2% for freedom from BOS after the same intervals.[23] This reflects the lungs as the far more susceptible organ to specific graft alteration following combined thoracic transplantation.

46.2.1 Perfusion of the Heart–Lung Donor Organ

Organ preservation on the cellular level might not differ considerably between transplantable organs, but three anatomical and physiological features discriminate the lungs from other solid organs: the airway system, the bronchial artery system, and the low-pressure pulmonary circulation. Studies revealed extension of ischemic tolerance by inflation or ventilation in contrast to deflation. The apprehension of harming the pulmonary vascular system physiologically exposed to low pressures by elevated perfusion pressures often resulted in low-flow flush perfusion compared to physiological blood flow.[26,27] During lung graft retrieval, the bronchial arterial system is not preserved selectively and consecutively inevitably interrupted. Although revascularization of the bronchial artery circulation during transplantation has been shown to be beneficial for airway healing in certain patient populations, this concept has not been widely accepted in lung transplantation.[28] Cold flush perfusion of the heart with subsequent cold storage had been shown as an adequate technique for sufficient prolonged ischemic times, allowing distant organ procurement.[29] Following the first successful human heart–lung transplantation at Stanford University in 1981, experimental research to improve pulmonary preservation was reinitiated and resulted in two main concepts. The antegrade cold flush perfusion via the pulmonary artery initially employed either cardioplegic solutions prior to Euro-Collins solution after its introduction in 1983 or donor blood-related cold flush perfusion in the clinical setting. The second concept involved donor core cooling using a portable extracorporeal circulation system.[30] Experimental data revealed comparable or better preservation of the combined graft after flush perfusion in contrast to core cooling by extracorporeal perfusion.[31] Combined donor organs preserved by autoperfusion for distant procurement were successfully transplanted, but the setting was lavish and unwieldy and therefore was not employed in broad clinical application.[32] Finally, antegrade flush perfusion to achieve adequate preservation of the pulmonary integrity was widely accepted as the standard technique for pulmonary grafts and for combined heart–lung preservation with separate solutions and routes of delivery.[33]

In the early 1990s, retrograde lung preservation via the left atrium was described to perfuse both the bronchial arteries supplying the intrapulmonary airways and the pulmonary circulation, thereby enhancing the preservation of airway structures. Improvement of the early clinical course could be accomplished.[34] Experimental results of this route of delivery revealed decreased residual blood and macroscopic clots remaining in the graft. After reperfusion, enhanced expansion of damaged epithelium and accentuated thickness of the air-blood barrier was seen in the antegrade preserved lung grafts compared to retrograde perfusion. In comparison to the accepted antegrade flush preservation, the grade of reperfusion edema and functional graft parameters were improved by retrograde perfusion.[35] Surfactant function, oxygenation index, and dynamic lung compliance was increased in a porcine single-lung transplantation model after 24 h of cold ischemia after retrograde perfusion.[36] The retrograde flush perfusion was applied in two ways: in situ retrograde preservation via the left atrial appendage and drainage through the pulmonary artery[37] or retrograde flush perfusion in situ followed by a second step of antegrade back-table perfusion of the excised bilateral lung graft.[38] Also, regular antegrade flush preservation in situ at the donor hospital combined with a retrograde flush perfusion of the grafts directly prior to transplantation in the recipient hospital revealed beneficial effects on early functional and diagnostic parameters.[39] Even with the simultaneous retrieval of the heart for transplantation, these techniques allowed adequate cardiac preservation and posttransplant cardiac function.[38,39] The additional retrograde flush preservation after topical cooling in non-heart-beating donors was beneficial for experimental posttransplant graft function compared to supplementary antegrade perfusion.[40] Retrograde perfusion is not broadly applied in the clinical setting today.

Experimental data suggest an amelioration of posttransplant graft function merely by using a second antegrade rinse prior to graft implantation after regular antegrade pulmonary preservation by a common solution in rats.[41]

To obtain sufficient preservation of the airway system and potentially reduce bronchial healing complications, semiselective perfusion of the bronchial arteries in addition to the regular antegrade pulmonary artery flush preservation has been described. This option has not achieved clinical relevance yet.[42]

46.2.2 Surgical Technique of Heart–Lung Procurement

There are numerous alterations in details that cannot be discussed at this juncture. The intention is to depict the principle technical issues of the en bloc heart–lung procurement as currently applied.

Previous to the surgical procedure, the conducting surgeon should scrutinize the most recent donor details (e.g., ventilatory, respiratory, and hemodynamic parameters; catecholamine support; fundamental history; blood gas check) and reports on the chest radiograph, electrocardiogram (ECG), echocardiograph, and coronary angiogram when available. Performing a routine bronchoscopy as an option to evaluate the central airway system for signs of chronic bronchitis, aspiration, secretion, and mucosal status provides additional information.

After median sternotomy, the anterior mediastinum is dissected. Opening the bilateral pleural cavities allows inspecting the lungs for macroscopic patterns, detecting dys- or atelectic regions of both lungs with the opportunity to gently reair those regions, dissect adhesions, and remove pleural effusions prior to ischemia. Pericardiotomy is followed by dissection of inferior and superior vena cavae within the pericardium.

The ascending aorta and the pulmonary artery are then separated. Measurement of in situ blood pressures of the right and left atrium and the pulmonary artery might reveal further information. Purse-string sutures at the aorta and the proximal pulmonary artery are for later insertion and securing of the perfusion cannulas. After administration of heparin (300 U/kg donor body weight) and ensured passage throughout the systemic vascular bed, cannulation of the aorta and pulmonary artery are performed. The tip of the pulmonary arterial cannula should not be inserted beyond the bifurcation to avoid uneven distribution of the lung flush. Supplementary medication (e.g., prostaglandins, prostacyclins, antioxidants) could be administered directly into the vessels. The superior vena cava is then ligated, the inferior vena cava is opened, and the tip of the left atrial appendage is cut off for biventricular venting of the heart in coordination with abdominal organ procurement performed by the general surgeon. The cavities of the heart are empty within some beats, and the preservation solutions for pulmonary and cardiac perfusion can be started separately. The lungs should remain moderately ventilated to avoid atelectasis.

For in situ retrograde lung perfusion, a pressure line should be inserted into the left atrium via the right pulmonary veins to ensure and permanently monitor atrial pressure during the retrograde flush; pressure should not extend 10–12 mmHg to prevent overdistension of the left ventricle. For retrograde preservation, the aorta should always be cross clamped even if the heart will not be retrieved.

When the preservation of the thoracic organs has finished, both vena cavae are cut intrapericardially to allow bicaval anastomosis for implantation. Both ligamenta pulmonale are incised up to the lower pulmonary veins. The posterior mediastinum is dissected ventral to the esophagus from the diaphragm up to the retrotracheal gullet, with both pleural membranes slashed at the matching level. The aortic arch and proximal descending aorta, including the ligamentum Botalli and bronchial arteries, are separated from the peritracheal tissue, paying attention not to expose the trachea itself for sparing the tracheal vasculature. Finally, the upper mediastinum containing the supra-aortal branches is dissected, the aorta is incised, and the trachea finally clamped in the proximal portion, leaving the lungs in moderate inflation status. After the trachea is cut between clamps, the heart–lung block can be removed from the thorax, followed by inspection of the graft and transport threefold packed in sterile containments at a temperature of 2–8°C.

46.2.3 Preservation Solutions

Various solutions for pulmonary preservation are available. Those commonly applied and their components are depicted in Table 46.1.

While Euro-Collins and University of Wisconsin (UW; high potassium content) solutions are intracellular types of preservation solution with a high potassium concentration, low-potassium dextran (LPD) solution, UW (low-potassium content), and Celsior are the extracellular type characterized by a low-potassium component. The high-potassium content of preservation solutions is responsible for vasoconstriction because of its property to depolarize smooth muscle cells, resulting in smooth muscle cell contraction. Vasoconstriction during pulmonary artery flush may lead to inhomogeneous distribution of the preservation solution and thereby might result in inadequate lung preservation.[43,44] To counteract the vasoconstrictive result of high-potassium solutions, prostanoids, mainly prostaglandin E_1 (predominantly employed in North America) or prostacyclin (PGI_2) (primarily used in Europe), are supplemented to the preservation solution due to their vasodilating effect, as a bolus administration intravenously, into the pulmonary artery prior to the regular pulmonary flush, or as an additive to the solution itself.[43,45] Prostanoids develop a variety of properties that also might ameliorate protection against I/R injury. Adhesion of leukocytes to the vascular endothelium,[46] neutrophil infiltration of the

Table 46.1 Commonly applied solutions for pulmonary preservation

Components	Euro-Collins (EC)	University of Wisconsin (UW)	LPD[a]	Celsior
Na^+ (mmol/L)	10	28	138	100
K^+ (mmol/L)	115	125 (9[b])	6	15
Cl^- (mmol/L)	15	0	142	42
Mg^{2+} (mmol/L)	0	5	0	13
Ca^{2+} (mmol/L)	0	0	0	0.25
HCO_3^- (mmol/L)	10	5	0	0
PO_4^- (mmol/L)	100	25	0.8	0
SO_4^- (mmol/L)	8	5	2	0
Lactobionate (mmol/L)	0	100	0	80
Glucose (g/L)	3.5	0	0.91	0
Glutathione (mmol/L)	0	3	0	3
Glutamate (mmol/L)	0	0	0	20
Histidine (mmol/L)	0	0	0	30
Adenosine (mmol/L)	0	5	0	0
Allopurinol (mmol/L)	0	1	0	0
Mannitol (mmol/L)	0	0	0	60
Dextran 40 (mmol/L)	0	0	50	0
Hydroxyethyls tarch (g/L)	0	50	0	0
Raffinose (mmol/L)	0	30	0	0
Osmolality (mosmol/L)	359	320	292	320

[a]LPD low-potassium dextran
[b]Low-potassium content formula of UW

graft, and vascular permeability are reduced by prostanoids.[47] Prostanoids decrease platelet aggregation,[48] and the inflammatory response after treatment with prostanoids might reflect a shift from pro- to anti-inflammatory cytokine release by declining levels of tumor necrosis factor alpha (TNF-α), interferon gamma (IFN-γ), or IL-12.[49] PGI_2 improved surfactant function in a preclinical single-lung transplantation model by maintaining its capacity to reduce the intra-alveolar surface tension after transplantation.[50]

Since its clinical introduction 1983, Euro-Collins solution has provided sufficient and safe preservation of pulmonary grafts for up to 6 h and probably longer, especially when supplemented with prostanoids, allowing distant procurement without the necessity of transportation of excessive equipment, such as extracorporeal circulation units.[27,30,31,51,52] Conversely, experimental reports of elevated incidences of posttransplant I/R injury after preservation with Euro-Collins solution, even when supplemented by prostanoids, are at hand.[53-55] Since the mid- and late 1980s, investigational results promoted reliable preservation and posttransplant graft function of allograft lungs flushed with a modified extracellular type of solution containing LPD.[56-58] LPD solution decreased the vascular permeability by enhanced conservation of the endothelial-epithelial barrier, resulting in superior functional quality of porcine lung grafts in comparison to Euro-Collins solution.[59] Both dextran and low-potassium content contribute to the beneficial effect of LPD solution for lung preservation.[60] LPD-based lung preservation advances the physiological function of type II pneumocytes in contrast to Euro-Collins solution. Type II pneumocytes are responsible for the synthesis and secretion of surfactant, the transepithelial transport of fluid and electrolytes, and proliferation in response to lung injury.[61] The properties of LPD solution lead to improved pulmonary preservation by amelioration of I/R injury and protection of surfactant function when compared to Euro-Collins solution.[62]

Since clinical reports reflected sufficient preservation of pulmonary grafts in human lung transplantation,[63-65] LPD turned into a standard solution for pulmonary preservation in Europe and North America.[66] Analysis of clinical transplant programs identified a comparable effect on early and midterm survival or incidence of BOS of patients receiving either LPD- or Euro-Collins-preserved lung grafts. Onset and adverse effects of pulmonary graft dysfunction are more frequent in lungs after Euro-Collins preservation. Elevated ischemic time may increase the incidence of rejection.[67,68] Early posttransplant functional data of lung grafts suggested a beneficial effect of LPD compared to Euro-Collins solution. The oxygenation ratio (PaO_2/FiO_2) within the initial 24 h after postoperative intensive care unit (ICU) admission was significantly improved, and duration of mechanical ventilatory support and length of ICU stay decreased after LPD lung preservation.[69] Employment of an extracellular type of preservation solution is associated with a decreased incidence of reimplantation edema or grade of pulmonary dysfunction.[70,71] Clinical data contrarily also did not reveal a benefit of LPD compared to Euro-Collins solution in terms of survival up to 1 year or 1 year of BOS-free survival. However, both solutions are employed in clinical lung preservation, with increased popularity of LPD.[68,72]

The UW solution developed by Belzer et al. has been shown to improve and extend the preservation of hepatic, renal, pancreatic, and cardiac allografts. UW solution had been initially used for pulmonary flush perfusion in the late 1980s. Compared to Euro-Collins flush perfusion or donor core cooling, UW solution in combination with PGI_2 provided enhanced oxygenation in an animal transplant model.[73] UW reduced I/R injury as assessed by the filtration coefficient in contrast to Euro-Collins, Wallwork, or LPD solutions.[74] Preclinical data revealed also a beneficial effect of pulmonary preservation by UW solution with or without supplementation of prostaglandin E_1 in comparison to Euro-Collins solution.[75] The extracellular formula of UW solution and LPD achieved equivalent results in terms of improved gas exchange, pulmonary artery pressures, and wet-to-dry weight ratios when compared to Euro-Collins or extracellular UW solution.[76] Ten years after the clinical introduction of UW solution for lung preservation, 13.5% of the transplant centers used UW for preservation in 1998, in contrast to Euro-Collins solution, which has been used by 77% of the centers. Eight percent of the participating centers provided pulmonary preservation by Papworth solution, and only one center employed donor core cooling in that particular survey.[77] More recent clinical data on UW solution are diminishing, reflecting a decline of employing the solution for pulmonary preservation.

Celsior was originally developed for cardiac preservation and is of extracellular composition. It combines the general principles of hypothermic organ preservation with prevention of cell swelling, oxygen-derived free radical injury, and energy exhaust.[78] I/R injury has been reduced by enhancing microvascular permeability compared to Wallwork blood-based preservation.[79] Celsior has been shown to be superior to Euro-Collins and UW solutions by means of decreasing reimplantation edema.[80] Celsior was clinically used for graft preservation in smaller human cohorts for cardiac, pulmonary, hepatic, renal, and pancreatic organ protection. It has been at least as sufficient and safe as the standard protocol for each graft organ.[70,81,82]

In conclusion, the quality of pulmonary graft preservation was a contributing factor to the development of I/R injury that influences long-term outcome. The technique of lung procurement has not changed genuinely within the past three decades.

46.3 FuturePer spectives

Gene delivery offers the potential of effective treatment to patients with several pulmonary diseases. Gene expression from viral and nonviral gene delivery systems to the lung has been problematic. Extra- and intracellular barriers as well as the immune system are limits to gene transfer. But in principle, it represents a feasible and safe method.[83] Gene transfer to experimental lung grafts has been shown to attenuate I/R injury and acute rejection. Therefore, intratracheal gene transfer has been demonstrated as an optimal route for providing significant expression, mild inflammation, and minimal systemic response.[84] Antioxidant gene transfer enhances the production of antioxidant scavengers to reduce the consequences of I/R injury and leads to improved quality and function of liver grafts.[85] Nuclear factor kappa B (NFκB) is an important rapid-response transcription factor that upregulates apoptosis and maximizes expression of proinflammatory mediators. The activity of NFκB is a central factor in the development of pulmonary inflammation and is essential in the pathogenesis of acute lung injury. NFκB was crucial in initiating I/R injury in a porcine lung transplant model. Consecutively, inhibition of NFκB activation by gene transfer of NFκB inhibitor (superrepressor form of the NFkB inhibitor, IκBSR) improved the graft oxygenation, decreased pulmonary edema and neutrophil sequestration, and reduced apoptotic cell death in a lung transplant rat model.[86]

The complex mechanisms of I/R injury in lung transplantation are not completely understood. A substantial contribution of neutrophil leukocyte extravasation to graft alteration is widely accepted, although the recruitment itself remains partially elusive. The family of ELR+ (multiple glutamic acid leucine-argine) CXC chemokines (cystein-X-cystein chemokines) involves potent neutrophil chemoattractants that interact with several CXCR (CXC-receptors) (G protein-coupled) sites on neutrophils, thereby promoting neutrophil sequestration by expression of CXCR. CXCR interactions have been identified as important for the mobilization of neutrophils from the bone marrow and homing in the bone marrow after aging. Some of these CXCR ligand interactions can be blocked by specific antibodies. Elevated levels of multiple ELR+ CXC chemokines were demonstrated in bronchoalveolar lavage (BAL) fluids from human patients with evident I/R injury after lung transplantation. Experimental inhibition of the CXCR2 ligand interactions resulted in remarkably reduced neutrophil sequestration and graft injury in rats after lung transplantation.[87,88]

Returning to the principle of continuous graft perfusion during transportation as experimentally employed by Demikhov 60 years ago or in the clinical setting during the early 1980s, permanent machine perfusion of donor hearts has been beneficial for endothelial vasomotor function and myocardial acidosis in a porcine model.[89] In addition, prolonged normothermic continuous perfusion in a Langendorff model compared to the established, shorter, static cold storage resulted in improved systolic function and accelerated lactate consumption, indicating that continuous perfusion might favorably support metabolism at physiologically essential levels.[90] Some groups have pointed at the beneficial effect of normothermic machine perfusion as a new perspective in organ preservation and transplantation.[91] Normothermic preservation might not only expand the donor pool by greater use of expanded criteria donors and improve or resuscitate organ function, but also facilitate organ immunomodulation.[92,93]

There is one system in early clinical use for normothermic cardiac machine perfusion in Europe and North America. To our knowledge, two companies are developing devices for normothermic pulmonary machine perfusion in the advanced experimental status. The synthesis of both cardiac and pulmonary machine perfusion combined in only one apparatus could be the challenge of medical engineering in the fieldo fo rganp reservation.

References

1. Rukosujev A, Fugmann M, Glyantsev SP, Scheld HH. W.P. Demikhov: significance of his experimental activity in the development of organ transplantation. *Thorac Cardiovasc Surg*.2008;56:317-322.
2. Konstantinov IE. A mystery of Vladimir P. Demikhov: the 50th anniversary of the first intrathoracic transplantation. *Ann Thorac Surg*.1 998;65:1171-1177.
3. Neptune WB, Cookson BA, Bailey CP, Appler R, Rajkowski F. Complete homologous heart transplantation. *Arch Surg.* 1953;6:174-178.
4. Lower RR, Stofer RC, Hurley EJ, Dong E, Cohn RB, Shumway NE. Successful homotransplantations of the canine heart after anoxic preservation for seven hours. *Am J Surg*.1962;104:302.
5. Shumway NE. Thoracic transplantation. *World J Surg.* 2000;24:811-814.
6. Schwartz R, Dameshek W. Drug-induced immunological tolerance. *Nature*.1 959;183:1682-1683.
7. Lower RR, Dong E, Shumway NE. Long-term survival of cardiac homografts. *Surgery*.1965; 58:110-119.
8. Nakae S, Webb WR, Theodorides T, Sugg WL. Respiratory function following cardiopulmonary denervation in dog, cat and monkey. *Surg Gynecol Obstet*.1967; 125:1285-1292.
9. Hardy JD, Webb WR, Dalton ML, Walker GR. Lung homotransplantations in man: report of the initial case. *JAMA*.1963;186:10 65-1074.
10. Wildevuur CR, Benfield JR. A review of 23 human lung transplantations by 20 surgeons. *Ann Thorac Surg.* 1970; 9:489-515.
11. Cooper JD, Ginsberg RJ, Goldberg M. Unilateral lung transplantation for pulmonary fibrosis. *N Engl J Med.* 1986; 314:1140-1145.
12. Lima O, Cooper JD, Peters WJ. Effects of methylprednisolone and azathioprine on bronchial healing following lung auto-transplantation. *J Cardiovasc Thorac Surg.* 1981;82:211-215.
13. Barnard C. Human cardiac transplantation: an evaluation of the first two operations performed at the Groote Schuur Hospital, Cape Town. *Am J Cardiol*.1968; 22:584-596.
14. Jamieson SW, Baldwin J, Stinson EB, et al. Clinical heart-lung transplantation. *Transplantation*.1984; 37:81-84.
15. Wichert P. Studies on the metabolism of ischemic rabbit lungs. *J Thorac Cardiovasc Surg*.1972; 63:284-291.
16. Castagne JT, Shors E, Benfield JR. The role of perfusion in lung preservation. *J Thorac Cardiovasc Surg.* 1972;63:521-526.
17. Otto TJ, Trenker M, Stopczyk A, Gawdzinski M, Chelstowska B. Perfusion and ventilation of isolated canine lungs. *Thorax.* 1968;23:645-651.
18. Siegelman SS, Sinha SBP, Veith FJ. Pulmonary reimplantation response. *Ann Thorac Surg*.1973; 177:30-36.
19. Green CJ, Allison AC. Extensive prolongation of rabbit kidney allograft survival after short-term cyclosporine-A treatment. *Lancet*.1978; 8075:1182-1183.
20. Calne RY, White DJG, Rolles K, Smith DP, Herbertson BM. Prolonged survival of orthotopic heart grafts treated with cyclosporine-A. *Lancet*.1978; 8075:1183-1185.
21. Reitz BA, Wallwork JL, Hunt SA, et al. Heart-lung transplantation – successful therapy for patients with pulmonary artery disease. *N Engl J Med*.1982; 306:557-564.
22. Haverich A, Scott WC, Jamieson SW. Twenty years of lung preservation – a review. *Heart Transplant*.1985; 4:234-240.
23. Christie JD, Edwards LB, Aurora P, et al. Registry of the International Society for Heart and Lung Transplantation: twenty-fifth official adult lung an heart/lung transplantation report – 2008. *J Heart Lung Transplant*.2008; 27:937-983.
24. Patterson GA, Cooper JD, Goldman B, et al. Technique of successful clinical double lung transplantation. *Ann Thorac Surg*.1988; 45:626-633.
25. Bhorade SM, Stern E. Immunosuppression for lung transplantation. *Proc Am Thorac Soc*.2009; 6:47-56.
26. Veith FJ, Sinha SBP, Graves JS, Boley SJ, Dougherty JC. Ischemic tolerance of the lung: effect of ventilation and inflation. *J Thorac Cardiovasc Surg*.1971; 61:804-810.
27. Haverich A, Aziz S, Scott WC, Jamieson SW, Shumway NE. Improved lung preservation using Euro-Collins solution for flush-perfusion. *Thorac Cardiovasc Surg.* 1986;34:368-376.
28. Nørgaard MA, Efsen F, Andersen CB, Svendsen UG, Pettersson G. Medium-term patency and anatomic changes after direct bronchial artery revascularisation in lung and heart-lung transplantation with the internal thoracic artery conduit. *J Thorac Cardiovasc Surg*.1997; 114:326-331.
29. Jamieson SW, Oyer PE, Reitz BA Cardiac transplantation at Stanford. *Heart Transplant*.1981; 1:86-91.
30. Haverich A, Wahlers T, Schäfers HJ, et al. Distant organ procurement in clinical lung and heart-lung transplantation: cooling by extracorporeal circulation or hypothermic flush. *Eur J Cardiothorac Surg*.1990; 4:245-249.
31. Wahlers T, Haverich A, Fieguth HG, Schäfers HJ, Takayama T, Borst HG. Flush perfusion using Euro-Collins solution vs. cooling by means of extracorporeal circulation in heart-lung preservation. *J Heart Transplant*.1986; 5:89-96.
32. Ladowski JS, Kapelanski DP, Teodori MF, Stevenson WC, Hardesty RL, Griffith BP. Use of autoperfusion for distant procurement of heart-lung allografts. *Heart Transplant.* 1985;4:330-337.
33. Harjula A, Baldwin JC, Starnes VA, et al. Proper donor selection for heart-lung transplantation – the Stanford experience. *J Thorac Cardiovasc Surg*.1987; 94:874-880.
34. Sarsam MAI, Yonan NA, Deiraniya AK, Rahman AN. Retrograde pulmonaryplegia for lung preservation in clinical transplantation: a new technique. *J Heart Lung Transplant*.1993; 12:494-498.
35. Chen CZ, Gallagher RC, Ardery P, Dykman W, Low HBC. Retrograde versus antegrade flush perfusion in canine left lung preservation for six hours. *J Heart Lung Transplant.* 1996;15:395-403.
36. Strueber M, Hohlfeld JM, Kofidis T, et al. Surfactant function in lung transplantation after 24 hours of cold ischemia: advantage of retrograde flush perfusion for preservation. *J Thorac Cardiovasc Surg*.2002; 123:98-103.
37. Varela A, Montero C, Cordoba M, et al. Clinical experience with retrograde lung preservation. *Transpl Int.* 1996;9(suppl 1):S296-S298.

38. Varela A, Cordoba M, Serrano-Fiz S, et al. Early lung allograft function after retrograde and antegrade preservation. *J Thorac Cardiovasc Surg*.1997; 114:1119-1120.

39. Venuta F, Rendina E, Bufi M, et al. Preimplantation retrograde pneumoplegia in clinical lung transplantation. *J Thorac Cardiovasc Surg*.1999; 118:107-114.

40. van de Wauwer C, Neyrinck AP, Geudens N, et al. Retrograde flush following topical cooling is superior to preserve non-heart-beating donor lung. *Eur J Cardiothorac Surg*. 2007; 31:1125-1133.

41. Serrick CJ, Jamjoum A, Reis A, Giaid A, Shennib H. Amelioration of pulmonary allograft injury by administering a second rinse solution. *J Thorac Cardiovasc Surg*. 1996; 112:1010-1016.

42. Gohrbandt B, Warnecke G, Fischer S, Haverich A, Strüber M. A novel technique for semi-selective in-situ bronchial artery perfusion in human lung retrieval. *J Thorac Cardiovasc Surg*.2005;129:456 -457.

43. Kimblad PO, Sjoberg T, Massa G, Solem JO, Steen S. High-potassium contents in organ preservation solutions cause strong pulmonary vasoconstriction. *Ann Thorac Surg*. 1991;52:523-528.

44. Sasaki S, McCully JD, Alessandrini F, LoCicero J. Impact of initial flush potassium concentration on the adequacy of lung preservation. *J Thorac Cardiovasc Surg*. 1995;109: 1090-1096.

45. Kimblad PO, Steen S. Eliminating the strong pulmonary vasoconstriction caused by Euro-Collins solution. *Ann Thorac Surg*.1994; 58:728-733.

46. Jones G, Hurley JV. The effect of prostacyclin on the adhesion of leucocytes to injured vascular endothelium. *J Pathol*. 1984;142:51-59.

47. Naka Y, Roy DK, Liao H, et al. cAMP-mediated vascular protection in an orthotopic rat lung transplant model: insights into the mechanism of action of prostaglandin E1 to improve lung preservation. *Circ Res*.1996; 79:773-783.

48. Pallapies D, Peskar BA. Effect of prostaglandin (PG) E1 and its initial metabolites on neutrophil-induced inhibition of human platelet aggregation. *Thromb Res*.1993; 71:217-225.

49. De Perrot M, Fischer S, Liu M, et al. Prostaglandin E1 protects lung transplants from ischemia-reperfusion injury: a shift from pro- to anti-inflammatory cytokines. *Transplantation*. 2001;72:1505-1512.

50. Gohrbandt B, Sommer SP, Fischer S, et al. Iloprost to improve surfactant function in porcine pulmonary grafts stored for twenty-four hours in low-potassium dextran solution. *J Thorac Cardiovasc Surg*.2005; 129:80-86.

51. Wu G, Zhang F, Salley RK, Robinson MC, Chien S. A systematic study of hypothermic preservation solution: Euro-Collins solution. *Ann Thorac Surg*.1996; 62:356-362.

52. Aoe M, Trachiotis GD, Okabayashi K, et al. Administration of prostaglandin E1 after lung transplantation improves early graft function. *Ann Thorac Surg*.1994; 58:655-661.

53. Keenan RJ, Griffith BP, Kormos RL, Armitage JM, Hardesty RL. Increased perioperative lung preservation injury with lung procurement by Euro-Collins solution flush. *J Heart Lung Transplant*.1991; 10:650-655.

54. Kukkonen S, Heikkila LJ, Verkkala K, Mattila SP, Toivonen H. Prostaglandin E$_1$ or prostacyclin in Euro-Collins solution fails to improve lung preservation. *Ann Thorac Surg*. 1995;60:1617-1622.

55. DeLima NF, Binns OAR, Buchanan SA, et al. Euro-Collins solution exacerbates lung injury in the setting of high-flow reperfusion. *J Thorac Cardiovasc Surg*. 1996;112: 111-116.

56. Fujimura S, Kondo T, Handa M. Successful 24-hour preservation of canine lung transplants using modified extracellular fluid. *Transplant Proc*.1985; 17:1466-1467.

57. Keshavjee SH, Yamazaki F, Cardoso PF, McRitchie DI, Patterson GA, Cooper JD. A method for safe 12-hour pulmonary preservation. *J Thorac Cardiovasc Surg*. 1989; 98:529-534.

58. Yamazaki F, Yokomise H, Keshavjee SH, et al. The superiority of an extracellular fluid solution over Euro-Collins' solution for pulmonary preservation. *Transplantation*. 1990; 49:690-694.

59. Schneuwly OD, Licker M, Pastor CM, et al. Beneficial effects of leukocyte-depleted blood and low-potassium dextran solutions on microvascular permeability in preserved porcine lung. *Am J Respir Crit Care Med*. 1999;160:689-697.

60. Keshavjee SH, Yamazaki F, Yokomise H, et al. The role of dextran 40 and potassium in extended hypothermic lung preservation for transplantation. *J Thorac Cardiovasc Surg*. 1992;103:314-325.

61. Maccherini M, Keshavjee SH, Slutsky AS, Patterson GA, Edelson JD. The effect of low-potassium-dextran versus Euro-Collins solution for preservation of isolated type II pneumocytes. *Transplantation*.1991; 52:621-626.

62. Strueber M, Hohlfeld JM, Fraund S, Kim P, Warnecke G, Haverich A. Low-potassium dextran solution ameliorates reperfusion injury of the lung and protects surfactant function. *J Thorac Cardiovasc Surg*.2000; 120:566-572.

63. Müller C, Fürst H, Reichenspurner H, Briegel J, Groh J, Reichart B. Lung procurement by low-potassium dextran and the effect on preservation injury. *Transplantation*. 1999;68:1139-1143.

64. Fischer S, Matte-Martyn A, De Perrot M, et al. Low-potassium dextran preservation solution improves lung function after human lung transplantation. *J Thorac Cardiovasc Surg*.2001; 121:594-596.

65. Strueber M, Wilhelmi M, Harringer W, et al. Flush perfusion with low potassium dextran solution improves early graft function in clinical lung transplantation. *Eur J Cardiothorac Surg*.2001; 19:190-194.

66. Date H. Current status and future of lung transplantation. *Intern Med*.2001; 40:87-95.

67. Ganesh JS, Rogers CA, Banner NR, Bonser RS. Does the method of lung preservation influence outcome after transplantation? An analysis of 681 consecutive procedures. *J Thorac Cardiovasc Surg*.2007; 134:1313-1321.

68. Nath DS, Walter AR, Johnson AC, et al. Does Perfadex affect outcomes in clinical lung transplantation? *J Heart Lung Transplant*.2005; 24:2243-2248.

69. Rabanal JM, Ibañez AM, Mons R, et al. Influence of preservation solution on early lung function (Euro-Collins vs. Perfadex). *Transplant Proc*.2003; 35:1938-1939.

70. Thabut G, Vinatier I, Brugière O, et al. Influence of preservation solution on early graft failure in clinical lung transplantation. *Am J Respir Crit Care Med*. 2001;164: 1204-1208.

71. Oto T, Griffiths AP, Rosenfeldt F, Levvey BJ, Williams TJ, Snell GI. Early outcomes comparing Perfadex, Euro-Collins

and Papworth solutions in lung transplantation. *Ann Thorac Surg*.2006;82:1842 -1848.

72. Aziz TM, Pillay TM, Corris PA, et al. Perfadex for clinical lung procurement: is it an advance? *Ann Thorac Surg*. 2003;75:990-995.

73. Hirt SW, Wahlers T, Jurmann M, Fiegtuh HG, Dammenhayn L, Haverich A. Improvement of currently used methods for lung transplantation with prostacyclin and University of Wisconsin solution. *J Heart Lung Transplant*. 1992;4:656-664.

74. Xiong L, Mazmanian M, Chapelier AR, et al. Lung preservation with Euro-Collins, University of Wisconsin, Wallwork, and low-potassium dextran solutions. *Ann Thorac Surg*. 1994;58:845-850.

75. Lin PJ, Hsieh MJ, Cheng KS, Kuo TT, Chang CH. University of Wisconsin solution extends lung preservation after prostaglandin E1 infusion. *Chest*.1994; 105:255-261.

76. Oka T, Puskas JD, Mayer E, et al. Low-potassium UW solution for lung preservation. *Transplantation*. 1991;52:984-988.

77. Hopkinson DN, Bhabra MS, Hooper TL. Pulmonary graft preservation: a worldwide survey of current clinical practice. *J Heart Lung Transplant*.1998; 17:525-531.

78. Menasché P, Termignon JL, Pradier F, et al. Experimental evaluation Celsior®, a new heart preservation solution. *Eur J Cardiothorac Surg*.1994; 8:207-213.

79. Reignier J, Mazmanian M, Chapelier A, et al. Evaluation of a new preservation solution: Celsior in the isolated rat lung. *J Heart Lung Transplant*.1995; 14:601-604.

80. Barr ML, Nishanian G, Sakamaki Y, Carey JN, Chang J, Starnes VA. A new organ preservation solution, Celsior, is superior to Euro-Collins and University of Wisconsin solutions in decreasing lung reperfusion injury. *Transplant Proc*. 1997;29:1357-1358.

81. Baron O, Fabre S, Haloun A, et al. Retrospective clinical comparison of Celsior solution to modified blood Wallwork solution in lung transplantation for cystic fibrosis. *Prog Transplant*.2002;13: 176.

82. Karam G, Compagnon P, Hourmant M, et al. A single solution for multiple organ procurement and preservation. *Transpl Int*.2005;1 8:657-663.

83. Ferrari S, Griesenbach U, Geddes DM, Alton E. Immunological hurdles to lung gene therapy. *Clin Exp Immunol*.2003; 132:1-8.

84. Kanaan SA, Kozower BD, Suda T, et al. Intratracheal adenovirus-mediated gene transfer is optimal in experimental lung transplantation. *J Thorac Cardiovasc Surg*. 2002; 124:1130-1136.

85. Wu J, Hecker JG, Chiamvimonvat N. Antioxidant enzyme gene transfer for ischemic diseases. *Adv Drug Deliv Rev*. 2009;61(4):351-363.

86. Ishiyama T, Dharmarajan S, Hayama M, Moriya H, Grapperhaus K, Patterson GA. Inhibition of nuclear factor κB by IκB superrepressor gene transfer ameliorates ischemia-reperfusin injury after experimental lung transplantation. *J Thorac Cardiovasc Surg*.2005; 130:194-201.

87. Martin C, Burdon PCE, Bridger G, Gutierrez-Ramos JC, Williams TJ, Rankin SM. Chemokines acting via CXCR2 and CXCR4 control the release of neutrophils from the bone marrow and their return following senescence. *Immunity*. 2003;19:583-593.

88. Belperio JA, Keane MP, Burdick MD, et al. CXCR2/CXCR2 ligand biology during lung transplant ischemia-reperfusion injury. *J Immunol*.2005; 175:6931-6939.

89. Hassanein WH, Zellos L, Tyrrell TA, et al. Continuous perfusion of donor hearts in the beating state extends preservation time and improves recovery function. *J Thorac Cardiovasc Surg*.1998; 116:821-830.

90. Poston RS, Gu J, Prastein D, et al. Optimizing heart outcome after prolonged storage with endothelial function analysis and continuous perfusion. *Ann Thorac Surg*. 2004;78:1362-1370.

91. Maathius MH, Leuvenink HGD, Ploeg RJ. Perspectives in organ preservation. *Transplantation*.2007; 83:1289-1298.

92. Jamieson RW, Friend PJ. Organ reperfusion and preservation. *Front Biosci*.2008; 13:221-235.

93. Cobert ML, West LM, Jessen ME. Machine perfusion for cardiac allograft preservation. *Curr Opin Organ Transplant*. 2008;13:526-530.

Principles of Pulmonary Protection DuringHear tSur gery

47

Chi-Huei Chiang and Fang-Yue Lin

47.1 Introduction

Blood supply to the lungs is through extensive connection in the pulmonary and bronchial circulation.[1] The bronchial circulation is responsible for approximately 1% of lung perfusion, and its main function is nutrition of the pulmonary structure.[2-4] Connections between the pulmonary and bronchial circulation are particularly important when the pulmonary arterial circulation is lacking. In the long term, the bronchial circulation may dilate and support the functions of the affected areas.[5-9]

The pulmonary dysfunction after heart surgery remains an important issue because it increases morbidity and mortality. The disturbance may be manifested as conditions ranging from subclinical functional changes in most patients to full-blown acute respiratory distress syndrome (ARDS) in fewer than 2% after cardiopulmonary bypass (CPB).[10-12] The mortality rate associated with ARDS is more than 50%,[10,11] not including the morbidity leading to prolonged postoperative recoveries and hospital stays.[12] "Postbypass lung" is characterized by increased intrapulmonary shunting, atelectasis, increased alveolar-arterial oxygen partial pressure difference $P(A-a)O_2$, increased extravascular lung water, and decreased compliance.[13-17] The etiology of pulmonary dysfunction after cardiac surgery is thought to be multifactorial, occurring as a result of combined effects. However, major causes of postbypass lung are reduced or absent blood flow through the lungs during CPB (partial CPB) and entry into the pleural spaces during surgery.[9,18] Therefore, ischemia-reperfusion (I/R) injury occurs during heart surgery in which CPB is used. Besides I/R lung injury, another important cause is a systemic inflammatory response through contact of blood with the artificial material of the CPB circuit, leading to contact activation of leukocytes and platelets, which results in the activation of leukocytes, complement, and endothelial cells and secretion of cytokines and other soluble inflammatory mediators.[9]

Despite years of research into this phenomenon, understanding of the complex pathophysiology of CPB-induced lung injury and how to protect against it remains incomplete. Based on previous literature and review articles,[1,19] we examine the current knowledge of this subject.

47.2 MajorFac torsC ontributing to Pulmonary Dysfunction of extra-CPB and intra-CPB

The etiology of pulmonary dysfunction after cardiac surgery is multifactorial, occurring as a result of combined effects. These include extra-CPB factors (general anesthesia, sternotomy, and breach of the pleura) and intra-CPB factors (blood contact with artificial material, administration of heparin-protamine, hypothermia, cardiopulmonary ischemia, and lung ventilatorya rrest).[20,21]

C.-H.C hiang(✉)
Pulmonary Division of Immunology and Infectious Diseases, ChestD epartment, TaipeiV eteransG eneralH ospital, Taipei, Taiwana nd
Yang-MingU niversity, Taipei, Taiwana nd
TaiwanSoc ietyof C riticalC areM edicine, Taipei, Taiwan
e-mail:c hiang01@vghtpe.gov.tw

E.A. Gabriel and T. Salerno (eds.), *Principles of Pulmonary Protection in Heart Surgery*,
DOI: 10.1007/978-1-84996-308-4_47, © Springer-Verlag London Limited 2010

47.2.1 General Anesthesia

It has been noticed that lung functional impairment is inevitable after any major surgery, a condition that most likely is related to the general anesthesia. Computed tomographic (CT) scanning showed that general anesthesia induces atelectasis in nearly all patients.[22] However, CPB appears to cause additional lung injury and to delay pulmonary recovery compared with other types of major surgery, generally believed to be due to the damaging effects of a systemic inflammatory response associated with CPB.[21,23] Yet, it is also noteworthy that the continuing refinement of CPB materials (i.e., the use of a membrane oxygenator instead of a bubble oxygenator) as well as an improvement in anesthetic management (i.e., early extubation, leading to fast-track recovery) have largely limited such additional lung injury.

47.2.2 Hypothermic Versus Normothermic CPB

The impact of temperature during CPB on lung function has been controversial. Birdi et al.[24] found that the perfusion temperature did not significantly influence gas exchange according to $P(A-a)O_2$ after coronary artery bypass grafting (CABG). However, reduced values of intrapulmonary shunt function, $P(A-a)O_2$, and alveolar-arterial CO_2 gradient were reported in the normothermic group in another study,[25] indicating that normothermia may preserve lung function after CPB.

47.2.3 On-Pump Versus Off-Pump CABG

Off-pump CABG is associated with a reduced cytokine response, fewer circulating neutrophils and monocytes, and a significantly lower level of neutrophil elastase compared to on-pump CABG.[26-28] In other observational studies and randomized trials, however, off-pump CABG was associated with fewer pulmonary complications, less oxygenation impairment, earlier extubation, shorter mechanical ventilation, and a lower incidence of pneumonia than on-pump CABG, but these observations remain largely unexplained.[29-37]

47.2.4 Polymorphonuclear Neutrophil Activation

It is well known that CPB primes and activates polymorphonuclear cells (PMNs) through mechanical shear stress[38,39] and contact with the artificial surfaces of the CPB circuit. Proinflammatory mediators can subsequently promote lung injury by augmenting neutrophil activation.[21,40] Several cytokines, including interleukin (IL) 1, IL-2, IL-6, IL-8, and tumor necrosis factor alpha (TNF-α) have been shown to promote neutrophil activation and recruitment.[41-45] In addition, platelet-activating factor, leukemia inhibitory factor, and the arachidonic acid derivative leukotriene (LT) B4 also can contribute to this process.[46]

Activated PMNs can further release a number of proteolytic enzymes and oxidative chemicals both into the systemic circulation and into local lung tissue. These substances include degrading matrix metalloproteinases (MMPs),[47] PMN elastase,[48] and oxygen-free radicals (i.e., myeloperoxidase, hydrogen peroxide, and superoxides).[38] These enzymes are instrumental in the development of post-CPB lung injury by breaking down the pulmonary ultrastructure, which results in increased pulmonary alveolar-endothelial permeability, thereby affecting gas exchange and lung mechanics.

47.2.5 Neutrophil Elastase

Peak systemic neutrophil elastase levels were observed at the end of CPB and have long been associated with postoperative pulmonary injury. Elastase is currently believed not only to be a marker of PMN activation[47] but also to be responsible for causing direct injury by its proteolytic activity on lung microvasculature and on endothelial cadherins.[49]

47.2.6 Free Radicals

Systemic[47] and bronchoalveolar lavage (BAL) fluid[50] myeloperoxidase levels have been reported to be highest at the end of CPB, but the contribution of myeloperoxidase to lung injury is still controversial. It has been proposed that increased free radical activity represents a potential risk for ARDS after CPB.

Hyperoxic CPB is widely used in cardiac operations, and there is concern about whether oxygenation may induce oxygen-derived free radicals. It has been suggested that hyperoxic CPB increases oxygen free radical damage to the lung, compared to normoxic CPB, which is reflected in lower vital capacity and reduced values of forced expiratory volume in the first second.[51]

47.2.7 Ischemia-Reperfusion Injury

The detail pathogenesis of I/R is still unclear. Hypoxia and mechanotransduction[52] (no blood flow) during ischemia induces macrophages, endothelial cells, or other cells to generate reactive oxygen species (ROS), activation of nicotinamide adenine dinucleotide phosphate (NADPH) oxidase, nuclear factor kappa B (NFκB), and calcium-/calmodulin-dependent nitric oxide synthase (NOS)[53-56] and proinflammatory cytokines[57-59] as well as upregulation of molecules on the cell surface membrane. During reperfusion (reoxygenation), cytokines and ROS mediate neutrophil activation, rolling, and adherence to endothelial cells, which further promote release of their oxygen radicals, cytokines, and other mediators, beginning a complex cascade that results in vascular injury and migration of neutrophils into interstitium and alveoli. This sequence is followed by recruitment of more inflammatory cells into the interstitial spaces and alveoli.[57]

Using an isolated and perfused rat lung model, we demonstrated that I/R lung injury produced permeability pulmonary edema, which was reflected by an increasing pulmonary capillary filtration coefficient (K_{fc}) and lung weight gain (LWG).[58-67] BAL contained an increasing protein concentration and neurotphil count. Cytokine (IL-1, TNF-α, and MIP2) macrophage inflammatory protein-2 upregulation occurred in I/R.[58-60,66,67] Acute I/R lung injury with immediate permeability pulmonary edema was associated with an increase in TNF-α production.[60] A significant correlation existed between TNF-α and K_{fc} and TNF-α and LWG, indicating that TNF-α is an important cytokine that modulates early I/R injury (Fig. 47.1).[60] Pathologic examination showed edema and inflammatory cell

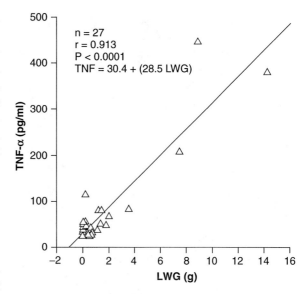

Fig. 47.1 Correlation between lung weight gain (LWG) and tumor necrosis factor alpha (TNF-α). A high linear correlation was noted between LWG and TNF-α. (From Chiang et al.[60])

infiltration in I/R. Our studies also showed perivascular, interstitial, and alveolar edema; focal intraalveolar hemorrhage; inflammatory cell infiltration; proteinous exudate; and intra-alveolar debris (Fig. 47.2).[59-64,66,67]

Our previous studies showed agents protective (Figs. 47.3–47.6) of I/R were prostaglandin E1 (PGE1), dexamethasone (Dex), U-74389G (an experimental drug of the lazaroid class), dibutyryl cyclic adenosine monophosphate (Bt_2-cAMP),[60] pentastarch (Penta),[64,66] anti-TNF-α,[63] anti-intercellular adhesion molecule 1 antibodies,[63] β_2-agonist,[66] and anti-NFκB antibody.[67] We also showed that N-acetylcysteine or apocynin (NADPH oxidase inhibitor) attenuated I/R (unpublished data). A combination of several known protective agents (such as Dex + PGE1, Dex + Bt_2-cAMP, PGE1 + Bt_2-cAMP, Penta + Dex, Penta + Bt_2-cAMP, Penta + β_2-agonist, Penta + Dex + Bt_2-cAMP, and Penta + Dex + β_2-agonist) act synergistically and greatly lessen or even prevent I/R injury.[61,66] Furthermore, we concluded that combined therapy with macromolecules that seal endothelial damage (Penta), an anti-inflammatory agent (Dex), and an agent that reabsorbs alveolar fluid (β_2-agonist or Bt_2-cAMP) would have additive ameliorating effects on I/R injury of the lung.[66]

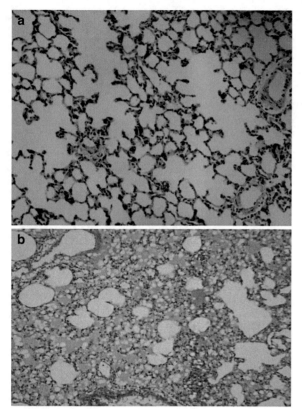

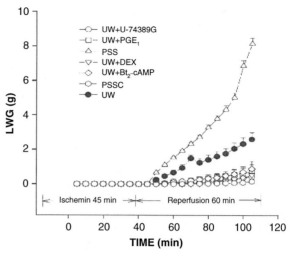

Fig. 47.3 Changes of lung weight gains (LWGs) during ischemia-reperfusion (I/R) lung injury. *PGE1* prostaglandin E1, *Dex* dexamethasone, *Bt₂-cAMP* dibutyryl adenosine 3′,5′-cyclic monophosphate, *PSSC* physiological salt solution control, *U-74389G* experimental drug of the lazaroid class. In PSS group, LWG was markedly increased during reperfusion. After I/R challenge, LWG in University of Wisconsin (UW) solution group was significantly less than that in PSS group. Modified UW groups showed further reduction in LWG. (From Chiang et al.[60])

Fig. 47.2 Light micrograph of rat lung tissue was stained with hematoxylin/eosin. (**a**) Normal control groups with no ischemia-reperfusion (I/R). (**b**) I/R group with isolated rat lung was challenged by 60 min of ischemia followed by 60 min of reperfusion. Perfusate was 0.9% normal saline. There was marked perivascular edema, focal interstitial and intra-alveolar leukocyte infiltration, and proteinous exudate. Original magnification ×200. (From Chiang et al.[66])

47.3 Therapeutic Interventions or Modifications to Avoid Lung Injury

47.3.1 Pharmaceuticals

The commonly scrutinized pharmacologic agents for treatment of pulmonary dysfunction are corticosteroids and aprotinin. Corticosteroid administration before CPB has been shown to reduce the release of proinflammatory mediators such as IL-6, IL-8, and TNF-α,[21] although there was little effect on complement activation.[68] In addition, methylprednisolone therapy can inhibit neutrophil CD11b expression[69] and neutrophil complement-induced chemotaxis,[70] thereby

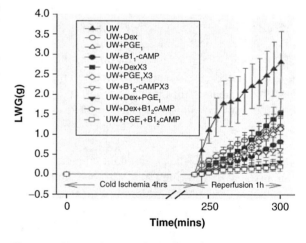

Fig. 47.4 Changes in lung weight gain (LWG) during ischemia-reperfusion (I/R) lung injury. In the University of Wisconsin (UW) group, LWG was markedly increased during reperfusion. LWG in all modified UW solutions was significantly less than that in the UW group. The LWG of UW+dexamethasone (Dex) +prostaglandin E1 (PGE1) was significantly lower than that in UW+Dex and UW+PGE1. Compared with UW+Dex and UW+dibutyryl adenosine 3′,5′-cyclic monophosphate (Bt₂-cAMP), the LWG of UW+Dex+Bt₂-cAMP was significantly lower. Compared with UW+PGE₁ and UW+Bt₂-cAMP groups, the LWG of UW+PGE1+Bt₂-cAMP was significantly lower. ×3 three times dosing. (From Chiang et al.[61])

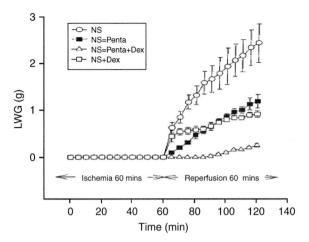

Fig. 47.5 The lung weight gain (LWG) in the various groups during ischemia-reperfusion (I/R) lung injury. *NS* normal saline, *Penta* pentastarch, *Dex* dexamethasone. Lungs were ischemic for the first 60 min and then reperfused with one of four solutions for the next 60 min. In the NS group, the LWG was markedly increased during reperfusion. After I/R challenge, the LWG in the NS + Dex and NS + Penta groups was significantly less than that in the NS group. Compared with the NS + Dex and NS + Penta groups, the NS + Penta + Dex group showed a further decrease in LWG. (From Chiang et al.[64])

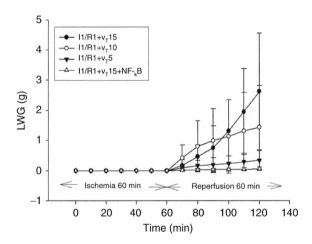

Fig. 47.6 Lung weight gain (LWG) change during the challenge with various lung injuries (ischemia-reperfusion [I/R] or I/R + ventilator-induced lung injury [VILI]) or pretreatment with anti-nuclear factor kappa B (NFκB) antibody. *I1/R1* ischemia 1 h then reperfusion 1 h; $V_T 5, 10, 15$ mechanical ventilation at tidal volume at 5, 10, or 15 mL/kg, respectively. Compared to the group with I/R lung injury (I1/R1 + V_T5) on ventilation with tidal volume (V_T) at 5 mL/kg, the LWG of combined 1/R and VILI groups with I1/R1 + V_T10 or I1/R1 + V_T15 was higher, but pretreatment with anti-NFκB antibody prevented lung edema. Therefore, combined I/R + VILI induced more lung injury, and anti-NFκB antibody attenuated both lung injuries. (From Chiang et al.[67])

decreasing neutrophil activation and post-CPB neutropenia.[45] However, it failed to limit PMN elastase activity.[71] In a porcine model,[72] post-CPB lung function, as indicated by P(A-a)O$_2$, pulmonary vascular resistance, and extracellular fluid accumulation, was better preserved after pretreatment with methylprednisolone. However, in a randomized clinical trial, patients who received methylprednisolone during a sternotomy or at the onset of CPB had similar or higher postoperative P(A-a)O$_2$ levels and pulmonary shunt function as well as longer intubation times compared with control subjects.[73,74] Furthermore, methylprednisolone therapy was unable to prevent poor postoperative lung compliance.[73,74]

Aprotinin is known to decrease lung injury by increasing neutrophil deformability and inhibiting the activity of adhesion molecules in neutrophils.[75] IL-8 levels in the BAL fluid and pulmonary neutrophil sequestration after CPB were inhibited after the use of aprotinin.[76] Aprotinin priming of the CPB circuit may result in reduced postoperative morbidity and shorter intensive care unit stay.[21]

47.3.2 Leukocyte Depletion

Leukocyte depletion during CPB may limit the postoperative inflammatory response, as measured by reduced IL-8 production, although its beneficial effects on post-CPB pulmonary function have been inconsistent.[77] In some studies, leukocyte depletion did not significantly improve postoperative Pao$_2$ levels and pulmonary hemodynamics.[77,78] In other reports, better preserved lung function and less free radical generation was associated with leukocyte-depleted CPB.[79-83]

47.3.3 Modification of CPB Circuit

Heparin-coated circuits are associated with reduced activation of leukocytes and release of cytokines, resulting in less inflammatory reaction following CPB.[84-86]

Compared with conventional circuits, heparin coating may improve lung compliance and pulmonary vascular resistance and may reduce intrapulmonary shunting.[87,88] However, such benefits can only be transient and might not be clinically significant.[89]

In addition, a comparison between the hollow-fiber and the flat-sheet membrane oxygenators has suggested that a greater pressure drop (which corresponds to shear stress) across the latter is associated with a more pronounced activation of leukocytes during clinical CPB and therefore should be avoided. Reduction of circuit surface area and the use of biocompatible surface-modified circuits might be useful and effective at attenuating the systemic inflammatory response to CPB and improving outcomes.

47.3.4 Continuous Hemofiltration

High-volume continuous hemofiltration, by removing potentially destructive and inflammatory substances from the circulation during CPB, can significantly reduce systemic edema and pulmonary hypertension, thereby improving lung function.[90] The combined use of balanced ultrafiltration and modified ultrafiltration can effectively concentrate the blood, modify the increase of some harmful inflammatory mediators, attenuate lung edema and inflammatory pulmonary injury, and mitigate the impairment of pulmonary function.

47.4 MaintainingMec hanical Ventilation During CPB

Hypoventilation during CPB is associated with the development of microatelectasis, hydrostatic pulmonary edema, poor compliance, and a higher incidence of infection.[91,92] Hence, some investigators[91-94] have hypothesized that mechanical ventilation during CPB may limit postoperative lung injury by preventing these complications. Moreover, the lungs are totally dependent on oxygen supply from the bronchial arteries in the period of cardiac arrest. Atelectasis is more important in postoperative lung gas exchange and ventilatory abnormalities than increased permeability edema.[95] The data agree with rapidly developing atelectasis during induction of anesthesia prior to surgery and may also explain the positive effect on postoperative lung function of continuous airway pressure or ventilation during surgery.[96,97]

To date, the evidence for the benefits of maintaining ventilation alone during CPB is inconsistent, with most studies showing no significant improvement of lung function. Continuous ventilation during CPB was shown to provide no significant improvement in pulmonary vascular resistance, cardiac index, or oxygen tensions in a pig model (102). Similarly, no differences in pulmonary epithelial permeability were found between ventilated and nonventilated patients undergoing CPB.[98] However, maintaining ventilation together with pulmonary artery (PA) perfusion during CPB may be advantageous. Friedman et al.[93] compared total CPB (i.e., no ventilation or PA perfusion) with partial CPB (i.e., with ventilation and PA perfusion) in a sheep model. They suggested that ventilation with PA perfusion during CPB may have a beneficial role in preserving lung function by limiting platelet and neutrophil sequestration and attenuating the thromboxane $B_2(TX\ B_2)$ response after CPB.[93]

Mechanical ventilation with larger tidal volume induced acute lung injury (Fig. 47.6). During CPB with mechanical ventilation, we suggest optimal tidal volume should be given to prevent ventilator-induced lung injury (VILI). Our results[67] from the pathology in response to VILI and cytokine upregulation further support the previous study that showed a mechanism for VILI in which the inciting factor, which may be mechanical, induces not only physical trauma (barotraumas and volutrauma) but also biotrauma (cytokine release and a number of cellular responses), leading to lung injury. If this is correct, this could lead to a paradigm shift in which therapies to prevent ventilator-induced lung injury are based not only on manipulating pressure or volume in the lung, but also on intervention for biotrauma.

47.5 MaintainingL ungPer fusion During CPB

Since the early days of open heart surgery, it has been recognized that CPB is associated with pulmonary I/R injury. However, as far as preventing tissue ischemia during CPB is concerned, the lungs remain one of the least-protected organs. The question remains whether maintaining pulmonary arterial perfusion during CPB could attenuate the deterioration of lung function. In animal models, CPB without pulmonary perfusion resulted in significantly higher pulmonary vascular resistance and PA-aO_2, with lower pulmonary compliance.[99] Liu and colleagues[75] have shown that use of a hypothermic anti-inflammatory solution for pulmonary perfusion may help to prevent lung injury, as measured by better post-CPB pulmonary histology and lung function, as well as lower plasma malondialdehyde levels. Richter and colleagues[100] reported an attenuated cytokine (IL-6, IL-8) response and better-preserved lung function (less pulmonary shunting, improved PA-aO$_2$ and respiratory indexes, and earlier extubation) in patients undergoing bilateral extracorporeal circulation (Drew–Anderson technique). In infants undergoing CPB, better-preserved lung function (i.e., an increased Pao$_2$/fraction of inspired oxygen ratio and shorter intubation time) was observed in a PA perfusion group compared with control subjects.[101] Another study in a canine model demonstrated that biventricular CPB helped to preserve lung function (reduced pulmonary vascular resistance and extravascular lung water, improved lung compliance) compared to conventional heart-lung bypass, which may further support the maintenance of PA perfusion during CPB.[102] Gabriel et al. showed that lung perfusion during CPB may improve pulmonary hemodynamic performance, optimize gas exchange, and maintain cellular integrity.[103] Rahman and colleagues[104] reported that malondialdehyde levels in lung tissue increased less in patients receiving aprotinin than in controls after PA clamping. This showed that PA clamping causes I/R injury in the lungs. Schlensak and colleagues[5] demonstrated in their experimental study that bronchial artery blood flow significantly decreased despite adequate perfusion pressure, and ischemia occurred during total CPB, causing ultrastructural changes. These severe ultrastructural changes highlight the importance of the pulmonary arterial circulation. Continuous PA perfusion with oxygenated blood during CPB can decrease lung injury.

In conclusion, although severe lung injury after CPB is uncommon, it remains a significant cause of morbidity and mortality with a major impact on health care expenditures. The etiology of pulmonary dysfunction after cardiac surgery is multifactorial; however, combined I/R during CPB and inflammatory mediators or activated inflammatory cells reperfused to the lung after CPB are major factors to induce pulmonary dysfunction, as supported by the ample experimental and clinical evidence. Despite advances in studies of acute lung injury, many molecular mechanisms remain unclear, and no pharmacologic agents targeting identified molecular pathways have been clinically effective. Some encouraging results have shown that maintaining lung ventilation and PA perfusion and modification of the CPB circuit during CPB potentially can minimize postoperative lung injury. However, we still need further elucidation of the underlying mechanism of CPB-induced lung injury to refine therapeutic strategies for patients who receive cardiac surgery.

References

1. Ng CS, Wan S, Yim AP, Arifi AA. Pulmonary dysfunction after cardiac surgery. *Chest*.2002; 121:1269-1277.
2. Mandel J, Taichman D. *Pulmonary vascular disease*. Philadelphia: Saunders; 2006.
3. Deffebach ME, Charan NB, Lakshminarayan S, Butler J. The bronchial circulation. Small, but a vital attribute of the lung. *Am Rev Respir Dis*.1987; 135:463-481.
4. Jamieson SW. Historical perspective: surgery for chronic thromboembolic disease. *Semin Thorac Cardiovasc Surg*. 2006;18:218-222.
5. Schlensak C, Doenst T, Preusser S, Wunderlich M, Kleinschmidt M, Beyersdorf F. Bronchial artery perfusion during cardiopulmonary bypass does not prevent ischemia of the lung in piglets: assessment of bronchial artery blood flow with fluorescent microspheres. *Eur J Cardiothorac Surg*.2001; 19:326-331.
6. Chai PJ, Williamson JA, Lodge AJ, et al. Effects of ischemia on pulmonary dysfunction after cardiopulmonary bypass. *Ann Thorac Surg*.1999; 67:731-735.
7. Guyton AC, Hall JE. Pulmonary circulation; pulmonary edema; pleural fluid. In: Guyton AC, Hall JE, eds. *Textbook of medical physiology*. 9th ed. Philadelphia: Saunders; 1996:491-499.
8. Wagner PD. Ventilation, pulmonary blood flow and ventilation perfusion relationships. In: Fishman AP, ed. *Fishiman's pulmonary disease and disorders*. 3rd ed. New York: McGraw-Hill;1998: 177-192.
9. Ege T, Huseyin G, Yalcin O, Us MH, Arar C, Duran E. Importance of pulmonary artery perfusion in cardiac surgery. *J Cardiothorac Vasc Anesth*.2004; 18:166-174.
10. Fowler AA, Hamman RF, Good JT, et al. Adult respiratory distress syndrome: risk with common predispositions. *Ann Intern Med*.1983; 98:593-597.
11. Messent M, Sullivan K, Keogh BF, et al. Adult respiratory distress syndrome following cardiopulmonary bypass: incidence and prediction. *Anaesthesia*.1992; 47:267-268.
12. Asimakopoulos G, Smith PL, Ratnatunga CP, et al. Lung injury and acute respiratory distress syndrome after cardiopulmonary bypass. *Ann Thorac Surg*.1999; 68:1107-1115.
13. Magnusson L, Zemgulis V, Wicky S, Tydén H, Hedenstierna G. Effect of CPAP during cardiopulmonary bypass on postoperative lung function. An experimental study. *Acta Anaesthesiol Scand*. 1998;42:1133-1138.
14. Tenling A, Hachenberg T, Tydén H, Wegenius G, Hedenstierna G. Atelectasis and gas exchange after cardiac surgery. *Anesthesiology*.1998; 89:371-378.

15. Berry CB, Butler PJ, Myles PS. Lung management during cardiopulmonary bypass: is continuous positive airway pressure beneficial? *Br J Anaesth*.1993; 71:864-868.

16. Boldt J, King D, Scheld HH, Hempelmann G. Lung management during cardiopulmonary bypass: influence on extravascular lung water. *J Cardiothorac Anesth*. 1990;4:73-79.

17. Ellis EL, Brown A, Osborn JJ, Gerbode F. Effect of altered ventilation patterns on compliance during cardiopulmonary bypass. *Anesth Analg*.1969; 48:947-952.

18. Ghia J, Andersen NB. Pulmonary function and cardiopulmonary bypass. *JAMA*.1970; 212:593-597.

19. Carvalho EMF, Gabriel EA, Salerno TA. Pulmonary protection during cardiac surgery: systemic literature review. *Asian Cardiovasc Thorac Ann*.2008; 16:1-5.

20. Picone AL, Lutz CJ, Finck C, et al. Multiple sequential insults cause post-pump syndrome. *Ann Thorac Surg*. 1999;67:978-985.

21. Wan S, LeClerc JL, Vincent JL. Inflammatory response to cardiopulmonary bypass: mechanisms involved and possible therapeutic strategies [review]. *Chest*. 1997;112:676-692.

22. Brismar B, Hedenstierna G, Lundquist H, Strandberg A, Svensson L, Tokics L. Pulmonary densities during anesthesia with muscular relaxation – a proposal of atelectasis. *Anesthesiology*.1985; 62:422-428.

23. Taggart DP, El-Fiky M, Carter R, Bowman A, Wheatley DJ. Respiratory dysfunction after uncomplicated cardiopulmonary bypass. *Ann Thorac Surg*. 1993;56:1123-1128.

24. Birdi I, Regragui IA, Izzat MB, et al. Effects of cardiopulmonary bypass temperature on pulmonary gas exchange after coronary artery operations. *Ann Thorac Surg*. 1996;61: 118-123.

25. Ranucci M, Soro G, Frigiola A, et al. Normothermic perfusion and lung function after cardiopulmonary bypass: effects in pulmonary risk patients. *Perfusion*. 1997;12:309-315.

26. Diegeler A, Doll N, Rauch T, et al. Humoral immune response during coronary artery bypass grafting: a comparison of limited approach, "off-pump" technique, and conventional cardiopulmonary bypass. *Circulation*. 2000;102(suppl 3):95-100.

27. Wan S, Izzat MB, Lee TW, Wan IY, Tang NL, Yim AP. Avoiding cardiopulmonary bypass in multivessel CABG reduces cytokine response and myocardial injury. *Ann Thorac Surg*.1999 ;68:52-57.

28. Ascione R, Lloyd CT, Underwood MJ, Lotto AA, Pitsis AA, Angelini GD. Inflammatory response after coronary revascularization with or without cardiopulmonary bypass. *Ann Thorac Surg*.2000; 69:1198-1204.

29. Weissman C. Pulmonary complications after cardiac surgery. *Semin Cardiothorac Vasc Anesth*.2004; 8:185-213.

30. Staton GW, Williams WH, Mahoney EM, et al. Pulmonary outcomes of off-pump vs. on-pump coronary artery bypass surgery in a randomized trial. *Chest*.2005; 127:892-901.

31. Van Dijk D, Nierich AP, Jansen EW, et al. Early outcome after off-pump versus onpump coronary bypass surgery: results from a randomized study. *Circulation*. 2001;104:1761-1766.

32. Angelini GD, Taylor FC, Reeves BC, Ascione R. Early and midterm outcome after off-pump and on-pump surgery in Beating Heart Against Cardioplegic Arrest Studies (BHACAS 1 and 2): a pooled analysis of two randomised controlled trials. *Lancet*. 2002;359:1194-1199.

33. Puskas JD, Williams WH, Duke PG, et al. Off-pump coronary artery bypass grafting provides complete revascularization with reduced myocardial injury, transfusion requirements, and length of stay: a prospective randomized comparison of two hundred unselected patients undergoing off-pump versus conventional coronary artery bypass grafting. *J Thorac Cardiovasc Surg*. 2003;125:797-808.

34. Syed A, Fawzy H, Farag A, Nemlander A. Comparison of pulmonary gas exchange in OPCAB versus conventional CABG. *Heart Lung Circ*.2004; 13:168-172.

35. Al-Ruzzeh S, George S, Bustami M, et al. Effect of off-pump coronary artery bypass surgery on clinical, angiographic, neurocognitive, and quality of life outcomes: randomised controlled trial. *Br Med J*. 2006;332:1365-1372.

36. Tschernko EM, Bambazek A, Wisser W, et al. Intrapulmonary shunt after cardiopulmonary bypass: the use of vital capacity maneuvers versus off-pump coronary artery bypass grafting. *J Thorac Cardiovasc Surg*. 2002; 124:732-738.

37. Berson AJ, Smith JM, Woods SE, Hasselfeld KA, Hiratzka LF. Off-pump versus on-pump coronary artery bypass surgery: does the pump influence outcome? *J Am Coll Surg*. 2004;199:102-108.

38. Tanita T, Song C, Kubo H, et al. Superoxide anion mediates pulmonary vascular permeability caused by neutrophils in cardiopulmonary bypass. *Surg Today*.1999; 29:755-761.

39. Gu YJ, Boonstra PW, Graaff R, et al. Pressure drop, shear stress, and activation of leukocytes during cardiopulmonary bypass: a comparison between hollow fiber and flat sheet membrane oxygenators. *Artif Organs*.2000; 24:43-48.

40. Wan S, LeClerc JL, Vincent JL. Cytokine responses to cardiopulmonary bypass: lessons learned from cardiac transplantation. *Ann Thorac Surg*.1997; 63:269-276.

41. Sullivan GW, Carper HT, Novick WJ Jr, Mandell GL. Inhibition of the inflammatory action of interleukin-1 and tumour necrosis factor (alpha) on neutrophil function by pentoxifylline. *Infect Immun*.1988; 56:1722-1729.

42. Abdullah F, Ovadia P, Feuerstein G, et al. The novel chemokine mob-1: involvement in adult respiratory distress syndrome. *Surgery*.1997; 122:303-312.

43. Ward NS, Waxman AB, Homer RJ, et al. Interleukin-6-nduced protection in hyperoxic acute lung injury. *Am J Respir Cell Mol Biol*.2000; 22:535-542.

44. Nathan N, Denizot Y, Cornu E, Jauberteau MO, Chauvreau C, Feiss P. Cytokine and lipid mediator blood concentrations after coronary artery surgery. *Anesth Analg*. 1997;85:1240-1246.

45. Jorens PG, De Jongh R, De Backer W, et al. Interleukin-8 production in patients undergoing cardiopulmonary bypass. *Am Rev Respir Dis*.1993; 148:890-895.

46. Martin TR, Pistorese BP, Chi EY, et al. Effects of leukotriene B4 in the human lung: recruitment of neutrophils into the alveolar spaces without a change in protein permeability. *J Clin Invest*.1989; 84:1609-1619.

47. Faymonville ME, Pincemail J, Duchateau J, et al. Myeloperoxidase and elastase as markers of leukocyte activation during cardiopulmonary bypass in humans. *Thorac Cardiovasc Surg*.1991; 102:309-317.

48. Tonz M, Mihaljevic T, von Segesser LK, et al. Acute lung injury during cardiopulmonary bypass: are the neutrophils responsible? *Chest*.1995; 108:1551-1556.

49. Carden D, Xiao F, Moak C, et al. Neutrophil elastase promotes lung microvascular injury and proteolysis of endothelial cadherins. *Am J Physiol*.1998; 275:H385-H392.

50. Zimmerman GA, Amory DW. Transpulmonary polymor-phonuclear leukocyte number after cardiopulmonary bypass. *Am Rev Respir Dis*.1982; 126:1097-1098.

51. Ihnken K, Winkler A, Schlensak C, et al. Normoxic cardio-pulmonary bypass reduces oxidative myocardial damage and nitric oxide during cardiac operations in the adult. *Thorac Cardiovasc Surg*.1998; 116:327-334.

52. Lansman JB. Endothelial mechanosensors: going with the flow. *Nature*.1988 ;331:481-482.

53. Fisher AB, Dodia C, Tan ZT, Ayene I, Eckenhoff RG. Oxygen-dependent lipid peroxidation during lung isch-emia. *J Clin Invest*.1991; 88:674-679.

54. Zhao G, Al Mehdi AB, Fisher AB. Anoxia-reoxygenation versus ischemia in isolated rat lungs. *Am J Physiol*. 1997; 273:L1112-L1117.

55. Al Mehdi AB, Zhao G, Dodia C, et al. Endothelial NADPH oxidase as the source of oxidants in lungs exposed to isch-emia or high K+. *Circ Res*.1998; 83:730-737.

56. Ishiyama T, Dharmarajan S, Hayama M, Hisao Moriya H, Grapperhaus K, Patterson GA. Inhibition of nuclear factor kappa B by I kappa B superrepressor gene transfer ameliorates ischemia-reperfusion injury after experimental lung transplantation. *J Thorac Cardiovasc Surg*. 2005; 130:194-201.

57. Perrot MD, Liu M, Waddell TK, Kesthavjee S. Ischemia-reperfusion induced lung injury. *Am J Respir Crit Care Med*.2003;167:49 0-511.

58. Chang DM, Hsu K, Ding YA, Chiang CH. Interleukin-1 in ischemia reperfusion acute lung injury. *Am J Respir Crit Care Med*.1997;1 56:1230-1234.

59. Chiang CH, Yu CP, Yan HC, Perng WC, Wu CP. Cytokine upregulation in ischemia-reperfused lungs perfused with University of Wisconsin solution and normal saline. *Clin Sci*.2001;101:285- 294.

60. Chiang CH, Hsu K, Yan HC, Harn HJ, Chang DM. Prostaglandin E1, dexamethasone, U74389G, or d-c AMP as an additive to promote the protection of ischemia-reper-fusion injury by University of Wisconsin solution. *J Appl Physiol*.1997;83:5 83-590.

61. Chiang CH, Wu K, Yu CP, et al. Protective agents used as additives to promote the protection of ischemia-reperfusion in university of Wisconsin solution (UW). *Clin Sci*. 1998;95:369-376.

62. Chiang CH, Wu K, Yu CP, Yan HC, Perng WC, Wu CP. Hypothermia and prostaglandin E1 produce synergistic attenuation of ischemia-reperfusion lung injury. *Am J Respir Crit Care Med*.1999; 160:1319-1323.

63. Chiang CH, Wu CP, Peerng WC, Yan HC. TNF-α antibody or 3-deazaadenosine as additives to promote protection by UW solution in I/R injury. *Clin Sci*.2000; 99:215-222.

64. Chiang CH, Wu CP, Peerng WC, Yan HC. Dexamethasone and pentastarch produce synergistic attenuation on ischemia-reperfusion lung injury. *Clin Sci*. 2000;99: 413-419.

65. Chiang CH. Effect of anti-tumor necrosis factor-α and anti-intercellular adhesion molecule-1 antibodies on ischemia/reperfusion lung injury. *Chin J Physiol*.2006; 5:1-9.

66. Liu SL, Chiang CH. Combined therapy of pentastarch, dexamethasone, and dibutyryl-cAMP or β2-agonist attenu-ates ischaemia/reperfusion injury of rat lung. *Injury*. 2008; 39:1062-1070.

67. Chiang CH, Pai HI, Liu SL. VILI promotes I/R lung injury and NF-κB antibody attenuated both injuries. *Resuscitation*. 2008;79:147-154.

68. Boscoe MJ, Yewdall VM, Thompson MA, et al. Complement activation during cardiopulmonary bypass: quantitative study of effects of methylprednisolone and pulsatile flow. *BMJ*.1983; 287:1747-1750.

69. Hill GE, Alonso A, Spurzem JR, et al. Aprotinin and meth-ylprednisolone equally blunt cardiopulmonary bypass-induced inflammation in humans. *Thorac Cardiovasc Surg*. 1995;110:1658-1662.

70. Tennenberg SD, Bailey WW, Cotta LA, et al. The effects of methylprednisolone on complement-mediated neutrophil activation during cardiopulmonary bypass. *Surgery*. 1986; 100:134-142.

71. Jansen NJ, van Oeveren W, van Vliet M, et al. The role of different types of corticosteroids on the inflammatory mediators in cardiopulmonary bypass. *Eur J Cardiothorac Surg*.1991; 5:211-217.

72. Lodge AJ, Chai PJ, Daggett CW, et al. Methylprednisolone reduces the inflammatory response to cardiopulmonary bypass in neonatal piglets: timing of dose is important. *Thorac Cardiovasc Surg*.1999; 117:515-522.

73. Chaney MA, Nikolov MP, Blakeman B, et al. Pulmonary effects of methylprednisolone in patients undergoing coro-nary artery bypass grafting and early tracheal extubation. *Anesth Analg*.1998; 87:27-33.

74. Chaney MA, Durazo-Arvizu RA, Nikolov MP, et al. Methylprednisolone does not benefit patients undergoing coronary artery bypass grafting and early tracheal extuba-tion. *Thorac Cardiovasc Surg*.2001; 121:561-569.

75. Liu Y, Wang Q, Zhu X, et al. Pulmonary artery perfusion with protective solution reduces lung injury after cardio-pulmonary bypass. *Ann Thorac Surg*.2000; 69:1402-1407.

76. Hill GE, Pohorecki R, Alonso A, et al. Aprotinin reduces interleukin-8 production and lung neutrophil accumulation after cardiopulmonary bypass. *Anesth Analg*. 1996;83: 696-700.

77. Gu YJ, de Vries AJ, Vos P, Boonstra PW, van Oeveren W. Leukocyte depletion during cardiac operation: a new approach through the venous bypass circuit. *Ann Thorac Surg*.1999; 67:604-609.

78. Mihaljevic T, Tönz M, von Segesser LK, et al. The influ-ence of leukocyte filtration during cardiopulmonary bypass on post-operative lung function: a clinical study. *J Thorac Cardiovasc Surg*.1995; 109:1138-1145.

79. Johnson D, Thomson D, Mycyk T, Burbridge B, Mayers I. Depletion of neutrophils by filter during aortocoronary bypass surgery transiently improves postoperative cardio-respiratory status. *Chest*.1995; 107:1253-1259.

80. Johnson D, Thomson D, Hurst T, et al. Neutrophil-mediated acute lung injury after extracorporeal perfusion. *J Thorac Cardiovasc Surg*.1994; 107:1193-1202.

81. Hachida M, Hanayama N, Okamura T, et al. The role of leukocyte depletion in reducing injury to myocardium and lung during cardiopulmonary bypass. *ASAIO J*. 1995; 41:M291-M294.

82. Morioka K, Muraoka R, Chiba Y, et al. Leukocyte and platelet depletion with a blood cell separator: effects on lung injury after cardiac surgery with cardiopulmonary bypass. *J Thorac Cardiovasc Surg*.1996; 111:45-54.

83. Bando K, Pillai R, Cameron DE, et al. Leukocyte depletion ameliorates free radical mediated lung injury after cardiopulmonary bypass. *J Thorac Cardiovasc Surg.* 1990;99:873-877.

84. Gu YJ, van Oeveren W, Akkerman C, Boonstra PW, Huyzen RJ, Wildevuur CR. Heparin-coated circuits reduce the inflammatory response to cardiopulmonary bypass. *Ann Thorac Surg.*1993 ;55:917-922.

85. Te Velthuis H, Baufreton C, Jansen PG, et al. Heparin coating of extracorporeal circuits inhibits contact activation during cardiac operations. *J Thorac Cardiovasc Surg.* 1997;114:117.

86. Wan S, LeClerc JL, Antoine M, DeSmet JM, Yim AP, Vincent JL. Heparin-coated circuits reduce myocardial injury in heart or heart-lung transplantation: a prospective, randomized study. *Ann Thorac Surg.*1999; 68:1230-1235.

87. Redmond JM, Gillinov AM, Stuart RS, et al. Heparin-coated bypass circuits reduce pulmonary injury. *Ann Thorac Surg.*1993 ;56:474-478.

88. Ranucci M, Cirri S, Conti D, et al. Beneficial effects of Duraflo II heparin-coated circuits on postperfusion lung dysfunction. *Ann Thorac Surg.*1996; 61:76-81.

89. Watanabe H, Miyamura H, Hayashi J, et al. The influence of a heparin-coated oxygenator during cardiopulmonary bypass on postoperative lung oxygenation capacity in pediatric patients with congenital heart anomalies. *J Card Surg.* 1996;11:396-401.

90. Nagashima M, Shin'oka T, Nollert G, Shum-Tim D, Rader CM, Mayer JE Jr. High-volume continuous hemofiltration during cardiopulmonary bypass attenuates pulmonary dysfunction in neonatal lambs after deep hypothermic circulatory arrest. *Circulation.* 1998;98(suppl 2):378-384.

91. Magnusson L, Zemgulis V, Tenling A, et al. Use of a vital capacity maneuver to prevent atelectasis after cardiopulmonary bypass. *Anesthesiology.*1998; 88:134-142.

92. Magnusson L, Wicky S, Tydén H, Hedenstierna G. Repeated vital capacity maneuvers after cardiopulmonary bypass: effects on lung function in a pig model. *Br J Anaesth.* 1998;80:682-684.

93. Friedman M, Sellke FW, Wang SY, Weintraub RM, Johnson RG. Parameters of pulmonary injury after total or partial cardiopulmonary bypass. *Circulation.* 1994;90:262-268.

94. Loeckinger A, Kleinsasser A, Lindner KH, Margreiter J, Keller C, Hoermann C. Continuous positive airway pressure at 10 cm H_2O during cardiopulmonary bypass improves postoperative gas exchange. *Anesth Analg.* 2000;91:522-527.

95. Verheij J, van Lingen A, Raijmakers PG, et al. Pulmonary abnormalities after cardiac surgery are better explained by atelectasis than by increased permeability oedema. *Acta Anaesthesiol Scand.*2005; 49:1302-1310.

96. Hedenstierna G, Edmark L. The effects of anesthesia and muscle paralysis on the respiratory system [review]. *Intensive Care Med.*2005; 31:1327-1335.

97. Reis Miranda D, Struijs A, Koetsier P, et al. Open lung ventilation improves functional residual capacity after extubation in cardiac surgery. *Crit Care Med.* 2005;33: 2253-2258.

98. Keavey PM, Hasan A, Au J, et al. The use of 99Tcm-DTPA aerosol and caesium iodide mini-scintillation detectors in the assessment of lung injury during cardiopulmonary bypass surgery. *Nucl Med Commun.*1997; 18:38-43.

99. Serraf A, Robotin M, Bonnet N, et al. Alteration of the neonatal pulmonary physiology after total cardiopulmonary bypass. *J Thorac Cardiovasc Surg.*1997; 114:1061-1069.

100. Richter JA, Meisner H, Tassani P, Barankay A, Dietrich W, Braun SL. Drew-Anderson technique attenuates systemic inflammatory response syndrome and improves respiratory function after coronary artery bypass grafting. *Ann Thorac Surg.*2000; 69:77-83.

101. Suzuki T, Fukuda T, Ito T, et al. Continuous pulmonary perfusion during cardiopulmonary bypass prevents lung injury in infants. *Ann Thorac Surg.*2000; 69:602-606.

102. Mendler N, Heimisch W, Schad H. Pulmonary function after biventricular bypass for autologous lung oxygenation. *Eur J Cardiothorac Surg.*2000; 17:325-330.

103. Gabriel EA, Locali RF, Matsuoka PK, et al. Lung perfusion during cardiac surgery with cardiopulmonary bypass: is it necessary? *Interact Cardiovasc Thorac Surg.* 2008;7: 1089-1095.

104. Rahman A, Ustünda B, Burma O, Ozercan IH, Cekirdekçi A, Bayar MK. Does aprotinin reduce lung reperfusion damage after cardiopulmonary bypass? *Eur J Cardiothorac Surg.* 2000;18:583-588.

Lung Perfusion: Reflections andPer spectives

48

Edmo Atique Gabriel and Tomas Salerno

Lung perfusion during heart surgery with cardiopulmonary bypass (CPB) is a breakthrough undertaking; therefore, it encourages heart surgeons to rethink their technical principles and physiologic concepts. When a heart surgeon decides to embrace that idea, he or she is starting to blaze a trail in which the final step will be paradigm change.

The development of CPB was a milestone achievement, by pioneers in the beginning of the era of cardiac surgery in the 1950s. As the evolution of cardiac surgery techniques continued, lung perfusion has surfaced as a useful adjunct to minimize pulmonary ischemia-reperfusion injury during heart surgeries requiring CPB.

To make new concepts reliable and safe is a hard task that requires. However, evidence and outcomes already exist regarding the benefits of lung perfusion during heart surgery with CPB. This book has presented several topics focusing on these benefits.

CPB consists of an assistance system in which the heart and lungs are bypassed. Nonetheless, it is intriguing to think that, for more than 50 years, heart surgeons concentrated their research and concerns only on myocardial protection. Bypassing the heart implies that no effective flow is provided to the coronary arteries. This issue encouraged heart surgeons to develop techniques of cardioplegia or coronary artery perfusion when the heart was not arrested. Likewise, why not to devise approaches for perfusing the pulmonary arteries, either when the heart is arrested, or when the heart is kept beating while empty? Maybe the there was

misconsumption over the years that bronchial arterial flow was sufficient to prevent pulmonary ischemia-reperfusion injury during CPB.

We have a thought-provoking question: What is most important during heart surgery with CPB: preventing ischemia-reperfusion injury or comfortable conditions for the heart surgeon? One more cannula (main pulmonary artery cannula) and the need for left atrial venting should not interfere with the procedure. Furthermore, we believe that the association between lung perfusion and lung ventilation during heart surgery with CPB, is feasible as well. We think that, one of the priorities during heart surgery with CPB should be to minimize the deleterious effects of pulmonary ischemia-reperfusion injury. For that purpose, lung perfusion and lung ventilation are necessary.

It is well known that there are many therapeutic agents and strategies to manage pulmonary hypertension. There are excellent chapters addressing different aspects of this topic in this book. However, if we start thinking about this topic, we will conclude that, the heart surgeon has worried only about pulmonary hypertension-related events taking place preoperatively and postoperatively. What about intraoperatively? What can the surgeon do to prevent the negative impact of pulmonary hypertension on cardiopulmonary physiology?

Lung perfusion – preferably controlled lung perfusion – is the immediate answer to these questions. That is a point that is emphasized in this book. The most effective lung perfusion is obtained when lung perfusion pressure is determined prior to cardiac surgery, taking into consideration physiologic levels for that variable. One of the basic principles of lung perfusion during heart surgery is not to cause additional injury to the pulmonary parenchyma. Controlled lung perfusion

E.A.G abriel (✉)
FederalU niversity ofSa oP aulo, SaoP aulo, Brazil
e-mail:e dag@uol.com.br

E.A. Gabriel and T. Salerno (eds.), *Principles of Pulmonary Protection in Heart Surgery*,
DOI: 10.1007/978-1-84996-308-4_48, © Springer-Verlag London Limited 2010

during heart surgery with CPB modulates and, sometimes reduces mean pulmonary artery pressure and pulmonary vascular resistance postoperatively.[1]

Despite evidence to use controlled lung perfusion during heart surgery with CPB, this approach should be further investigated via new clinical trials.

Areas for new research on lung protection during heart surgery include:

1. New extracorporeal circuit pathways for lung perfusion
2. Dual system for lung perfusion: antegrade plus retrograde
3. Lungpe rfusionus ingv enousblood
4. Lungpe rfusiona ssociatedw ithlungv entilation
5. Testingofd ifferents olutionsforlungpe rfusion
6. Lung perfusion in a continuous or intermittent manner
7. Revisitingth eD rewte chnique
8. Various strategies for controlling perfusion pressure within the pulmonary parenchyma
9. Strategies for lung perfusion in minimally invasive cardiacs urgery
10. Lung perfusion and extracorporeal membrane oxygenation(EC MO)

Lung perfusion is not ahead of our time. Lung perfusion has brought new trends, controversies, issues, and especially benefits for heart surgery with CPB. It is hoped that surgeons will further investigate it.

Reference

1. Gabriel EA, Locali RF, Matsuoka PK, et al. Lung perfusion during cardiac surgery with cardiopulmonary bypass: is it necessary? *Interact Cardiovasc Thorac Surg*. 2008;7: 1089-1095.

Index

A

Acute respiratory distress syndrome (ARDS), 251
Acute type A aortic dissection (AAAD), 401–404
Adenosine,207
Adhesionm olecules,130
Afferents, in ventilatory control
    central chemoreceptors, 39–40
    peripheral chemoreceptors, 38–39
    peripheralme chanoreceptors,40
Airway
    fluids, 34
    resistance,18,19
Alveolar-capillarym embrane,28–30
Alveolarc ells,35
Alveolare dema,140
Alveolarg asp ressures
    alveolar oxygen pressure, 20
    carbon dioxide equation, 20
    partial pressure of oxygen, 19
    respiratory exchange ratio, 20
    respiratory quotient (R), 20
    ventilation, distribution of, 20–21
Alveolarinte rstitial space,138
Alveolarma crophages(AM),35
Alveolarv entilation
    dead space, 10–11
    lungv olumes,11–1 2
Ambrisentan,152–153,199
Anatomicde ads pace,10
Anesthetic management, pulmonary arterial hypertension
    (PAH),20 3–204
Angiography, for chronic thromboembolic pulmonary
    hypertension,1 63
ANP. *See* Atrial natriuretic peptide
Anticoagulants
    DIC,189
    pathways,i nhibition,182–183
Antifibrinolytic agents, for DIC
    aprotinin,190
    prohemostatica gents,190–191
Antioxidants. *See* Glutathione (GSH), ischemia-reperfusion injury
Aortic surgery, lung perfusion
    AAAD treatment, 401–404
    CPB,397
    CRP,397–398
    hypothermic circulatory arrest, 397

    Kazui technique, brain and pulmonary function, 399–400
    pulmonary artery (PA) flushing, 399–401
    pulmonary perfusion, 398
    thoracoabdominal perfusion (TP), 401
Aprotinin,190
    cellular mechanisms, 76–77
    immune system, 76
    and lung transplantation surgery, 76–78
    randomizedt rial,75
ARDS. *See* Acute respiratory distress syndrome
L-Arginine,i schemia-reperfusioni njury
    exogenous, effects of
        lungi nflammatory injury, mitigated, 102–103
        lung surfactant integrity, 103
        microvascular permeability and PVR, 102
    and NO pathway disturbance of, lung insult, 100
        depletion of, CPB, 100
        lung ischemia, 101–102
        NOS enzymes, 100–101
    NO pathway, lung physiology regulation
        microvascular endothelial function, 98–99
        neutrophil adhesion inhibition and transmigration, 99
        platelet aggregation and thrombosis formation, 99–100
        vascular resistance, 98
    practicalc onsideration
        inducible (iNOS), inhibition of, 104
        perfusion with, during lung ischemia, 104
        timingf or,103–104
Arterial blood gas analysis, 298, 305, 370
Arterial oxygen content (CaO_2),9–10
Atrial natriuretic peptide (ANP)
    apoptosis evaluation, immunohistochemistry, 360, 364
    experimental protocols, 360, 362
    histologic evaluation, reperfused lungs, 360, 363
    pulmonary vascular resistance (PVR), 360, 362
Atrials eptostomy(AS),153

B

Balancedul trafiltration (BUF), 255–256
Beatinghe artt echnique,131–132
Beraprost,201
Bilateral extracorporeal circulation (ECC)
    clinical and experimental models, 388
    perfusion and ventilation, lungs, 387–388
Bioengineeringbi omaterials. *See* Extracorporeal circulation
    (ECC) circuit *vs*.bi oengineeringbi omaterials

Bleeding and thrombotic manifestations, in DIC, 180
BNP. *See* Brain natriuretic peptide
Bohr'sc quation,10
Bosentan,152,199
Boyle'sla w,13
Brain natriuretic peptide (BNP)
    β-actin, genic amplification curves, 359, 360
    change in plasm, 359, 361
    postoperative, 359, 360
    preoperative plasma, 359, 361
    vs. total pulmonary resistance, 359, 361
Breathing, gradient pressures. *See*Pul monaryv entilation
Bronchus-associated lymphoid tissue (BALT), 34
BUF. *See* Balanced ultrafiltration

C

CABG. *See* Coronary artery bypass graft
Calciumc hannelbl ockers,198–199
Capacitancec oefficient,10
Capillarype rmeability,i ncreased,142
Cardiac catheterization, for chronic thromboembolic
        pulmonary hypertension, 163
Cardiac conditions and pulmonary VEGF, 70
Cardiacs urgery,223–224
    extracorporealc irculation,125–126
Cardiogenicpul monarye dema,140–142
Cardioplegic and organ preservation solutions, endothelial
        dysfunction,57–59
Cardioplegic arrest/beating heart group, 335, 338
Cardiopulmonary bypass (CPB), 223–226
    L-arginine, depletion of, 99–100
    beating heart technique, 131–132
    clinical heart-lung surgery, 407
    gas exchange features
        Drew-Anderson techniques, 241
        endothelium-dependent relaxation, 240, 241
        lung dysfunctional mechanism, 240
        oxygen tension values, 240
        protective ventilatory strategies, 239
        pulmonary artery perfusion, 239
        respiratory abnormalities, 239, 240
        respiratorybe nefits, 241, 242
        respiratory variables, 239
    hemodynamic performance, 295
    hemodynamicv ariables
        biventricular approaches, 235
        controlled pulmonary reperfusion, 237
        lung perfusion effects, 236
        physiological impacts, 235
        reperfusion injury, 236
        strategies,236
        uncontrolled lung perfusion, 237
    hemofiltration (HF)
        in adult patients, 266–267
        in animal experiments, 264–265
        in pediatric patients, 265–266
        prime solution, 263–264
    ischemia-reperfusion injury, 130–131
    lung perfusion, 349–350, 351, 441, 442
        components,27 9–280
    lung protection, carbon monoxide inhalation

anti-inflammatory agent, 380
    heat shock proteins, 378, 379
    inflammation and dysfunction, 378
    protective effects, 378
pathogenesis
    adhesion molecules, 130
    cytokines,129–130
    endotoxin,130
    nuclear factor kappa B, 130
postreperfusion pulmonary vascular resistance, 237, 238
pulmonary injury mechanism
    atelectasis,368–369
    inflammatory response, 368
    ischemia-reperfusion injury, 368
    mucin accumulation, 368–369
technical strategies, 131
ultrafiltration (UF), pulmonary function, 251–252
Cathelicidins,34
Cellular therapy, for IPH, 155
Celsior®,82
Chcmoreceptors
    central,39–40
    peripheral,38–39
Chestr adiography
    chronic thromboembolic pulmonary hypertension, 162
    Eisenmengers yndrome
        unrepaired atrial septal defect and left pulmonary artery
            angiogram, 175
        ventricular septal defect, 174
    thorax,45–46
Chest wall compliance, pulmonary ventilation, 17
Closed-circuitpe rfusion,280,283
Closing volume (CV), pulmonary ventilation, 17–18
Coagulation inhibitors, DIC, 185–186, 189–190
Colloid osmotic pressure, decreased, 143
Combination therapy, for IPH, 153
    evidence-based treatment algorithm for, 154
    interventional therapy for, 153–154
Complements ystem,215
    Computed tomography, of thoraxair bronchograms,
            consolidation area, 48
    air trapping, lower lobes, 48
    anterior mediastinal lesion with fat density, teratoma, 50
    lower density areas, emphysema, 49
    multiple round pulmonary opacities, 48
    postcontrast, sagittal oblique reformation, 50
    trachea,47
Congenital heart disease surgery
    cardiopulmonary bypass (CPB), 407
    continuous lung perfusion, total CPB, 408–410
    future perspective, 410–411
    history,408
    intermittent lung perfusion, 410
Continuousl ungpe rfusion,408–410
Controlledpe rfusion,335,340
Controlled pulmonary reperfusion, 237, 275
Conventionalul trafiltration (CUF), 253–254
Coronary artery bypass graft (CABG), 239, 266–267
Coronarype rfusion,349–350
CPB. *See*C ardiopulmonarybypa ss
CUF. *See* Conventional ultrafiltration

CXC-receptors(CXCR),424
Cytokines and cellular adhesion molecules
    cycle threshold (CT), 326–328
    genetic expression, 323
    intercellular adhesion molecule 1 (ICAM-1)
        genetica mplification curves, 326, 328, 329
        pre and postoperative values, 326, 330
    interleukin 4 (IL-4)
        genetica mplification curves, 326, 328, 329
        pre and postoperative values, 326, 330
    postoperativemR NA
        subgroup IA and IB, 323, 324
        subgroups IA and IC, 323, 324
        subgroups IB and IC, 323, 325
        subgroups IIA and IIB, 323, 325
        subgroups IIA and IIC, 323, 326
        subgroups IIB and IIC, 323, 326
    preoperative and postoperative mRNA
        subgroup IA, IB and IC, 323, 324
        subgroup IIA, IIB and IIC, 323, 325
    tumor necrosis factor alpha (TNF-a)
        genetica mplification curves, 326, 328, 329
        pre and postoperative values, 326, 330
    Western blot analysis, 326, 331

D
Dalton'sla w,12
Defensins,34
Desmopressin,190–19 1
DIC. See Disseminated intravascular coagulation
Dipyridamole,205
Disseminated intravascular coagulation (DIC)
    bleeding and thrombotic manifestations, 180
    classification
        acute/decompensated,183
        chronic/compensated,183–184
    clinical manifestation, 184
    definition, 179
    diagnosis
        coagulation factors and inhibitors, 185–186
        increasedfi brinolysis, markers of, 186
        intravascularfi brin formation and fibrin degradation
            products, 185
        laboratory tests, 185
        platelet count, 185
        scoring system, 187–188
        thrombin generation, markers of, 185
    etiology and incidence, 180–181
    andi nflammation, 183
    management
        anticoagulants, 189
        antifibrinolytic agents, 190–191
        coagulation inhibitors, 189–190
        platelet and plasma replacement therapy, 188–189
    pathogenesis of, 181
        defectivefi brinolysis, 183
        physiological anticoagulant pathways, inhibition of,
            182–183
        thrombin generation, 181–182
    prognosis,191
Dobutamine,207

Drew–Andersont echniques,241
Dysoxia,9

E
ECC. See Bilateral extracorporeal circulation
Echocardiograms,196–197
Echocardiography,t ransthoracic,1 62
Eisenmengers yndrome
    causes of, 171
    chest radiograph of
        unrepaired atrial septal defect and left pulmonary
            artery angiogram, 175
        ventricular septal defect, 174
    cyanosis and hypoxemia, 174–175
    death, causes of, 175
    definition, 171
    evaluation,176
    follow-up,176
    normal lung, elastic Van Gieson stain (EVG), 172
    prognosis for, 175
    pulmonary hypertension severity, grades of, 173
    pulmonary vascular resistance (PVR), 172
    treatmentof ,177
Elastance,17
Elastic Van Gieson stain (EVG), of normal lung, 172
Electrocardiogram(EKG),196
Embryology and lung development, 4
EndothelialN OS(eNOS)
    densitometric assessment of, 109
    and hypoxic preconditioning in, 109–110
    immunohistochemical expression of, 108
Endothelin(ET)
    actions of, 91, 93
    IPAH, pathogenesis of, 148
    in ischemia/reperfusion lung injury, 93–94
    pathways for, 91
    pulmonary vascular tone balance, factors on, 92
    receptor antagonist, 94–96, 151–153, 199–200
    structure of, 92
    synthesis of, protein-cleavage, 93
Endothelium
    anticoagulant pathways, 182
    damage in heart and lung surgery, mechanisms, 55–56
    dysfunction
        EDRFs,57–58
        ischemia-reperfusion,56–57
        K^+,58
        Mg^{2+},58–59
        procaine,59
    microvascular function, maintenance of, 98–99
    neutrophil adhesion inhibition and, 99
    protection, in heart surgery and lung transplantation
        cardioplegic/organ preservation solutions, additives,
            60–61
        postconditioning,59
        preconditioning,59
    and smooth muscle interaction alteration, 61
Endothelium-derived hyperpolarizing factor (EDHF), 57–58
    analogs,60
Endotoxin,130
Epoprostenol,151,200

Ethyleneo xide(EO),2 18

Euro-Collins®,82

Excrcise tolerance testing, pulmonary arterial
        hypertension,1 97

ExhaledN O,110–111

Extra-alveolarinte rstitials pace,138

Extracorporealc irculation(ECC)
    cardiac surgery, 125–126
    circuit vs. bioengineering biomaterials
        biocompatibility,2 16
        complement system, 215
        development in, 220
        negative outcomes, 215
        oxygenators,217
        patient pathway, 216
        plastics, advantages of, 217–220
        prodedures and definition, 217
        synthetic surface, exposure to, 217

Extracorporeallungc ircuit,280,284

F

Fibrin degradation products (FDPs), 185

Fibrinolysis,de fective,183

Fick'se quation,25

Fick'sla w,24

Fluoroscopy,of t horax,46

G

Gamma-glutamyltra nsferase(GGT),116

Gasdif fusion
    oxygen-diffusing capacity, 25
    rate of diffusion, 24
    transferf actor,24

Gase xchangequa lity
    alveolar-arterial gradient, 298, 304, 305
    arterial blood gas analysis, 298, 305
    postoperative times, gasometric variables
        subgroups IA and IB, 297, 300
        subgroups IA and IC, 297, 300
        subgroups IB and IC, 297, 301
        subgroups IIA and IIB, 297, 303
        subgroups IIA and IIC, 297, 303
        subgroups IIB and IIC, 297, 304
    pre-and postoperative times, gasometric variables
        subgroup IA, 297, 298
        subgroup IB, 297, 299
        subgroup IC, 297, 299
        subgroup IIA, 297, 301
        subgroup IIB, 297, 302
        subgroup IIC, 297, 302

Glutathione (GSH), ischemia-reperfusion injury
    antioxidants,119
        functions,115
        glutathione-S-transferase (GST) super family, 116
        harmful molecules and protective effect of, 116
        mechanism of, 118
        peroxidases,116
        protective role of, 114–115
        structure of, 115
    oxidative stress, role of
        myocardial stunning, 114
        pathophysiologic and therapeutic implications, 115
        peroxynitrite,114

Glutathione peroxidises (GP), 116, 117

Glutathione-S-transferase (GST) super family, 116

Graham'sl aw,24

Growthf actors ynthesis,i nhibitors,155

H

HE. SeeH ematoxylin-eosin

Heart histopathology, in ischemia-reperfusion injury
    cardiac surgery, extracorporeal circulation, 125–126
    causes of, 124
    cell death, 121
    morphological patterns, myocardial infarction, 121, 122
    myocardial reperfusion, consequences of, 123
    pathologicalfi ndings
        preconditioning and postconditioning, 124
        ultramicrography,m itochondria,1 25

Heart-lung donor organ perfusion, 420–421

Heart-lung procurement, surgical technique, 421–422

Heart-lungt ransplantation
    clinicals tatus
        heart-lung donor organ perfusion, 420–421
        heart-lung procurement, surgical technique, 421–422
        International Society of Heart and Lung Transplantation
            (ISHLT), 419–420
        preservation solutions, 422–424
    CXC-receptors (CXCR), 424
    endothelialpr otection
        EDHF analogs, 60
        K+ channel openers (KCOs), 60
        NO substrates/donors, 60
        oxygen-derived free radicals, scavengers of, 60
        PGI$_2$ analogs, 60
        sodium-hydrogen ion exchange (NHE) inhibitors, 60
        substances in, 60
        postconditioning,59
        preconditioning,59
    gene expression and transfer, 424
    history,417–419
    nuclear factor kappa B (NFkB), 424

Heatpr econditioning,l ungs,229–230

Heat shock proteins, 378, 379
    Hsp27,335,339

Hematoxylin-eosin (HE), 333, 336, 337

Hemodilution,U F,252

Hemodynamicpa rameters
    arterial/alveolar (a/A) ratio, 276
    controlled pulmonary reperfusion, 275
    CPBt ime
        subgroups IA, IB, IC, 273
        subgroups IIA, IIB, IIC, 273, 274
    crystalloidsv olume
        subgroups IA, IB, IC, 273
        subgroups IIA, IIB, IIC, 273, 274
    experimental groups and subgroups, 271, 272
    great vessels and cannulae, 271, 273
    lung reperfusion benifits, 276, 277
    monitor of, 271, 272
    pulmonary compliance, 276
    pulmonarype rfusion

subgroups IA, IB, IC, 273, 274
 subgroups IIA, IIB, IIC, 273, 274
pulmonary vascular resistance (PVR), 276
pumpfl ow
 subgroups IA, IB, IC, 273
 subgroups IIA, IIB, IIC, 273, 274
Swan–Ganz catheter, 271, 272
urinaryout put
 subgroups IA, IB, IC, 273
 subgroups IIA, IIB, IIC, 273, 274
Hemodynamicpe rformance
 cardiopulmonary bypass (CPB), 295
 parameters,294
 postoperativetime s
  subgroups IA and IB, 287, 289
  subgroups IA and IC, 287, 290
  subgroups IB and IC, 287, 290
  subgroups IIA and IIB, 287, 292
  subgroups IIA and IIC, 287, 293
  subgroups IIB and IIC, 287, 293
 pre and postoperative times
  subgroup I, 287, 288
  subgroup IA, 287, 288
  subgroup IC, 287, 289
  subgroup IIA, 287, 291
  subgroup IIB, 287, 291
  subgroup IIC, 287, 292
 pulmonary vascular resistance (PVR), 287, 295
Hemofiltration (HF), CPB
 in adult patients, 266–267
 in animal experiments, 264–265
 in pediatric patients, 265–266
 primes olution,263–264
Henry'sla w,24
HF. SeeH emofiltration,C PB
Hyperoxia-inducedlun gi njury,68–69
Hypoxia,10

I
ICAM-1. See Intercellular adhesion molecule 1
Idiopathic pulmonary hypertension (IPH)
 cellular therapy, 155
 clinicalc lassification, 148
 combinationt herapy
  evidence-based treatment algorithm for, 154
  interventional therapy for, 153–154
 endothelin receptor antagonists, 151–153
 growth factor synthesis, inhibitors of, 155
 managementof
  calcium channel blockers, 151
  conventional therapy, 151
  general measures, 151
  specific therapy, 151, 152
  targets for, 152
 pathogenesisof
  diagnostic approach, 150
  endothelin-1,14 8
  nitric oxide, 149–150
  prostacyclin,148
 pathology of, 147, 149
 phosphodiesterase 5 inhibitors, 153

 prostacyclin analogs, 151
 Rho kinase inhibitors, 154–155
 serotonin receptor and transporter function, 154
 vasoactive intestinal polypeptide (VIP), 154
Iloprost,151,201
Inflammatory cardiac lesion, 341, 344, 345
Inflammatory cell markers
 intercellular adhesion molecule 1 (ICAM-1)
  genetica mplification curves, 326, 328, 329
  pre and postoperative values, 326, 330
 interleukin 4 (IL-4)
  genetica mplification curves, 326, 328, 329
  pre and postoperative values, 326, 330
 leukosequestration and neutrophilic sequestration
  subgroups IA and IB, 307, 320
  subgroups IA and IC, 307, 320
  subgroups IB and IC, 307, 320
  subgroups IIA and IIB, 307, 320
  subgroups IIA and IIC, 307, 321
  subgroups IIB and IIC, 307, 321
 platelet concentration ratios, 321, 322
 postoperativec orellations
  subgroups IA and IB, 307, 311
  subgroups IA and IC, 307, 312
  subgroups IB and IC, 307, 313
  subgroups IIA and IIB, 307, 317
  subgroups IIA and IIC, 307, 318
  subgroups IIB and IIC, 307, 319
 pre and postoperative corellations
  subgroup IA, 307, 308
  subgroup IB, 307, 309
  subgroup IC, 307, 310
  subgroup IIA, 307, 314
  subgroup IIB, 307, 315
  subgroup IIC, 307, 316
 tumor necrosis factor alpha (TNF-a)
  genetica mplification curves, 326, 328, 329
  pre and postoperative values, 326, 330
 white blood cell ratios, 307, 321
Inhaled nitroprusside and nitroglycerin, 206
Inhaled NO, 110, 205, 207
Inotropicdr ugs,204
Intercellular adhesion molecule 1 (ICAM-1)
 genetica mplification curves, 326, 328, 329
 pre and postoperative values, 326, 330
Interleukin4(IL-4)
 genetica mplification curves, 326, 328, 329
 pre and postoperative values, 326, 330
Intermittentl ungpe rfusion,410
International Society of Heart and Lung Transplantation
  (ISHLT),419–420
International Society on Thrombosis and Haemostasis (ISTH),
  179, 186, 187
Interstitialpr essure,de creased,143
Intravenousv asodilators,205
IPC. SeeI schemicpr econditioning
Ischemia,27
Ischemia-reperfusion injury, 130–131, 245–246, 370–371,
  433–435
 aprotinin,75–78
 endothelial dysfunction, 56–57

endothelin(ET)
    biological effects of, 94
    immunoreactivity, 93, 95
    pathophysiology of, 94
    receptor antagonist treatment, 94–96
glutathione,113–119
heart and lung surgery, endothelium damage in, 55
heart histopathology in, 121–127
L-arginine,97–104
mechanism of, 81–82
nitric oxide (*see* Nitric oxide (NO), ischemia-reperfusion
    injury)
VEGF and lung Injury, 70
Ischemic preconditioning (IPC) and lung preservation
    cardiopulmonary bypass (CPB), 223–226
    lunginjury
        cardiac surgery, 223–224
        transplantation,224–225
    lung protection techniques, 225–226
    potential mechanisms, 231, 232
    preconditioning
        heat,229–230
        ischemic/hypoxic,2 26–228
        pharmacological,228–229
        remote,230
Isoproterenol,207

J

Japanese Association for Acute Medicine (JAAM) scoring
    system for DIC, 188

K

Kazui technique, brain and pulmonary function, 399–400
K^+ channel openers (KCOs), 60
K^+ effect, endothelial dysfunction, 58

L

Laplace'sl aw,14,1 40
Leukocytede pletion,435
Lightmic roscopy,371,372
Lipopolysaccharide,69–70
Low-frequency ventilation (LFV), mechanical
    electron microscopy, 371, 373
    experimental model, LFV, 369
        arterial blood gas analysis, 370
        histopathological examinations, 371–374
        ischemia-reperfusion injury reduction, 370–371
    histopathological changes, 371, 374
    light microscopy, 371, 372
    limitation and controversy, 372, 374
    pulmonary injury mechanism, CPB, 367
        atelectasis,368– 369
        inflammatory response, 368
        ischemia-reperfusion injury, 368
        mucina ccumulation,368–369
Lungpe rfusion
    arterial blood, 349
    arterial oxygen pressure, 352
    cardiopulmonary bypass (CPB), 351
    clinical aortic surgery
        AAAD treatment, 401–404

        CPB,397
        CRP,397–398
        hypothermic circulatory arrest, 397
        Kazui technique, brain and pulmonary function,
            399–400
        pulmonary artery (PA) flushing, 399–401
        pulmonary perfusion, 398
        thoracoabdominal perfusion (TP), 401
    in clinical heart-lung surgery
        cardiopulmonary bypass (CPB), 407
        continuous lung perfusion, total CPB, 408–410
        future perspective, 410–411
        history,408
        intermittent lung perfusion, 410
    clinical heart-lung transplantation
        CXC-receptors (CXCR), 424
        gene expression and transfer, 424
        heart-lung donor organ perfusion, 420–421
        heart-lung procurement, surgical technique, 421–422
        history,417–419
        International Society of Heart and Lung Transplantation
            (ISHLT), 419–420
        Nuclear factor kappa B (NFkB), 424
        preservation solutions, 422–424
    clinical mitral valve surgery
        malondialdehyde, 393, 394
        mechanical ventilation time, 393, 395
        oxygen index, 393, 395
        pulmonary vascular resistance (PVR), 393, 394
    closed-circuit perfusion, 280, 283
    continuous or intermittent, 349–350
    and coronary artery bypass graft
        cardiac surgery, 388–390
        clinical and experimental models, 388
        CPB and lung function, 385
        overt postoperative respiratory failure treatment, 389
        pathophysiology, CPB, 385–386
        perfusion and ventilation, ECC, 387–388
    CPB components, 279–280
    Drew technique, evidences, 352–356
    experimentalm odel
        arterial blood, 279, 281
        venous blood, 279, 282
    extracorporeal lung circuit, 280, 284
    isolated working lung apparatus, 280, 284
    maintanence,436–437
    pulmonary artery pressure, 352
    pulmonary ischemia reperfusion injury, 441
    pulmonary parenchyma, 442
    pulmonary trunk perfusion, 279, 282
    scheme of, 279, 283
    strategies of, 349–350
    venousbl ood,349
Lung reperfusion, hemodynamic parameters, 276, 277
Lungs
    aprotinin, transplantation surgery, 76–78
    carbon monoxide inhalation, protection
        anti-inflammatory agent, 380
        heat shock proteins, 378, 379
        inflammation and dysfunction, 378
        protective effects, 378

in cardiac disease, histological features of
    alveolar-capillary membrane, 28–30
    cardiac arrest, 30, 31
    compensatory measures, 30
    ischemia,27
    multifocal lesion of, 30
    organic impairment of, 27
    pulmonary congestion, 29
    pulmonary edema, 28
    reperfusion lesion, 28
cardiopulmonary bypass (CPB), 223–226
cellular and molecular aspects of
    airway smooth muscle, integrins, 37, 38
    alveolar cells, 35
    cell-matrix adhesions and downstream regulation,
        model of, 36
    cytoskeletal processes, shortening and tension
        development in, 39
    defense mechanisms, 33–35
    ion channel pathway, activation of, 36
    mechanical forces, 35
    mechanotransduction in, 37
    physical forces, response to, 35–37
compliance,16–17
conducting airways to alveoli
    bronchioles,5
    Jackson-Huber pulmonary segmental classification, 5
    pulmonary lobule, 5–6
dysfunctional mechanism, 240
edema,257
embryology and development, 4
fluid movement, physical forces
    endothelium,13 8
    pulmonary capillary hydrostatic pressure, 138
    Starling's equation, 138, 139
history of, 3
inflammatory injury, mitigated, 102–103
injury
    cardiac surgery, 223–224
    transplantation, 224–225
innervation of, 7
ischemia, reperfusion, 101–102
lymphatic drainage of, 7
microstructures of, 137–138
normal, elastic Van Gieson stain (EVG), of, 172
perfusion(see Lung perfusion)
preconditioning
    heat,229–230
    ischemic/hypoxic,2 26–228
    pharmacological,228–229
    remote,230
preservation
    composition of, 83
    flush solution for, 82–84
    intracellular and extracellular solutions, 82
    ischemia-reperfusion injury, mechanism of, 81–82
    nitroglycerin in, 84–85
    prostaglandins in, 84
    pulmonoplegia and additives, 85–86
protection techniques, 225–226
pulmonary vascular system, 6–7

recoil, causes of
    elastic,13
    surface tension, 14–15
surfactant integrity, 103
trachea,4–5
transplantation,153–154
tumor, MRI, 50
uncontrolled perfusion, 237
vascular resistance maintenance, NO pathway, 98
and VEGF, 68
volumes
    functional residual capacity (FRC), 11
    standard volumes and capacities, 11
Lymphaticdr ainage
of lung, 7
reduced,142–143

M
Macroscopical and microscopical finding
    beating heart subgroups, 333, 335
    cardioplegic arrest/beating heart group, 335, 338
    cardioplegic arrest subgroups, 333, 335
    controlled perfusion, 335, 340
    heat shock protein 27 (Hsp27), 335, 339
    hematoxylin-eosin (HE), 333, 336, 337
    inflammatory cardiac lesion, 341, 344, 345
    pre and postoperative cardiac histologic variable
        subgroup IA and IB, 341, 342
        subgroup IC and IIA, 341, 343
        subgroup IIB and IIC, 341, 344
    pre and postoperative histologic variables
        subgroup IA, IB and IC, 333, 334
        subgroup IIA, IIB and IIC, 333, 334
    pre and postoperative immunohistochemical analysis
        within groups I and II, 335, 337
        per subgroup, 333, 337
    pulmonary concomitant analysis, 333, 335
    tomographic features, 335, 341
Magnetic resonance imaging (MRI), of thorax
    angiography, coarctation area, 51
    lung tumor, pericardium, 50
Malondialdehyde,3 93,3 94
Mechanical ventilation, 395, 436. See also Lung perfusion;
        Low-frequency ventilation (LFV), mechanical
Mg^{2+} effect, endothelial dysfunction, 58–59
Microstructures,of l ung,137–138
Milrinone,205,207
Minutev entilation,10
Mitralv alves urgery
    cardiopulmonary bypass (CPB), 393–395
    lungpe rfusion
        malondialdehyde, 393, 394
        mechanical ventilation time, 393, 395
        oxygen index, 393, 395
        pulmonary vascular resistance (PVR), 393, 394
Modified ultrafiltration (MUF), 254–255
Mucociliary clearance, defense mechanisms
    airwayfl uids, action and control of, 34
    defensins and cathelicidins, 34
    periciliaryfl uid, 34
    production and composition, 33–34

Mucosal associated lymphoid tissue (MALT), 34
MUF. *See*M odified ultrafiltration
Multiplcinfl ammatory repercussions
  apoptosis and acute inflammation, 245
  depletion and control groups, 247
  inflammatory mediator, 248
  ischemia-reperfusion injury, 245–246
  ribonuclease protection assay densitometry, 246, 247
  warm ischemia period, 245
  Western blot analysis, 246
Myocardialre perfusion,123

N
Natriureticpe ptides. *See* Pulmonary hemodynamic profile
Neurogenicpulmona rye dema,143–144
Neutrophile lastase,432
NFkB. *See* Nuclear factor kappa B
Nitric oxide (NO), 149–150. *See also* L-Arginine, ischemia-reperfusion injury
  effect, endothelial dysfunction, 57
  in ischemia-reperfusion injury
    endothelial NOS (eNOS), protective role of, 107–109
    exhaled NO, 110–111
    hypothermic protection, 109
    and hypoxic preconditioning in, eNOS in, 109–110
    inhaled nitric oxide and, 110
    nitric oxide synthase (NOS), 107
  substrates/donors, 60Nitric oxide synthase (NOS), 97, 100–101,10 7
Nitroglycerin,206
  in lung preservation, 84–85
Nuclearf actorka ppa-B(NF-kB),56,130,424

O
Obstructive sleep apnea (OSA), 198
Off-pump coronary artery bypass (OPCAB), 251
Ohm'sla w,12
OPCAB. *See* Off-pump coronary artery bypass
Oxidative stress, ischemia-reperfusion injury, 113–114
Oxygen-derived free radicals, scavengers, 60
Oxygen-diffusingc apacity,25
Oxygen
  index, 393, 395
  respiratoryp hysiology
    delivery,9–10
    functionof,9

P
PAfl ushing. *See* Pulmonary artery flushing
PAH. *See* Pulmonary arterial hypertension
Parasympathetic innervation, of lung, 7
Perfadex®,82
Perfusion,21
Periciliaryfl uid,34
Peripheralm echanoreceptors,40
Pharmacologicalpr econditioning,l ungs,228–229
Phosphodiesterase 5 inhibitors, 153, 200
Physiologicald eads pace,1 0
Plastics advantages, in bioengineering
  ethylene oxide (EO), 218
  medical device biological evaluation, 220
  plastificants, 218
  polyvinyl chloride (PVC), 218
  selectionof ,219
Platelet
  aggregation inhibition and thrombosis formation, 99–100
  DIC
    count, in, 185
    and plasma replacement therapy, 188–189
Poiseuille'sl aw,18
Polymorphonuclearne utrophila ctivation,432
Polyvinylc hloride(PVC),218
Pre-Bötzingerc omplex,40
Procaine,e ndothelialdys function,59
Prostacyclin,148,2 05–206
  analogs,151
  PGI_2
    analogs,60
    effect, endothelial dysfunction, 57
Prostaglandins, in lung preservation, 84
Prostanoids,200–201,207
ProteinC ,190
Pulmonary arterial hypertension (PAH)
  classification of
    clinical evaluation, 196
    definition, 195
    echocardiograms,196–197
    electrocardiogram (EKG), 196
    exercise tolerance testing, 197
    function testing, 197
    laboratory evaluation, 196
    patient-related risk factors, 198
    right heart catheterization, 197
  genetics of, 147
  outpatient treatment of
    calcium channel blockers, 198–199
    diuretics and digoxin, 198
    endothelin (ET) receptor antagonists, 199–200
    hypoxemia,1 98
    phosphodiesterase inhibitors, 200
    prostanoids,200–201
    treatment based on, 201
    warfarin,198
  perioperativem anagement
    anesthetic management, 203–204
    assessment,203
    dipyridamole,205
    inhaled nitroprusside and nitroglycerin, 206
    inhaled NO, 205
    intravenous vasodilators, 205
    milrinone,205
    prostacyclins,205– 206
  postoperative management of
    agents, 207, 208
    goals in, 206–207
    mechanical therapies, 207–208
  preoperative management of, 201–203
Pulmonary artery (PA) flushing,399–401
Pulmonarya rterype rfusion,239
Pulmonary concomitant analysis, 333, 335
Pulmonary congestion, histological features, 29
Pulmonarydys functionf actors

anesthesia,432
    free radicals, 432–433
    hypothermic *vs.* normothermic CPB, 432
    ischemia-reperfusion injury, 433–435
    neutrophil elastase, 432
    on-pump *vs.* off-pump CABG, 432
    polymorphonuclear neutrophil activation, 432
Pulmonarye dema
    fluid movement, physical forces, 138–139
    histological features, 28
    lung microstructures, in normal fluid circulation
        alveolar interstitial space, 138
        arterioles,137
        extra-alveolar interstitial space, 138
    pathogenesisof
        capillary permeability, increased, 142
        cardiogenic,141–142
        clinical conditions with, 142
        colloid osmotic pressure, decreased, 143
        high-altitude,14 3
        interstitial pressure, decreased, 143
        lymphatic drainage, reduced, 142–143
        neurogenic,143 –144
        noncardiogenic,142
        schematic representation of, 141
        transfusion-related acute lung injury (TRALI), 144
        types,140
    pathophysiology
        histology of, 139
        Laplace's law, 140
        radiographic appearance of, 140
Pulmonarye mbolism, 159
Pulmonarye ndarterectomy,163
Pulmonarye nergyme tabolism
    apoptosis and acute inflammation, 245
    depletion and control groups, 247
    inflammatory mediator, 248
    ischemia-reperfusion injury, 245–246
    ribonuclease protection assay densitometry, 246, 247
    warm ischemia period, 245
    Western blot analysis, 246
Pulmonaryhe modynamicpr ofile
    atrial natriuretic peptide (ANP)
        apoptosis evaluation, immunohistochemistry, 360, 364
        experimental protocols, 360, 362
        histologic evaluation, reperfused lungs, 360, 363
        pulmonary vascular resistance (PVR), 360, 362
    brain natriuretic peptide (BNP)
        β-actin, genic amplification curves, 359, 360
        change in plasm, 359, 361
        postoperative, 359, 360
        preoperative plasma, 359, 361
        vs. total pulmonary resistance, 359, 361
Pulmonary hemodynamic variables, CPB
    biventricular approaches, 235
    controlled pulmonary reperfusion, 237
    lung perfusion effects, 236
    physiological impacts, 235
    reperfusion injury, 236
    strategies,236
    uncontrolled lung perfusion, 237

Pulmonary hypertension, 252, 258
    clinicalc lassification, 148
    severity, grades of, 173
Pulmonaryi njury
    mechanism,C PB
        atelectasis,368–369
        inflammatory response, 368
        ischemia-reperfusion injury, 368
        mucin accumulation, 368–369
    andV EGF,67–71
Pulmonaryi schemia,441
Pulmonaryp arenchyma,4 42
Pulmonary perfusion, 273, 274, 398
Pulmonarypr otectionpr inciples
    coronary artery bypass grafting (CABG), 266–267
    hemofiltration (HF), CPB
        in adult patients, 266–267
        in animal experiments, 264–265
        in pediatric patients, 265–266
        prime solution, 263–264
    lung perfusion maintenance, 436–437
    mechanical ventilation maintanence, 436
    pulmonary dysfunction factors
        anesthesia,432
        free radicals, 432–433
        hypothermic *vs.* normothermic CPB, 432
        ischemia-reperfusion injury, 433–435
        neutrophil elastase, 432
        on-pump *vs.* off-pump CABG, 432
        polymorphonuclear neutrophil activation, 432
    therapeutici nterventions
        continuoushe mofiltration, 436
        CPB circuit modification, 435–436
        leukocyte depletion, 435
        pharmaceuticals,434–435
    ultrafiltration (UF), 263
Pulmonary thromboembolism, retrograde pulmonary perfusion
    conventional pulmonary embolectomy defects, 413–414
    goals,415
    pulmonary angioscopy, 414
    surgicalt echnique,414–415
Pulmonary thromboendarterectomy (PTE), for chronic
            thromboembolic pulmonary hypertension
    adverse effects, 167
    clinical presentation, 161–162
    diagnostics tudies
        angiography,1 63
        cardiac catheterization, 163
        chest radiography, 162
        radioisotope ventilationperfusion (V/Q), 163
        tansthoracic echocardiography, 162
    history,160–161
    incidence of, 160
    indications for, 163–164
    operation
        principles for, 164
        surgical specimen, and types of, 165
        technique,164–167
    pathophysiology,1 61
    results,167–168
Pulmonaryt issuer esistance,18

Pulmonary trunk perfusion, 279, 282
Pulmonary vascular resistance (PVR), 102
   atrial natriuretic peptide (ANP), 360, 362
   cardiopulmonary bypass, 237, 238
   Eisenmenger syndrome, 172
   hemodynamic parameters, 276
   hemodynamic performance, 287, 295
   lung perfusion, 393, 394
Pulmonaryv asculars ystem,6–7
Pulmonaryv entilation
   alveolar gas pressures, 19–21
   breathing, forces involved in
      airways resistance, 18, 19
      alveolar pressure, 13
      barometric pressure (PB),12–13
      chest wall compliance, 17
      closing volume (CV), 17–18
      expiration,12
      inspirations,12
      lung compliance, 16–17
      lung recoil, causes of, 13–15
      maximal inspiratory and expiratory pressure, mouth, 13
      Ohm's law, 12
      pleural (intrapleural) pressure, 15
      pressure gradient, 12
      pulmonary tissue resistance, 18
      respiratory muscles and, 15–16
      specific compliance (sC), 17
      transdiaphragmatic pressure, 13
      volume, pressure, and airflow changes, respiratory cycle, 12
      work of breathing (WOB), 19
   gas diffusion, 24–25
   lungv olumes
      functional residual capacity (FRC), 11
      sitting pressure-volume curve, 11
      standard volumes and capacities, 11
   to perfusion, unequal distribution of
      alveolar vessels, recruitment and distention of, 22
      pulmonary vascular resistance (PVR), 21
      radial traction, on blood vessels, 21
      ratios, lung regions with, 23
      regional perfusion changes, gravity, 22, 23
   shunt/venousa dmixture
      absolute,24
      anatomic (extrapulmonary), 23
      physiological,2 4
Pulmonoplegia, for lung preservation, 85–86
   compositionof ,86
PVR. SeePulmona ryv ascularr esistance

R
Radioisotope ventilationperfusion (V/Q), for chronic thromboembolic pulmonary hypertension, 163
Remotepr econditioning,l ungs,230
Reperfusioni njury,l ungs,236
Reperfusionl esion,28
Respiratoryp hysiology
   alveolarv entilation
      dead space, 10–11
      forces, gradient pressures

      lung volumes, 11–12
   oxygen
      delivery,9–10
      function of, 9
   pulmonaryv entilation
      alveolar gas pressures, 19–21
      breathing, forces involved in, 12–19
      gas diffusion, 24–25
      lung volumes, 11–12
      to perfusion, unequal distribution of, 21–23
      shunt/venousa dmixture,23–24
Respiratorys ystem
   abnormalities, 239, 240
   control and regulation of
      effectors in, 41
      ventilatory control, afferents in, 37–40
      ventilatory pattern, 40–41
   defensem echanisms
      alveolar macrophages (AM), 35
      mucociliary clearance, 33–34
   variablcs,239
Retrograde pulmonary perfusion. SeeP ulmonary thromboembolism, retrograde pulmonary perfusion
Rhoki nasei nhibitors,154–155
Righthe artc atheterization,197

S
Scientific and Standardisation Committee (SSC) scoring system for overt DIC, 186
Sepsis-inducedl ungi njury,69–70
Serotonin receptor and transporter function, 154
Sitaxsentan,153,199–200
Sodium-hydrogen ion exchange (NHE) inhibitors, 60
Starling'se quation,138
Surfacet ension,l ung,14–15
Surfactant,14
Swan–Ganzc atheter,271,272
Sympathetic innervation, of lung, 7
Systemici nflammatory response syndrome, 215

T
Tadalafil,20 0
Thoracoabdominalpe rfusion(TP),401
Thorax,i maginge valuation
   chest radiography, 45–46
   computedt omography
      air bronchograms, consolidation area, 48
      air trapping, lower lobes, 48
      anterior mediastinal lesion with fat density, teratoma, 50
      lower density areas, emphysema, 49
      multiple round pulmonary opacities, 48
      postcontrast, sagittal oblique reformation, 50
      trachea,47
   fluoroscopy, 46
   magnetic resonance imaging (MRI), 50–51
   ventilation-perfusions can,49
Thrombin generation, in DIC
   markers of, 185
   pathogenesisof ,181–182
Thromboembolic pulmonary hypertension, chronic. See

Pulmonary thromboendarterectomy (PTE), for
chronic thromboembolic pulmonary hypertension
Thrombosisf ormation,99–100
Tidalv olume,10
TNF-a. *See* Tumor necrosis factor alpha
TP. *See*Thora coabdominalpe rfusion
Trachea,4–5
Transfusion-related acute lung injury (TRALI), 144
Transthoracic echocardiography, for chronic thromboembolic
pulmonary hypertension, 162
Treprostinil,151,200–201
Tumorne crosisf actora lpha(TNF-a)
genetica mplification curves, 326, 328, 329
pre and postoperative values, 326, 330

U
UF. *See*U ltrafiltration, pulmonary function
Ultrafiltration (UF), pulmonary function, 263
acute respiratory distress syndrome (ARDS), 251
benefits of, 256–257
CPB and pulmonary injury, 251–252
current use of
balancedultra filtration (BUF), 255–256
conventionalulultr afiltration (CUF), 253–254
modified ultrafiltration (MUF), 254–255
hemodilution,252
inflammatory reaction, 252
mechanism
inflammatory reaction, 257–258
lung edema, 257
pulmonary hypertension, 258
off-pump coronary artery bypass (OPCAB), 251

pulmonary hypertension, 252
transmembrane pressure (TMP) gradient, 253
University of Wisconsin solution®,82

V
Vascular endothelial growth factor (VEGF) and pulmonary
injury
biology, receptors, and regulation, 67
cardiac conditions and, 70
and hyperoxia-induced lung injury, 68–69
ischemia-reperfusion-induced lung injury, 70
lipopolysaccharide and sepsis-induced lung injury, 69–70
and lung, 68
phasic role of, 71
ventilation and hyperoxia-induced lung injury, 69
Vasoactive intestinal polypeptide (VIP), 154
Vasodilators,197
Vasopressors,204
Ventilation
distribution of, alveolar gas pressures, 20–21
pattern
automatic pattern, 40
dorsal and ventral group, 41
effectors in, 41
VEGF and hyperoxia-induced lung injury, 69
Ventilation-perfusion scan, of thorax, 49
Ventricular septal defect (VSD), chest radiograph, 174
Viscoelasticm ucus, 33

W
Warfarin,198
Westernbl ota nalysis,i nterleukin,246